CLINICAL APPLICATIONS OF
NURSING
DIAGNOSIS

**Adult Health, Child Health,
Women's Health, Mental Health,
Home Health**

CLINICAL APPLICATIONS OF
NURSING DIAGNOSIS

Adult Health, Child Health, Women's Health, Mental Health, Home Health

Helen C. Cox, R.N., Ed.D.
Associate Dean for Continuing Nursing Education, Professor of Nursing

Mittie D. Hinz, R.N.,C., M.S.N.
Assistant Professor of Nursing

Mary Ann Lubno, R.N., Ph.D., C.N.A.A.
Associate Dean for Undergraduate Program, Associate Professor of Nursing

Susan A. Newfield, R.N., M.S.N., C.S.
Associate Professor of Clinical Nursing

Nancy A. Ridenour, R.N., Ph.D., C.F.N.C.
Associate Dean for Practice Program/Practice Development, Associate Professor of Nursing

Kathryn L. Sridaromont, R.N.,C., M.S.N.
Assistant Professor of Clinical Nursing

Texas Tech University Health Sciences Center School of Nursing
Lubbock, Texas

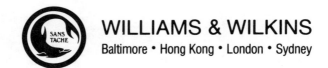

WILLIAMS & WILKINS
Baltimore • Hong Kong • London • Sydney

Editor: Susan M. Glover
Associate Editor: Marjorie Kidd Keating
Copy Editor: Thomas Lehr
Design: Joanne Janowiak
Production: Anne Seitz

Copyright © 1989
Williams & Wilkins
428 East Preston Street
Baltimore, Maryland 21202, USA

Accurate indications, adverse reactions, and dosage schedules for drugs are provided in this book, but it is possible that they may change. The reader is urged to review the package information data of the manufacturers of the medications mentioned.

Printed in the United States of America

Library of Congress Cataloging-in-Publication Data

Clinical applications of nursing diagnosis.

Includes bibliographies and index.
1. Diagnosis. 2. Nursing. I. Cox, Helen C. [DNLM:
1. Nursing Assessment. 2. Nursing Process.
WY 100 C6403]
RT48.C57   1989   610.73   88-33790
ISBN 0-683-02153-2

89 90 91 92 93
1 2 3 4 5 6 7 8 9 10

To the administration, faculty, students, and staff of
Texas Tech University Health Sciences Center School of Nursing
for support and encouragement above and beyond the usual.

FOREWORD

Clinical Applications of Nursing Diagnosis represents a significant step forward in the development and application of nursing diagnoses to clinical practice. It utilizes Gordon's functional health patterns as the typology to categorize the North American Nursing Diagnosis Association (NANDA) nursing diagnoses.

Specifically, this book gives the reader concise information on each functional health pattern. Information includes not only the *pattern* description and assessment, but also conceptual and developmental aspects. This is the only book that collects all of the information in one place. This approach will aid nurses in conceptualizing nursing care more readily in terms of *nursing* diagnosis rather than medical diagnosis.

In addition to providing comprehensive information about each functional health pattern, *Clinical Applications of Nursing Diagnosis* also gives generic care plans for each NANDA nursing diagnosis. Moreover, generic care plans are provided not only for adult medical-surgical applications, but also for the specialty areas of children's, women's, mental, and home health. This coverage will enable specialists, educators, students, and practitioners to use this one book as they work in different clinical areas.

The evaluation component of the care plans deserves special attention. Written in the form of an algorithm, the evaluation process is presented in a step-by-step format. This specificity allows the reader to differentiate each of the various steps, which in turn aids in the transfer of that learning to subsequent objectives.

Nursing diagnosis has had the greatest impact on nursing since Florence Nightingale. It is an evolving concept, and *Clinical Applications of Nursing Diagnosis* represents a milestone in this evolution.

Margo C. Neal, R.N., M.N.
Malibu, California

PREFACE

The North American Nursing Diagnosis Association (NANDA) has been identifying, classifying, and testing diagnostic nomenclature since the early '70s. In our opinion, use of nursing diagnosis helps to define the essence of nursing and to give direction to care that is uniquely nursing care.

If nurses (in all instances we are referring to registered nurses) enter the medical diagnosis of acute appendicitis in the patient problem or assessment area of the care plan, they have met defeat before a start can be made. A nurse cannot intervene for this medical diagnosis; intervention requires a medical practitioner who can perform an appendectomy. However, if the nurse enters the nursing diagnosis, "Alteration in Comfort: Pain, related to surgical incision," then a number of nursing interventions come to mind.

Several previously published books use nursing diagnosis to contribute to nursing care plans. However, these books focus outcome and nursing interventions on the related factors; that is, nursing interventions deal with resolving, to the extent possible, the causative and contributing factors that result in the nursing diagnosis. We have chosen to focus nursing intervention on the nursing diagnosis. To focus on the nursing diagnosis promotes the use of concepts in nursing rather than worrying about a multitude of specifics; for example, there are common nursing measures that can be used to relieve pain regardless of the etiologic pain factor involved. Likewise, the outcomes focus on the nursing diagnosis. The main outcome nurses want to achieve when working with the nursing diagnosis, "Alteration in Comfort: Pain," is control of the pain to the extent possible. Again, the outcome allows the use of a conceptual approach rather than a multitude-of-specifics approach. To clarify further, we ask you to look again at the medical diagnosis of appendicitis. The physician's first concern is not related to whether the appendicitis is caused by a fecalith, intestinal helminths, or *Escherichia coli* run amok. The physician focuses first on intervening for the appendicitis, which usually results in an appendectomy. The physician will deal with etiologic factors following the appendectomy, but the appendectomy is the first level of intervention. Likewise, the nurse can deal with the related factors through nursing orders, but the first level of intervention is toward the nursing diagnosis. Additionally, there is continuing debate among NANDA members as to whether the current list of diagnoses that are accepted for testing are nursing diagnoses or are lists of diagnostic categories or concepts. We therefore have chosen to focus on concepts. Using a conceptual approach allows focus on independent nursing functions and helps avoid focusing on medical intervention. This book has been designed to serve as a guide to completing nursing care plans that use nursing diagnosis as a base. The plans are not meant to serve as standardized care plans but rather as handy references in promoting the visibility of the contribution by nursing to health care.

A change in vocabulary will be required. Rather than "Patient/Client Problem or Assessment" as is usual in the first column of a care plan, we use the term "Nursing Diagnosis." The book does not deal with problems that are not nursing diagnoses. The second column, "Patient Objectives," should be stated in terms of patient behavior or action that is measurable. We chose to use the term "Objectives" rather than "Outcomes" simply because this is the term used on many nursing care plan formats. The second column also contains the "Target Date." "Intervention" or "Implementation" is the usual heading for the third column; we use the term "Nursing Orders." The fourth column will remain "Evaluation." Thus, the nursing care plan would appear as follows:

NURSING DIAGNOSIS	OBJECTIVES AND TARGET DATE	NURSING ORDERS	EVALUATION

For the sake of printing considerations the information presented in this book is in a vertical rather than a horizontal format. Readers will find it easy to transcribe the information to the horizontal format.

Marjory Gordon's "Functional Health Patterns" are used as an organizing framework. The functional health patterns allow grouping of the nursing diagnoses into mutually inclusive groupings which, in our opinion, promotes a conceptual approach to assessment and formulation of a nursing diagnosis. Use of the functional health patterns also serves to highlight which author needed to be the initial author of each chapter. For example, the functional health pattern "Coping-Stress Tolerance" calls for an author with specialization in mental health-psychiatry.

Chapter 1 serves as the overview-introductory chapter and gives expanded content related to the nursing care plan format as well as information regarding the relationship between nursing models, nursing process, and nursing care plans. Titles for Chapters 2 through 12 are taken from the functional patterns. Included in each of these chapters is a pattern description, pattern assessment, conceptual information, and developmental information related to the pattern. Each nursing diagnosis within the pattern is then introduced with accompanying information of definition, defining characteristics, related factors, and differential diagnosis. Following differential diagnosis are care plans specific to the nursing diagnosis in the areas of adult health, child health, women's health, mental health, and home health. In all instances, the authors have used the definitions, major and minor defining characteristics, and related factors that have been accepted by NANDA for testing. All of these materials may be found in the NANDA publication, *Taxonomy I—Revised 1989* ($10.00 from NANDA, St. Louis University School of Nursing, 3525 Caroline Street, St. Louis, MO 63104).

On initial drafts, each separate care plan (adult health, child health, etc.) had its own set of objectives and its own evaluative statement. In reviewing these drafts, we found a great deal of duplication; therefore, the format was changed to show one set of objectives for each diagnosis. The objectives are connected by the words "and/or," signifying that readers may choose to use only one of the objectives or to use both of the objectives. Readers might also choose to design their own client-specific objectives using these objectives as guidelines.

In each instance the adult health nursing orders serve as the generic nursing orders. Each subsequent set of nursing orders (child health, women's health, mental health, and home health) shows only the nursing orders that are different from the generic nursing orders. The different nursing orders make each set specific for the target population, but must be used in connection with the generic nursing orders to be complete.

Because evaluation of the care plan is based on the degree of progress toward achieving the objectives, there is an evaluation flowchart for each objective. The flowcharts provide minimum information, but demonstrate the decision-making process that must be used.

Target dates are given in reference to short-term care. For home health, particularly, the target date would be in terms of weeks and months rather than days.

In some instances, additional information is included following a specific care plan. The additional information includes material that either needed to be highlighted or did not logically fall within the defined outline areas.

Throughout the nursing orders we have used "patient" and "client" interchangeably. The terms refer to the system of care and include the individual as well as the family and other social support systems.

We have written this book for any nurse or nursing student who is beginning to work with nursing diagnosis. We hope to promote the use of nursing diagnosis to the end that nursing itself is advanced. If you, our readers, begin to feel more comfortable with using nursing diagnosis nomenclature and begin to use nursing diagnosis more in your practice, then our hope will have become reality.

Helen Cox, R.N., Ed.D.

ACKNOWLEDGMENTS

The publication of a book necessitates the involvement of many persons beyond the authors. We wish to acknowledge the support and assistance of the following persons who indeed made this book possible:

Our families, who supported our taking time away from family activities.

Margo Neal and Rose Mary Carroll-Johnson, who helped us clarify and refine so that this book became even more than we had envisioned it could be.

Sue Glover, Nursing Editor, of Williams & Wilkins, who was willing to take on a book with multiple authors and support us in our ideas.

Marilyn Buchanan, who patiently typed many drafts and revisions.

Please accept our deepest gratitude and appreciation.

CONTENTS

CHAPTER FOUR

Elimination Pattern 157

CHAPTER FIVE

Activity-Exercise Pattern 199

CHAPTER SIX

Sleep-Rest Pattern 327

CHAPTER SEVEN

Cognitive-Perceptual Pattern 339

CHAPTER EIGHT

Self-Perception and Self-Concept Pattern 399

CHAPTER NINE

Role-Relationship Pattern 455

CHAPTER TEN

Sexuality-Reproductive Pattern 541

CHAPTER ELEVEN

Coping–Stress Tolerance Pattern 573

CHAPTER TWELVE

Value-Belief Pattern 623

CHAPTER ONE

Overview

Introduction

Nursing care plans have been the bane of many practicing nurses for years. The reasons for completing and using care plans have been enumerated dozens of times; however, evidence suggests that nursing care plans often are neither fully completed nor fully used. In addition, various reasons for not doing care plans have been discussed numerous times. One common theme is that the care plan is not readily usable in practice.

All of us can recall writing long, detailed care plans as nursing students. Although it did serve as a significant teaching-learning method, this type of care plan is not usable in practice. Day-to-day practice demands a pragmatic document with a holistic viewpoint.

The care plans promoted by this book are pragmatic. They give a practical, readily usable, easily adaptable approach. Through the use of nursing diagnoses, they offer a holistic approach that addresses the patient's physical, emotional, cognitive, family, social, and cultural needs.

The care plans presented in this book demonstrate adaptation for adult health, child health, mental health, women's health, and home health. Each column on the nursing care plan represents a product of a phase of the nursing process. The care plans represent the end product of the nursing process.

The Nursing Process and Nursing Care Plans

The nursing process represents the cognitive, psychomotor, and affective skills and abilities used by the nurse to derive a nursing care plan. Figure 1.1 is a graphic representation of the relationship between the process and the plan. Even though the nurse may use a wide range of skills and may gather a wide variety of data, there is no need for all of this to be entered on the care plan. Only those things that directly affect care delivery are written on the care plan. The remainder of the assessment is entered in the chart as documentation of how the care plan originated.

A care plan has four basic components: assessment, planning, implementation, and evaluation (Yura & Walsh, 1983). To emphasize the unique nature of nursing and to clarify the difference between the nursing process and nursing care plans we have chosen to use terms representing outcomes: nursing diagnosis, objectives, nursing orders, and evaluation.

Nursing Diagnosis

The North American Nursing Diagnosis Association (NANDA), formerly the National Conference Group for Classification of Nursing Diagnosis, has been meeting since 1973 to identify, develop, and classify nursing diagnoses. The group has been meeting every other year since 1980. Setting forth a nursing diagnosis nomenclature articulates nursing language, thus promoting the identification of nursing's contribution to health. In addition, the use of nursing diagnosis provides a clear distinction between nursing diagnosis and medical diagnosis as well as providing clear direction for the remaining aspects of the care plan.

NANDA has yet to accept and approve a definition of nursing diagnosis. Discussion regarding the need for such a definition arose several times during the Eighth Conference in St. Louis.

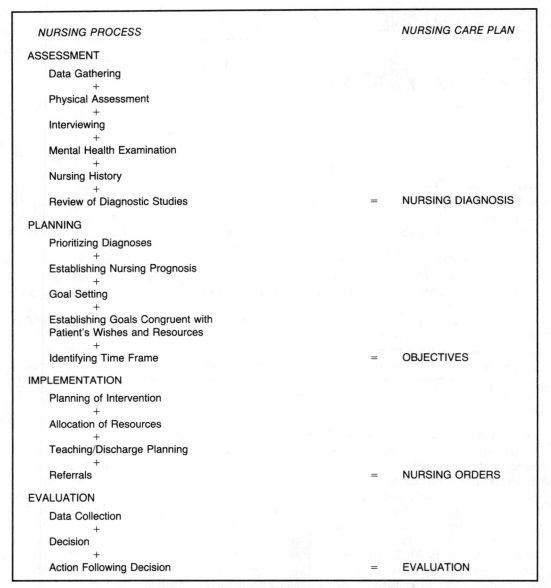

Figure 1.1   Relationship between nursing process and nursing care plan.

Moritz's (1982) adaptation of Gordon's definition of nursing diagnosis is used in this book: "Nursing diagnoses are responses to actual or potential health problems which nurses by virtue of their education and experience are able, licensed, and legally responsible and accountable to treat."

The definition of nursing diagnosis distinguishes the primary ways nursing diagnosis differs from medical diagnosis. Another way nursing diagnosis is different from medical diagnosis is in the area of focus. Nursing diagnoses focus on patient response while medical diagnoses focus on the disease process (Sorensen & Luckmann, 1979). As indicated by the definition of nursing diagnosis, nurses also identify potential problems while physicians place primary emphasis on identifying the current problem.

Nursing diagnosis and medical diagnosis are similar in that the same basic procedures are used to derive the diagnosis (i.e., physical assessment, interviewing). Likewise, both types of diagnoses are designed for essentially the same reason—planning care for a patient (Sorensen & Luckmann, 1979).

NURSING DIAGNOSIS STATEMENTS

According to the literature, complete nursing diagnostic statements include, at a minimum, the unhealthy response and an indication of the factors contributing to the response. Tartaglia (1985) presents a good rationale for the two-part statement:

Each nursing diagnosis, when correctly written, can accomplish two things. One, by identifying the unhealthy response, it tells you what should change. . . . And two, by identifying the probable cause of the unhealthy response, it tells you what to do to effect change.

While there is no consensus on the phrase that should be used to link the response and etiologic factors, perusal of current literature indicates that the most commonly used phrases are:

related to
secondary to
due to

The phrase "related to" is gaining the most acceptance because it does not imply a direct cause-and-effect relationship. Using the phrases "due to" and "secondary to" could reflect such a cause and effect relationship which could be hard to prove (Kieffer, 1984). Thus a complete nursing diagnostic statement would read:

Comfort, Altered: Pain related to Anxiety.

Gordon (1976) identifies three structural components of a nursing diagnosis statement: The problem (P), the etiology (E), and signs and symptoms (S). The problem describes the patient's response or current state. The etiology describes the cause or causes of the response, and the symptoms delineate the defining characteristics or observable signs and symptoms demonstrated or described by the patient. The S component can be readily connected to the P and E statements through the use of the phrase "as evidenced by." Using this format a complete nursing diagnostic statement would read:

Comfort, Altered: Pain related to Anxiety as evidenced by oral comments and body posture.

As discussed in the Preface, the authors of this book recommend starting with stating the nursing diagnosis only. Therefore, the nursing diagnosis would be listed on the care plan in the same manner as it is given in the nomenclature:

Comfort, Altered: Pain.

These nursing diagnosis statement examples reflect the existence of an actual problem. Professional nurses are strong supporters of preventive health care—cases in which a problem does not yet exist and measures can be taken to ensure that the problem does not arise. In such instances the nursing diagnostic statement can be prefaced by the word "potential." Carpenito (1985) advises the use of "potential" when factors exist that could place the patient at risk for the development of a problem. For example, a patient may not have an actual fluid volume deficit but because of age, weight, pathophysiology (vomiting, diarrhea), presence of catheters, and the like has a high probability of developing fluid volume deficit if appropriate measures are not taken to prevent it. Note that potential problems do not have etiologic factors but have risk factors instead.

Carpenito (1985) describes another term that can be used to alert nurses to gather further data. The term Carpenito suggests is "possible." This term is used when there are not enough data to support the use of "potential" or when an actual problem does not exist.

In this book only the actual and potential diagnoses accepted by NANDA for testing will be used. Probable related factors (formerly etiologic factors) will be grouped, as will signs and symptoms, under each specific nursing diagnosis. The care plan will reflect a conceptual approach rather than a specific (to etiology or signs and symptoms) approach. To illustrate this approach, let us use the diagnosis Comfort, Altered: Pain. There are common nursing orders related to the incidence of pain regardless of whether the pain is caused by surgery, labor, or trauma. You can take this conceptual approach and make an individualized adaptation according to the etiologic factors affecting your patient and the reaction your patient is exhibiting to pain.

CONCEPTUAL FRAMEWORKS

NURSING MODELS

Many practicing nurses do not see a direct relationship between nursing models (nursing theories) and nursing care plans, but a direct relationship does exist. Nursing models present a systematic method for assessing and directing nursing practice through promoting organization and integration of what is known about man, health, illness, and nursing. Nursing models are based on purposeful orientations; therefore, the nursing process is the action phase of a nursing model (Flynn & Heffron, 1984). In short, nursing models guide the use of the nursing process (Yura & Walsh, 1983) and, as previously stated, the nursing care plan is presented in this book as one outcome of the nursing process.

For further clarification, let us look at a few examples. If you are a supporter of Levine's conservation model, you would assess your patient in keeping with this model and then design your care plan to reflect prioritizing of the nursing diagnoses and nursing orders in a manner that would best promote conservation principles. Likewise, if you are a proponent of Roy's adaptation model, you would assess the four adaptation modes, then prioritize your diagnoses in an order that would best promote adaptative responses. In summation, current nursing models affect the nursing care plan in terms of assessment and prioritizing of nursing diagnoses rather than requiring different diagnostic statements and different nursing orders.

PATTERNS

Two typologies have emerged as a result of the work done with nursing diagnosis. The typologies are representative of another step in theory development and are designed to facilitate the use of nursing diagnosis. The typologies provide an organizational framework that enables the nurse to focus on the pattern description and assessment rather than trying to remember all the details of individual diagnoses. The nurse can easily locate the individual diagnoses by being familiar with the patterns.

Functional Health Patterns

Gordon (1982) writes that the functional health patterns were identified, circa 1974, to assist in the teaching of assessment and diagnosis at Boston College School of Nursing. The functional health patterns organize the individual diagnoses into categories, thus standardizing data collection. Figure 1.2 lists the functional health patterns along with a brief description of each pattern (Gordon, 1985). The titles of the patterns are, in essence, self-explanatory. Because the titles are self-explanatory, the functional health patterns are easy to use. The chapters in this book are organized using the functional health patterns and each chapter will include more detail regarding each functional health pattern as introductory information for the specific chapter.

Patterns of Unitary Persons

Patterns of Unitary Persons was first presented at the Fourth National Conference of NANDA. A group of nursing theorists met in between, as well as during, conferences to design a framework for classification of nursing diagnoses (Roy, 1982, 1984). The NANDA Taxonomy Committee and Special Interest Group on Taxonomy, chaired by Phyllis Kritek, reviewed and clarified the patterns and relabeled the patterns as Human Response Patterns. These revisions were presented at the Fifth and Sixth National Conferences (Kritek, 1984). According to Newman (1984), the patterns proposed by the theorist group describe clustering factors that represent person-environment interaction. The Unitary Persons categories were not mutually exclusive; that is, one nursing diagnosis might relate to one, two, or even three of the patterns. From the Fifth through the Eighth

PATTERN	DESCRIPTION
Health Perception–Health Management	The patient's awareness of personal health and well-being; health practices; understanding of how health practices contribute to health status.
Nutritional–Metabolic	The patient's description of food and fluid intake; relationship of intake to metabolic needs; includes indicators of ineffectual nutrition on metabolic functioning, e.g., healing.
Elimination	Description of all routes and routines of output. Includes any aids to excretion.
Activity-Exercise	Patient's overall activities of daily living, including recreational activity.
Sleep-Rest	Patient's 24-hour routine of rest, relaxation, and sleep.
Cognitive-Perceptual	Cognitive functional performance and sensory performance.
Self-Perception–Self-Concept	Patient's self-assessment; attitudes, ability, worth; verbal and nonverbal communication.
Role-Relationship	Patient's assessment of all roles, related responsibilities, and interrelatedness between these factors and other people.
Sexuality-Reproductive	Satisfaction-dissatisfaction with sexuality. Any dysfunction in sexuality or reproduction.
Coping–Stress Tolerance	Effectiveness or noneffectiveness in dealing with difficult situations; how handles; reaction to; support available.
Value-Belief	Ideas held in esteem by patient. Guiding principles for overall life-style.

Figure 1.2   Functional health patterns (Gordon, 1985, pp. 10–13).

National Conferences refinement of the Human Response Patterns has continued. At the Seventh National Conference the Human Response patterns were presented as the framework for "NANDA Nursing Diagnosis Taxonomy I" and was endorsed by NANDA members attending this conference.

This endorsement indicated acceptance of the Taxonomy I as a working document that would require further testing, revision, refinement, and expansion. Additional input regarding Taxonomy I was solicited at the Eighth National Conference. Much of the discussion at the Eighth Conference focused on the various levels of the taxonomy with specific questioning of the clinical usefulness of level I.

The first level of abstraction in Taxonomy I is the Human Response Patterns. The second level is alterations in functions. Levels II through V become increasingly concrete, with levels IV and V reflecting the diagnostic labels. Figure 1.3 lists the Human Response Patterns with accompanying brief definitions. In this book we have focused on level II and include levels IV and V in the conceptual information and differential diagnosis areas.

Following completion of the assessment data base and formulation of the nursing diagnoses, the same assessment data base that was used to establish the nursing diagnosis is immediately used again. This time the assessment is used in completing the next column on the care plan form: Objectives.

Objectives

As indicated by Figure 1.1, patient care objectives represent the outcome of the planning phase of the nursing process. Briefly defined, patient care objectives are "the day-to-day levels of performance which the patient must reach in order to eventually attain his long range goals"

PATTERN	DESCRIPTION
Exchanging	Involves mutual giving and receiving. Includes alterations in nutrition, physical regulation, elimination, circulation, oxygenation, and physical integrity.
Communicating	Involves sending messages. Includes alterations in communication.
Relating	Involves establishing bonds. Includes alterations in socialization and role as well as altered sexuality patterns.
Valuing	Involves the assigning of relative worth. Includes alteration in spiritual states.
Choosing	Involves the selection of alternatives. Includes alternatives in coping and participation.
Moving	Involves activity. Includes alterations in activity, rest, recreation, ADL, self-care, growth, and development.
Perceiving	Involves the reception of information. Includes attention in self concept, meaningfulness, and sensory-perceptual alteration.
Knowing	Involves the meaning associated with knowing. Includes alterations in knowledge, learning, and thought process.
Feeling	Involves the subjective awareness of information. Includes alterations in comfort and emotional integrity.

Figure 1.3. Human response patterns (NANDA, 1987).

(Sorensen & Luckmann, 1979, P. 293). Formulating good patient care objectives requires two separate steps.

Step 1 focuses on establishing patient care objectives. This means the objectives are written in a behavioral fashion that focuses on patient behavior, not nursing behavior.

Step 2 consists of establishing a target date. The target date does not mean the objective must be totally achieved by that time; instead, the target date signifies the evaluation date.

BEHAVIORAL OBJECTIVES

Clinically useful patient care objectives are (Kozier, 1972; Sorensen & Luckmann, 1979; Cox, 1982):

1. Clearly stated in terms of patient behavior or observable assessment factors.

   Example: POOR Will increase fluid balance.
   GOOD Will increase oral fluid intake to 1500 ml per 24 hours.

2. Realistic, achievable, safe, and acceptable from the patient's viewpoint.

   Example: Mrs. Braxton is a 28-year-old female who has delayed healing of a surgical wound. She is to receive discharge instructions regarding a high-protein diet. She is a widow with three children under the age of 10. Her only source of income is Social Security.

   Example: POOR Will eat at least two 8-oz. servings of steak daily [unrealistic, etc.].
   GOOD Will eat at least two servings from the following list each day:
   Lean ground meat
   Eggs
   Cheese
   Pinto beans
   Peanut butter
   Fish
   Chicken

3. Written in specific, concrete terms depicting patient action.

   Example: POOR Maintains fluid intake.
   GOOD Will drink at least 8 oz of fluid every hour from 7 AM to 10 PM

4. Directly observable by use of at least one of the five senses.

   Example: POOR Understands how to self-administer insulin.
   GOOD Accurately return demonstrates self-administration of insulin.

5. Patient-centered rather than nurse-centered.

   Example: POOR Teaches how to measure blood pressure.
   GOOD Accurately measures own blood pressure.

SETTING TARGET DATES

Writing a target date at the end of the objective statement facilitates the nursing care plan in several ways (Kozier, 1972; Sorensen & Luckmann, 1979):

1. Assists in "pacing" the care plan. Pacing helps keep focus on the patient's progress.
2. Serves to motivate both patients and nurses toward accomplishing the objective.
3. Helps patient and nurse to see accomplishments.
4. Alerts nurses when to evaluate care plan.

Target dates can be realistically established by paying attention to the usual progress and prognosis connected with the patient's medical and nursing diagnoses. Additional review of the data collected during the initial assessment will help indicate individual factors to be considered in establishing the date. For example, one of the previous objectives was stated as: Self-administer insulin injection.

The progress or prognosis according to the patient's medical and nursing diagnosis will be immaterial. The primary factor will be whether diabetes mellitus is a new diagnosis for the patient or is a recurring problem for a patient who has had diabetes mellitus for several years.

For the newly diagnosed patient we would probably want our deadline day to be 5–7 days from the date of learning the diagnosis. For the recurring problem we might establish the target date to be 2–3 days from the date of diagnosis. The difference is, of course, the patient's basic knowledge base.

Now, look at an example related to the progress issue. Mr. Kit is a 19-year-old college student who was admitted early this morning with a medical diagnosis of acute appendicitis. He has just returned from surgery following an appendectomy. One of the nursing diagnoses for Mr. Kit would, in all probability, be: Comfort, Altered: Pain. The objective could be: Will have decrease in number of requests for analgesics by (date). In reviewing the general progress of a young patient with this medical and nursing diagnosis, we know that generally analgesic requirements start decreasing within 48–72 hours. Therefore, we would want to establish our target date as 2 or 3 days following the day of surgery. This would result in the objective reading (assume date of surgery was 11/1): Will have decrease in number of requests for analgesics by 11/3.

To further emphasize the target date, it is suggested that the date be underlined, highlighted by using a different-colored pen, or circled to make it stand out. Pinpointing the date in such a manner emphasizes that evaluation of the progress toward achievement of the objective should be made on that date. In assigning the dates be sure you do not schedule all of the diagnoses and objectives for evaluation on the same date. This would require a total revision of the care plan which could contribute to not keeping the care plan current. Being able to revise single portions of the care plan facilitates using and updating the care plan.

Once the objective column has been completed, the nurse is then ready to focus on the next phase—implementation. As previously indicated, the title supported by this book for the third column is "Nursing Orders."

Nursing Orders

Nursing orders represent the outcome of the implementation phase of the nursing process (refer to Figure 1.1). Nursing orders are defined as:

Nursing behavior and actions that serve to help the patient achieve the stated objectives.

Nursing orders include both independent and collaborative (interdependent) activities; for example, implementing a physician's order or referring to a dietitian. Nursing orders function to guide both actual patient care and proper documentation.

Nursing orders differ from physician orders in depth. A nursing order should be more detailed and exact than what is generally found in physician orders. For example, a physician writes the order, "Increase ambulation as tolerated," for a patient who has been immobile for 2 weeks. The nursing orders should reflect specified increments of ambulation as well as ongoing assessment:

11/2   1.   a.   Prior to activity assess BP, P, and R. After activity assess: (1) BP, P, R; (2) Presence/absence of vertigo; (3) circulation; (4) presence/absence of pain.
           b.   Assist to dangle on bedside for 15 minutes at least 4 times a day on 11/2.
           c.   If BP, P, or R change significantly or vertigo present or impaired circulation present or pain present, return to supine position immediately. Elevate head of bed 30° for 1 hour; then to 45° for 1 hour; then to 90° for 1 hour. If tolerated with no untoward signs or symptoms, initiate order 1b again.
           d.   Assist up to chair at bedside for 30 minutes at least 4 times a day on 11/3.
           e.   Assist to ambulate to bathroom and back at least 4 times a day on 11/4.
           f.   Supervise ambulation of one-half length of hall at least 4 times a day on 11/5 and 11/6.
           g.   Supervise ambulation of length of hall at least 4 times a day on 11/7.

S.J. Smith, R.N.

Nursing orders further differ from physician orders in that the patient's response is directly related to the implementation of the order. It is rare to see a physician's order that includes alternatives if the first order has minimal, negative, or no effect on the patient.

A complete nursing order incorporates the following five components (Sorensen & Luckmann, 1979):

1. Date the order was written.
2. A specific action verb that tells what the nurse is to do (e.g., "assist," "supervise").
3. A prescribed activity (e.g., ambulation).
4. Specific time units (e.g., for 15 minutes at least 4 times a day).
5. Signature of the nurse who writes the order (i.e., accepting legal and ethical accountability).

A nursing order should not be implemented unless all five components are present. A nurse would not administer a medication if the physician's order read, "Give Demerol"; neither should a nurse be expected to implement a nursing order that reads, "Increase ambulation gradually."

Additional criteria that should be remembered to ensure complete, quality nursing orders, include:

1. Consistency between the orders, the nursing diagnosis, and objectives (including numbering). For example:
   Nursing Diagnosis—1. Impaired physical mobility, level 2.
   Objective—1. Will ambulate length of hall by 11/8.
   Nursing Orders—11/2

    1a.   Prior to activity assess BP, P, and R. After activity assess: (1)BP, P, R; (2) presence/absence of vertigo; (3) circulatory check; (4) presence/absence of pain.
    1b.   Assist to dangle on bedside for 15 minutes at least 4 times a day on 11/2.
    1c.   If BP, P, R change significantly or vertigo present or impaired circulation present or pain present, return to supine position immediately. Elevate head of bed 30° for 1 hour; then to 45° for 1 hour; then to 90° degrees for 1 hour. If tolerated with no untoward signs or symptoms, initiate order 1b again.

1d. Assist up to chair at bedside for 30 minutes at least 4 times a day on 11/3.
1e. Assist to ambulate to bathroom and back at least 4 times a day on 11/4.
1f. Supervise ambulation of one-half length of hall at least 4 times a day on 11/5 and 11/6.
1g. Supervise ambulation of length of hall at least 4 times a day in 11/7.

S.J. Smith, R.N.

2. Consideration of both patient and facility resources. It would be senseless to order referral to services such as P T and O T if these were not available. Likewise, from the patient's resource viewpoint, it would be foolish to teach him and his family how to manage his care in a hospital bed if this bed would not be available to the patient at home.
3. Careful scheduling to include the patient's significant others and to incorporate his usual activities of daily living (i.e., rest, meals, sleep, and recreation).
4. Incorporation of patient teaching and discharge planning from the 1st day of care.
5. Individualization and updating in keeping with the patient's condition and progress.

Including the key components and validating the quality of the order helps to promote improved documentation. In essence, the nursing orders can give an outline for documentation.

Properly written nursing orders demonstrate to the nurse not only what actions are to be done, but also the charting to be done. Referring to the example on page 8, we can see that the nurse responsible for this patient's care should chart the patient's BP, P, and R rates prior to the activity, the patient's BP, P, and R rates after the activity, the presence or absence of vertigo, the presence or absence of pain, and the results of a circulatory check. Additionally, the nurse knows to chart that the patient dangled, sat up, or ambulated for a certain length of time or distance. Further, the nurse has guidelines of what to do and chart if an untoward reaction occurs in initial attempts at ambulation.

> *Example*: 1000—BP $^{132}/_{82}$, P 74, R 16. Up on side of bed for 5 minutes. Complained of vertigo and nausea. Returned to supine position with head of bed elevated to 30° angle. BP $^{100}/_{68}$, P 8, R 24.
> 1100—BP $^{122}/_{74}$, P 76, R 18. No complaints of vertigo or nausea. Head of bed elevated from 30° to 45° angle.

Writing nursing orders in such a manner automatically leads to reflection of the nursing care plan in the chart. Demonstrating implementation of the care plan in the chart meets Joint Commission on Accreditation of Health Care Organizations (formerly JCAH) criteria and, as a quick review of this section on nursing orders will show, it was not difficult at all.

To complete the first care plan cycle and, depending on its outcome, perhaps start another cycle, the final phase of the care plan must be done. The last part of the care plan is evaluation.

Evaluation

Evaluation simply means assessing what progress has been made toward meeting the stated objectives. The evaluation phase is the feedback and control part of the nursing care plan. Evaluation requires continuation of assessment that was begun in the initial nursing diagnosis phase. In this instance, assessment is the data collection form we use to measure patient progress.

DATA COLLECTION

The data collection should initially be aimed at collecting the specific data needed to measure the progress made toward achieving the stated objective. As an example, let us return to the objective written for Mr. Kit, the 19-year-old college student who had an appendectomy. The objective read, "Will have decrease in number of requests for analgesics by 11/3." It is now 11/3, the nurse caring for Mr. Kit notes the date and initiates evaluation of the objective. She first checks the chart and counts the number of complaints of pain, number of analgesics given, and Mr. Kit's response to the pain medication. She looks for any change in medication or a change in Mr. Kit's condition. She then interviews Mr. Kit regarding his perception of pain acuity and level of relief. At the same time the nurse will be completing other assessments such as wound condition, ease of ambulation, or presence of any other untoward signs or symptoms. The nurse then studies the data to see what action is necessary.

ACTION FOLLOWING DATA COLLECTION

Action following data collection simply means making a nursing judgment of what modification in the nursing care plan is needed. There are essentially only three judgments that can be made:

1. Resolved
2. Revise
3. Continue

Resolved means that the evaluative data indicates the health care problem reflected in the nursing diagnosis and its accompanying objective no longer exist; that is, the objective has been met. The nurse reflects, in the evaluation column, the data collected and records the judgment Resolved. To illustrate, let us return to Mr. Kit.

The nurse first reviews the chart. She finds that Mr. Kit requested pain medication every 3–4 hours for the first 18 hours after surgery. The nurses taught Mr. Kit relaxation exercises and turned him, positioned him, and gave him a backrub after each analgesic. Mr. Kit has requested only one analgesic in the last 24 hours. No changes in orders or in Mr. Kit's condition were reflected on the chart. During the subsequent interview Mr. Kit indicates the pain medication fully relieved his pain and he has had no pain in the last 12 hours. He can return demonstrate relaxation exercises and states he has only a mild "twinge" when he gets out of bed. He is looking forward to returning to school next week.

The nurse returns to the care plan and records the following: "11/3 Data—1 analgesic in last 24 hours. Ambulates without pain; states having no pain. Resolved." She then will draw one line through the nursing diagnosis, related objective, and nursing orders to show they have been discontinued.

Revise can indicate two actions. In one instance, the initial nursing diagnosis was not correct so the diagnosis is revised. For example, the nurse may have made an initial diagnosis of Self-Esteem Disturbance. Upon collecting evaluation data, the patient and his family share further information that indicates the more appropriate diagnosis is Powerlessness: moderate. The nursing care plan is then modified to reflect the change in the nursing diagnosis. In the evaluation column on the nursing care plan, the nurse again records the data and the word, "Revised." She then adds the new nursing diagnosis and marks one line through the initial nursing diagnosis.

In the second instance, while the nurse is collecting evaluation data for one nursing diagnosis and objective, she finds assessment factors that show another problem has arisen. She simply records the appropriate judgment for the initial diagnosis and objective (e.g., Resolved), and revises the plan to include the new nursing diagnosis with its appropriate objective and nursing orders.

Continue indicates that the objective has not been met. The nurse again collects the appropriate data and, based on the data, makes the nursing judgment that the objective has not been met. She records the data and adds the phrase, "Continue, reevaluate on (date)." She then modifies the care plan by going back to the objective column, marking one line through the date, and adding a new date.

With evaluation, the cycle is completed. Another cycle can begin with both the nurse and the patient being sure that quality care is being given and received.

Valuing Care Plans

Another major reason, besides not being pragmatic, that care plans have not been completed and used is that value has not been attached to care plans. All of us will make time or a place for those things that are of value to us. It is only recently that completing and evaluating the quality of care plans have begun to show up on employee evaluation forms. Likewise, it is still rare to see "complete nursing care plan" or "update care plan" on the patient assignment form.

With the changes that are occurring in health care, due to federal and state legislated mandates, completion and use of nursing care plans are going to increase in importance. Several insurance companies now audit charts, care plans, and the like in detail. No documentation of care means no reimbursement for care. Likewise, one of the first places a lawyer looks when hunting evidence for health-related court cases is the patient's chart. The basic principle in lawsuits has been, "not charted; not done." Designing the care plan, as proposed by this book, would furnish additional documentation that reasonably prudent care was given as well as providing a guideline for better charting.

Use of nursing diagnosis helps ensure that teaching and discharge planning are considered from the start of care. As we increase our knowledge and begin to think in terms related to nursing nomenclature, a natural nursing order for many of the diagnoses is going to relate to teaching and planning for home care.

Many of the standards supported by the Joint Commission on Accreditation of Health Care Organizations, the American Nurses' Association, and state boards of nursing are automatically implemented when nursing care plans are completed and used. A review of these standards by the reader will show that the nursing care plan can meet several standards through the utilization of just this one nursing tool.

It is not uncommon to hear, "I don't do care plans because I don't have time to do them." It is true there is an investment of time in designing a care plan, but in the long-range view, care plans actually save time. To illustrate, one nurse we know works full time in nursing education but works part time at a local hospital to keep her clinical skills current. One afternoon she went to work at the hospital, received her patient assignments and a brief report, then began to implement patient care. One nursing order read, "Change dressing as needed." Assessment of the dressing showed a change was needed. In the patient's room were all kinds of dressings, fluids, and ointments. There were no instructions for changing the dressing on the care plan nor on the patient's chart. The nurse then requested information from the patient who stated, "I don't like to look at it, so I don't know." The nurse then began to search for a staff member who had cared for this patient and could teach her the routine for the special dressing change. After 30 minutes, she finally found a nurse who had cared for the patient. Learning the proper dressing change took only a few minutes. The nurse then went back to the care plan, and in 3 minutes recorded the way to change the dressing under nursing orders. Comparing the time it took to locate the information and the time it took to record the information gives a graphic example of how time can be saved by completing the care plan. Consider the time saved if the nursing orders are used as an outline for charting, or the time that could be saved in between-shift reports if care plans were complete. Lastly, consider the time that could be saved by not having to go to court when questions arise over reasonably prudent care. Making time to complete care plans, because we can see their value to us, actually saves us time in the long run.

Summary

Nursing care plans that are complete and utilized provide a quality tool for nurses. Designing the care plan with the format of nursing diagnosis, objectives, nursing orders, and evaluation makes the plans more pragmatic and reflective of the true nature of nursing.

REFERENCES

Carpenito, L. J. (1985). Actual, potential, or possible. *American Journal of Nursing, 85*(4), 458.
Cox, H. C. (1982). *Developing nursing care plan objectives: A programmed unit of study.* Lubbock, TX: Texas Tech University, Health Sciences Center, School of Nursing, Continuing Nursing Education Program.
Flynn, J. M., & Heffron, P. B. (1984). *Nursing: From concept to practice.* Bowie, MD: Brady Communication.
Gordon, M. (1985). *Manual of nursing diagnosis: 1984–1985.* New York: McGraw-Hill.

Gordon, M. (1976). Nursing diagnosis and the diagnostic process. *American Journal of Nursing, 76* (8), 1298–1300.

Gordon, M. (1982). *Nursing diagnosis: Process and application*. New York: McGraw-Hill.

Kieffer, J. S. (1984). Nursing diagnosis can make a critical difference. *Nursing Life, 4* (3), 18–21.

Kozier, B., & Dugas, B. W. (1972). *Introduction to patient care: A comprehensive approach to nursing*. Philadelphia: W. B. Saunders.

Kritek, P. B. (1984). Report of the group who worked on taxonomies. In M. J. Kim, G. K. McFarland, & A. M. McLane (Eds.), *Classification of nursing diagnosis: Proceedings of the fifth national conference* (pp. 46–58). St. Louis: C. V. Mosby.

Moritz, D. A. (1982). Nursing diagnosis in relation to the nursing process. In M. J. Kim & D. A. Moritz (Eds.), *Classification of nursing diagnosis: Proceedings of the third and fourth national conferences* (pp. 53–57). St. Louis: McGraw-Hill.

Newman, M. A. (1984). Looking at the whole. *American Journal of Nursing, 84*(12), 1496–1499.

North American Nursing Diagnosis Association. (1987). *Taxonomy I with complete diagnoses*. St. Louis: Author.

Roy, C., Sr. (1982). Historical perspective of the theoretical framework for the classification of nursing diagnosis (1980). In M. J. Kim & D. A. Moritz (Eds.), *Classification of nursing diagnosis: Proceedings of the third and fourth national conferences* (pp. 235–245). St. Louis: McGraw-Hill.

Roy, C., Sr. (1984). Framework for classification system development: Progress and issues. In M. J. Kim, G. K. McFarland, & A. M. McLane (Eds.), *Classification of nursing diagnosis: Proceedings of the fifth national conference* (p. 29). St. Louis: C. V. Mosby.

Sorensen, K., & Luckmann, J. (1979). *Basic nursing: A psychophysiologic approach*. Philadelphia: W. B. Saunders.

Tartaglia, M. J. (1985). Nursing diagnosis: Keystone of your care plan. *Nursing 85, 15* (3), 34–37.

Yura, H., & Walsh, M. B. (1983). *The nursing process: Assessing, planning, implementing, evaluating* (4th ed.). East Norwalk, CT: Appleton-Century-Crofts.

CHAPTER TWO

Health Perception– Health Management Pattern

Pattern Description

Nurses care for patients who may have altered perceptions of health or difficulties in maintaining their health management programs. Some people may seek assistance in altering health habits and environmental conditions in order to achieve optimal health. The alteration in health perception– health management pattern may be recognized by the patient or the patient's family and may be the reason for seeking care. The nurse may identify the pattern alteration while working with a patient who is receiving care for other nursing diagnoses. Whether the alteration is identified by the patient, by his or her family, or by the nurse, care needs to be individualized to meet the specific alteration in health perception–health management pattern according to the patient's needs.

This pattern includes the individual's and the family's perception and understanding of health status and how perception and understanding are incorporated into life-style, including plans for future health planning and life-style decisions.

Pattern Assessment

1. Patient description of health status.
2. Family description of health status.
3. Patient description of usual health management strategies, health care behaviors, and preventive practices.
4. Family description of usual health management strategies, health care behaviors, and preventive practices.
5. Nursing observations of health behaviors.
6. Congruence between patient and family description; congruence between descriptions and nursing observations.

Conceptual Information

A person who practices health management techniques and adequately perceives the level of personal health status will identify techniques to maintain health and accurately report the level of health status. Alterations in health status will also be identified and steps taken to correct the alteration to increase movement toward optimal health. Measures to prevent further alterations in health status will be initiated.

Various factors influence a person's capability to achieve optimal health perception and health management patterns. Sensory organs provide information to the individual regarding the environment. An intact nervous system provides for optimal processing of sensory, motor, and cognitive activities. An accurate cognitive-perceptual pattern and self-perception–self-concept pattern are necessary to achieve the optimal level of health perception and health management pattern. Knowledge related to health promotion, disease prevention, and healthy living is essential. Cultural, societal, and familial values and beliefs also influence the capacity to achieve optimal health perception and health management patterns. Values and beliefs will also influence what is identified as optimal health.

The Health Belief Model (Rosenstock, 1974) provides a framework in which to study actions taken by individuals to avoid illness. A basic assumption of the model is that the subjective state of the individual is more important in determining actions than is the objective reality of the situation. The health belief model states that for an individual to take action to avoid a disease she or he needs to believe the following:

1. That she or he is personally susceptible to disease;
2. That the occurence of the disease will have at least moderate severity on some part of her or his life;
3. That taking action will be beneficial;
4. That such action will not involve overcoming psychological barriers such as cost, pain, or embarrassment.

These variables can be described under the headings of perceived susceptibility and severity as well as the variables that define perceived benefits and barriers to taking action. Because these variables do not account for the activation of the behavior, the originators of the health belief model have added another class of variable called cues to action. The individual's level of readiness provides the energy to act, and the perception of benefits provides a preferred manner of action which offers the path of least resistance. A cue to action is required to set off this appropriate action. The model suggests that by manipulating any combination of variables affecting action, the inclination to seek preventive care can be altered.

The Health Belief Model does not contain concepts related to knowledge of disease as a potential factor determining an individual's inclination to engage in preventive behavior. Several authors point out that knowledge of health consequences has only a limited relationship to the occurrence of the desired health behavior (Arya & Bennett, 1974; Sackett & Haynes, 1976; Ridenour, 1983). Yet, quite often, imparting knowledge about diseases to the patient, in an effort to encourage future preventive behavior, is the main method employed by nurses.

The Health Belief Model is disease specific. The model is not adequate to explain positive health actions designed to maximize wellness, fulfillment, and self-actualization. Although the Health Belief Model is useful in predicting preventive behavior, it does not explain behavior motivated by health promotion (Pender, 1987). More research is needed to identify the determinants of health-promoting behavior.

Pender (1987) points out that while health promotion and disease prevention are complementary concepts, they are not congruent. Health promotion is directed toward growth and improvement in well-being, while disease prevention conceptually operates to maintain status quo (Brubaker, 1983).

The Health Promotion Model as developed by Pender (1987) provides the framework for nursing research and practice. This model emphasizes the importance of cognitive perceptual factors in behavior regulation. Cognitive perceptual factors such as importance of health, definition of health, perceived self-efficacy, and perceived control of health are primary motivational mechanisms for health-promoting behavior.

The Health Belief Model does provide the nurse with the conceptual notion that by working with the patient's perception of the situation, increasing an individual's cues to action, and decreasing an individual's barriers to action, the nurse can enhance the possibility that the patient will engage in disease prevention and early detection activities.

The concepts of primary, secondary, and tertiary prevention (Stanhope, 1988) are also useful to the nurse when assessing the health management pattern. It is important for the nurse to recognize that a focus on the patient's strengths and not just on the patient's problems is an integral part of health promotion (Gleit & Tatro, 1981).

Primary Prevention: Consists of activities that prevent a disease from occurring.

1. Maintains up-to-date immunizations.
2. Has adequate water supply and sanitation facilities.
3. Uses seat belts and infant car seats and properly stores household poisons to minimize accident fatalities.
4. Eliminates tobacco products.
5. Maintains adequate nutrition, elimination, exercise, social, and personal relationships, etc.
6. Employs regular oral care and dental examinations.
7. Demonstrates safe sun exposure.
8. Maintains weight within normal range for age, sex, and height.
9. Maintains environment free of chemical, biological, and physical hazards.
10. Maintains regular sleep and rest patterns.
11. Practices healthy nutritional intake (e.g., low salt, sugar, and fat intake with balanced intake of basic four food groups and total calories as appropriate for age, sex, and condition).
12. Maintains regular relaxation, recreation, and exercise activities.

Secondary Prevention: Activities designed to detect disease before symptoms are recognized.

1. Glaucoma screening.
2. Hypertensive screening.
3. Hearing and vision testing.
4. Pap smears.
5. Breast examinations.
6. Prostate and testicle examinations.
7. Well-baby examinations.
8. Colon and rectal examinations.

Tertiary Prevention: Treatment, care, and rehabilitation of current illness.

1. Adheres to medical and nursing treatments.
2. Makes life-style changes necessitated by condition.
3. Seeks consultation from experts in area requiring intervention.

Developmental Considerations

Care providers can encourage the teaching of responsibility for health-promoting activities and adherence to agreed-on treatment plans as appropriate for the developmental capabilities of the individual.

Sensorimotor State (Birth–24 Months)

Since the neonate is dependent on others for care, it is the primary caregiver who is entrusted with carrying out the therapeutic interventions. As the infant grows and develops, self-care abilities increase. The following information outlines developmental milestones from birth to approximately 24 months as described by Piaget's Sensorimotor stage of cognitive development (Schuster & Ashburn, 1986). During this period of development the individual must be protected from hazards in the environment, and the primary caregiver must assume major responsibility for compliance with the treatment program.

Providing a safe environment includes the following accident prevention strategies: (a) turning pot handles away from edge of stove; (b) storing medicines, matches, alcohol, plastic bags, and house and garden chemicals in child-proofed areas (c) using cold-water, not hot-water, humidifier; (d) avoiding heating formula in microwave (e) using protection screens on heaters, fireplaces, and electrical outlets; (f) using nonflammable clothing (g) protecting stairways and windows; (h) supervising children at play, while bathing, in car, or in shopping cart; (i) controlling pets or stray animals; (j) avoiding items hung around neck; (k) providing a smoke-free environment; (l) avoiding small objects that can be inserted in mouth or nose; (m) avoiding pillows and plastic in crib; (n) removing poisonous plants from house and garden; (o) removing lead-based paint.

Children should be screened at birth for congenital anomalies, phenylketonuria (PKU), thyroid function, cystic fibrosis, vision, and hearing. A newborn assessment should be performed, and anticipatory guidance should be provided for patients regarding growth and development, safety, health promotion, and disease prevention.

Well-baby examinations and developmental assessments are recommended every 2–3 months. These should include diphtheria, pertussis, tetanus (DPT) and trivalent oral polio vaccine (TOPV) at 2, 4, and 6 months; tuberculin test at 12 months; measles, mumps, and rubella (MMR) vaccine at 15 months, and DPT and TOPV repeated at 18 months. Information regarding oral, perineal, and perirectal hygiene, sensory stimulation, nutrition, and safety and accident prevention is important during this period.

Host factors such as age and behavior will affect the susceptibility to infectious disease. In general, most infectious diseases produce the greatest morbidity and mortality in the very old and the very young (Baron & Tafuro, 1985). It is also important to note that the normal newborn will have a white blood cell count that is higher than that of the normal adult. The normal white blood cell count decreases gradually throughout childhood until reaching the adult norms (Schuster, 1977). The nurse is advised to learn the norms for the target population.

During fetal life, the fetus has been protected by maternal antibodies (assuming the mother has developed antibodies to these diseases) to such things as diphtheria, tetanus, measles, and polio infections. This temporary immunity lasts 3–6 months. Colostrum contains antibodies that provide protection against enteric pathogens. Some infections can cross the placental barrier, leading to congenital infections. Syphilis and rubella are examples of such infections. Pathogenic organisms such as herpes simplex may be acquired during passage through the birth canal. Because the infant does not begin to produce its own immuno-globulins until 2–3 months after birth, it is susceptible to infections for which it has not gained passive immunity.

TORCH infections (toxoplasmosis, hepatitis B, rubella, cytomegalovirus, herpes) can be of serious concern during the perinatal period (Devore, Jackson, & Piening, 1983). When caring for a pregnant female or a newborn it is important to teach techniques to prevent acquisition and transmission of these disorders and to recognize early signs and symptoms so that early interventions can be instituted.

Child care practices must include hygienic disposal of soiled diapers and cleaning of the perineum. Proper handwashing technique is required of the care provider. Proper formula preparation and storage are also critical if the newborn is to be bottle fed. Anatomically the newborn and infant's eustachian tube facilitates the traffic of infection-causing organisms into the middle ear. It is important for care providers not to prop bottles but rather to hold the newborn or infant while feeding. Passive exposure to tobacco smoke irritates the bronchial tree and increases the possibility of respiratory infection.

The infant may respond to an infection with a high fever. Care providers should be instructed in taking axillary temperatures, providing hydration to an ill infant, giving tepid baths when fever is elevated, and seeking professional evaluation when an infant has febrile illness.

During the preoperational period, children learn how to teach themselves through the development of trial and error, exploration, and repetition. From age 2–4 years the child is egocentric, using himself or herself as a standard for others; he or she can categorize on the basis of a single characteristic. Because of the child's curiosity and exploration of the environment, it is important for the care provider to provide a safe environment. During this period the concepts of "no," "hot," "sharp," and "hurt" should be repeatedly introduced and reinforced by the care provider. Safety rules should be taught and reinforced repeatedly.

From ages 4–7 years the child can begin to see simple relationships and has the beginning ability to think in logical classes. The child can learn his or her own address and can follow directions of three steps. Rules need to be reinforced. The child can be responsible for personal hygiene with instruction and coaching.

Strategies used to provide a safe environment for the infant should also be employed during childhood. Discipline, accident prevention, and the development of self-care proficiency related to eating, dressing, bathing, and dental hygiene are important areas of concern. Annual developmental assessments with emphasis on hearing, vision, and speech development are recommended. DPT and TOPV should be given at 18 months and MMR at 15 months. Anticipatory guidance should be given to parents regarding the growth and development of the preschooler, including the development of initiative, guilt, and preconceptual, preoperational thought (Schuster & Ashburn, 1986).

As the child begins to explore the environment and put objects and foods into his or her mouth, it is important to ensure that contact with infectious pathogens or foreign bodies is controlled. Foreign-object-induced infection should be considered in childhood infections of the external ear, nose, and vagina, for example.

If the preschooler has been exposed to other children, he or she most likely will have experienced several middle ear, gastrointestinal, and upper respiratory tract infections. If the child has not been around other children, he or she will likely experience such infections when entering preschool or kindergarten.

The DPT and TOPV vaccinations are given between 4 and 5 years of age. The child will require assistance with toileting hygiene until 4–5 years of age. Handwashing techniques can be introduced along with toilet training and followed with consistent role modeling by the adults and older children with assistance to the child.

Prevention of injury will also assist in prevention of infection.

The adenoidal and tonsillar lymphoid tissue may normally enlarge in early school years. Proper dental hygiene is important to prevent tooth and gum infections.

Bubble baths and other scented soaps and toilet tissue may irritate the urethra in the female and lead to urinary tract or vaginal infections. Such items should be avoided.

Concrete Operations (7–11 Years)

This period is characterized by developing logical approaches to concrete problems; the concepts of reversibility and conservation are developed, and the child can organize objects and events into classes and arrange in order of increasing values. The child can be responsible for personal hygiene and simple household tasks. The child will need assistance when ill, but can be taught self-care activities as required such as insulin injections or taking medications on a regular basis. The child can distinguish and describe physical symptoms and report them to the appropriate caregiver, and can follow instructions. Strategies employed by care providers to provide a safe environment, prevent disease, and promote health can be taught to the child. The child can perform many of these functions with supervision. Emphasis is placed on health education of the child in safety and accident prevention, nutrition, substance abuse, and anticipated changes with puberty. Developmental assessments are performed with emphasis on language, vision, and hearing. DPT and TOPV boosters are given between 4 and 6 years. Anticipatory guidance for parents and child should include the development of industry and inferiority. Intuitive, preoperational thought begins to develop into concrete operational thinking (Schuster & Ashburn, 1986).

Formal Operations (11–15 Years–Adolescence)

True logical thought is developed. Abstract concepts are manipulated. A scientific approach to problem solving can be planned and implemented. The adolescent can develop, with guidance, responsibility for total self-care. With experience the adolescent requires less guidance and can assume full decision making responsibility and total responsibility for self-care.

Emphasis is placed on health education of the adolescent in healthful living habits, safe driving, sex education, skin care, substance abuse, career choices, relationships, dating and marriage, self breast examination for females, and self testicular examination for males. Screening for pregnancy, sexually transmitted diseases, depression, high blood pressure, and substance abuse can be done. Anticipatory guidance for parents and adolescent should include the development of identity and role confusion and formal operational thought (Schuster & Ashburn, 1986).

The hormonal changes of puberty may lead to acne vulgaris. If severe, proper hygiene and dermatologic evaluation will prevent serious complications. The changes in the vaginal tissue secondary to hormonal changes provide an environment conducive to yeast infections. If the adolescent is engaging in sexual activity, he or she is at risk for exposure to sexually transmitted diseases. Irritants such as soap, bubble bath, etc. may increase the possibility of urinary tract infection in females. Improper genital hygiene also predisposes the female to urinary tract infection.

A diphtheria and tetanus vaccination (Td) should be given at age 14–15. Adolescents may be living in group settings as in a dormitory. Increased risk of communicable disease is present in such living arrangements. Good personal hygiene is important to decrease this risk.

Risk-taking behavior of adolescents may increase the risk of infection and accidents (e.g., IV drug use; use of tobacco; traumatic injury which breaks the skin, allowing a portal of entry for pathogenic organisms; fad diets or other activities which decrease the overall health status; improper technique or equipment in water sports; motor vehicle accidents; running a vehicle or other combustion engines when not properly ventilated; substance abuse; choking on food; smoke inhalation; improper storage and handling of guns, ammunition, and knives; excessive risk-taking behavior; smoking in bed; improper use or storage of flammable items, hazardous tools, and equipment; drug ingestion; playing or working around toxic vegetation; improper preparation and storage of food; improper precautions and use of insecticides, fertilizers, cleaning products, medications, alcohol, and other toxic substances).

Formal Operations (Adulthood)

Adult thought is more refined than adolescent thought in that experience and education allow the adult to differentiate among many points of view and potential outcomes in an objective and realistic manner. The adult can consider more options and can apply inductive as well as deductive approaches to problem solving. The adult assumes total responsibility for the care of a child. In middle adult years, the adult may also care for an elder parent.

The adult is concerned about many of the same health-promotion and disease-prevention issues as is the adolescent. Emphasis is placed on life-style counseling related to family planning, parenting, stress management, career advancement, relationship enhancement, hazards at work, and development of intimacy and generativity. Regular self breast examination and Pap smear (female) and self testicular examination (male) should be done. Screening for glaucoma, high blood pressure, and colon, endometrial, oral, or breast cancer should be done if the patient is in a risk category.

As the body develops more and more antibodies to pathogens, the adult may find that he or she does not have as many colds as he or she used to. Some viral infections (mumps for example) may present serious consequences to adults (men in this case). The adult female is as susceptible to genitourinary infections as the adolescent. Sexually active adults are at risk for sexually transmitted diseases.

Formal Operations (Elderly)

In the absence of illness affecting cognitive functioning, the elderly person maintains formal operational abilities. The elder person can assume total responsibility for decision making and self-care. The elder adult also often assumes responsibility for the care of others, for example children or grandchildren. As with other developmental levels, illness or physical disability can alter the cognitive functioning and lead to self-care deficits.

Emphasis is on health education related to grandparenting, retirement, and home safety. Anticipatory guidance is related to the development of ego-integrity. Self breast examination, Pap smear, mammography (female), self testicular examination (male) should be done. Glaucoma, blood pressure, and colon cancer screening should also be done. Podiatry care should be given as needed.

The elderly person may have decreased ability to remove himself or herself from hazardous situations due to decreased mobility, and decreased ability to recognize smoke inhalation or gas-related hazards due to decreased olfactory sense. Sensory, motor, and perceptual deficits and orthostatic hypotension may increase the potential for injury and increase self-care deficits.

Elderly persons may experience a decline in the immunologic response, making them more susceptible to infections. Skin changes may provide easier access to infecting organisms. (Increased dryness and thinning of the dermis may make the skin more injury prone.) Susceptible elderly persons should be vacinnated for influenza and pneumonia. Many older people are also not adequately protected against tetanus.

There is an increase in frequency and severity of infections with aging. Normally the immunologic defenses decline with aging (Baron & Tafuro, 1985). Mechanical and chemical defenses also are diminished with increasing age.

Mechanical. Motility and secretion decrease in the GI tract. Esophageal and gastric peristalsis are decreased. Renal filtration, absorption, and excretion diminish. Incomplete emptying of the bladder provides a medium for the growth of organisms. The respiratory muscles are weaker and there is decreased elasticity of lung tissue. Diminished cough and gag reflexes may increase the possibility of aspiration. The skin becomes thinner and less elastic. Poor circulation related to vascular insufficiency, peripheral neuropathy, and the increased fragility of the skin increase the possibility of tissue trauma and resulting invasion by microorganisms.

Chemical. Hydrochloric acid secretion diminishes.

Internal. There is decreased production of T-lymphocytes leading to impaired ability to destroy infectious organisms. The production of antibodies by β-lymphocytes is also decreased. These changes make the elderly more susceptible to infection and unable to recover as quickly as when they were younger; some may not develop immunity after an infection.

Chronic illness and hospitalization or nursing home placement additionally increase the risk of infection (Baron & Tafuro, 1985). The elderly adult may not demonstrate an increased body temperature in response to an infection.

Applicable Nursing Diagnoses

Health Maintenance, Altered

DEFINITION

Inability to identify, manage, or seek out help to maintain health (North American Nursing Diagnosis Association [NANDA], 1987, p. 86).

(Note: Carpenito [1987] recommends that this diagnostic category be used for an asymptomatic person. It may also be employed to assist a person with a chronic disease to achieve a higher level of wellness.)

DEFINING CHARACTERISTICS (NANDA, 1987, p. 86)

The nurse will review the initial pattern assessment for the following defining characteristics to determine the diagnosis of health maintenance alteration:

1. Major defining characteristics
   a. Demonstrated lack of knowledge regarding basic health practices.
   b. Demonstrated lack of adaptive behaviors to internal/external environmental changes.
   c. Reported or observed inability to take responsibility for meeting basic health practices in any or all functional pattern areas.
   d. History of lack of health seeking behavior.
   e. Expressed interest in improving health behaviors.
   f. Reported or observed lack of equipment, financial, and/or other resources.
   g. Reported or observed impairment of personal support systems.
2. Minor defining characteristics
   None given.

RELATED FACTORS (NANDA, 1987, p. 86)

1. Lack of, or significant alteration in communication skills (written, verbal, and/or gestural).
2. Lack of ability to make deliberate and thoughtful judgements.
3. Perceptual/cognitive impairment (completed/partial lack of gross and/or fine motor skills).
4. Ineffective individual coping.
5. Dysfunctional grieving.
6. Unachieved developmental tasks.
7. Ineffective family coping.
8. Disabling spiritual distress.
9. Lack of material resources.

DIFFERENTIATION

Several other nursing diagnoses may need to be considered in the differential. Perhaps the patient is experiencing difficulty with the Value-Belief Pattern. Differentiation is based on assessment of the patient's description of individual values, goals, or beliefs which guide personal decision making. If conflict exists in areas other than or in addition to the area of health maintenance, the nurse should assess the Value-Belief Pattern of the patient.

Individual Coping, Ineffective or Family Coping, Ineffective could be suspected if there are major differences between the patient and family reports of health status, health perception, and health care behavior. Verbalizations by the patient or family regarding inability to cope also indicate this differential nursing diagnosis. Through observing family interactions and communication the nurse may assess that Family Process, Altered is a consideration. Rigidity of family functions and roles, poorly communicated messages, and failure to accomplish expected family developmental tasks are a few observations to alert the nurse to this possible diagnosis.

The nursing diagnoses of Activity Intolerance or Self-Care Deficit should be considered if the nurse observes or validates reports of inability to complete the required tasks because of insufficient energy or because of the patient's inability to feed, bathe, toilet, dress, and groom him or her self.

The nursing diagnosis of Powerlessness is considered if the patient reports or demonstrates having little control over situation, expresses doubt about ability to perform, or is reluctant to express feelings to health care providers.

A Knowledge Deficit may exist if the patient or family verbalizes less-than-adequate understanding of health management or recalls inaccurate health information.

The nursing diagnosis of Noncompliance should be explored if the patient or family fails to maintain a therapeutic plan.

Potential for Injury should be assessed if the patient is at risk for bodily harm.

Home Maintenance Management, Impaired is demonstrated by the inability of the patient or family to provide a safe living environment.

OBJECTIVES

1. Will describe at least (number) contributing factors which lead to health maintenance alteration and at least one measure to alter each factor by (date).

AND/OR

2. Will design a positive health maintenance plan by (date).

TARGET DATE

Assisting patients to adapt their health maintenance will require a significant investment of time and will also require close collaboration with home health caregivers. For these reasons it is recommended the target date be no less than 4 days from the date of admission.

NURSING ORDERS

ADULT HEALTH

1. Assist patient to identify factors contributing to health maintenance alteration through:
   a. One-to-one interviewing;
   b. Value clarification strategies.
2. Teach patient appropriate information to improve health maintenance (e.g., hygiene, diet, medication administration, relaxation techniques, coping strategies).
3. Have patient return demonstrate health management procedures at least once a day for at least 3 days before discharge.
4. Review activities of daily living (ADL) with patient. Incorporate these activities into the design for a health maintenance plan. (*Note: May have to either increase or decrease ADL.*)
5. Assist patient to design a monthly calendar that reflects the daily activities needed to succeed in health maintenance.
6. Have patient identify at least two support persons. Arrange for these persons to come to the unit and participate in designing the health maintenance plan.
7. Refer patient to appropriate community health agencies or follow-up care (e.g., visiting nurse service, Meals on Wheels, transportation service, social service). Be sure referral is made at least 3–5 days before discharge to ensure the service can complete their assessment and initiate operations before patient is discharged from the hospital.
8. Schedule appropriate follow-up appointments for patient before discharge. Notify transportation service and support persons of these appointments. Write appointments on brightly colored cards for attention. Include date, time, appropriate name (physician, physical therapist, nurse practitioner, etc.), address, telephone number, and name and telephone number of person who will provide transportation.

CHILD HEALTH

(*Note: Obviously there will be a range of needs represented for health maintenance for the pediatric population. Beginning with neonates who are totally dependent on others for care, the gradual assumption of self-care should be fostered to culminate in adolescent self-care. Developmental consideration should always guide the health maintenance planned for the child patient. Also, identification of primary defects is stressed to reduce the likelihood of secondary and tertiary delays.*

Special considerations will also be necessary for the infant or child with major deficits in terms of required time and effort. The important notion is that a realistic potential ought to be identified irrespective of obstacles encountered. Safety needs must be properly addressed. Self-care may be unrealistic in a general sense for some children; even so, special care in helping parents and primary caregivers attain and maintain relative optimum health for the patient is essential.)

1. Teach patient and family essential information to establish and maintain health according to age, development, and status.
2. Assist patient and family in designing a calendar to monitor progress in meeting goals (may suggest the use of colored stickers related to child's hobbies).

WOMEN'S HEALTH

1. Assist the patient to describe her perception and understanding of health maintenance as it relates to her life-style.
2. Develop with the patient a list of stress-related problems within her work situation.
3. Develop with the patient a list of stress-related problems within her home situation.
4. Assist the patient in describing how she manages her responsibilities as a mother and a working woman.
5. Develop with the patient a list of assets and deficits as she perceives them.
6. From this list (#5) list the life-style adjustments that need to be made.
7. Identify possible solutions, modifications, etc. to cope with each adjustment.
8. Develop a plan with the patient which shows the short-term goals (specify time to be completed) and long-term goals (specify time to be completed).
9. Plan a mutually agreed time to review the goals and assess the progress of the patient and reformulate goals if necessary.
10. Identify significant others in patient's social network.
11. Involve significant others, if so desired by patient, in discussion and problem solving activities regarding life-style adjustments.
12. Provide an atmosphere that allows the patient to discuss freely her partner choice, whether it be heterosexual, homosexual, or bisexual.
13. Assist the patient in identifying life-style adjustments to each different cycle of reproductive life.
14. Record accurate menstrual cycle, obstetric, and sexual history.
15. Provide factual information to the patient about menstrual cycle patterns throughout the life span. (This should include prepubertal, menarcheal, menstrual, perimenopausal, menopausal, and post-menopausal phases.)
16. Describe the changes seen in estrogen-dependent tissues, such as the pelvic organs, breasts, mucosa, bones, and skin in the post-menopausal stage.
17. Emphasize the importance of life-style changes necessary to cope with these post-menopausal changes in the body, such as estrogen replacement therapy, calcium supplements, good balanced diet, routine exercise program, and at least 7–8 hours of sleep per night.
18. Discuss pregnancy and the changes that will occur during pregnancy.
19. Stress the importance of a physical examination *before* becoming pregnant to include:
    a. Pap smear;
    b. Rubella titer;
    c. AIDS profile;
    d. Genetic workup (if indicated by family history).
20. Assist the patient in listing ways to reduce fatigue during pregnancy.

21. Describe dietary requirements and adjustments needed to maintain well-being for mother and fetus.
22. Discuss childbirth and the changes that will occur:
    a. Prenatal
       (1) Stress the importance of early prenatal care.
       (2) Encourage attending childbirth education classes in preparation for birthing experience.
       (3) Provide factual information regarding the birthing experience.
       (4) Involve the significant other (spouse, boyfriend, etc.) in prenatal preparation for birth.
    b. Labor/delivery
       (1) Provide factual information about the labor and birth process.
       (2) Provide support during labor process.
       (3) Assist significant others in providing support and comfort to the patient during the labor process.
    c. Postpartum
       (1) Provide factual information about the involution process.
       (2) Teach proper hygiene and care of episiotomy and breasts after delivery.
23. Provide information and support for breastfeeding mothers.
24. Provide factual information about breastfeeding and bottle feeding.
25. Refer to appropriate reference groups for support and encouragement (i.e., La Leche League, parenting groups, etc.)
26. Teach terminology and factual information related to spontaneous abortion or the interruption of pregnancy.
27. Allow expression of feelings by woman and significant others.
28. Allow verbal expressions of grief.
29. Provide referrals to appropriate support groups within the community.
30. Provide women with factual information and describe different methods of contraception and their advantages and disadvantages. Include the following methods in your discussion:
    a. Mechanical
       (1) Condom
       (2) Diaphragm
       (3) Intrauterine device (IUD)
    b. Chemical
       (1) Spermicides
       (2) Pill
    c. Behavioral
       (1) Abstinence
       (2) Temperature, ovulation, cervical mucus (Billing's Method)
       (3) Coitus interruptus
    d. Sterilization
       (1) Vasectomy
       (2) Tubal ligation
       (3) Hysterectomy
31. Teach the patient the importance of routine physical assessments throughout the reproductive life cycle.
    a. Breast self-examination;
    b. Routine Pap smear examination.

MENTAL HEALTH

1. Assist patient and significant others to develop a list of *potential* strategies that would assist in the development of the life-style changes necessary for health maintenance. (This list should be a brainstorming process and include those solutions that appear to be very unrealistic as

well as those that appear most realistic). After the list is developed, review each item with the patient, combining and eliminating strategies when appropriate.

2. Develop with the patient a list of the benefits and disadvantages of behavior change. Discuss each item with the patient as to the strength of motivation that each item has.
3. Develop a behavior change contract with the patient, allowing the patient to identify appropriate rewards and consequences. Remember to establish modest goals and short-term rewards. Note reward schedule here.
4. Provide the patient with the information necessary to alter the identified behavior.
5. Set a time to reassess with the patient progress toward the established goals (this should be on a frequent schedule initially and can then gradually decrease as the patient demonstrates mastery).
6. Provide time to practice home maintenance skills. This should be at least 30 minutes every day. Times and types of skills to be practiced should be noted here.
7. Include the patient in group therapy to:
   a. Provide positive role models;
   b. Provide peer support;
   c. Permit assessment of goals;
   d. Expose to differing problem solutions;
   e. Provide socialization and social skill learning.
8. Provide the patient with appropriate positive feedback on goal achievement. Remember to keep this behaviorally oriented and specific.
9. Communicate the established plan to the collaborative members of the health care team.

HOME HEALTH

1. Assist the patient in identifying life-style changes that may be required:
   a. Stopping smoking;
   b. Ceasing drug and alcohol use;
   c. Establishing exercise patterns;
   d. Following good nutritional habits;
   e. Using stress management techniques;
   f. Using family and community support systems;
   g. Using over-the-counter medications;
2. Teach the patient and family health promotion and disease prevention activities:
   a. Relaxation techniques;
   b. Nutritional habits to maintain optimal weight and physical strength;
   c. Techniques for developing and strengthening support networks (e.g., communication techniques, mutual goal setting);
   d. Physical exercise to increase flexibility, cardiovascular conditioning, and physical strength and endurance;
   e. Control of harmful habits (e.g., control of substance abuse);
3. Involve the patient and family in planning, implementing, and promoting a health maintenance pattern through:
   a. Helping to establish family conferences;
   b. Teaching mutual goal setting;
   c. Teaching communication;
   d. Assisting family members in specified tasks as appropriate (e.g., cooking, cleaning, transportation, companionship, support person for exercise program).
4. Refer to other appropriate assistive resources as indicated:
   a. Outpatient clinics;
   b. Physician, dentist, physical therapist, occupational therapist, nutritionist, etc.;
   c. Job or education counselor;
   d. Home health aid;

  e. Stop smoking clinics;
  f. Alcoholics Anonymous;
  g. YMCA/YWCA or other health facilities;
  h. Stress reduction classes;
  i. Time management classes;
  j. Financial counselor;
  k. Family counselor;
  l. Religious counselor;
5. Assist the patient and family to identify home management factors that can be modified to promote health maintenance (e.g., ramps instead of steps, tacking down throw rugs, etc.).

EVALUATION
OBJECTIVE 1

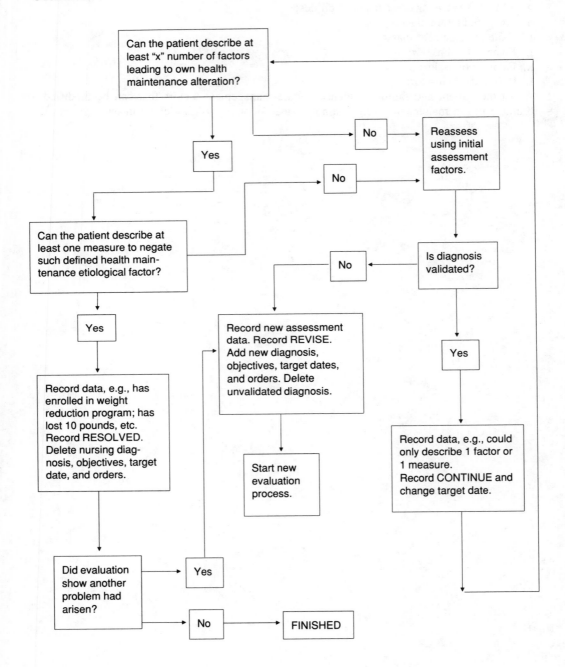

OBJECTIVE 2

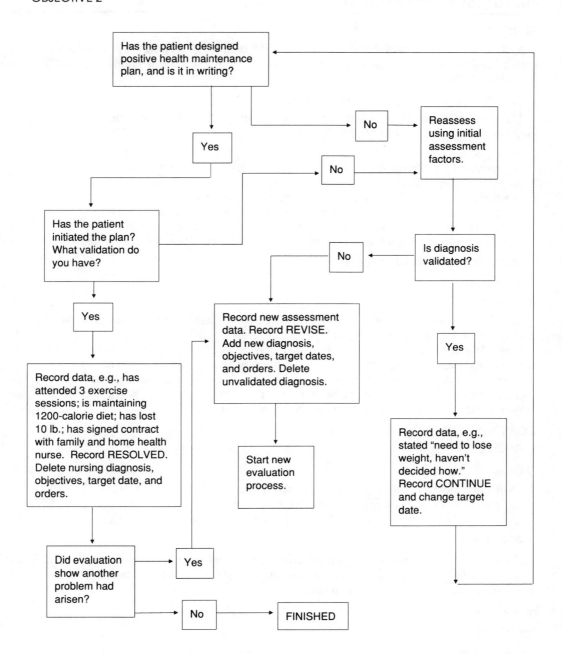

Has the patient designed positive health maintenance plan, and is it in writing?

No → Reassess using initial assessment factors.

Yes

No

Has the patient initiated the plan? What validation do you have?

Is diagnosis validated?

No

Yes

Record new assessment data. Record REVISE. Add new diagnosis, objectives, target dates, and orders. Delete unvalidated diagnosis.

Yes

Record data, e.g., has attended 3 exercise sessions; is maintaining 1200-calorie diet; has lost 10 lb.; has signed contract with family and home health nurse. Record RESOLVED. Delete nursing diagnosis, objectives, target date, and orders.

Start new evaluation process.

Record data, e.g., stated "need to lose weight, haven't decided how." Record CONTINUE and change target date.

Did evaluation show another problem had arisen?

Yes

No → FINISHED

Health Seeking Behaviors (SPECIFY)

DEFINITION

A state in which an individual in stable health[a] is actively seeking ways to alter personal health habits, and/or the environment in order to move toward a higher level of health. (NANDA, 1988)

DEFINING CHARACTERISTICS (NANDA, 1988)

The nurse will review the initial pattern assessment for the following defining characteristics to determine the diagnosis of Health Seeking Behaviors.

1. Major defining characteristics
   a. Expressed or observed desire to seek a higher level of wellness
2. Minor defining characteristics
   a. Stated or observed unfamiliarity with wellness community resources
   b. Demonstrated or observed lack of knowledge in health promotion behavior
   c. Expressed or observed desire for increased control of health practice
   d. Expression of concern about current environmental conditions on health status

RELATED FACTORS (NANDA, 1988)

None given

DIFFERENTIATION

Health Maintenance, Altered should be considered if the individual is not able to identify, manage, or seek out help to maintain health.

Home Maintenance Management, Impaired may be operating if the individual or family is unable to independently maintain a safe, growth-promoting immediate environment.

If the client expresses the perception of lack of control or influence over the situation and potential outcomes, or does not participate in care or decision-making when opportunities are provided, the diagnosis of Powerlessness should be investigated.

OBJECTIVES

1. Will describe or write realistic plans to modify (name) habit by (date).

AND/OR

2. Will (increase/decrease) (habit) by (amount) by (date).
   Examples: Will decrease smoking by 75% by (date).
   Will increase exercise by walking 2 miles 3 times/week by (date).

TARGET DATE

Changing a habit involves a significant investment of time and energy, regardless of whether the change involves starting a new habit or stopping an old habit. Therefore the target dates should be expressed in terms of weeks and months.

NURSING ORDERS

ADULT HEALTH

1. Teach patient about activities for promotion of health and prevention of illness (e.g., well-balanced diet, including restricted sodium and cholesterol intake; need for adequate rest and exercise; effects of air pollutants, including smoking; stress management techniques; etc.).
2. Give and review pamphlets about wellness community resources.

---

[a]Stable health status is defined as age appropriate illness prevention measures achieved, the client reports good or excellent health, and signs and symptoms of disease, if present, are controlled.

3. Support patient in his or her health seeking behavior; advocate for the patient when necessary.
4. Review patient's problem-solving abilities and assist patient to identify various alternatives, especially in terms of altering his or her environment.
5. Teach assertiveness to patient.

CHILD HEALTH

1. Assess child and family for perceived value of health and personal and family needs.
2. Initiate discharge plans soon after admission to facilitate post-hospital follow-up.
3. Assist child and family to identify appropriate health maintenance needs and resources to include:
   a. Immunizations;
   b. Nutrition;
   c. Daily hygiene;
   d. Basic safety;
   e. How to obtain medical services when needed, including health education;
   f. How to take temperature on an infant;
   g. Basic skills and care for health problems;
   h. Health insurance, Medicaid, Crippled Childrens' Services.
4. Note potential risk factors that should be dealt with regarding actual health status (e.g., financial status, coping strategies, resources).
5. Provide appropriate teaching to assist child and family in becoming confident in self-seeking health care behavior.
6. Help child and family develop a basic plan for high-level wellness with individualization which reflects the necessary components of health.
7. Allow for questions before dismissal to affirm plans for follow-up.
8. Assist child and family in understanding appropriate long-term benefits of appropriate high-level wellness and health seeking behavior.

WOMEN'S HEALTH

(Note: These orders are similar in nature to those described in Health Maintenance, Altered and in Adult Health except for the following.)

1. Refer to appropriate childbirth teaching groups in the community.
2. Refer to community groups that participate in exercise programs during pregnancy, such as swimming classes at the YWCA.
3. Refer eligible clients to food supplement programs available in the community. (This will vary from state to state and county to county; for a listing of the supplement food programs for pregnant women and infants in your area, contact your Department of Human Resources.)

MENTAL HEALTH

(Note: The objectives and nursing orders for the mental health client will be the same as those described for adult health. The following nursing orders are specific considerations for the mental health client.)

1. Assign client a primary care nurse.
2. Primary care nurse will spend 30 minutes twice a day with client (note times here). The focus of these interactions will conform to the following schedule:
   a. Interaction 1—Have the client identify *specific* areas of concern. List the identified concerns on the care plan. Also identify the primary source of this concern (i.e., client, family member, member of the health care team or other members of the client's social system).
   b. Interaction 2—List *specific* goals for each concern the client has identified. These goals should be achievable within a 2–3 day period. (One way of setting realistic, achievable goals is to divide the goal described by the client by 50%.)

   c. Interaction 3—Have the client identify steps that have been taken to address the concern previously.

   d. Interaction 4—Determine the client's perceptions of abilities to meet established goals and areas where assistance may be needed. (If client indicates a perception of inability to pursue goals without a great deal of assistance, the alternative nursing diagnoses of Powerlessness and Knowledge Deficit may need to be considered.)

   e. All future interactions will be spent assisting the client in developing strategies to achieve the established goals, developing action plans and evaluating the outcome of these plans, and then revising future actions.

3. Provide positive verbal reinforcement for client's achievements of goals. This reinforcement should be specific to the client's goals. Note those things that are rewarding to the client here with the kind of behavior to be rewarded.

4. Refer the client to appropriate resources for increasing knowledge. This could include books, community support groups, clinical nurse specialists, educational programs, or other professionals in the community who specialize in the area of the client's concerns. Note the resources here with any information necessary for the nursing staff to facilitate the client's obtaining the information. Note times and dates of client's appointments with resource persons here.

HOME HEALTH

1. Assist the client in identifying required life-style changes. Assist the client to develop potential strategies that would assist in the life-style changes required.

2. Help the client identify his or her personal definition of health, perceived personal control, perceived self-efficacy, and perceived health status.

3. Refer to Health Maintenance, Altered for additional orders that would also be applicable here.

EVALUATION
OBJECTIVE 1

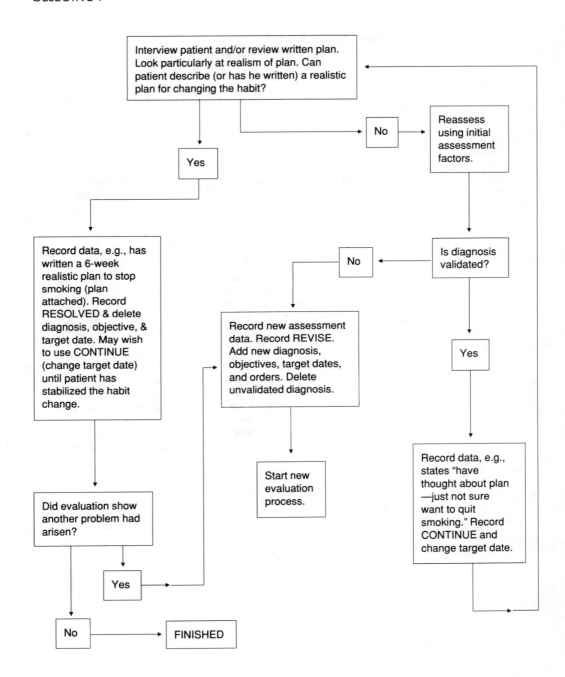

OBJECTIVE 2

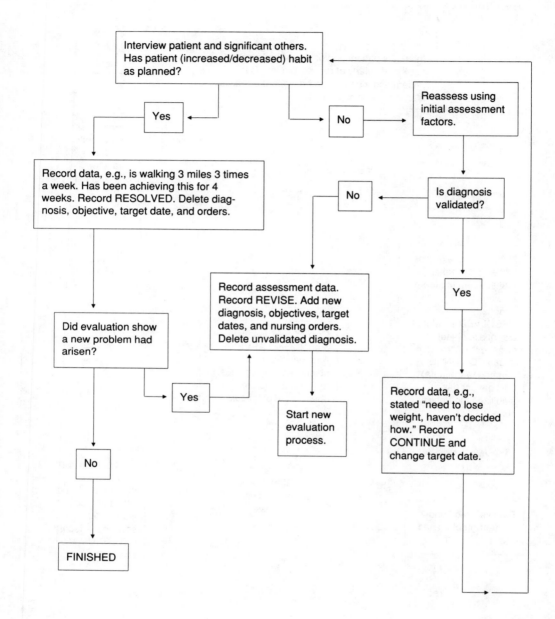

NONCOMPLIANCE

DEFINITION

A person's informed decision not to adhere to a therapeutic recommendation (NANDA, 1987, p. 79).

DEFINING CHARACTERISTICS (NANDA, 1987, p. 79)

The nurse will review the initial pattern assessment for the following defining characteristics to determine the diagnosis of Noncompliance:

1. Major defining characteristics
   a. Behavior indicative of failure to adhere (by direct observation or by statements of patient or significant others)
   b. Objective tests (physiologic measures, detection of markers)
   c. Evidence of development of complications
   d. Evidence of exacerbation of symptoms
   e. Failure to keep appointments
   f. Failure to progress
2. Minor defining characteristics
   None given.

RELATED FACTORS (NANDA, 1987, p. 79)

1. Patient value system: health beliefs, cultural influences, spiritual values.
2. Client-provider relationships.

DIFFERENTIATION

Knowledge Deficit may exist if the patient or family verbalizes less-than-adequate understanding of health management or recalls inaccurate health information.

Individual Coping, Ineffective or Family Coping, Ineffective is suspected if there are major differences between the patient and family reports of health status, health perception, and health care behavior. Verbalizations by the patient or family regarding inability to cope also indicate this differential nursing diagnosis. Through observing family interactions and communication, the nurse may assess that Family Processes, Altered is a consideration. Poorly communicated messages, rigidity of family functions and roles, and failure to accomplish expected family developmental tasks are a few observations to alert the nurse to this possible diagnosis.

The nursing diagnoses of Activity Intolerance or Self-Care Deficit should be considered if the nurse observes or validates reports of inability to complete the tasks required because of insufficient energy or because of inability to feed, bathe, toilet, dress, and groom self.

If the patient exhibits impaired attention span; impaired ability to recall information; impaired perception, judgment, and decision making; or impaired conceptual and reasoning abilities, the nursing diagnoses of Thought Process, Altered should be considered.

The nursing diagnosis of Health Maintenance, Altered should be explored when a patient or family fails to adhere to a therapeutic plan.

Home Maintenance Management, Impaired is demonstrated by the inability of the patient or family to provide a safe living environment.

ADDITIONAL INFORMATION

(Note: Some nursing authors object to the term Noncompliance [Ridenour, 1986; Hagey & McDonough, 1984; Edel, 1985; Breunig, Brutwitzk, Schulte, Crane, Schroeder, & Lutze, 1986].)

Compliance can become the basis for a power-oriented relationship in which one is judged and labeled compliant or noncompliant based on the hierarchical position of the professional in relation to the patient. Carpenito (1987, p. 408) attempts to deal with this potential problem of professional labeling by indicating that "the nurse is cautioned against using the diagnosis of noncompliance to describe an individual who has made an informed autonomous decision not to comply." The diagnosis of Noncompliance, then, is to be used for those patients who wish to comply with the therapeutic recommendations but are prevented from doing so by the presence of certain factors. The nurse can in such situations strive to lessen or eliminate the factors which preclude the willing patient from complying with recommendations.

The principles of informed consent and autonomy (Beauchamp & Childress, 1983) are critical to the appropriate use of this diagnosis. A person may freely choose not to follow a treatment plan. The nursing diagnosis Noncompliance should not carry a connotation of the ability of the patient to obey, but rather, the patient has attempted the prescribed plan and has found it difficult to do so. The area of noncompliance must also be specified. A patient may follow many aspects of a treatment program very well and only find a small part of the plan difficult to manage. Such a patient is noncompliant only in the area of difficulty.

OBJECTIVES

1. Will identify barriers to compliance and devise at least one way to overcome each barrier by (date).

AND/OR

2. Will return demonstrate appropriate technique or procedures for self-care by (date).

TARGET DATE

The specific target dates for these objectives will be directly related to the barriers identified, the patient's entering level of knowledge, and the comfort the patient feels in expressing satisfaction or dissatisfaction. The target date could range from 1 to 5 days following the date of admission.

NURSING ORDERS

ADULT HEALTH

1. Help the patient identify potential areas of conflict (e.g., values, religious beliefs, cultural mores, cost, etc.)
2. Start instructions for self-care within 24 hours of admission.
3. Teach the patient and significant others knowledge and skills needed to comply (e.g., measuring blood pressure, counting calories, administering medications, weighing self, etc.)
4. Have the patient and significant others return demonstrate or restate principles at least daily for at least 3 consecutive days prior to discharge.
5. Design a chart to assist the patient to visually see the effectiveness of therapeutic regimen (e.g., weight loss chart, days without smoking, blood pressure measurements). Begin the chart in hospital within 1 day of admission.
6. Contract with the patient and significant others for specifics regarding compliance. Follow-up 1 week after discharge; recheck 6 weeks following discharge.
7. If the idea of stopping smoking, etc. is too overwhelming, help patient design a personal adaptive program; for example, change to a lower tar and nicotine cigarette, time smoking (only one cigarette per 30 or 60 minutes), stabilize, then make further reductions.
8. Teach the patient and significant others assertive techniques that can be used to deal with dissatisfaction with caregivers.
9. Allow time for the patient to verbalize fears related to therapeutic regimen (e.g., body image, cost, side effects, pain, dependency).
10. Assist in correction of sensory, motor, etc. deficits to the extent possible through referrals to appropriate consultants (e.g., occupational therapist, physical therapist, ophthalmologist, audiologist).

11. To increase the patient's sense of control, have him or her design home care plan. Assist him or her to modify the plan as necessary. Forward the plan to home health service, social service, physician, etc.
12. Relate any information regarding dissatisfaction to appropriate caregiver (e.g., to physician— problems with the time spent in waiting room, cultural needs, privacy needs, costs, need for generic prescriptions).
13. Make follow-up appointments prior to the patient's leaving the hospital. Do it from the patient's room to demonstrate how, etc. Put appropriate information regarding appointment on brightly colored card (i.e., name, address, time, date, telephone number).
14. Refer the patient to appropriate follow-up personnel (e.g., nurse practitioner, visiting nurse service, social service, transportation service). Make referral at least 3 days prior to discharge to allow home care assessment and initiation of service.
15. Request follow-up personnel to remind the patient of appointments via card or telephone.
16. For the last 2–3 days of hospitalization let the patient perform all his or her own care. Supervise performance, critique, reteach as necessary.

CHILD HEALTH

(Note: the general plan is as noted for adult health.)

1. Assist in developing health values of compliance before the birth of the infant.
2. Allow for the infant's or child's schedule in appointment scheduling (e.g., respect for naps).
3. Involve the family in the process of dealing with the desired plan for care.
4. Assist the child and parents in identifying factors that actually or potentially may impede desirous plan for compliance.
   a. Sense of control
   b. Language barriers
   c. Cultural concerns
   d. Financial constraints
   e. Knowledge deficit
   f. Time constraints
5. Allow opportunities for the family to vent feelings about compliance.
6. Reward progress in the appropriate manner for age and development.
7. Begin plans for discharge soon after admission.
8. Provide appropriate follow-up for progress.

WOMEN'S HEALTH

This section is the same as Adult Health with the following additions:

1. Assist in the development of a schedule that will allow the patient to keep appointments and not miss work.
2. Assist the patient in developing time-management skills to incorporate time for relaxation and exercise.
3. Design techniques that encourage the patient's compliance, such as setting single, easy-to-accomplish, short-term goals first and progressing to long-term goals as the short-terms goals are met.
4. Design a plan for follow-up with the patient and family.
5. Assist patient in identifying potential areas of conflict (i.e., economics, entry to the health care system, cultural mores, religious beliefs, etc.).
6. Allow patient to-verbally express concerns with her sense of control or loss of control.
7. Provide an atmosphere that allows the patient to express her concerns with her language barrier.
8. Provide translators.
9. Assign nursing personnel who speak the patient's language.

10. Keep a list of nursing personnel who speak different languages in case of emergency.
11. Develop a sensitivity for cultural differences of women's roles and the impact on their compliance with nursing orders.
12. Design a plan that will allow incorporation of nursing orders within the cultural norms of the patient.

MENTAL HEALTH

(Note: It is important to remember that the mental health patient is influenced by a larger social system and that this social system plays a crucial role in the patient's ongoing participation with the health care team. The conceptualization that may be most useful in intervention and assessment of the patient who does not follow the recommendations of the health care team in this area may be system persistence. Hoffman [1983] uses this concept to communicate the idea that the system is signaling that it desires to continue in its present manner of organization. This could present a situation in which the individual patient indicates to the health care team that he or she desires change, and yet change is not demonstrated due to the constraints placed on the individual by the larger social system [i.e., the family]. This places the responsibility on the nurse to initiate a comprehensive assessment of the patient system when the diagnosis of Noncompliance is considered.)

1. Involve the patient system in discussions on the treatment plan. This should include:
   a. Family
   b. Individuals the patient identifies as important in making decisions related to health (i.e., cultural healers, social institutions such as probation officers, public welfare workers, officials in the school system, etc.)
2. Discuss with the identified system those factors that inhibit system reorganization:
   a. Knowledge and skills related to necessary change
   b. Resources available
   c. Ability to use these resources
   d. Belief system about treatment plan
   e. Cultural values related to the treatment plan
3. Assist the system in making the appropriate adjustments in system organization:
   a. Enhance current patterns that facilitate system re-organization
   b. Make small changes in those patterns that inhibit system change (i.e., ask the patient to talk with the family in the group room instead of in an open public area on the unit or ask the patient who washes his or her hands frequently to use a special soap and towel and then gradually introduce more changes in the patterns)
4. Advise the patient to make changes slowly. It is important not to expect too much too soon.
5. Provide the appropriate positive verbal feedback to all parts of the system involved in assisting with the changes. It is important not to focus on the demonstration of old patterns of behavior at this time. The smallest change should be recognized.
6. Communicate the plan to all members of the health care team.
7. Refer to appropriate assistive resources as indicated:
   a. Family counselor
   b. Stress reduction classes
   c. Spiritual counselor
   d. Job or vocational rehabilitation counselor
   e. Financial counselor
   f. Health care providers that adjust for those identified barriers, etc.

HOME HEALTH

1. Involve the patient and family in planning, implementing, and promoting treatment plan through:
   a. Assisting with family conferences;

  b. Coordinating mutual goal setting;

  c. Promoting increased communication;

  d. Assigning family members specific tasks as appropriate to assist in maintaining desired compliance (e.g., support person for patient, transportation, companionship in meeting mutual goals, etc.).

2. Assist the patient to delineate factors contributing to noncompliance by helping the patient to assess:

  a. Level of knowledge and skill related to treatment plan;

  b. Resources available to meet treatment plan objectives;

  c. Appropriate use of resources to meet treatment plan objectives;

  d. Complexity of treatment plan;

  e. Current response to treatment plan;

  f. Use of nonprescribed interventions;

  g. Barriers to compliance.

3. Help the patient and family to write life-style adjustment plan (e.g., dieting, rearrangement of furniture, etc.).

4. Reteach the patient and family appropriate therapeutic activities as need arises.

5. Support the patient in eliminating barriers to compliance by:

  a. Helping patient to find a private area in the home;

  b. Referring to services (e.g., church, home health volunteer, transportation service);

  c. Alerting other health care providers of the problem that long waiting period in waiting room is causing;

  d. Providing interpreter resource in instances of language barrier;

  e. Assigning one health care provider, as much as possible, to avoid lack of continuity in care provision.

6. Refer to the appropriate assistive resources as indicated:

  a. Family counselor

  b. Stress reduction classes

  c. Religious counselor

  d. Time management classes

  e. Job or education counselor

  f. Self-help groups

  g. Financial counselor

  h. Health care provider or facilities which have eliminated barriers to compliance

EVALUATION
OBJECTIVE 1

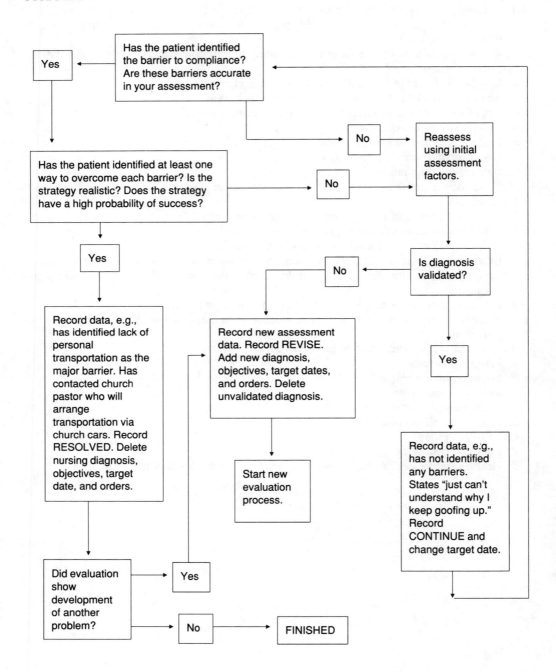

OBJECTIVE 2

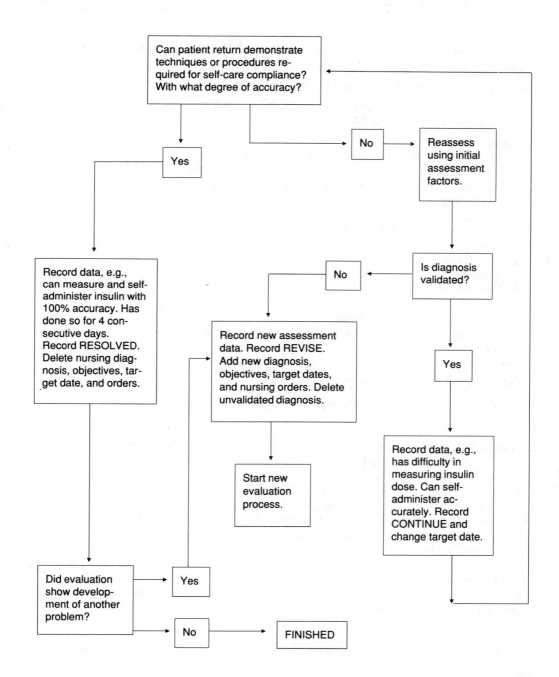

Infection, Potential for

DEFINITION

The state in which an individual is at increased risk for being invaded by pathogenic organisms (NANDA, 1987, p. 17).

DEFINING CHARACTERISTICS (NANDA, 1987, p. 17)

The nurse will review the initial pattern assessment for the following risk factors to determine the diagnosis of Infection, Potential for:

1. Major risk factors
   a. Inadequate primary defenses (broken skin, traumatized tissue, decrease in ciliary action, stasis of body fluids, change in pH secretions, altered peristalsis)
   b. Inadequate secondary defenses (e.g., decreased hemoglobin, leukopenia, suppressed inflammatory response) and immunosuppression
   c. Inadequate acquired immunity
   d. Tissue destruction and increased environmental exposure
   e. Chronic disease
   f. Invasive procedures
   g. Malnutrition
   h. Pharmaceutical agents
   i. Trauma
   j. Rupture of amniotic membranes
   k. Insufficient knowledge to avoid exposure to pathogens
2. Minor risk factors
   None given.

RELATED FACTORS (NANDA, 1987, p. 17)

The risk factors given previously also serve as the related factors.

DIFFERENTIATION

Several other nursing diagnoses may need to be considered in the differential:

Self-Care Deficit especially in the areas of toileting, feeding, and bathing-hygiene may need to be considered if improper handwashing, personal hygiene, toileting practices, or food preparation and storage have increased the risk of infection.

Skin Integrity, Impaired; Tissue Integrity, Impaired; Nutrition, Altered: Less Than Body Requirements; or Oral Mucous Membranes, Altered may be predisposing the client to infection.

Physical Mobility, Impaired should be considered if skin breakdown leading to infection is related to impaired mobility.

Body Temperature, Altered: Potential or Hyperthermia should be considered when body temperature increases above normal.

Noncompliance may be occurring in cases of inappropriate antibiotic usage or inadequate treatment of wounds or chronic diseases.

OBJECTIVES

1. Will return demonstrate measures to decrease the potential for infection by (date).

AND/OR

2. Will not develop an infection by (date).

TARGET DATE

An appropriate target date would be within 3 days of the date of diagnosis.

NURSING ORDERS

ADULT HEALTH

1. Teach the patient about the infectious process, routes, pathogens, environmental and host factors, and aspects of prevention.
2. Maintain adequate nutrition and fluid and electrolyte balance—well-balanced diet with increased amounts of vitamin C, sufficent iron, and 2400–2600 ml of fluids daily.
3. Wash hands and skin carefully and thoroughly.
4. Protect the patient from exposure to pathogens by using reverse or protective isolation if necessary.
5. Use sterile technique when changing dressings or for invasive procedures.
6. Turn every 2 hours; cough and deep breathe every 2 hours; perform passive or have patient perform active range of motion (ROM) exercises every 2 hours.

CHILD HEALTH

1. Monitor axillary temperature every 2–4 hours as ordered and as required.
2. Check for signs and symptoms of infection every 2–3 hours and as required.
3. Monitor contributory factors for potential for infection, including:
   a. Surgical wound;
   b. Entry of drainage tube into body cavity or orifice, Foley, IV;
   c. Immunosuppression;
   d. Administration of steroids;
   e. Nonsocomial infection;
   f. Break in isolation technique.
4. Monitor appropriately the administration of antibiotics for maintenance of blood levels and assess for side effects, including diarrhea.
5. Collaborate with physician regarding spinal fluid or other specimen reports for culture and sensitivity.
6. Address related primary nursing care needs, such as fluid and electrolyte needs.
7. Appropriately answer questions of child and parents regarding procedures, treatments, or care.
8. Provide educational offerings for care, especially related to isolation or sterile technique if applicable.
9. Maintain a neutral thermal environment.
10. Maintain appropriate handwashing between patients.
11. Provide appropriate sterile technique in maintenance of IVs, wound care, etc.
12. Encourage patient and parents to verbalize fears, concerns, or feelings related to infection.
13. In instances of immuno-suppression, provide appropriate information to patient and parents regarding isolation technique and rationale.
14. Allow for decreased tolerance of activity.
15. Encourage patient and parental input in planning for care when possible and appropriate.

WOMEN'S HEALTH

(Note: The orders for women are the same as for adult health in any surgical situation, except for the following special events.)

Newborn

1. In presence of meconium in amniotic fluid, immediately clear airway of infant by suctioning (preferably done by physician immediately upon delivery of infant's head).
2. Suction gastric contents.
3. Observe for sternal retractions, grunting, trembling, jitters, or pallor; if any of these signs are present notify the physician at once.
4. Wash hands before and after each time baby is handled.

5. Avoid wearing sharp jewelry which could scratch baby.
6. Keep umbilical cord clean and dry by cleansing at each diaper change or at least every 2 hours.
7. Assess site of circumcision for swelling, odor, or bleeding every diaper change or at least every 2 hours.
8. Demonstrate how to take baby's temperature, and allow time for return demonstration by mother and father.
9. Demonstrate to mother proper care of cord and circumcision before discharge, and allow time for return demonstration.

Pregnancy

10. In the presence of ruptured membranes, assess for signs of infection every 4 hours (i.e., elevated temperature, odor of vaginal discharge).
11. Instruct mother not to take tub baths, only showers.
12. Instruct mother how to assess her temperature and record it every 4 hours.

Labor and Delivery

13. During labor, use aspectic technique when performing vaginal examinations.
14. Limit the number of vaginal examinations during labor.
15. Keep linens and underpads clean and changed as necessary during labor.

Postpartum

16. Assess incision (C-section) for any signs of redness, drainage, oozing, loss of approximation, or odor.
17. Assess episiotomy (vaginal delivery) for any signs of redness, drainage, oozing, hematoma, or loss of approximation.
18. Assess fundal height.
19. Note any signs of foul-smelling lochia.
20. Note any signs of uterine tenderness.
21. Note increased temperature.

Abortion

22. Assess abdomen, and note swelling and tenderness.
23. Assess temperature.
24. Note any signs of foul-smelling vaginal discharge.
25. Obtain complete obstetric history.

MENTAL HEALTH

(Note: The nursing orders for the mental health client will be the same as those described for adult health and women's health. The following nursing orders are specific considerations for the mental health client.)

1. Monitor the temperature of clients receiving antipsychotic medications twice a day and report any elevations to physician. Note times for temperature evaluations here. (These clients are at risk for developing agranulocytosis. The greatest risk is 3–8 weeks after therapy has begun.)
2. Monitor the client for the presence of a sore throat in the absence of a cold or other flu-like symptoms. Report any occurrence. (This could be a symptom of agranulocytosis.)
3. Teach the client to report temperature elevations and sore throats in the absence of other symptoms to the physician.
4. During the first 8 weeks of treatment with an antipsychotic, report any signs of infection in the client to the physician for assessment of white cell count.
5. Review the client's CBC before antipsychotics are started and report any abnormalities on subsequent CBCs to the physician.
6. Teach the client and family measures to prevent or decrease potential for infection:

   a. Handwashing technique
   b. Nutrition
   c. Appropriate antibiotic use
   d. Hazards of substance abuse
7. Consult with appropriate assistive resources as indicated:
   a. Infection control department
   b. City or state health department
   c. Physician

HOME HEALTH

1. Monitor for factors contributing to the potential for infection.
2. Involve the patient and family in planning, implementing, and promoting reduction in the potential for infection.
   a. Family conference
   b. Mutual goal setting
   c. Communication
3. Teach the patient and family measures to prevent or decrease potential for infection.
   a. Handwashing technique
   b. Personal hygiene and health habits
   c. Nutrition
   d. Immunization schedule
   e. Proper food storage and preparation
   f. Elimination of environmental hazards such as rodents or insects
   g. Proper sewage control and trash collection
   h. Appropriate antibiotic use
   i. Hazards of substance abuse
   j. Preparation and precautions when traveling to areas in which infections diseases are endemic
   k. Signs and symptoms of infectious diseases for which patient and family are at risk
   i. Preparation for disaster (water storage, canned or dried food, emergency waste disposal)
4. Teach patient and family measures to prevent transmission of infectious disease to others. Assist patient and family with life-style changes that may be required.
   a. Handwashing
   b. Isolation as appropriate
   c. Proper disposal of infectious waste (e.g., bagging)
   d. Proper use of disinfectants
   e. Appropriate medical intervention (e.g., antibiotics, antipyretics, etc.)
   f. Immunization
   g. Signs and symptoms of infection
   h. Treatment for lice and removal of nits
   i. Asepsis for wound care
     (Note: Items can be sterilized at home by immersing in boiling water for 10 minutes. The water needs to be boiling for the entire 10 minutes.)
5. Consult with appropriate assistive resources as indicated:
   a. City or State Health Department
   b. Centers for Disease Control
   c. Physician
   d. Visiting nurse or homemaker

EVALUATION
OBJECTIVE 1

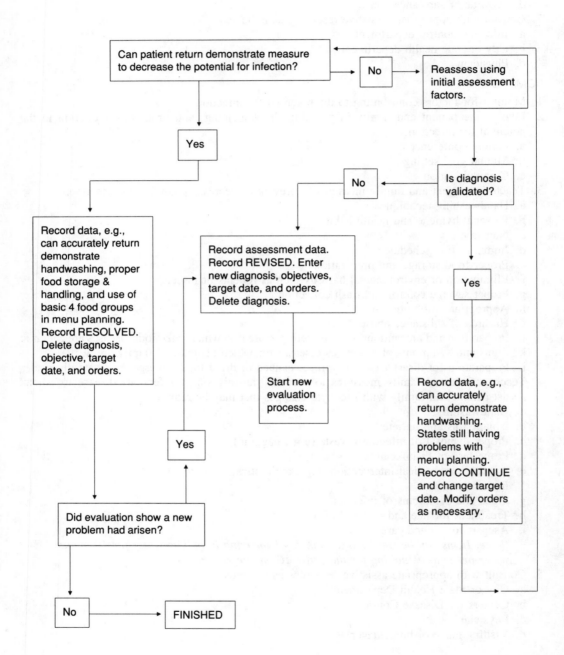

OBJECTIVE 2

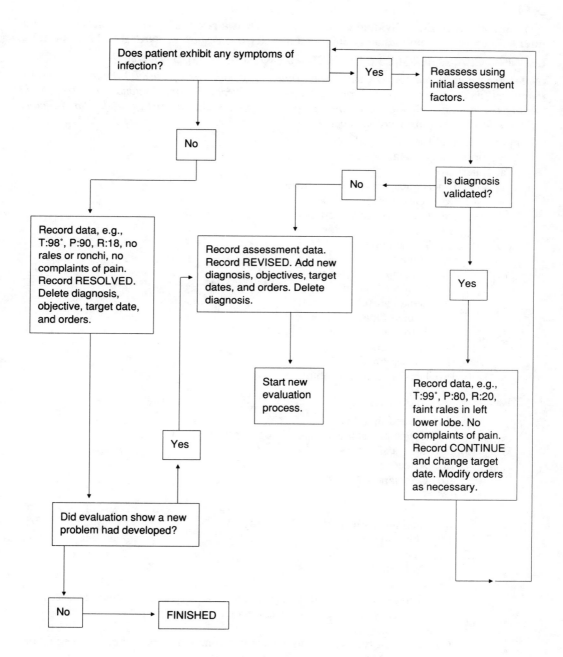

Injury, Potential for

DEFINITION

A state in which the individual is at risk of injury as a result of environmental conditions interacting with the individual's adaptive and defensive resources (NANDA, 1987, p. 45).

DEFINING CHARACTERISTICS (RISK FACTORS—NANDA, 1987, pp. 45–51.)

(Note: According to the NANDA Taxomony, Injury, Potential for is a level 3 diganosis. Level 4 diagnoses under Injury, Potential for are Suffocating, Poisoning, and Trauma. To assist you in making the most specific diagnosis, the definitions, defining characteristics, and related factors for these level 4 diagnoses are included.)

A. Injury, Potential for
1. Major defining characteristics
   a. Internal
      (1) Biochemical, regulatory function
         (a) Sensory dysfunction
         (b) Integrative dysfunction
         (c) Effector dysfunction
         (d) Tissue hypoxia
         (e) Malnutrition
         (f) Immuno-autoimmune
         (g) Abnormal blood profile
         (h) Leukocytosis, leukopenia
         (i) Altered clotting factors
         (j) Thrombocytopenia
         (k) Sickle cell
         (l) Thalassemia
         (m) Decreased hemoglobin
      (2) Physical
         (a) Broken skin
         (b) Altered mobility
         (c) Developmental age—physiologic, psychosocial
      (3) Psychological
         (a) Affective
         (b) Orientation
   b. External
      (1) Biological
         (a) Immunization level of community
         (b) Microorganism
      (2) Chemical
         (a) Pollutants
         (b) Poisons
         (c) Drugs—pharmaceutical agents, alcohol, caffeine, nicotine, preservatives, cosmetics and dyes, nutrients (vitamins, food types)
      (3) Physical
         (a) Design, structure, and arrangement of community, building, and/or equipment
         (b) Mode of transport or transportation
      (4) People or provider
         (a) Nosocomial agent
         (b) Staffing patterns
         (c) Cognitive, affective, and psychomotor factors

    2. Minor defining characteristics
      None given.
B. Injury, Potential for: Suffocating
    1. Definition—Accentuated risk of accidental suffocation (inadequate air available for inhalation) (NANDA, 1987, p. 47).
    2. Major defining characteristics
      a. Internal (individual)
        (1) Reduced olfactory sensation
        (2) Reduced motor abilities
        (3) Lack of safety education
        (4) Lack of safety precautions
        (5) Cognitive or emotional difficulties
        (6) Disease or injury process
      b. External (environmental)
        (1) Pillow placed in an infant's crib
        (2) Propped bottle placed in an infant's crib
        (3) Vehicle warming in closed garage
        (4) Children playing with plastic bags
        (5) Discarded or unused refrigerator or freezer without removed doors
        (6) Children left unattended in bathtub or pool
        (7) Household gas leak
        (8) Smoking in bed
        (9) Use of fuel-burning heater not vented to outside
        (10) Low-strung clothesline
        (11) Pacifier hung around infant's head
        (12) Eating large mouthfuls of food
    3. Minor defining characteristics
      None given.
C. Injury, Potential for: Poisoning
    1. Definition—Accentuated risk of accidental exposure to or ingestion of drugs or dangerous products in doses sufficient to cause poisoning (NANDA, 1987, p. 48).
    2. Major defining characteristics
      a. Internal (individual)
        (1) Reduced vision
        (2) Verbalization of occupational setting without adequate safeguards
        (3) Lack of safety or drug education
        (4) Lack of proper precaution
        (5) Cognitive or emotional difficulties
        (6) Insufficient finances
      b. External (environmental)
        (1) Large supplies of drugs in house
        (2) Medicines stored in unlocked cabinet accessible to children or confused persons
        (3) Dangerous products placed or stored within the reach of children or confused persons
        (4) Availability of illicit drugs potentially contaminated by poisonous additives
        (5) Flaking, peeling paint or plaster in presence of young children
        (6) Chemical contamination of food and water
        (7) Unprotected contact with heavy metals or chemicals
        (8) Paint, lacquer, etc. in poorly ventilated areas or without effective protection
        (9) Presence of poisonous vegetation
        (10) Presence of atmospheric pollutants

3. Minor defining characteristics
   None given.
D. Injury, Potential for: Trauma
   1. Definition—Accentuated risk of accidental tissue injury such as wound, burn, or fracture (NANDA, 1987, p. 49).
   2. Major defining characteristics
      a. Internal (individual)
         (1) Weakness
         (2) Poor vision
         (3) Balancing difficulties
         (4) Reduced temperature or tactile sensation
         (5) Reduced large or small muscle coordination
         (6) Reduced hand-eye coordination
         (7) Lack of safety education
         (8) Lack of safety precautions
         (9) Insufficient finances to purchase safety equipment or effect repairs
         (10) Cognitive or emotional difficulties
         (11) History of previous trauma
      b. External (environmental)
         (1) Slippery floors (e.g., wet or highly waxed)
         (2) Snow or ice collected on stairs, walkways
         (3) Unanchored rugs
         (4) Bathtub without handgrip or antislip equipment
         (5) Use of unsteady ladders or chairs
         (6) Entering unlighted rooms
         (7) Unsteady or absent stair rails
         (8) Unanchored electric wires
         (9) Litter or liquid spills on floors or stairways
         (10) High bed
         (11) Children playing without a gate at the top of the stairs
         (12) Obstructed passageways
         (13) Unsafe window protection in homes with young children
         (14) Inappropriate call-for-aid mechanisms for bedresting patient
         (15) Pot handles facing toward front of stove
         (16) Bathing in very hot water (e.g., unsupervised bathing of young children)
         (17) Potential igniting gas leaks
         (18) Delayed lighting of gas burner or oven
         (19) Experimenting with chemical or gasoline
         (20) Unscreened fires or heaters
         (21) Wearing plastic apron or flowing clothes around open flame
         (22) Children playing with matches, candles, cigarettes
         (23) Inadequately stored combustibles or corrosives, (e.g., matches, oily rags, lye)
         (24) Highly flammable children's toys or clothing
         (25) Overloaded fuse boxes
         (26) Contact with rapidly moving machinery, industrial belts, or pulleys
         (27) Sliding on coarse bed linen or struggling within bed restraints
         (28) Faulty electrical plugs, frayed wires, or defective appliances
         (29) Contact with acids or alkalis
         (30) Playing with fireworks or gunpowder
         (31) Contact with intense cold
         (32) Overexposure to sun, sunlamps, or radiotherapy

(33) Use of cracked dinnerware or glasses
(34) Knives stored uncovered
(35) Guns or ammunition stored unlocked
(36) Large icicles hanging from roof
(37) Exposure to dangerous machinery
(38) Children playing with sharp-edged toys
(39) High-crime neighborhood and vulnerable clients
(40) Driving a mechanically unsafe vehicle
(41) Driving after partaking of alcoholic beverages or drugs
(42) Driving at excessive speed
(43) Driving without necessary visual aid
(44) Children in the front seat in car
(45) Smoking in bed or near oxygen
(46) Overloaded electrical outlets
(47) Grease waste collected on stoves
(48) Use of thin or worn potholders
(49) Unsafe road or road-crossing conditions
(50) Play or work near vehicle pathways (e.g., driveways, laneways, railroad tracks)
(51) Nonuse or misuse of seat restraint or misuse of necessary headgear for motorized cyclists or young children carried on adult bicycles

3. Minor defining characteristics
None given.

RELATED FACTORS (NANDA, 1987, pp. 45–51)

1. Interactive factors between individual and environment which impose a risk to the defensive and adaptive resources of the individual.
2. Internal factors (host): biological, chemical, physiological, psychological perception, developmental.
3. External factors (environment): biological, chemical, physiological, psychological, people/provider.

DIFFERENTIATION

Several other nursing diagnoses may need to be considered in the differential.

Activity Intolerance should be considered if the nurse observes or validates reports of the patient's inability to complete required tasks because of insufficient energy. Physical Mobility, Impaired is appropriate if the patient has difficulty with coordination, range of motion, muscle strength and control, or activity restrictions related to treatment.

Uncompensated Sensory Deficit is of concern when a loss of acuity, vision, touch, smell, hearing, or balance is assessed.

A Knowledge Deficit may exist if the client or family verbalizes less-than-adequate understanding of injury prevention.

Home Maintenance Management, Impaired is demonstrated by the inability of the patient or the family to provide a safe living environment.

If the patient exhibits impaired attention span; impaired ability to recall information; impaired perception, judgment, and decision making; or impaired conceptual reasoning abilities, the nursing diagnosis of Thought Process, Altered should be considered.

The nursing diagnosis of Health Maintenance, Altered should be explored when a patient or family fails to adhere to a therapeutic plan.

The Potential for Violence exists if there are risk factors present for self-inflicted or other-directed physical trauma (e.g., self-destructive behavior, substance abuse, rage, hostile verbalizations, etc.)

OBJECTIVES

1. Will identify hazards contributing to potential for injury and at least one corrective measure for each hazard by (date).

AND/OR

2. Will have no incidences of injury by (date).

TARGET DATE

While preventing injury may be a lifelong activity, establishing a mindset to avoid injury can be begun rapidly. An appropriate target date would be within 2 days of admission.

NURSING ORDERS

ADULT HEALTH

1. Assist in correcting, to the extent possible, any sensory-perceptual problems through appropriate referrals.
2. Keep bed wheels locked and bed in low position. Keep head of bed elevated at least 30° at all times.
3. Pad siderails and keep siderails up when patient is in bed.
4. Make sure handrails are in place in the bathroom and that safety strips are in tub and shower. Do not leave patient unattended in bathtub or shower.
5. Keep the patient's room free of clutter.
6. Orient the patient to time, person, place, and environment at least once a shift.
7. Assist the patient with all transfer and ambulation. If the patient requires multiple pillows for rest or positioning, tape the bottom layer of pillows to prevent dislodging.
8. Teach patient and significant others:
   a. Alteration in life-style that may be necessary (e.g., stopping smoking, stopping alcohol ingestion, decreasing or ceasing drug ingestion, ceasing driving);
   b. Use of assistive devices (e.g., walkers, canes, crutches, wheelchairs);
   c. Heimlich maneuver;
   d. CPR;
   e. Recognition of signs and symptoms of choking and carbon monoxide poisoning;
   f. Necessity of chewing food thoroughly and cutting food into small bites.
9. Provide night light.
10. Check on patient at least once an hour. If high potential for injury exists, do not leave patient unattended. Schedule sitters around the clock.
11. Carefully check temperature of food and bath water before allowing patient to eat or bathe.
12. Check respiratory rates, depth, and chest sounds at least every 4 hours.
13. Do not leave medications, solutions, or any type of liquids in the room. Use only paper cups and containers that can be disposed of immediately in patient's room. Use "Mr. Yuk" on bottle labels of poisonous substances. Teach patient and famly to use this type of labeling at home.
14. Keep continuous check on airway patency. Keep suctioning equipment, ventilation equipment, and lavage setup on standby.
15. Refer to appropriate agency for safety check of home. Make referral at least 3 days prior to discharge to allow time for correction of problem areas.
    a. Utility companies
    b. Fire department
    c. Visiting Nurse Service
    d. Public health department
    e. City health department
16. Teach patient and family safety measures for use at home:

   a. Use nonskid rugs or tack down throw rugs
   b. Use handrails
   c. Install ramps
   d. Use color contrast for steps, door knobs, electrical outlets, and light switches
   e. Avoid surface glare (e.g., floors, table tops)
   f. Change physical position slowly
   g. Use covers for electrical outlets
   h. Position pans with handles toward back of stove
   i. Have family post poison control number for ready reference
   j. Provide extra lighting in room

CHILD HEALTH

1. Maintain appropriate contact with infant at all times. Allow for respite time for parents. Do not leave infant unattended.
2. Keep siderails of crib up, and monitor appropriate safety checks of all attachments for crib or infant's bassinet.
3. Keep infant free of scalding or chilling by checking temperature of water before bathing, and formula or food before feeding.
4. Maintain contact at all times during bathing—infants unable to sit must be held constantly. Older children should be monitored as well, with special attention given mental or physical needs for handicapped.
5. Ensure appropriate environmental safety, including:
   a. Provide adequate lighting and night lights
   b. Maintain clean, non-skid floors
   c. Keep rooms and halls free of clutter
   d. Keep electrical equipment in working order, with outlets covered
   e. Keep beds of ambulatory patients in locked position and at height suited for patient
   f. Ensure proper disposal of needles, and use caution with glass objects and eating utensils
   g. Keep windows and doors locked in halls
   h. Store plastic bags in cabinet out of child's reach
   i. Do not cover mattress or pillows of infant or child with plastic
   j. Make certain crib design follows federal regulations and that mattress has appropriate fit with crib frame
   k. Discourage sleeping in bed with infant
   l. Avoid use of homemade pacifiers (use only those of one-piece construction with loop handle)
   m. Do not tie pacifier around infant's neck
   n. Untie bibs, bonnets, or other garments with snug fit around neck of infant before sleep
   o. Never leave infant or toddler alone in bathtub
   p. Inspect toys for removable parts and check for safety approval
   q. Do not feed infant foods which do not readily dissolve such as grapes, nuts, popcorn, etc.
   r. Keep doors of large appliances, especially refrigerators, closed at all times
   s. Maintain fence and constant supervision with swimming pool
   t. Exercise caution while cleaning with attention to pails of water and cleaning solutions
   u. As infant or child is able, encourage swimming lessons with supervision and foster water safety
6. Teach patient, parents, and significant others:
   a. All of the aforementioned as it relates to creating a safe home environment and the need to foster safety;
   b. Alteration in life-style that may be necessary;
   c. Caution in exposure to sun for periods greater than 10 minutes at a time;

    d. Use of appropriate seat belts and care seats according to weight and development;

    e. Need to keep matches and pointed objects, such as knives, in a safe place out of child's reach;

    f. Use of lead-free paint in child's furniture and environment;

    g. To keep toxic substances locked in cabinet and out of child's reach;

    h. To hang plants and avoid placement on floor and tables;

    i. To discard used poisonous substances;

    j. Not to store toxic substances in food or beverage containers;

    k. To administer medication as a drug, not as candy;

    l. To use child-proof medication containers;

    m. Appropriate use of Syrup of Ipecac;

    n. Heimlich maneuver for age of client;

    o. CPR for client's age;

    p. Recognition of signs and symptoms of choking;

    q. As applicable, use of any special monitoring equipment;

    r. Caution in cutting food into small bites and monitoring eating;

    s. Need for appopriate meal-time safety to prevent aspiration with giggling.

7. Investigate any signs and symptoms that warrant potential child protective service referral.

8. Be aware of potential for young children to answer to any name. Validate identification for procedures in all young children.

9. Assist in referrals necessary for sensory or motor deficits related to potential for suffocation (e.g., speech therapy for follow-up or feeding therapy post operatively in cleft palate repair).

10. Place infant on abdomen with face turned to one side or the other until capable of rolling from side to side.

11. Have bulb syringe available in case of need to suction oropharynx. If regular equipment for suctioning is required, make appropriate safety checks.

12. Provide appropriate follow-up as needed (Visiting Nurse Service,etc.). If client is hospitalized, arrange for referrals before discharge.

WOMEN'S HEALTH

1. Teach patient and family the potential for injury to the fetus when the pregnant woman:

    a. Smokes or is exposed to smoke;

    b. Engages in substance abuse.

      (1) Alcohol

      (2) Drugs

        (a) Over-the-counter

        (b) Legal (i.e., prescription drugs, tranquilizers, etc.)

        (c) Illegal (i.e., cocaine, heroin, marijuana, etc.)

2. Report to proper authorities any suspicion of family violence. (See Chapter 9 and 10 for more detailed careplans.)

    a. Refer patient to appropriate assistance and resources such as:

      (1) Medical intervention

      (2) Police intervention

      (3) Psychologic intervention

      (4) Women's shelter (abused women)

      (5) Rape crisis center

3. Provide atmosphere that allows the patient considering abortion to relate her concerns and experiences.

4. Obtain detailed information of the method of abortion considered or used by the patient.

    a. Self-induced abortion

(1) Provide atmosphere that allows patient to relate her experience
(2) Obtain detailed information on method of abortion used by patient
   (a) Abortifacients
      [1] Castor oil
      [2] Turpentine
      [3] Other solutions (lye, ammonia, etc.)
   (b) Mechanical means
      [1] Coat hangers
      [2] Knitting needles
      [3] Broken bottle
      [4] Knives
b. Elective abortion
  (1) Encourage questions and verbalization of patient's life expectations
  (2) Provide information on options available to patient
  (3) Assist patient in identifying life-style adjustments that decision could entail
  (4) Involve significant others, if so desired by patient, in discussion and problem-solving activities regarding life-style adjustments
c. Obtain history from patient to include:
  (1) Date of last menstrual period
  (2) Method of contraception, if any
  (3) Previous obstetric history
  (4) Known allergies to anesthetics, analgesics, antibiotics, or other drugs
  (5) Current drug usage
  (6) Past medical history
d. Note patient's mental state: is she anxious, frightened, or ambivalent?
e. Perform physical assessment with special notice of:
  (1) Amount and character of vaginal discharge
  (2) Temperature elevation
  (3) Pain
  (4) Bleeding: consistency, amount, and color

5. Teach client importance of proper storage of birth control pills, spermicides, and medications (away from small children).
6. Assist patient in identifying drugs that are teratogenic to the fetus.
7. Assist patient in becoming aware of environmental hazards when pregnant, such as:
  a. X-rays
  b. People with infections
  c. Cats (litter boxes)
  d. Hazards on the job (surgical gases, industrial hazards)

MENTAL HEALTH

1. Orient patient to person, place, and time on each interaction.
2. Provide appropriate assistance to patient as he or she moves about the environment.
3. Assess level of consciousness every 15 minutes when the patient is acutely disoriented following special treatments or when consciousness is affected by drugs or alcohol. If level of consciousness is impaired, place patient on side to prevent aspiration of vomitus, and withhold solid food until level of consciousness improves.
4. Do not allow patient to smoke without supervision when disoriented or when consciousness is clouded.
5. Provide supervision for patients using new tools that could precipitate injury in special activities such as occupational therapy.

6. Teach client and support system:
   a. Risks associated with excessive use of drugs and alcohol;
   b. Appropriate methods for compensating for sensory-perceptual deficits (e.g., use of pictures or colors to distinguish environmental cues when ability to read is lost).
7. Remove all environmental hazards (e.g., personal grooming items that could produce a hazard, cleaning agents, foods that produce a hazard when taken with certain medicines, plastic bags, clothes hangers, belts and ties, shoestrings. Remove unnecessary pillows and blankets from the bed).
8. Maintain close supervision of patient (see care plan for Violence, Potential for [Chapter 9] for specific interventions).
9. Check patient's mouth carefully after oral medicines are given for any amounts that might be held in the mouth to be used at a later date.
10. If patient is at risk for holding pills in the mouth to be used later, consult with physician to have doses changed to liquids or injections.
11. Keep lavage setup and airway and oxygen equipment on standby.
12. Talk with patient and support system about situations that increase the potential for poisoning and develop a list of these situations.
13. Refer to appropriate persons or agencies for modification of the contributing factors to increased risk.
14. Label all medicines and poisonous substances appropriately.

HOME HEALTH

1. Assist patient and family to identify factors contributing to the potential for injury (e.g., items listed under common etiologies section with special emphasis on headings labeled household, occupational, community, fire hazards and vehicular hazards).
2. Involve patient and family in planning, implementing, and promoting reduction in the potential for injury:
   a. Arranging family conferences
   b. Assisting family to define mutual goals
   c. Promoting communication
   d. Assisting family members with specific tasks as appropriate to reduce the potential for injury (e.g., picking up objects that may be blocking pathways, removing unsafe or improperly stored chemicals, weapons, cooking utensils, and appliances; safe use and storage of toxic substances; certification in first aid and CPR; proper storage of food; knowledge of poisonous plants; learning to swim; removing fire hazards from environment; designing and practicing an emergency plan for action if fire occurs; proper use of machines using petroleum products; etc.)
3. Assist patient and family in life-style adjustments that may be required.
4. Teach patient and family injury prevention activities as appropriate:
   a. Proper lifting techniques
   b. Back exercises to prevent back injury
   c. Removal of hazardous environmental conditions such as improper storage of hazardous substances, improper use of electrical appliances, smoking in bed, open heaters and flames, congested walkways, etc.
   d. Proper ventilation when using toxic substances
   e. First aid for poisoning
   f. Proper labeling, storage, and disposal of toxic materials such as household cleaning products, lawn and garden chemicals, and medications
   g. Proper food preparation and storage
   h. Proper skin, lung, and eye protection when using toxic substances
   i. Toxic substances out of reach of infants and young children

j. Recognition of toxic plants and removal from environment as indicated
k. Plan of action if accidental poisoning occurs
5. Refer to appropriate assistive resources as indicated:
   a. Community home extension service for information regarding safe home environment
   b. Professional electricians
   c. Professional heating and air conditioning contractors
   d. Financial counselor
   e. Community action services such as police, fire officials, city and county commissioners, traffic control officers, school officials, and occupational health and safety officials to alter community hazards
   f. Poison control center
   g. First aid and CPR classes

EVALUATION
OBJECTIVE 1

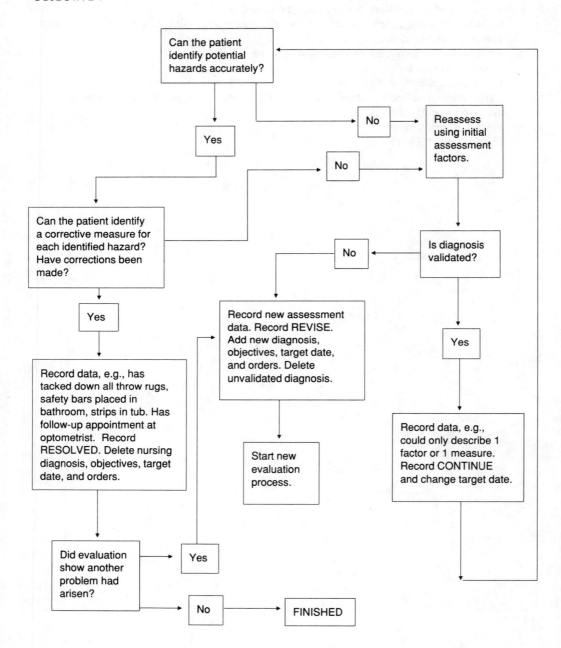

OBJECTIVE 2

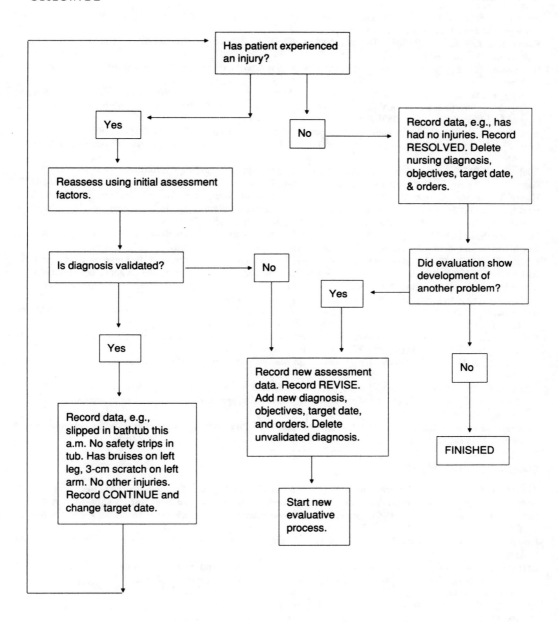

REFERENCES

Arya, O., & Bennett, P. (1974). Venereal disease control: Case study of university students in Uganda. *International Journal of Health Education, 17,* 53–65.

Baron, M., & Tafuro, P. (1985). The extremes of age: The newborn and the elderly. *Nursing Clinics of North America, 20,* 181–190.

Beauchamp, T., & Childress, J. (1983). *Principles of biomedical ethics* (2nd ed.). New York: Oxford University Press.

Breunig, K., Brutwitzk, G., Schulte, J., Crane, L., Schroeder, P., & Lutze, J. (1986). Noncompliance as a nursing diagnosis: Current use in clinical practice. In M. Hurley (Ed.), *Classification of nursing diagnoses. Proceedings of the sixth conference* (pp. 387–395). St. Louis: C. V. Mosby.

Brubaker, B. (1983). Health promotion: A linguistic analysis. *Advances in Nursing Science, 5*(3), 1–14.

Devore, N., Jackson, V., & Piening, S. (1983). TORCH infections. *American Journal of Nursing, 83,* 1660–1665.

Edel, M. (1985). Noncompliance: An appropriate nursing diagnosis? *Nursing Outlook, 33,* 183–185.

Gleit, C., & Tatro, S. (1981). Nursing diagnoses for healthy individuals. *Nursing & Health Care, 32,* 151–157.

Hagey, R., & McDonough, P. (1984). The problem of professional labeling. *Nursing Outlook, 32,* 151–157.

Hoffman, L. (1983). A co-evolutionary framework for systemic family therapy. In B. P. Keeney (Ed.), *Diagnosis and assessment in family therapy* (pp. 35–62). Rockville, MD: Aspen Systems.

North American Nursing Diagnosis Association. (1987). *Taxonomy I with complete diagnosis.* St. Louis: Author.

North American Nursing Diagnosis Association. (1988). *Proposed nursing diagnoses.* St. Louis: Author.

Pender, N. (1987). *Health promotion in nursing practice* (2nd ed.). East Norwalk, CT: Appleton-Century-Crofts.

Ridenour, N. (1983). Health beliefs, preventive behavioral intentions and knowledge of gonorrhea: Predictors of recidivism? In Monograph 1983 Proceedings of 2nd Annual Sigma Theta Tau Conference, *The world of work: Research in nursing practice.* Indianapolis, IN: Sigma Theta Tau.

Ridenour, N. (1986). *View of illness and approaches to therapy: Paradigm and paradox.* Unpublished manuscript, Texas Tech University Health Sciences Center School of Nursing, Lubbock, TX.

Rosenstock, I. (1974). Historical origins of the health belief model. In M. Becker (Ed.), *The health belief model and personal behavior.* Thorofare, NJ: Charles B. Slack.

Sackett, D., & Haynes, B. (1976). *Compliance with therapeutic regimens.* Baltimore: Johns Hopkins University Press.

Schuster, C. (1977). Normal physiological parameters through the life cycle. *Nurse Practitioner, 2,* 25–28.

Schuster, C., & Ashburn, S. (1986). *The process of human development: A holistic lifespan approach* (2nd ed.). Boston: Little, Brown.

Stanhope, M. (1988). Economics of health care delivery. In M. Stanhope & J. Lancaster (Eds.), *Community health nursing: Process and practice for promoting health* (pp. 44–65). St. Louis: C. V. Mosby.

SUGGESTED READINGS

Adams, A. (1985). External barriers to infection. *Nursing Clinics of North America, 20,* 145–149.

American Nurses' Association. (1986). *Standards of home health nursing practice.* Kansas City, MO: Author.

Baretich, D., & Anderson, L. (1987). Should we diagnose strengths? No: Stick to the problems. *American Journal of Nursing, 87,* 1211–1212.

Benenson, A. (1985). *Control of communicable diseases in man.* Washington, DC: American Public Health Association.

Carpenito, L. J. (1987). *Nursing diagnosis: Application to Practice* (2nd ed.). Philadelphia: J. B. Lippincott.

Centers for Disease Control. (1984). *CDC guideline for isolation precautions in hospitals.* Washington, DC: U.S. Government Printing Office.

Clark, C. (1986). *Wellness nursing.* New York: Springer.

Coralli, C. (1985). Promoting health in international travel. *Nurse Practitioner, 10,* 28–43.

Crittenden, R. (1983). *Discharge planning.* Bowie, MD: Robert J. Brady.

Dixon, J., & Dixon, J. P. (1984). An evolutionary-based model of health and viability. *Advances in Nursing Science, 6* (3), 1–18.

Dracup, K., & Meleis, A. (1987). Compliance: An interactionist approach. *Nursing Research, 31,* 31–36.

Edelman, C., & Mandle, C. (1986). *Health promotion throughout the lifespan.* St. Louis: C. V. Mosby.

Fogel, C., & Wood, N. (1981). *Health care of women: A nursing perspective.* St. Louis: C. V. Mosby.

Feuer, L. (1987). Discharge planning: Home caregivers need your support too. *Nursing Management, 18,* 58–59.

Gettrust, K. V., Ryan, S. C., & Engleman, D. S. (1985). *Applied nursing diagnosis.* New York: John Wiley & Sons.

Gordon, M. (1987). *Manual of nursing diagnosis 1986–1987*. New York: McGraw-Hill.

Greene, C. (1987). Blood and immunology. In C. Greene (Ed.), *Handbook of adult primary care*. New York: John Wiley & Sons.

Gurevich, I. (1985). The competent internal immune system. *Nursing Clinics of North America, 20*, 151–161.

Guyton, A. (1986). *Medical physiology* (7th ed). Philadelphia: W.B. Saunders.

Hadeka, M. (1987). *Clinical judgment in community health nursing*. Boston: Little, Brown.

Hall, B., & Allan, J. (1986). Sharpening nursing's focus by focusing on health. *Nursing and Health Care, 7* (6), 315–329.

Hilbert, G. (1985). Accuracy of self-reported measures of compliance. *Nursing Research, 34*, 319–320.

Howes, A. (1984). Nursing diagnoses and care plans for ambulatory care patients with AIDS. *Topics in Clinical Nursing, 6* (2), 61–66.

Humphrey, C. (1986). *Home care nursing handbook*. East Norwalk, CT: Appleton-Century-Crofts.

Jackson, M. (1984). Infection control. *American Journal of Nursing, 84*, 208–211.

Jaffe, M., & Skidmore-Roth, L. (1988). *Home health nursing care plans*. St. Louis: C. V. Mosby.

Johnson-Saylor, M. (1980). Seize the moment: Health promotion for the young adult. *Topics in Clinical Nursing, 2* (2), 9–19.

Kemp, H., Silver, H., & O'Brien, D. (1984). *Current pediatric diagnosis and treatment* (8th ed.). Los Altos, CA: Lang.

Laffrey, S., Loveland-Cherry, C., & Winkler, S. (1986). Health behavior: Evolution of two paradigms. *Public Health Nursing, 3* (2), 92–100.

Lenz, E. (1984). Information seeking: A component of client decisions and health behavior. *Advances in Nursing Science, 6* (3), 59–72.

McClelland, E., Kelly, K., & Buckwalter, K. (1984). *Continuity of care: Advancing the concept of discharge planning*. Orlando, FL: Grune & Stratton.

National League for Nursing. (1986). *Policies and procedures*. New York: Author.

National League for Nursing. (1988). *Accreditation program for home care and community health: Criteria and standards*. New York: Author.

Nowakowski, L. (1980). Health promotion/self care programs for the community. *Topics in Clinical Nursing, 2* (2), 21–27.

O'Ryan, P., & Falco, S., (1985). A pilot study to validate the etiologies and deferring characteristics of the nursing diagnosis noncompliance. *Nursing Clinics of North America, 20*, 685–695.

Popkess-Vawter, S., & Pinnell, N. (1987). Should we diagnose strengths? Yes: Accentuate the positive. *American Journal of Nursing, 87*, 1211–1216.

Ridenour, N. (1987). *A dialogical paradigm for holistic discourse in nursing*. Unpublished doctoral dissertation, Texas Tech University, Lubbock, TX.

Rinke, L. (1988). *Outcome standards in home health*. New York: National League for Nursing.

Rosenstock, I. (1974a). Historical origins of the health belief model. *Health Education Monographs, 2*, 328–335.

Rosenstock, I, (1974b). The health belief model and preventive health behavior. *Health Education Monographs, 2*, 354–386.

Sennott-Miller, L., & Miller, J. (1987). Difficulty: A neglected factor in health promotion. *Nursing Research, 36*, 268–272.

Steffi, B., & Eide, I. (1978). *Discharge planning handbook*. New York: Charles B. Slack.

Turner, J. (1988). Communicable diseases and infection control practices in community health. In M. Stanhope & J. Lancaster (Eds.), *Community health nursing: Process and practice for promoting health* (2nd ed.). St. Louis: C. V. Mosby.

Valanis, B. (1986). *Epidemiology in nursing and health care*. East Norwalk, CT: Appleton-Century-Crofts.

Walker, S., & Sechrist, K. (1987). The health promoting lifestyle profile: Development and psychometric characteristics. *Nursing Research, 36*, 76–81.

Walsh, J., Persons, C., & Wieck, L. (1987). *Manual of home health care nursing*. Philadelphia: J. B. Lippincott.

Woods, N. (1984). *Human sexuality in health and illness*. St. Louis: C. V. Mosby.

CHAPTER THREE

Nutritional-Metabolic Pattern

Pattern Description

The nutritional-metabolic pattern considers the food and fluid intake of the patient and the indicators of how this intake is used in meeting the body's functional needs. Problems in nutritional-metabolic functioning may arise from a physiologic, psychologic, or sociologic base. Physiologic problems may be primary in nature, (e.g., vitamin deficiency) or may arise secondary to another pathophysiologic state such as peptic ulcer. Psychosocial factors, such as eating to cope with stress, may result in an alteration in the nutritional-metabolic pattern. Sociocultural factors such as low income, inadequate storage, and cultural food preferences may result in an altered nutritional-metabolic state.

The nutritional-metabolic pattern includes both the what and when of intake, the use of dietary supplements (dieting aids, vitamins, etc.), and the body's use of the intake (healing, weight, etc.). A popular saying is "you are what you eat." This is a truism; what we eat is converted to our cellular structure and its functioning. The nutritional-metabolic pattern allows us to look at the whole of this relationship.

Pattern Assessment

1. Patient's description of daily food and fluid intake
   a. Number of meals and snacks each day
   b. Type of food intake—are basic four food groups included?
   c. Type of fluid intake—milk, water, caffeinated fluids, carbonated fluids, alcohol (Ask specifically about beer. Numerous persons do not consider beer to be alcohol, i.e., "hard liquor.")
   d. Personal food and fluid likes and dislikes
   e. Where meals are usually eaten—at desk, at home, in fast food restaurant
   f. Resources for food purchase, storage, and preparation
   g. Approximation of output—urine, feces, perspiration, respiratory rate
2. Weight
   a. Relationship to normal range for age, sex, and height
   b. Gain or loss
   c. Activity level
   d. Amount of body fat—measure skin fold with caliper
   e. Abdominal girth
3. Ingestion factors
   a. Appetite
   b. Discomfort, indigestion dysphagia
   c. Alterations in taste or smell

   d. Alterations in teeth or oral mucosa
   e. Any dietary restrictions or food allergies—what is allergic response (e.g., rash, drowsiness, nausea, diarrhea)?
   f. Bowel sounds—listen for at least 5 minutes before judging bowel sounds are absent
4. Health status
   a. Trauma, infections, illnesses
   b. Medications
   c. Healing rate
   d. Skin problems
   e. Nausea or vomiting
   f. Position and size of abdominal organs—palpation and percussion
5. Related factors
   a. Educational background
   b. Religious, ethnic, or cultural influences
   c. Developmental level

Conceptual Information

The nutritional-metabolic pattern requires looking at four separate but closely aligned aspects: nutrition, fluid balance, the skin, and thermoregulation. All four functionally interrelate to maintain the integrity of the overall nutritional-metabolic functioning of the body.

Food and fluid intake provides carbohydrates, proteins, fats, vitamins, and minerals which are metabolized by the body to meet energy needs, maintain intracellular and extracellular fluid balances, prevent deficiency syndromes, and act as catalysts for the body's biochemical reactions (Potter & Perry, 1985).

Nutrition

Nutrition refers to the intake, assimilation, and use of food for energy, maintenance, and growth of the body (Flynn & Heffron, 1984, p. 191). Assisting the patient in maintaining a good nutritional-metabolic status facilitates health promotion and illness prevention and provides dietary support in illness (Potter & Perry, 1985).

Many factors affect a person's nutritional status. Included in these factors are food availability; food cost; the meaning food has for the individual; cultural, social, and religious mores; and physiologic states that might alter the individual's ability to eat (Mitchell & Loustau, 1981).

In essence, we are initially concerned with the adequacy or inadequacy of the patient's nutritional state. If the diet is adequate, there is no major reason for concern; but we must be sure that all are defining adequacy in a similar manner.

Most people probably define an adequate diet as lack of hunger; however, professionals look at an adequate diet as being one in which nutrient intake balances with body needs. The diet is adequate if it meets either MDR (minimum daily requirements) or RDA (recommended dietary allowances) standards. The MDR standards are lesser in amount than the RDA standards but do provide enough nutrients to prevent deficiency problems. The RDA standards are the ones most widely used and are the ones that provide us the well-known basic four food groups (Mitchell & Loustau, 1981). The basic four food groups are the best standards to use in assessing dietary adequacy and call for:

Meat Group	Meat, eggs, fish, poultry. Two or more 2-to 3-ounce servings per day.
Milk and Dairy Product Group	Milk, ice cream, yogurt, cheese.
	Adults—equivalent of two 8-ounce glasses of milk per day.
	Children—equivalent of two to three 8-ounce glasses of milk per day.
Bread and Cereals Group	Enriched or whole-grain products.
	At least four servings daily.

Fruit and Vegetables   At least four servings daily, including at least one vitamin C source
group   daily and a dark green or deep yellow vegetable at least three times
                        a week

An inadequate nutritional state may be reflective of intake (calories) or use of the intake (metabolism) or a change in activity level. Underweight and overweight are the most commonly seen conditions that reflect alteration in nutrition (Murray & Zentner, 1985).

Underweight can be caused by inadequate intake of calories. In some instances, the intake is within recommended daily allowances but there is malabsorption of the intake. The malabsorption or inadequate intake can be due to physiologic reasons (pathophysiology), psychologic reasons (anorexia, bulimia), or cultural factors (lack of resources, religious proscriptions) (Murray & Zentner, 1985).

Overweight is rarely due to a physiologic disturbance, although a genetic predisposition may exist. Overweight is most commonly due to an imbalance between food and activity habits, (i.e., increased intake and decreased activity) (Murray & Zentner, 1985). However, recent research is indicating there is a metabolic set point and in actuality, overweight people may be eating less than normal-weight people.

Either underweight or overweight may be a sign of malnutrition (inadequate nutrition) with the result of the patient exhibiting signs and symptoms of more than body requirements or less than body requirements. In either instance, the nurse must assess carefully for the overall concept of malnutrition.

Fluid Volume

Fluid volume incorporates the aspects of actual fluid amount, electrolytes, and metabolic acid-base balance. Regardless of how much or how little a patient's intake is or how much or how little a patient's output is, the fluid, electrolyte, and metabolic acid-base balances are maintained within a relatively narrow margin. This margin is essential for normal functioning in all body systems and so it must receive close attention in providing care.

Approximately 60% of an adult's weight is body fluid (liquid plus electrolytes plus minerals plus cells) and approximately 70% of an infant's weight is body fluid. These various parts of body fluid are taken in daily through food and drink and are formed through the metabolic activities of the body (Mitchell & Loustau, 1981; Potter & Perry, 1985). The body fluid distribution includes intracellular (within the cells), interstitial (around the cells), and intravascular (in blood vessels) fluids. The combination of interstitial and intravascular is known as extracellular (outside the cells) fluid. Distribution of body fluid is influenced by both the fluid volume and the concentration of electrolytes. Body fluid movement, between the compartments, is constant and occurs through the mechanisms of osmosis, diffusion, active transport, and osmotic and hydrostatic pressure (Mitchell & Loustau, 1981; Potter & Perry, 1985).

Body fluid balance is regulated by intake (food and fluid), output (kidney, gastrointestinal tract, skin, and lungs) and hormonal control (antidiuretic hormone, glucocorticoids, and aldosterone). The largest amount of fluid is located in the intracellular compartment, with the volume of each compartment being regulated predominantly by the solute (mainly the electrolytes).

Electrolytes are either positively or negatively charged particles (ions). The major positively charged electrolytes (cations) are sodium (the main extracellular electrolyte), potassium (the most common intracellular electrolyte), calcium, and magnesium. The major negatively charged electrolytes (anions) are chloride, bicarbonate, and phosphate. The electrolyte compositions of the two extracellular compartments (interstitial and intravascular) are nearly identical. The intracellular fluid contains the same the number of electrolytes as the extracellular fluid does, but the intracellular electrolytes carry opposite electrical charges from the electrolytes in the extracellular fluid. This difference between extracellular and intracellular electrolytes is necessary for the electrical activity of nerve and muscle cells (Mitchell & Loustau, 1981 Potter & Perry, 1985). Therefore, the electrolytes help regulate cell functioning as well as the fluid volume in each compartment.

Usually the body governs intake through thirst and output through increasing or decreasing body fluid excretion via the kidneys, gastrointestinal tract, and respiration. Because of the way the body governs intake and output, in addition to the effects of pathophysiologic conditions such as shock, hemorrhage, diabetes, and vomiting on intake and output, the patient may enter a state of metabolic acidosis or alkalosis.

Acid-base balance reflects the acidity or alkalinity of body fluids and is expressed as the pH. In essence, the pH is a function of the bicarbonate: carbonic acid ratio (Mitchell & Loustau, 1981).

Acid-base balance is regulated by chemical, biologic, and physiologic mechanisms. The chemical regulation involves buffers in the extracellular fluid, while the biologic regulation involves ion exchange across cell membranes. The physiologic regulation is governed in the lungs by carbon dioxide excretion and in the kidneys through metabolism of bicarbonate, acid, and ammonia (Potter & Perry, 1985).

Metabolic acidosis is caused by situations in which the cellular production of acid is excessive (e.g., diabetic ketoacidosis), high doses of drugs have to be metabolized (e.g., aspirin), or excretion of the produced acid is impaired (e.g., renal failure) (Mitchell & Loustau, 1981). Weight reduction practices can contribute to the development of acidosis (fad diets, diuretics) as can chemical substance abuse (Potter & Perry, 1985).

Fluid volume is affected by regulatory mechanisms, body fluid loss, or increased fluid intake. Because fluid volume is so readily affected by such a variety of factors, continuous assessment for alterations in fluid volume must be made.

The Skin

The integrity of the skin is extremely important in the promotion of health since the skin is the body's first line of defense. The skin also plays a role in temperature regulation and in excretion.

The skin acts as protection through its abundant supply of nerve receptors that alert the body to the external environment (e.g., temperature, pressure, pain). The skin also acts as a barrier to pathogens, thus protecting the internal environment from these organisms (Mitchell & Loustau, 1981).

The skin's superficial blood vessels and sweat glands assist in thermoregulation. As the body temperature rises, the superficial blood vessels dilate and the sweat glands increase secretion. These two actions result in increased perspiration which, through evaporation, cools the body. During instances of excessive perspiration, water, sodium chloride, and nonprotein nitrogen are excreted through the skin; this affects fluid volume and osmotic balance. As the body temperature drops, the opposite reactions occur; there is vessel constriction and decreased sweat gland secretion, so that body heat is retained internally.

To fulfill its protective function the skin must be intact. Any change in skin integrity can allow pathogen invasion and will also allow fluid and electrolyte loss. Skin integrity relies on adequate nutrition and removal of metabolic wastes internally and externally, cleanliness, and proper positioning. Any factor that compromises nutrition, fluid, or electrolyte balance can result in impairment of skin integrity or, at least, the potential for impairment of skin integrity.

Thermoregulation

Thermoregulation refers to the body's ability to adjust its internal core temperature within a narrow range. The core temperature must remain fairly constant for metabolic activities and cellular metabolism to function for the maintenance of life. The core temperature rarely varies more than 1°C (less than 2°F). In fact, the range of temperature that is compatible with life ranges only from approximately 32.2° to 40° C (90° to 104° F).

Both the hypothalamus and the thyroid gland are involved in thermoregulation. The hypothalamus regulates temperature by responding to changes in electrolyte balances. Both the extracellular cations sodium and calcium affect the action potential and depolarization of cells. When there is an imbalance of sodium and calcium within the hypothalamus, hypothermia or hyperthermia can result. The thyroid gland regulates core body temperature by increasing or decreasing metabolic activities and cellular metabolism, thus altering heat production.

Many factors influence thermoregulation. The skin has previously been mentioned as a thermoregulatory organ. Heat is gained or lost to the environment by evaporation, conduction, convection, and radiation.

Evaporation occurs when body heat transforms the liquid on a person's skin to vapor. Conduction is the loss of heat to a colder object through direct contact. When heat is lost to the surrounding cool air, it is called convection. Radiation occurs when heat is given off to the environment, helping to warm it.

A person generally loses approximately 70% of heat from radiation, convection, and conduction. Another 25% is lost through insensible mechanisms of the lungs and evaporation from the skin, and about 5% is lost in urine and feces. When the body is able to produce and dissipate heat within a normal range, the body is in "heat balance" (Guyton, 1981).

The interrelationship of nutrition, fluid balance, thermoregulation, and skin integrity explains the nursing diagnoses that have been accepted in the nutritional-metabolic pattern. Indeed, if there is an alteration in any one of these four factors, it would be wise for the nurse to assess the other three to ensure a complete assessment.

Developmental Considerations

Infant

Swallowing is a reflex present before birth, since during intrauterine life the fetus swallows amniotic fluid. Following the transition to extrauterine life, the infant learns very rapidly (within 12–24 hours) to coordinate sucking and swallowing. There are really no developmental considerations of the act of swallowing since it is a reflex.

The normal process for swallowing involves both the epiglottis and the true vocal cords. These two structures move together to close off the trachea and to allow saliva or solid and liquid foods to pass into the esophagus. The respiratory system is thus protected from foreign bodies.

Salivation is adequate at birth to maintain sufficient moisture in the mouth. However, maturation of many salivary glands does not occur until the 3rd month and corresponds with the baby's learning to swallow at other than a reflex level (Schuster & Ashburn, 1986). Tooth eruption begins at about 6 months of age and stimulates saliva flow and chewing. The infant has a small amount of the enzyme ptyalin, which breaks down starches.

Water constitutes the greatest proportion of body weight of the infant. Approximately 75–78% of an infant's body weight is water with about 45% of this water found in the extracellular fluid. The newborn infant loses water through insensible water loss (approximately 35–45%) because of relatively greater body surface area to body weight.

The respiratory rate is approximately two times that of the adult. Therefore, the infant is also losing water through insensible loss from the lungs.

The newborn also loses water through direct excretion in the urine (50–60%) and through fairly rapid peristalsis due to the immature GI tract.

The newborn is unable to concentrate urine well and so is more sensitive to inadequate fluid intake or uncompensated water loss (Korones, 1981). The body fluid reserve of the infant is less than that of the adult, and since the infant excretes a greater volume per kilogram of body weight than the adult, infants are very susceptible to fluid volume deficit. The infant needs to consume water equal to 10–15% of body weight. Fluid and electrolyte requirements for the newborn are 70–100 ml/kg/24 hr, 2 mEq of Na and K^+ per kilogram per 24 hr and 2–4 mEq of Cl^- per kilogram per 24 hr.

The kidney function of the infant does not reach adult levels until 6 months to 1 year of age (Korones, 1981). The functional capacity of the kidneys is limited, especially during stress. In addition, the glomerular filtration rate is low, tubular reabsorption or secretory capacity is limited, sodium reabsorption is decreased, and the metabolic rate is higher. Therefore, there is a greater amount of metabolic wastes to be excreted. The infant kidney is less able to excrete large loads of solute-free water than is the more mature kidney (Driscoll & Heird, 1973).

Feeding behavior is important not only for fluid but also for food. The caloric need of the infant is 117 calories/kg of body weight (Murray & Zentner, 1985).

Breast milk contains adequate nutrients and vitamins for approximately 4–6 months of life. Some formulas prepared for the bottle are overly high in carbohydrates and fat (especially cholesterol) which may lead to a potential for increasing fat cells.

The introduction of solid foods should not occur until 4–6 months of age. Studies have indicated that there is a relationship between the early introduction of solid food (less than 3 months of age) and overfeeding of either milk or food leading to infant and adult obesity (Murray & Zentner, 1985). The infant should be made to feel secure, loved, and unhurried at feeding time. Skin contact is very important for the infant for both physiologic and psychologic reasons.

The skin of an infant is functionally immature and thus the baby is more prone to skin disorders. Both the dermis and the epidermis are loosely connected and both are relatively thin, which easily leads to chafing and rub burns (Schuster & Ashburn, 1986). Epidermal layers are permeable, resulting in greater fluid loss. Sebaceous glands, which produce sebum, are very active in late fetal life and early infancy, causing milia and cradle cap which goes away at about 6 months of age. Dry, intact skin is the greatest deterrent to bacterial invasion. Sweat glands (eccrine or apocrine) are not functional in response to heat and emotional stimuli until a few months after birth and function remains minimal through childhood. The inability of the skin to contract and shiver in response to heat loss causes ineffective thermal regulation (Murray & Zentner, 1985). Also, the infant has no melanocytes to protect against the rays of the sun. This is true of dark-skinned infants as well as light-skinned infants.

Core body temperature in the infant ranges from 97° to 100° F. Temperature in the infant fluctuates considerably because the regulatory mechanisms in the hypothalamus are not fully developed. (It is not considered abnormal for the newborn infant to lose 1°–2°F immediately after birth.) The infant is unable to shiver to produce heat, nor does the infant have much subcutaneous fat to insulate the body.

However, the infant does have several protective mechanisms by which he or she is able to conserve heat to keep the body temperature fairly stable. These mechanisms include vasoconstriction so that heat is maintained in the inner body; an increased metabolic rate which increases heat production; a closed body position (the so-called fetal position) which reduces the amount of exposed skin; and the metabolism of adipose tissue.

This particular adipose tissue is called "brown fat" because of the rich supply of blood and nerves. Brown fat composes 2–6% of body weight of the infant. This brown fat aids in adaptation of thermoregulation mechanisms (Schuster & Ashburn, 1986).

The ability of the body to regulate temperature at the adult level matures at approximately 3–6 months of age.

Toddler and Preschooler

By the end of the 2nd year, the child's salivary glands are adult size and have reached functional maturity (Schuster & Ashburn, 1986). The toddler is capable of chewing food, so it stays longer in his or her mouth and the salivary enzymes have an opportunity to begin breaking down the food. The saliva also covers the teeth with a protective film that helps prevent decay. Drooling no longer occurs, since the toddler easily swallows saliva.

Dental caries occur infrequently in children under 3 years; but rampant tooth decay in very young children is almost always related to prolonged bottle feeding at nap time and bedtime (bottle mouth syndrome). The toddler should be weaned from the bottle or at least not allowed to fall asleep with the bottle in his or her mouth (Chinn & Leonard, 1980). Parents should be taught that the adverse effects of bedtime feeding are greater than thumb sucking or the use of pacifiers.

Affected teeth remain susceptible to decay after nursing stops. If deciduous teeth decay and disintegrate early, spacing of the permanent teeth is affected, and immature speech patterns develop. Discomfort is felt and emotional problems may result (Chinn & Leonard, 1980).

The first dental examination should be between the ages of 18 and 24 months. Dental hygiene should be started when the first tooth erupts by cleansing the teeth with gauze or cotton moistened with hydrogen peroxide and flavored with a few drops of mouthwash. After 18 months, the child's teeth may be brushed with a soft or medium toothbrush (Chinn & Leonard, 1980). Fluoride supplements are believed to prevent caries.

In the toddler there is beginning to be the appropriate proportion of body water to body weight (62% water) (McCrory, 1972). The extracellular fluid is about 26%, whereas the adult has about 19% extracellular fluid. Toddlers have less reserve of body fluid than adults and lose more body water daily, both from sensible and insensible loss. This age group is highly predisposed to fluid imbalances (Masiak, Naylor, & Hayman, 1985). These imbalances relate to the fact that the kidney still is immature so water conservation is poor and the toddler still has an increased metabolic rate and therefore greater insensible water loss than the adult. However, GI motility slows so this age group is better able to tolerate fluid loss through diarrhea. The 2–3 year old needs 1100–1200 ml (4–5 8-oz glasses) of fluid every 24 hours, whereas the preschooler needs 1300–1400 ml fluid every 24 hours.

The caloric need in the toddler is 1000 cal/day or 100 cal/kg at 1 year and 1300–1500 cal/day at 3 years. A child should not be forced to "clean the plate" at mealtime and food should not be viewed as a reward or punishment. Instead, caloric intake should be related to the growing body and energy expenditures.

The caloric need of the preschooler is 85 cal/kg. Eating assumes increasing social significance and continues to be an emotional as well as a physiologic experience (Murray & Zentner, 1985). Frustrating or unsettled mealtimes can influence caloric intake, as can manipulative behavior on the part of the child or parent. The child may also be eating empty calories between meals.

In the toddler functional maturity of skin creates a more effective barrier against fluid loss; the skin is not as soft as the infant's and there is more protection against outside bacterial invasion. The skin remains dry because sebum secretion is limited. Eccrine sweat gland function remains limited, eczema improves, and the frequency of rashes declines.

Skin, as a perceptual organ, experiences significant development during this period. Children like to "feel" different objects and textures and like to be hugged; melanin is formed during these years and thus the toddler, preschooler, and school-age child is more protected against sun rays (Schuster & Ashburn, 1986).

In addition, small capillaries in the periphery become more capable of constriction and thus thermoregulation. Also, the child is able to sense and interpret that he or she is hot or cold and can voluntarily do something about it.

School-Age Child

The child at this age begins losing baby teeth as permanent teeth erupt. The child should not be evaluated for braces until after all 6-year molars have come in. The permanent teeth are larger than the baby teeth and appear too large for the small face, causing some embarrassment. Good oral hygiene is important.

For the school-age child, the percentage of total body water to total body weight continues to decrease until about 12 years of age when it approaches adult norms (Masiak, Naylor, & Hayman, 1985). Changes occur in extracellular fluid from 22% at 6 years to 17.5% at age 12 due to the proportion of body surface area to mass, increasing muscle mass and connective tissue, and increasing percentage of body fat.

Water is needed for excretion of the solute load. Balance is maintained through mature kidneys leading to mature concentration of urine and acidifying capacities. Fluid requirements can be calculated by height, weight, surface area, and metabolic activity. The school-age child needs about 1.5–3 quarts of fluid a day. Additionally, the child needs a slightly positive water balance. The electrolyte values are similar to those for the adult except for phosphorus and calcium (due to bone growth).

The caloric need of the school-age child is greater that that of an adult (approximately 80 cal/ kg or 1600–2200 cal/day). The ages of 10–12 reflect the peak ages of caloric and protein needs of the school-age child (need 50–60 cal/kg) due to the accelerated growth, muscle development, and bone mineralization. "The school age child reflects the nutritional experiences of early childhood and the potential for adulthood" (Murray & Zentner, 1985).

Adolescent

By age 21, all 32 permanent teeth have erupted. The adolescent needs frequent dental visits because of cavities and also for orthodontic work that may be in progress.

There is a growth spurt and sexual changes. A total increase in height of 25% and a doubling of weight are normally attained (Stone & Church, 1968). Muscle mass increases and total body water declines with increasing sexual development (Young, Bogan, Roe, & Lutwak, 1968). The adolescent needs 34–45 cal/kg and tends to have eating patterns based on external environmental cues rather than hunger. Eating becomes more of a social event. There is a high probability of eating disorders such as anorexia and bulimia arising during this age period.

The basal metabolic rate increases, lung size increases, and maximal breathing capacity and forced expiratory volume increase leading to increased insensible loss of fluid through the lungs. Total body water decreases from 61% at age 12 to 54% by age 18 due to an increase in fat cells. Fat cells do not have as much water as tissue cells (Young et al., 1968). The water intake need of the adolescent is about 2200–2700 ml/24 hr.

Sebaceous glands become extremely active during adolescence and increase in size. Eccrine sweat glands are fully developed and are especially responsive to emotional stimuli (are more active in males); and apocrine sweat glands also begin to secrete in response to emotional stimuli (Chinn & Leitch, 1979). Stopped-up sebaceous glands lead to acne, and the adolescent's skin is usually moist.

Young Adult

The amount of ptyalin in the saliva decreases after 20 years of age; otherwise the digestive system remains fully functioning. The appearance of "wisdom teeth" or third molars occurs at 20–21 years. There are normally four third molars, although some individuals may not fully develop all four. Third molars can create problems for the individual. Eruptions are unpredictable in time and presentation, and molars may come in sideways or facing any direction. This can force other teeth out of alignment which makes chewing difficult and painful. Often these molars need to be removed to prevent irreparable damage to proper occlusion of jaws. Even normally erupting third molars may be painful. The young adult must see a dentist regularly.

Total body water in the young adult is about 50–60%. There is a difference between males and females due to the difference in the number of fat cells. Most water in the young adult is intracellular with only about 20% of fluid being extracellular. Growth is essentially finished by this developmental age.

Adult

Ptyalin has sharply decreased by age 60 as well as other digestive enzymes. Total body water is now about 47–54.7%. Diet and activity indirectly influence the amount of body water by directly altering the amount of adipose tissue.

In the adult the activity level is stable or is beginning to decline. The basal metabolic rate gradually decreases along with a reduced demand for calories. The adult needs to reduce calorie intake by approximately 7.5% (Mitchell, Runbergen, Anderson, & Dibble, 1982).

Tissues of the integumentary system maintain a healthy, intact, glowing appearance until age 50 or 55 if the individual is receiving adequate vitamins, minerals, other nutrients, and fluids, and maintains good personal hygiene. Wrinkles do become more noticeable, however, and body water (from integumentary tissues) decreases leading to thinner, drier skin that bruises easier. Fat increases, leading to skin that is not as elastic and will not recede with weight loss so bags develop readily under the eyes (Schuster & Ashburn, 1986). Also, skin wounds heal more slowly because of decreased cell regeneration.

Older Adult

In the older adult the mouth undergoes changes associated with aging which can affect nutrition. Tooth decay, loss of teeth, degeneration of jaw bone, progressive gum recession, and increased reabsorption of the dental arch can make eating and chewing a difficult task for the elderly person if good dental health has not been maintained. Reduced chewing ability, decrease in salivation, and perhaps poorly fitting dentures compound the problem of poor nutrition of the aged. Aging causes an atrophy of olfactory organs and a loss of taste buds. Usually salt and sweet taste buds are lost first with bitter and sour taste buds remaining intact; therefore, food has little flavor. This leads to aged persons having a characteristic unpleasant bitter taste in their mouths called dysgeusia (Shafer, 1965).

Loss of taste is compounded by gum disease, poor teeth, or dentures. Fifty percent of the elderly have lost their teeth. Ninety percent who have natural teeth have periodontal disease (Kopac, 1983). The aged are especially vulnerable to oral carcinoma (Murray & Zentner, 1985).

Total body water of the older adult is about 45–50%. Although values are within normal, the elderly cannot tolerate extremes of temperature well because of slower response time to adapt to change. Excess heat and overexertion are not tolerated well by the older adult. The older adult naturally has drier, wrinkled skin so assessment of skin in the elderly for alteration in fluid volume needs to be interpreted carefully. There is a decreased number of body cells and adipose tissue leading to a decrease in total body water. However, cell size increases.

Serum protein (albumin) production is decreased but globulin is increased. Therefore, there is not much difference in blood volume. However, the nurse needs to consider the proportion of blood volume to body weight.

There is a decrease in tubular functioning, which affects removal of waste, urine concentration, and dilution. This in turn leads to a decrease in specific gravity and urine osmolarity. There is decreased bladder capacity leading to nocturia. Therefore the elderly may limit fluid in the evening to offset nocturia, but limiting fluids may lead to nocturnal dehydration.

Sodium and chloride levels remain constant but potassium decreases. In the older adult the blood level and excretion of aldosterone decreases 50% if sodium is depleted (Cugini, Scavo, Halberg, Schramm, Pusch, Franke, 1982).

Gonadal hormones may influence fluid and electrolyte balance in terms of sodium and water retention. Therefore, with the loss of hormones with aging, there is a decrease in sodium and water retention.

Many changes are occurring in the gastrointestinal tract (decreased enzyme secretion, general gastric irritation, decreased nutrient and drug absorption, decreased HCl secretion, decreased peristalsis and elimination, and decreased sphincter muscle tone) of the older adult that make nutrition a primary concern (Murray & Zentner, 1985). The older adult needs decreased calories but needs an increase in vitamins and trace elements as well as an adequate intake of protein, fat, carbohydrates, bulk, and electrolytes (Na^+, K^+, Ca^{++}, Mg^{++}). However, financial concerns may lead the elderly to buy inappropriate foods containing empty calories.

The skin of the older adult becomes drier and thinner; skin lesions of discoloration and scaliness (keratosis) may appear. Integumentary changes in the older adult are readily noticeable because of our society's emphasis on youth and beauty (Schuster & Ashburn, 1986). The older adult has wrinkles, mostly in the face; exposure to the sun also produces and hastens formation of wrinkles. Fatty layers are lost in the trunk, face, and extremities leading to the appearance of increased joint size throughout the body. The skin is nonelastic and may lose water to the air in low-humidity situations, which results in chapping.

Extremes of temperature are difficult for the elderly. Body temperature may increase because of a decrease in size, number, and functioning of the sweat glands; or the person may need a sweater because of decreased fat and peripheral circulation. Fragile blood vessels lead to bruising. The older adult loses melanocytes leading to pale, light skin; hair turns grey and the elderly lose hair. Older women may have hair on the face or chin due to androgen-estrogen imbalances.

There is an absolute decrease in intracellular water and a decrease in both sebaceous and sweat glands. With age, skin becomes less effective as a tactile organ (touch, pressure, pain, local temperature changes) because of the slowing of impulses to the brain and a decrease in the number of receptors (Carnevali & Patrick, 1979). Therefore, elderly persons may burn or have frostbite and not be cognizant of the problem.

Applicable Nursing Diagnoses

Body Temperature, Altered: Potential

DEFINITION

The state in which the individual is at risk for failure to maintain body temperature within the normal range. (North American Nursing Diagnosis Association ([NANDA], 1987, p. 18).

DEFINING CHARACTERISTICS (RISK FACTORS) (NANDA, 1987, p. 18)

The nurse will review the initial pattern assessment for the following risk factors to determine the diagnosis of Body Temperature, Altered: Potential.

1. Extremes of age
2. Extremes of weight
3. Exposure to cold/cool or warm/hot environment
4. Dehydration
5. Inactivity or vigorous activity
6. Medications causing vasoconstriction or vasodilation
7. Altered metabolic rate
8. Sedation
9. Inappropriate clothing for environmental temperature
10. Illness or trauma affecting temperature regulation.

RELATED FACTORS (NANDA, 1987, p. 18)

The risk factors also serve as the related factors for this nursing diagnosis.

DIFFERENTIATION

Body Temperature, Altered: Potential needs to be differentiated from Hypothermia, Hyperthermia, and Thermoregulation, Ineffective.

Hypothermia is the condition under which a person maintains a temperature lower than normal for him or her. This means that the body is probably dissipating heat normally but is unable to produce heat normally. In Body Temperature, Altered: Potential, both heat production and heat dissipation are potentially nonfunctional.

Hyperthermia is the condition under which a person maintains a temperature higher than normal. This means that the body is probably producing heat normally but is unable to dissipate the heat normally. Both heat production and heat dissipation are potentially nonfunctional in Body Temperature, Altered: Potential.

Thermoregulation, Ineffective means that a person's temperature fluctuates between being too high and too low. There is nothing wrong, generally, with heat production or heat dissipation. However, the thermoregulatory systems in the hypothalamus or the thyroid are dysfunctional.

OBJECTIVES

1. Will have no alteration in body temperature by (date).

AND/OR

2. Will describe at least (number) measures to keep body temperature within a range of 98° to 99° F by (date).

TARGET DATE

Initial target dates would be stated in hours. After stabilization, target dates could be extended to 2–3 days.

NURSING ORDERS

ADULT HEALTH

1. Monitor temperature (rectally) at least every 2 hours on (odd or even) hour.
2. Maintain consistent room temperature.
3. Teach patient to wear appropriate clothing:
   a. Close-knit undergarments in winter to prevent heat loss
   b. Hat and gloves in cold weather because heat is lost from head and hands
   c. Wool in preference to synthetic fibers, because wool provides better insulation
   d. Socks or stockings at night
   e. Light, loose, but protective clothing in hot weather
   f. Hat in hot weather to protect head
4. Encourage use of sheet blankets rather than regular sheets.
5. Encourage patient to stay indoors on windy days.
6. Give frequent, small meals and warm liquids.
7. Assist patient to learn to assess biorhythms—generally early morning is the period of lowest body metabolic activity; add extra clothes until food and physical movement stimulate increased cellular metabolism and circulation.
8. Alternate physical and sedentary activity.
9. Avoid sedatives and tranquilizers that depress cerebral function and circulation.
10. Encourage patient to work outdoors in early morning and to work for limited periods of time.

CHILD HEALTH

1. Monitor temperature as ordered, or at least every 4 hours.
2. Note pattern of temperature from past 48 hours if possible.
3. If temperature is less than 97° F (or as parameters dictate per physician), take appropriate measures for maintaining temperature:
   a. Infants—radiant warmer or isolette
   b. Older child—thermoblanket
   c. Administration of medications as ordered
4. If temperature is above 101° F (or as dictated per physician), take appropriate measures to bring temperature back to normal range:
   a. Administer antibiotics or Tylenol as ordered per physician.
   b. Note related symptoms, especially delirium or loss of consciousness in high fever or reduced tolerance of fever.
5. Be alert for possible febrile seizures, and check for history of same.
6. If child has reduced threshold for seizures during times of fever, be prepared to treat seizures with anticonvulsants, maintain airway, and provide for safety from injury.
7. Provide appropriate teaching to child and parents related to fever and its treatment.
8. Monitor skin integrity and potential for alteration in mucous membranes, and maintain fluid and electrolyte balance.
9. Follow up with cultures for identification of causative organisms if infection is present.

WOMEN'S HEALTH

This nursing diagnosis will pertain to women the same as to any other adult. The reader is referred to the other sections (Adult Health, Home Health, and Mental Health) for specific nursing orders and objectives pertaining to women and potential alteration in temperature.

MENTAL HEALTH

(Note: The objectives and nursing orders for the mental health client will be the same as those described for adult health. The following nursing orders are specific considerations for the mental health client.)

1. Clients receiving neuroleptic drugs may experience a decrease in their ability to sweat and therefore experience difficulty in reducing body temperature in warm weather. They should be observed for signs and symptoms related to hyperthermia when involved in outdoor activities. Teach clients these symptoms and caution them to decrease their outdoor activities in the warmest part of the day and to maintain adequate hydration, especially if they are receiving lithium carbonate with these drugs.
2. Clients receiving antipsychotics and antidepressants can experience a loss of thermoregulation. The elderly client, especially, should be monitored for this side effect. Provide the client with extra clothing and blankets to maintain comfort. Protect this client from contact with uncontrolled hot objects such as space heaters and radiators. Heating pads and electric blankets can be used with supervision. These clients are at risk for thermal injuries because of the drug's effects on the client's learned avoidance behavior and possible clouded consciousness.
3. Teach client to use heating pads and electric blankets in a safe manner.
4. Do not provide electric heating devices to the client who is on suicide precautions or who has alterations in thought processes.
5. Fever in clients receiving antipsychotic agents, especially chlorpromazine and thioridazine should be carefully evaluated for agranulocytosis. This risk is greatest 3–8 weeks after therapy has begun. Clients who have had this side effect should not receive the drug again since a repeat episode is highly possible. Notify physician if client has an elevation in temperature or flu-like symptoms
6. Review client's CBC before drug is started and report any abnormalities on subsequent CBCs to the physician.
7. Phenothiazines can produce hyperthermia, which can be fatal. This is due to a peripheral autonomic effect. These clients should be monitored for hot, dry skin, CNS depression, and rectal temperatures up to 108° F. Monitor client's temperature three times a day while awake (note times here). Notify physician of alterations.
8. A hyperpyretic crisis can be produced in clients receiving tricyclic antidepressants (TCAs) and the monoamine oxidase inhibitors (MAOIs). Monitor clients receiving TCAs and MAOIs for alterations in temperature three times a day while awake (note times here). Notify physician of any alterations.
9. Refer to nursing diagnosis Hypothermia or Hyperthermia for interventions related to these situations once the alteration has occurred.

HOME HEALTH

1. Monitor for factors contributing to the potential for alteration in body temperature (Refer to Risk Factors).
2. Involve patient and family in planning, implementing, and promoting reduction or elimination of the potential of alteration in body temperature by establishing family conferences to set mutual goals and to improve communication.
3. Teach patient and family measures to decrease or eliminate potential for alterations in body temperature.
   a. Wearing appropriate clothing
   b. Taking appropriate care of underlying disease
   c. Avoiding exposure to extremes of environmental temperature
   d. Maintaining temperature within norms for age, sex, and height
   e. Ensuring appropriate use of medications
   f. Ensuring proper hydration
4. Assist patient and family to identify life-style changes that may be required.
   a. Learn survival techniques if client works or plays outdoors
   b. Measure temperature in a manner appropriate for the developmental age of the person
   c. Maintain ideal weight

  d. Avoid substance abuse
5. Consult with appropriate assistive resources as indicated:
  a. YMCA/YWCA for classes on outdoor recreation and survival
  b. Nurse
  c. Physician
  d. Nutritionist
  e. Drug and alcohol counselor

EVALUATION
OBJECTIVE 1

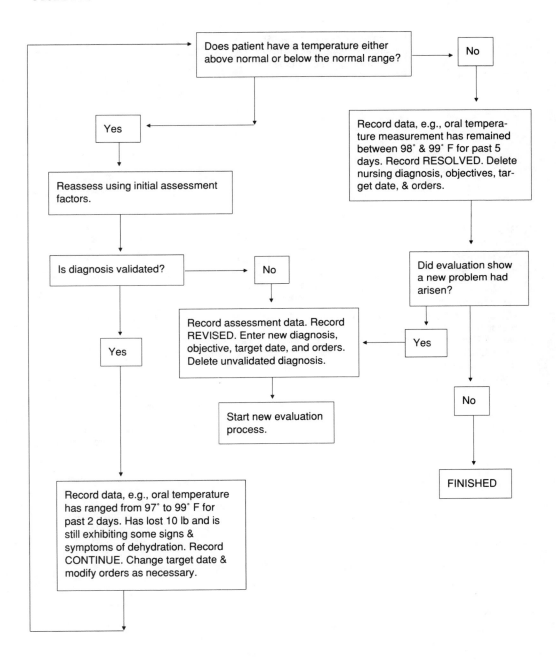

OBJECTIVE 2

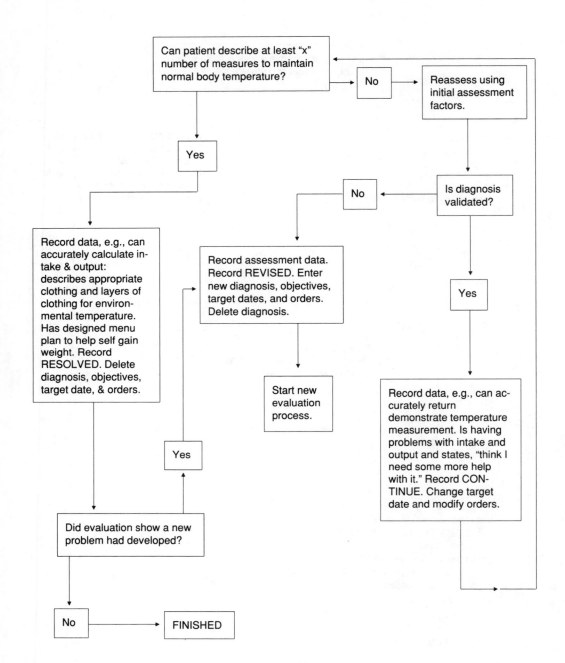

Can patient describe at least "x" number of measures to maintain normal body temperature?

No → Reassess using initial assessment factors.

Yes

Is diagnosis validated?

No

Yes

Record data, e.g., can accurately calculate intake & output: describes appropriate clothing and layers of clothing for environmental temperature. Has designed menu plan to help self gain weight. Record RESOLVED. Delete diagnosis, objectives, target date, & orders.

Record assessment data. Record REVISED. Enter new diagnosis, objectives, target dates, and orders. Delete diagnosis.

Start new evaluation process.

Record data, e.g., can accurately return demonstrate temperature measurement. Is having problems with intake and output and states, "think I need some more help with it." Record CONTINUE. Change target date and modify orders.

Yes

Did evaluation show a new problem had developed?

No → FINISHED

Breastfeeding, Ineffective

DEFINITION

The state in which a mother, infant, or child experiences dissatisfaction or difficulty with the breastfeeding process (NANDA, 1988).

DEFINING CHARACTERISTICS (NANDA, 1988)

The nurse will review the initial pattern assessment for the following defining characteristics to determine the diagnosis of Breastfeeding, Ineffective.

1. Major defining characteristics
   a. Unsatisfactory breastfeeding process.
2. Minor defining characteristics
   a. Actual or perceived inadequate milk supply.
   b. Inability of infant to attach on to maternal breast correctly.
   c. No observable signs of oxytocin release.
   d. Observable signs of inadequate infant intake.
   e. Nonsustained sucking at the breast.
   f. Insufficient emptying of each breast per feeding.
   g. Persistence of sore nipples beyond the 1st week of breastfeeding.
   h. Insufficient opportunity for sucking at the breast.
   i. Infant fussiness and crying within the 1st hour after breastfeeding; unresponsiveness to other comfort measures.
   j. Infant arching and crying at the breast; resisting latching on.

RELATED FACTORS (NANDA, 1988)

1. Prematurity.
2. Infant anomaly.
3. Maternal breast anomaly.
4. Previous breast surgery.
5. Previous history of breastfeeding failure.
6. Infant receiving supplemental feedings with artificial nipple.
7. Poor infant sucking reflex.
8. Nonsupportive partner or family.
9. Knowledge deficit.
10. Interruption in breastfeeding.
11. Maternal anxiety or ambivalence.

DIFFERENTIATION

Breastfeeding, Ineffective should be differentiated from the patient's concern over whether she wants to breastfeed or not. Although a mother who does not want to breastfeed will more than likely be ineffective in her breastfeeding attempts, ineffective breastfeeding can be related to other problems than just the unwillingness to breastfeed. Other diagnoses which might need to be differentiated include:

- Anxiety—Defined as a vague, uneasy feeling, the source of which is often nonspecific or unknown to the individual. If an expression of perceived threat to self-concept, health status, socioeconomic status, role functioning, or interaction patterns is made, this would constitute the diagnosis of Anxiety.
- Parenting, Altered—Defined as the inability of the nurturing figures to create an environment which promotes optimum growth and development of another human being. Adjustment to parenting, in general, is a normal maturation process following the birth of a child.

- Growth and Development, Altered: Self-Care Skills—Defined according to a demonstrated deviation from age-group norms for self-care. Inadequate caretaking would be defined according to specific behavior and attitudes of the individual mother or infant.
- Individual Coping, Ineffective—Defined as the inability of the individual to deal with situations which require coping or adaptation to meet life's demands and roles.

OBJECTIVES

1. Will verbalize increased satisfaction with breastfeeding process by (date).

AND/OR

2. Infant will require no supplemental feedings by (date).

TARGET DATE

Because ineffective breastfeeding can be physically detrimental to the infant as well as emotionally detrimental to the mother, an initial target date of 2 days would be best.

NURSING ORDERS

ADULT HEALTH

1. Allow for uninterrupted breastfeeding.
2. Determine ways to make abnormal breast structure amenable for breastfeeding.
3. Discourage supplemental feedings with artificial nipple.
4. Explain and demonstrate methods to increase infant sucking reflex.
5. Teach and reinforce breastfeeding technique knowledge.
6. Determine partner and family perceptions of breastfeeding process.
7. Refer to La Leche League or other community support groups.
8. Encourage maternal affiliation behavior.

CHILD HEALTH

1. Monitor for contributory factors related to infant's ability to suck.
   a. Structural abnormalities (e.g., cleft lip or palate)
   b. Altered level of consciousness, seizures, CNS damage
   c. Mechanical barriers to sucking (e.g., endotracheal tube or ventilator)
   d. Pain or underlying altered comfort or medication
   e. Prematurity with diminished sucking ability
2. Determine the effect the altered or impaired breastfeeding has on mother and infant.
3. To the degree possible, provide emotional support for infant in instances of temporary inability to breastfeed, as with gavage feedings; allow for sucking of pacifier if possible, etc.
4. Coordinate actual visitation of mother, father, and infant to best facilitate successful breastfeeding with respect to rest, natural hunger cycles, and comfort of all involved.
5. Assist with plans to manage impaired breastfeeding to best provide support to all involved (e.g., breast-pumping for period of time with verbal acknowledgment of the value of this effort until breastfeeding can be successful, or support for choice for alternate plans of feeding according to situation).

WOMEN'S HEALTH

1. Assess mother's desire to breastfeed infant.
2. List the advantages and disadvantages of breastfeeding for the mother.
3. Obtain a breastfeeding and bottle feeding history from the mother (i.e., did she breastfeed before, successfully or unsuccessfully, etc.).
4. Observe mother with infant during breastfeeding.

5. Demonstrate to mother various positions for breastfeeding and how to alternate positions with each feeding to prevent nipple soreness.
   a. Sitting up
   b. Lying down
   c. Using football hold
   d. Holding baby "tummy-to-tummy"
   e. Using pillows for mother's comfort
   f. Using pillows for supporting baby
6. Ascertain mother's need for privacy during breastfeeding.
7. Monitor the baby's position on the breast (correct or incorrect).
8. Assess mother's support for breastfeeding from
   a. Husband;
   b. Patient's mother;
   c. Doctors (obstetrician and pediatrician);
   d. Nurses (on postpartum units).
9. Discuss infant's needs and frequency of feedings.
10. Assist mother in planning a day's activities when breastfeeding, ensuring that mother gets plenty of rest.
11. Discuss diet for the breastfeeding mother, listing important food groups and necessary calories to adequately maintain milk production.
12. Encourage advance planning for the working mother if she intends to breastfeed.
13. Assist the working mother in the proper methods of expressing milk and storing it properly.
14. Reassure mothers that it takes time to establish breastfeeding (usually a month).
15. Be available for support and consultation.
16. Check for poor or dysfunctional sucking by checking:
    a. Position mother is holding the baby (see nursing order 5 above);
    b. Baby's mouth position on areola and nipple;
    c. Position of baby (i.e., hyperextension of head).
17. If baby is separated from mother, such as in NICU, involve baby's nurses in planning with mother routines and times for breastfeeding infant.
18. Refer mother to breastfeeding support groups.
    a. Childbirth educator
    b. Lactation consultant
    c. La Leche League International, Inc.
       9616 Minneapolis Avenue
       Franklin Park, IL 60131
    d. Hospital nursery, mother-baby units.
19. Demonstrate various hand pumps, battery-operated pumps, and electric pumps for the mother.
20. Demonstrate and allow mother to return demonstrate hand expression of breast milk.
21. Place a pillow over abdomen of cesarean mother to assist in keeping pressure off incision while breastfeeding.
22. Assist the mother of a premature baby to pump breasts routinely to begin milk production.
23. Demonstrate proper storage and transportation of breast milk for the premature baby.
24. Assist mother when weaning premature baby from tube feeding to breastfeeding.
    a. When ready allow infant to nipple, if possible several times a day and while tube feeding.
    b. Allow mother time to hold, cuddle, and interact with infant during tube feedings.
    c. Allow mother and infant privacy to begin interaction with breastfeeding.
    d. Be available to assist with infant during breastfeeding interaction.
    e. Reassure mother it might take several attempts before baby begins to breastfeed.
25. Provide educational materials for breastfeeding mothers on request.

26. If unable to breastfeed because of infant physical deformity, assist with pumping breasts and feeding breast milk in bottles with special nipples.

MENTAL HEALTH

Refer to Women's Health nursing orders for interventions related to this diagnosis.

HOME HEALTH

1. Teach patient and family measures to promote effective breastfeeding.
    a. Quiet environment
    b. Adequate nutrition and hydration
    c. Appropriate technique
    d. Family support
2. Assist patient and family in identifying risk factors pertinent to the situation.
    a. Premature infant
    b. Infant anomaly
    c. Maternal breast dysfunction
    d. Infection
    e. Previous breast surgery
    f. Supplemental bottle feedings
    g. Nonsupportive family
    h. Lack of knowledge
    i. Anxiety
3. Consult with or refer to appropriate resources as indicated.
    a. La Leche League
    b. Pediatrician
    c. Obstetrician
    d. Breastfeeding education
    e. Family support group
    f. Stress reduction

EVALUATION
OBJECTIVE 1

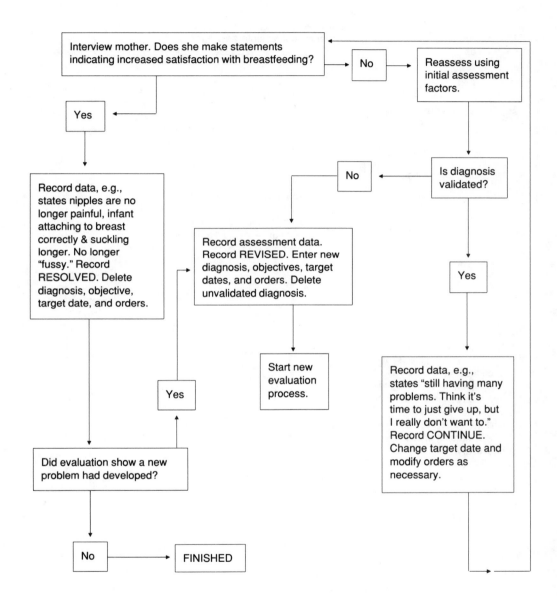

OBJECTIVE 2

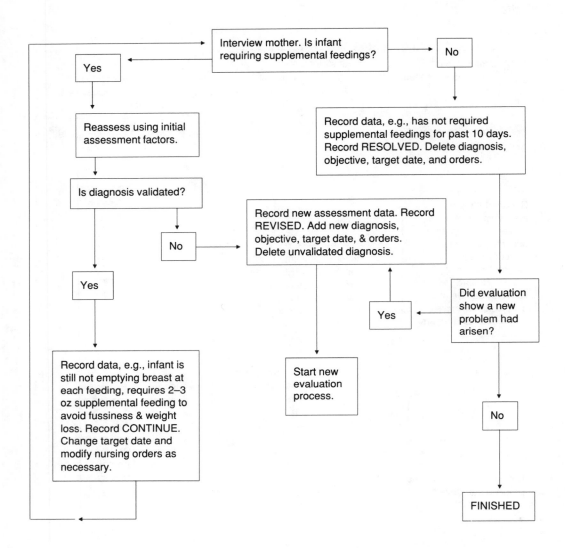

Interview mother. Is infant requiring supplemental feedings?

No

Yes

Reassess using initial assessment factors.

Record data, e.g., has not required supplemental feedings for past 10 days. Record RESOLVED. Delete diagnosis, objective, target date, and orders.

Is diagnosis validated?

Record new assessment data. Record REVISED. Add new diagnosis, objective, target date, & orders. Delete unvalidated diagnosis.

No

Yes

Did evaluation show a new problem had arisen?

Yes

Record data, e.g., infant is still not emptying breast at each feeding, requires 2–3 oz supplemental feeding to avoid fussiness & weight loss. Record CONTINUE. Change target date and modify nursing orders as necessary.

Start new evaluation process.

No

FINISHED

Fluid Volume, Altered: Deficit (Potential or Actual [1 and 2])

DEFINITION

The state in which an individual is at risk of experiencing or is experiencing vascular, cellular, or intracellular dehydration (NANDA, 1987, pp. 38–40)[a]

DEFINING CHARACTERISTICS (NANDA, 1987, pp. 38–40)

The nurse will review the initial pattern assessment for the following defining characteristics to determine the diagnosis of Fluid Volume, Altered: Deficit (Potential or Actual [1 or 2]).

A. Fluid Volume, Altered: Deficit (Potential)
  1. Major defining characteristics
    a. Increased output
    b. Urinary frequency
    c. Thirst
    d. Altered intake
  2. Minor defining characteristics
    None given.
B. Fluid Volume, Altered: Deficit (Actual [1])
  1. Major defining characteristics
    a. Dilute urine
    b. Increased urine output
    c. Sudden weight loss
  2. Minor defining characteristics
    a. Possible weight gain
    b. Hypotension
    c. Decreased venous filling
    d. Increased pulse rate
    e. Decreased skin turgor
    f. Decreased pulse volume or pressure
    g. Increased body temperature
    h. Dry skin
    i. Dry mucous membrane
    j. Hemoconcentration
    k. Weakness
    l. Edema
    m. Thirst
C. Fluid Volume, Altered: Deficit (Actual [2])
  1. Major defining characteristics
    a. Decreased urine output
    b. Concentrated urine
    c. Output greater than intake
    d. Sudden weight loss
    e. Decreased venous filling
    f. Hemoconcentration
    g. Increased serum sodium
  2. Minor defining characteristics
    a. Hypotension
    b. Thirst

---

[a]The primary means of distinguishing the various deficits is the related factor.

    c. Increased pulse rate
    d. Decreased skin turgor
    e. Decreased pulse volume or pressure
    f. Change in mental state
    g. Increased body temperature
    h. Dry skin
    i. Dry mucous membrane
    j. Weakness

RELATED FACTORS (NANDA, 1987, pp. 38–40)

A. Fluid Volume, Altered: Deficit (Potential)
    1. Extremes of age
    2. Extremes of weight
    3. Excessive losses through normal routes (e.g., diarrhea)
    4. Loss of fluid through abnormal routes (e.g., indwelling tubes)
    5. Deviations affecting access to intake or absorption of fluids (e.g., physical immobility)
    6. Factors influencing fluid needs (e.g., hypermetabolic state)
    7. Knowledge deficiency related to fluid volume
    8. Medications (e.g., diuretics)
B. Fluid Volume, Altered: Deficit (Actual [1])
    1. Failure of regulatory mechanisms
C. Fluid Volume, Altered: Deficit (Actual [2])
    1. Active loss

DIFFERENTIATION

Fluid Volume, Altered: Deficit (Potential or Actual) would need to be differentiated from several other nursing diagnoses. For example, Oral Mucous Membrane, Altered and Nutrition, Altered: Less than Body Requirements may be the primary nursing diagnosis. The person may not be able to ingest food or fluid because of primary problems in the mouth, or the person just may not be ingesting enough food from which the body can absorb fluids. Elimination, Altered: Diarrhea or Urinary Elimination, Impaired: Incontinence or Altered Elimination Pattern may be causing an extreme loss of fluid before it can be absorbed and used by the system.

Skin Integrity, Impaired could also be the primary problem. For example, the patient who has been burned has grossly impaired skin integrity. The skin is supposed to regulate the amount of fluid lost from it. If there is relatively little skin intact, the skin is unable to perform its regulatory function and there is much loss of fluid and electrolytes.

In the infant or young child, the problem may be primarily a Self-Care Deficit or Parenting, Altered. The infant or young child is not able to obtain the fluid he or she wants and must depend on others. If the parents are unable to recognize or meet these needs then the infant or young child may have a potential or actual fluid volume deficit. Even in an adult, the primary nursing diagnosis may be Self-Care Deficit. Again, if the adult is unable to obtain the fluid he or she wants because of some pathophysiologic problem, then he or she may have a potential or actual fluid volume deficit.

OBJECTIVES

1. Intake and output will balance within 200 ml by (date).

AND/OR

2. Will describe (number) factors influencing adequate hydration and methods to prevent fluid volume deficit by (date).

TARGET DATE

Normally, intake and output will approximately balance only every 72 hours; thus, an appropriate target date would be 3 days.

NURSING ORDERS

ADULT HEALTH

1. Measure and record total intake and output every shift:
    a. Check intake and output hourly.
    b. Observe and document color and consistency of all urine, stools, and vomitus.
    c. Check urine specific gravity every 4 hours at (state time here).
2. Force fluids to a minimum of 2000ml daily:
    a. Ascertain patient's fluid likes and dislikes (list here).
    b. Offer small amount of fluid (4–5 oz) at least every hour while awake and at every awakening during night.
    c. Offer fluids at temperature that is most acceptable to patient (e.g., warm, cool).
    d. Interspace fluids with high-fluid-content foods (e.g., popsicles, gelatin, pudding, ice cream).
3. Monitor intravenous fluids carefully. (See Nutrition, Altered: Less than Body Requirements—Additional Information.)
4. Take vital signs every 2 hours on (odd/even) hour and include apical pulse.
5. Weigh daily at (state time here). Teach patient to weigh at same time each day in same-weight clothing.
6. Assist patient to eat and drink as necessary.
7. Turn and properly position patient at least every 2 hours on (odd/even) hour:
    a. Encourage patient to alter position frequently.
    b. Provide active and passive range of motion every 4 hours while awake.
8. Administer or assist with complete oral hygiene at least twice a day.
9. Schedule at least 1 hour total rest periods for patient at least four times a day.
10. Monitor:
    a. Skin turgor at least every 4 hours while awake;
    b. Electrolytes, blood urea nitrogen, hematocrit, and hemoglobin. Collaborate with physician regarding frequency of lab tests;
    c. Central venous pressure every hour (if appropriate);
    d. Mental status and behavior at least every 2 hours;
    e. For signs and symptoms of shock at least every 4 hours (e.g., weakness, diaphoresis, hypotension, tachycardia, tachypnea).
11. If temperature elevation arises:
    a. Maintain cool room temperature;
    b. Offer cool, clear liquids;
    c. Administer ordered antipyretics;
    d. Give tepid sponge bath;
    e. Remove heavy and excess clothing and bed covers.
12. If gastric tube is present:
    a. Use only normal saline for irrigation;
    b. Monitor amount of oral intake of water and ice chips. Avoid if at all possible. Offer commercial electrolyte replenishment solutions if permitted (e.g., Gatorade).
13. Administer medications as ordered (e.g., antidiarrheal, antiemetics). Monitor medication effects.
14. Teach patient to increase fluid intake at home during:
    a. Elevated temperature episodes;
    b. Periods infections are present;

   c. Periods of exercise;
   d. Hot weather.
15. Refer to other health care professionals as necessary:
   a. Home health
   b. Dietitian
   c. Dentist
   d. Social services

CHILD HEALTH

1. Measure and record total intake every shift:
   a. Check intake and output hourly (may require weighing diapers).
   b. Check urine specific gravity every 2 hours or every voiding otherwise ordered.
2. Force fluids to a minimum appropriate for size: infants, 70–100 ml/kg in 24 hr (e.g., 3-kg infant needs 240–300 ml/24 hr) toddler, 120–135 ml/kg in 24 hr (e.g., 9.5-kg toddler needs 1150–1300 ml/24 hr) school-age child, 100–110 ml/kg in 24 hr (e.g., school-age child of 16.2 kg requires 1600–1800 ml/24 hr).
3. Weigh patient daily at same time on same scale. (Weigh infants without clothes, children in underwear.)
4. Assist patient in eating as necessary; offer option of allowing parents to feed infant.

WOMEN'S HEALTH

1. Assist client to identify life-style factors which could be contributing to symptoms of nausea and vomiting.
   a. Identify client's support system.
   b. Monitor client's feelings (positive or negative) about pregnancy.
   c. Evaluate social, economic, and cultural conditions.
   d. Involve significant others in discussion and problem solving activities regarding physiologic changes of pregnancy that are affecting work habits and interpersonal relationships (e.g., nausea and vomiting).
2. Teach client measures that can help alleviate physiologic pathologic changes of pregnancy.
   a. In collaboration with dietitian:
      (1) Obtain dietary history;
      (2) Assist patient in planning diet which will provide adequate nutrition for her and her fetus' needs.
   b. Teach methods of coping with gastric upset, nausea, and vomiting.
      (1) Eat bland, low-fat foods (no fried foods or spicy foods).
      (2) Increase carbohydrate intake.
      (3) Eat small amounts of food every 2 hours (avoid empty stomach).
      (4) Eat dry crackers or toast before getting up in morning.
      (5) Take vitamins and iron with night meal before going to bed (Vitamin B,50 mg can be taken twice a day—never on an empty stomach).
      (6) Drink high-protein liquids (e.g., soups, eggnog) (Neeson & May, 1986).
   c. Monitor client for:
      (1) Variances in appetite;
      (2) Vomiting first 16 weeks (beyond 12 weeks) of pregnancy;
      (3) Weight loss;
      (4) Intractable nausea and vomiting.
3. In collaboration with physician assess lab work for:
   a. Electrolyte imbalance
      (1) Hemoconcentration
      (2) Ketosis with ketonuria

       (3) Hyponatremia

       (4) Hypokalemia

   b. Dehydration *(Note: "During pregnancy, gastric acid secretion normally is reduced because of increased estrogen stimulation. This places the woman at risk for alkalosis rather than the acidosis that usually occurs in an advanced stage of dehydration." [Neeson & May, 1986, p. 494].)*

   c. Hydrate patient, establish electrolyte balance, and provide vitamin supplements in collaboration with physician.

   d. Restrict oral intake and provide parenteral administration of fluids and vitamins in collaboration with physician. *(Note: "Vitamin B_6 has been found effective and safe for use in nausea and vomiting of pregnancy." [Neeson & May, 1986, p. 495].)*

4. Monitor and record intake and output (urinary and vomitus) at least once per shift.
5. Provide good oral hygiene before each meal and at bedtime.
6. Provide quiet, restful environment.
7. Provide nonjudgmental atmosphere.
8. Allow expression of feelings and encourage verbalization of fears and questions by scheduling at least 30 minutes with client at least once per shift.
9. Provide client and family with information and appropriate referrals (e.g., dietitian, physician).
10. Provide client and family with diet information for the breastfeeding mother to prevent dehydration.
    a. Increase daily fluid intake.
       (1) Drink at least 2500 ml of fluid daily.
       (2) Extra fluid can be taken just before each breast feeding (e.g. water, fruit juices, decaffeinated tea, milk).
    b. Eat well-balanced meals to include four basic food groups.
11. Encourage and support the working woman who wishes to continue breastfeeding.
    a. Assist client by providing information and ideas on breastfeeding and working.
       (1) Establishing a home milk supply (pumping breasts)
       (2) How to pump
          (a) At home
          (b) At work
       (3) How to store breast milk
          (a) Freezing
          (b) Refrigerating
          (c) Dating and labeling
       (4) Transporting breast milk
       (5) Equipment needed
       (6) Preparation of stored breast milk for feeding
12. For the newborn or neonate in the first 6 months:
    a. Give vitamin supplements as recommended by physician.
       (1) Vitamin D.
       (2) Fluoride
       (3) If indicated, iron
    b. Teach patient intake for infant. Infant should be taking in approximately 420 ml soon after birth and building to 1200 ml at the end of 3 months.
13. Monitor for fluid deficit and teach patients to monitor via following factors:
    a. "Fussy baby," especially immediately after feeding
    b. Constipation (remember breast-fed babies have less stools than formula-fed babies)
    c. Weight loss or slow weight gain
       (1) Closely assess baby, mother, and nursing routine.
       (2) Is baby getting empty calories (e.g., a lot of water between feedings)?

    (3) Nipple confusion—from switching baby from breast to bottle and vice versa many times

    (4) Count number of diapers per day (should have 6–8 really wet diapers per day)

  d. Intolerance to mother's milk or bottle formula

  e. Monitor baby for illness or lactose intolerances

  f. Monitor how often mother is nursing infant (infrequent nursing can cause slow weight gain)

MENTAL HEALTH

1. If client is confused or is unable to interpret signs of thirst, place on intake and output measurement and record this information every shift.
2. Evaluate potential for fluid deficit resulting from medication or medication interactions (e.g., lithium and diuretics). If this presents a risk, place client on intake and output measurement every shift.
3. Evaluate mental status every shift.
4. Teach client how to measure, record, and evaluate intake and output.
5. Assist client in consuming 2000 ml of fluids per day by:
   a. Providing fluids client likes (note those here);
   b. Offering small amounts of fluid at least every hour while awake and at every awakening during the night;
   c. Providing foods with high fluid content such as popsicles, gelatin, pudding, ice cream, watermelon (note preferences here).
6. Teach client measures to ensure adequate hydration, such as:
   a. Need to increase fluids during exercise, fever, hot and dry climate;
   b. Need to drink fluids before feeling of thirst is experienced;
   c. How to recognize signs and symptoms of dehydration such as dry skin, dry lips, excessive sweating, dry tongue, and decreased skin turgor.

HOME HEALTH

1. Teach patient and family measures to ensure adequate hydration, such as:
   a. Need to increase fluids during exercise, fever, hot and dry climate;
   b. How to recognize signs and symptoms of dehydration (e.g., dry, cracked lips, dry skin or excessive sweating, dry tongue, decreased skin turgor).
2. Assist patient and family in identifying life-style changes that may be required (e.g., avoiding excessive use of caffeine, alcohol, laxatives, diuretics, salt tablets, exercise without electrolyte replacement, antihistamines, fasting, and high-protein diets).
3. Assist patient and family in identifying risk factors pertinent to the situation (e.g., diabetes, protein malnourishment, elderly, excessive vomiting or diarrhea, medications for fluid retention or high blood pressure, confusion or lethargy, fever, excessive blood loss, wound drainage and inability to obtain adequate fluids because of pain, immobility, or difficulty in swallowing).
4. Teach patient and family how to measure, record, and evaluate intake and output.
5. Offer fluids frequently. Include foods high in fluid content (gelatin, popsicles, ice chips, sherbet, ice cream).
6. Refer to appropriate assistive resources as indicated (e.g., visiting nurse, nutritionist, physician).

EVALUATION
OBJECTIVE 1

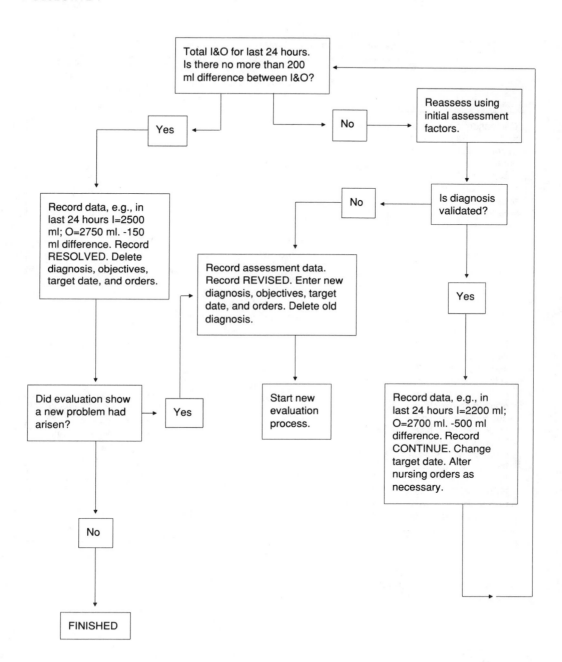

OBJECTIVE 2

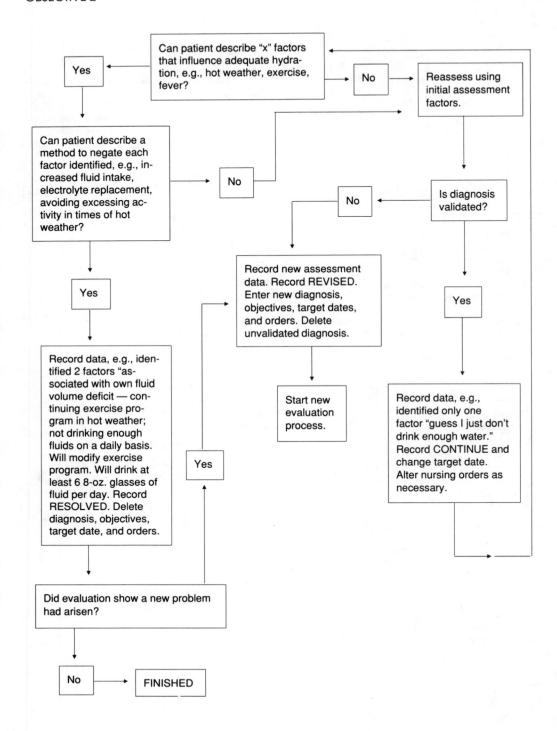

Fluid Volume, Altered: Excess

DEFINITION

A condition in which the individual experiences increased fluid retention and edema (NANDA, 1987, p. 37).

DEFINING CHARACTERISTICS (NANDA, 1987, p. 37)

The nurse will review the initial pattern assessment for the following defining characteristics to determine the diagnosis of Fluid Volume, Altered: Excess.

1. Major defining characteristics
   a. Edema
   b. Effusion
   c. Anasarca
   d. Weight gain
   e. Shortness of breath
   f. Orthopnea
   g. Intake greater than output
   h. S_3 heart sound
   i. Pulmonary congestion (chest x-ray)
   j. Abnormal breath sound
   k. Rales (crackles)
   l. Change in respiratory pattern
   m. Change in mental status
   n. Decreased hemoglobin and hematocrit
   o. Blood pressure changes
   p. Central venous pressure changes
   q. Pulmonary artery pressure
   r. Jugular vein distention
   s. Positive hepatojugular reflex
   t. Oliguria
   u. Specific gravity changes
   v. Azotemia
   w. Altered electrolytes
   x. Restlessness
   y. Anxiety

RELATED FACTORS (NANDA, 1987, p. 37)

1. Compromised regulatory mechanisms
2. Excess fluid intake
3. Excess sodium intake

DIFFERENTIATION

Fluid Volume Altered: Excess should be differentiated from Cardiac Output, Altered: Decreased; Gas Exchange, Impaired; Physical Mobility, Impaired; Nutrition, Altered: More than Body Requirements; and Urinary Elimination, Impaired: Retention.

The body depends on both appropriate gas exchange and adequate cardiac output to oxygenate tissues and circulate nutrients and fluid for use and disposal. If either of these is altered, then the body will suffer in some way. One of these ways will be in the circulation of fluid in the body. Fluid will be left in tissue and not be able to be absorbed into the general circulation to be redistributed or eliminated.

Nutrition, Altered: More than Body Requirements could be the primary problem. The person ingests more food and fluid than the body can handle and the result is excess fluid volume as well as other changes in the body's physiology.

Fluid volume excess must also be differentiated from Urinary Elimination, Impaired: Retention. One way the body compensates fluid balance is through urinary elimination. If the body cannot properly eliminate fluids then the system "backs up," so to speak, and excess fluid remains in the tissues.

Besides appropriate gas exchange and adequate cardiac output, the body also needs movement of muscles to assist in transporting food and fluids to and from the tissues. Mobility, Impaired may lead to an alteration in this movement of food and fluids. Waste products of metabolism and excess fluid are allowed to remain in tissues, creating a fluid volume excess.

OBJECTIVES

1. Intake and output will balance within 200 ml by (date).

(Note: may want difference to be only 50 ml for a child.)

AND/OR

2. Will not exhibit any signs or symptoms of fluid volume excess by (date).

TARGET DATE

In a healthy person, intake and output reach an approximate balance over a span of 72 hours. An acceptable target date would then logically be the 3rd day of admission.

NURSING ORDERS

ADULT HEALTH

1. Measure and record total intake and output every shift.
   a. Check intake and output hourly.
   b. Observe and document color and character of urine, vomitus, and stools.
   c. Check urine specific gravity at least every 4 hours at (state times here).
2. Collaborate with the physician regarding limiting intake:
   a. Amount
   b. Type (e.g., clear fluids only, intravenous only)
3. Take vital signs every 2 hours at (state times here) and include apical pulse.
4. Check lung, heart, and breath sounds every 2 hours on (odd/even) hour.
5. Weigh daily at (state times here).
6. Turn and properly position patient at least every 2 hours on (odd/even) hour.
   a. Check dependent parts for edema (e.g., ankles, sacral area, buttocks.
   b. Protect edematous skin from injury:
      (1) Avoid shearing force
      (2) Powder or cornstarch to avoid friction
      (3) Pillows, foam rubber pads, etc. to avoid pressure
   c. Encourage patient to alter position frequently.
   d. Provide active/passive range of motion every 4 hours while awake at (state times here).
7. Administer medications (e.g., diuretics) as ordered. Monitor medication effects.
8. Administer or assist with complete oral hygiene at least twice a day and as required.
9. Monitor:
   a. Skin turgor at least every 4 hours while awake
   b. Electrolytes, hemoglobin, and hematocrit. Collaborate with physician regarding frequency of lab tests
   c. Mental status and behavior at least every 2 hours on (odd/even) hour.
10. Teach patient to monitor own intake and output at home.

11. Refer to other health care professionals as appropriate:
    a. Home health
    b. Social services
    c. Dietitian

Additional Information

Fluid volume excess can occur as a result of water excess, sodium excess, or water and sodium excess. The nurse needs to recognize the difference in precipitating causes.

Edema: mild or 1+ means that the skin can be depressed 0–¼inch; moderate or 2+ means that the skin can be depressed ¼–½ inch; severe or 3+ means that the skin can be depressed ½–1 inch; and deep pitting edema or 4+ means that the skin can be depressed more than 1 inch and it takes longer than 30 seconds to rebound.

CHILD HEALTH

1. Measure and record total intake every shift:
   a. Check intake and output hourly, weigh diapers.
   b. Check urine specific gravity every 2 hours on (odd/even) hour or every voiding unless otherwise ordered.
2. Collaborate with physician regarding limiting intake:
   a. Amount
   b. Type of fluids to be allowed, including route (in some instances, such as renal failure, intake may be dictated by urinary output of the previous 8 hours)
3. Reposition as tolerated every ½ hour.
4. Elevate head of bed to facilitate breathing.
5. Weigh patient daily at same time on same scale (weigh infants without clothes, children in underwear).
6. Monitor skin turgor and on infant, anterior fontanel for bulging every 2–4 hours.
7. Teach patient and family to monitor fluid intake and output at home according to the specific needs of the situation.

WOMEN'S HEALTH

1. Review client's history for factors associate with pregnancy-induced hypertension (PIH):
   a. Family history
   b. Diabetes
   c. Multiple gestation
   d. Polyhydramnios
   e. Persistent hypertension
   f. Hydatidiform mole
   g. R H incompatibility
2. Monitor client for signs of PIH.
   a. Prenatal
      (1) Weight
      (2) BP
      (3) Presence of edema
      (4) Proteinuria
   b. Preeclampsia
      (1) Headaches
      (2) Visual changes such as blurred vision
      (3) Increased edema of face and pitting edema of extremities
      (4) Oliguria
      (5) Hyperreflexia
      (6) Nausea or vomiting

(7) Epigastric pain
c. Eclampsia
(1) Convulsions
(2) Coma
3. Monitor, at least once per shift, for edema:
a. Swelling of hands, face, legs, or feet.
(1) Caution: may have to remove rings.
(2) May need to wear loose shoes or a bigger shoe size.
(3) Schedule rest breaks during day where she can put her feet up.
(4) When lying down—lie on left side to promote placental perfusion and prevent compression of vena cava.
4. In collaboration with dietitian:
a. Obtain nutritional history;
b. Begin high-protein diet (80–100 gm protein);
c. Reduce sodium intake (not above 6 gm daily or below 2.5 gm daily).
5. Monitor at least every 4 hours:
a. Intake and output (urinary output not less than 30 ml/hr or 120 ml/4 hr).
b. Effect of magnesium sulfate ($MgSO_4$) and hydralizine hydrochloride (Apresoline) therapy. Have antidote for $MgSo_4$—Calcium gluconate—available at all times during $MgSo_4$ therapy.
c. Deep tendon reflexes (DTR).
d. Respiratory rate, pulse, and BP as often as needed.
e. Seizure precautions.
f. Bed rest and reduction in noise level in patient's environment.
g. Fetal heart rate and well-being.
6. Provide client and family factual information and support as needed.

MENTAL HEALTH

(Note: The nursing orders for the mental health client will be the same as those described for adult health. The following nursing orders are specific considerations that need to be added for the mental health client.)

1. Teach client to:
a. Remove constrictive clothing.
b. Avoid crossing legs.
c. Elevate edematous limb.
2. Assist client to identify risk factors (e.g., heart disease, kidney disease, diabetes mellitus, liver disease, pregnancy, and immobility).
3. Assist client in identifying life-style changes that may be required (e.g., avoid standing or sitting for long periods of time, avoid excess salt); teach to read labels for sodium content, using spices other than salt with cooking, and maintaining adequate protein intake.
4. Teach client purposes and side effects of medications.

HOME HEALTH

1. Teach patient and family signs and symptoms of fluid excess (e.g., peripheral and dependent edema, shortness of breath, taut and shiny skin).
2. Assist patient and family in identifying risk factors pertinent to the situation (e.g., heart disease, kidney disease, diabetes mellitus, liver disease, pregnancy, and immobility).
3. Assist patient and family in identifying life-style changes that may be required.
a. Avoid standing or sitting for long periods of time, elevate edematous limb.
b. Avoid crossing legs.
c. Avoid constrictive clothing (girdles, garters, knee-highs, rubber bands to hold up stockings, etc.).

     d. Consider antiembolism stockings.
     e. Avoid excess salt: teach to read labels for sodium content; avoid canned and fast foods.
     f. Use spices other than salt with cooking.
     g. Ensure adequate protein.
     h. Avoid lying in one position for longer than 2 hours.
     i. Raise head of bed or sit in chair if having difficulty breathing.
     j. Restrict water if required (e.g., liver or kidney disease).
     k. Weigh daily wearing the same clothes, using the same scale, and at the same time of day.
4. Teach patient and family methods to protect edematous tissue.
     a. Practice body alignment.
     b. Use pillows, pads, etc. to relieve pressure on dependent parts.
     c. Avoid shearing force when moving in bed or chair.
     d. Alter position a minimum of every 2 hours.
5. Teach purposes and side effects of medications (diuretics, cardiac medications, etc.).
6. Assist patient and family to set criteria to help them to determine when a physician or other intervention is required.
7. Refer to appropriate assistive resources as indicated (e.g., nutritionist, physician, social services).

EVALUATION
OBJECTIVE 1

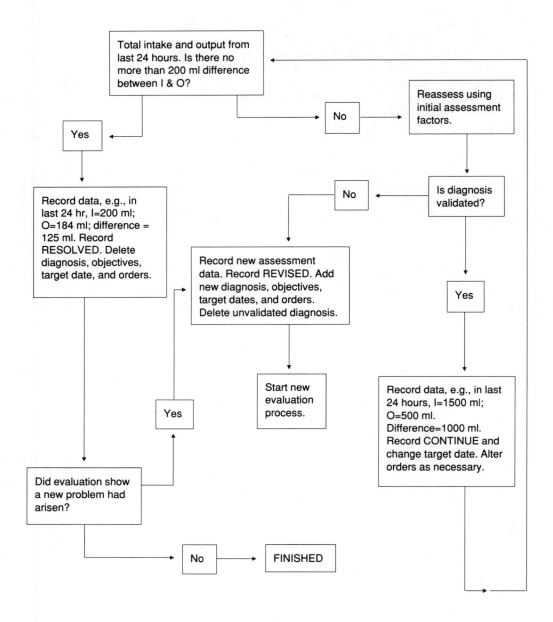

OBJECTIVE 2

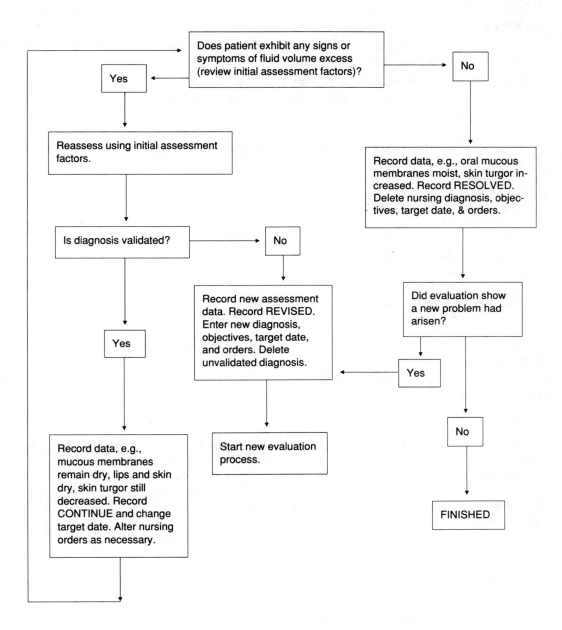

Hyperthermia

DEFINITION

A state in which an individual's body temperature is elevated above his or her normal range (NANDA, 1987, p. 20).

DEFINING CHARACTERISTICS (NANDA, 1987, p. 20)

The nurse will review the initial pattern assessment for the following defining characteristics to determine the diagnosis of hyperthermia.

1. Major defining characteristics
   a. Increase in body temperature above normal range
2. Minor defining characteristics
   a. Flushed skin
   b. Warm to touch
   c. Increased respiratory rate
   d. Tachycardia
   e. Seizures or convulsions

RELATED FACTORS (NANDA, 1987, p. 20)

1. Exposure to hot environment
2. Vigorous activity
3. Medications or anesthesia
4. Inappropriate clothing
5. Increased metabolic rate
6. Illness or trauma
7. Dehydration
8. Inability or decreased ability to perspire

DIFFERENTIATION

Hyperthermia needs to be differentiated from Body Temperature, Altered: Potential and Thermoregulation, Ineffective.

Body Temperature, Altered: Potential indicates that the person is potentially unable to regulate heat production and dissipation within a normal range. In Hyperthermia, the patient's ability to produce heat is not imparied. Heat dissipation is impaired to the degree that Hyperthermia results.

Thermoregulation, Ineffective means that the body temperature fluctuates between being too high and being too low. In Hyperthermia, the temperature does not fluctuate, it remains high.

OBJECTIVES

1. Will return to normal body temperature range by (date).

AND/OR

2. Will identify at least (number) measures to use in correcting hyperthermia.

TARGET DATE

Because hyperthermia can be so life-threatening, initial target dates should be in terms of hours. After the patient has demonstrated some stability toward a normal range, the target date can be increased to 2–4 days.

NURSING ORDERS

ADULT HEALTH

1. Sponge patient with cool water *or* rubbing alcohol, *or* apply cold packs continuously, *or* place patient in a tub of cool water until temperature is lowered to at least 102° F. (Be careful not to overchill the patient.) Dry patient off. Keep dry and clean.

2. Use a fan or place in front of an air conditioner to promote cooling. Cool environment to no more than 70° F.
3. Do not give stimulants.
4. Give sips of salt water if conscious and not vomiting.
5. Encourage fluid up to 3000 ml every 24 hours.
6. Give antipyretic drugs as ordered. Monitor effects and record.
7. Give skin, mouth, and nose care at least every 4 hours.

CHILD HEALTH

1. Monitor temperature every 30 minutes as ordered (rectal is most accurate).
2. Monitor and use equipment according to manufacturer's guidelines and policies of unit, especially cooling blanket.
3. Observe for seizures and note history of same.
4. Administer antipyretics and/or seizure or antibiotic medications as ordered with precaution for:
   a. Maintenance of IV line
   b. Drug safe range and therapeutic effects
   c. Potential untoward response
   d. IV compatibility
   e. Infant's or child's renal, hepatic, and GI status
   f. Underlying reason or etiology for fever
   g. Other contributory factors (e.g., blood administration)
5. Gather data relevant to underlying contributory factors.
6. Provide health care teaching regarding:
   a. Need for frequent temperature checks;
   b. Related medical or nursing care;
   c. Safety needs, especially with electric cooling blanket;
   d. How parents can assist in care;
   e. Importance of hydration;
   f. Possible fear or altered comfort of child with fever due to discomfort, fast heart rate, dizziness, and general feeling of illness;
   g. Possible seizure activity.
7. Provide padding to siderails of crib or bed to prevent injury in event of possible seizures.
8. Ensure that airway maintenance is addressed by appropriate suctioning and airway equipment according to age.
9. Carry out appropriate infection control in the event or potential event of infectious disease process according to actual or suspect organisms.
10. Assist in promoting a quiet environment to allow for essential sleep and rest needs.
11. Maintain cautious skin care to prevent breakdown.
12. Carry out sponging only as ordered. If alcohol is used, exercise caution by placing bottle outside of patient's room.
13. Carry out appropriate documentation of all aspects of care.

WOMEN'S HEALTH

Newborn

1. Observe the infant for increased redness and sweating.
2. Check heat source frequently (overhead or isolettes).
3. Replace lost fluids by offering the infant water or formula.
4. Check for urination.
5. Check for dehydration or infection.
6. Monitor rectal temperature every hour.

Pregnancy

7. Avoid use of hot tubs or saunas.
    a. During 1st trimester—concerns about possible central nervous system defects in fetus and failure of neural tube closure (Olds, London, & Ladewig, 1988, p. 306).
    b. During 2nd and 3rd trimesters—concerns about cardiac load for mother.
8. Provide fans during labor.
9. Keep labor room cool for mother's comfort.
10. Provide cool fans for patient on MgSO₄therapy.
11. Give cool, tepid sponge bath.

MENTAL HEALTH

(Note: The objectives and nursing orders for the mental health client will be the same as those described for adult health. The following nursing orders are specific considerations for the mental health client.)

1. Monitor clients receiving neuroleptic drugs for decreased ability to sweat by observing for decreased perspiration and an increase in body temperature with activity, especially in warm weather. Note alterations in the client's plan of care and initiate the following orders:
    a. Client should not go outside in the warmest part of the day during warm weather.
    b. Maintain client's fluid intake up to 3000 ml every 24 hours by (this is especially important for clients who are also receiving lithium carbonate; lithium levels should be carefully evalutated):
        (1) Having client's favorite fluids on the unit;
        (2) Having client drink 240 ml (8-oz glass) of fluids every hour while awake and 240 ml with each meal. If necessary the nurse will sit with the client while the fluid is consumed;
        (3) Maintaining record of client's intake and output.
    c. Dress client in light, loose clothing.
    d. If client is disoriented or confused, provide one-on-one observation.
    e. Decrease client's activity level by:
        (1) Decreasing stimuli;
        (2) Sitting with client and talking quietly or involving client in a table game or activity that requires little large muscle movement (note activities that client enjoys here);
        (3) Assigning room near nurse's station and day room areas.
    f. Monitor client's mental status every hour.
    g. Do not provide clients with alterations in mental status with small electrical cooling devices unless they receive constant supervision. (Note any special considerations and equipment here.)
    h. Give client as much information as possible about his or her condition and measures that are implemented to decrease temperature.
    i. Teach client and family measures to decrease or eliminate potential for hyperthermia (see Home Health for teaching information).
    j. Consult with appropriate assistive resources as indicated:
        (1) Clinical specialist
        (2) Community health nurse
        (3) Physician
        (4) Occupational therapist
        (5) Physical therapist

HOME HEALTH

1. Monitor for factors contributing to hyperthemia (e.g., infection, myocardial infarction, pulmonary embolism, injuries to head and spinal cord, rheumatoid arthritis, hyperthyroidism, leukemia, heat stroke, radiation, sickness, anaphylactic reactions, dehydration, acidosis).

2. Involve patient and family in planning, implementing, and promoting reduction or elimination of the potential for hyperthermia.
3. Teach patient and family measures to decrease or eliminate potential for hyperthermia.
   a. Wearing appropriate clothing
   b. Taking appropriate care of underlying disease
   c. Avoiding exposure to hot environments
   d. Preventing dehydration
   e. Using antipyretics
   f. Performing early intervention with gradual cooling
4. Assist patient and family to identify life-style changes that may be required.
   a. Measure temperature using appropriate method for developmental age of person.
   b. Learn survival techniques if patient works or plays outdoors
   c. Ensure proper hydration
   d. Transport to health care facility
   e. Use emergency transport system
5. Teach patient and family signs and symptoms of hyperthermia.
   a. Flushed skin
   b. Increased respiratory rate
   c. Increased heart rate
   d. Increase in body temperature
   e. Seizure
6. Consult with appropriate assistive resources as indicated.
   a. YMCA or YWCA for classes on outdoor recreation and survival
   b. Nurse
   c. Physician
   d. Occupational health nurse if work-related

EVALUATION
OBJECTIVE 1

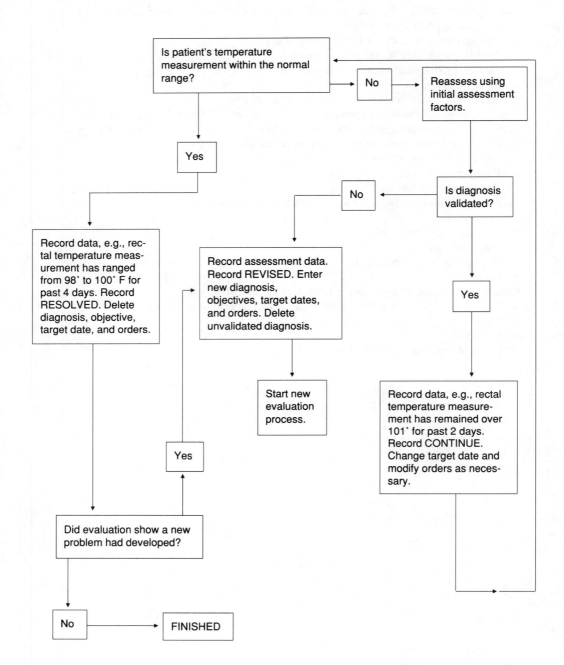

OBJECTIVE 2

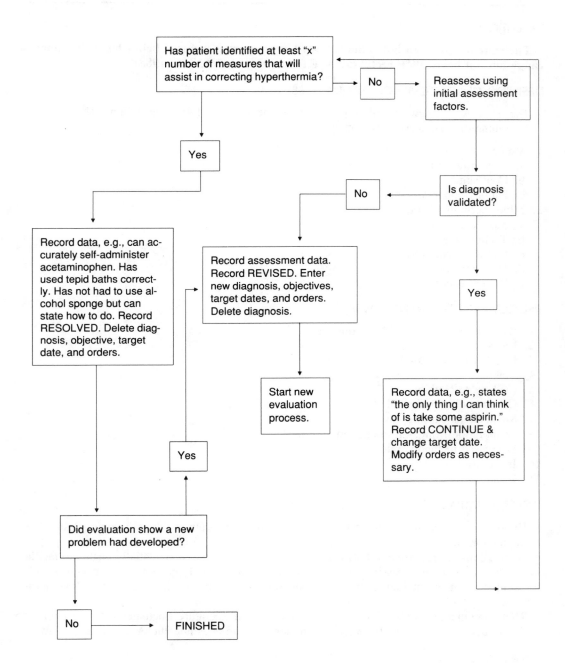

Hypothermia

DEFINITION

The state in which an individual's body temperature is reduced below his or her normal range but not below 96°F rectal (97.5° F for newborn) (NANDA, 1988).

DEFINING CHARACTERISTICS (NANDA, 1988)

The nurse will review the initial pattern assessment for the following defining characteristics to determine the diagnosis of Hypothermia.

1. Major defining characteristics
   a. Shivering (mild)
   b. Cool skin
   c. Pallor (moderate)
2. Minor defining characteristics
   a. Slow capillary refill
   b. Tachycardia
   c. Cyanotic nail beds
   d. Hypertension
   e. Piloerection

RELATED FACTORS (NANDA, 1988)

1. Exposure to cool or cold environment
2. Illness or trauma
3. Inability or decreased ability to shiver
4. Malnutrition
5. Inadequate clothing
6. Consumption of alcohol
7. Medications causing vasodilation
8. Evaporation from skin in cool environment
9. Decreased metabolic rate
10. Inactivity
11. Aging

DIFFERENTIATION

Hypothermia needs to be differentiated from Body Temperature, Altered: Potential and Thermoregulation, Ineffective.

Body Temperature, Altered: Potential indicates that the person is potentially unable to regulate heat production and heat dissipation within a normal range. In Hypothermia, the patient's ability to dissipate heat is not impaired. Heat production is impaired to the degree that Hypothermia results.

Thermoregulation, Ineffective means that the body temperature fluctuates between being too high and being too low. In Hypothermia, the temperature does not fluctuate; it remains low.

OBJECTIVES

1. Will return to normal body temperature range by (date).

AND/OR

2. Will identify at least (number) measures to use in correcting hypothermia.

TARGET DATE

Hypothermia can be extremely life-threatening; therefore, initial target dates should be in terms of hours. After the patient has demonstrated some stability toward a normal range target dates can be increased to 2–4 days.

NURSING ORDERS

ADULT HEALTH

1. Warm the patient quickly. Use warm blankets, warm water (102°–105°F), extra clothing, warm drinks, warm room. Do not use a heat lamp or hot water bottles.
2. Prevent injury. Gently massage body to stimulate circulation; however, *do not* rub a body part if frostbite is evident, as rubbing may lead to tissue death and gangrene.
3. Once the patient is rewarmed, he or she may increase activity or exercise body parts as tolerated.
4. Give fluids such as salt and soda solution. Have client sip slowly (if conscious and not vomiting). Do not give alcohol.
5. Maintain respiratory rate and depth. Provide for airway suctioning and positioning as needed.
6. Measure temperature at least every 2 hours on (odd/even) hour until stabilized for 24 hours.
7. Maintain consistent room temperature.

CHILD HEALTH

1. Monitor for contributory etiologic factors.
2. Measure and record vital signs, especially temperature, at least every 2 hours on (odd/even) hour or via continuous monitor.
3. Provide for maintenance of body temperature, by hat (stockinette for infant), open radiant warmer, isolette, or heating blanket.
4. Prevent drafts in room.
5. Maintain ambient room temperature at 80° F.
6. Bathe with appropriate protection and covering.
7. Address skin protective needs by frequent monitoring for breakdown or altered circulation.
8. Provide for other primary health needs related to hypothermia.
9. Obtain detailed history regarding:
   a. Onset;
   b. Related trauma;
   c. Duration of hypothermia;
   d. Previous weight;
   e. Previous health history;
   f. Allergies;
   g. Details surrounding onset.
10. Provide opportunities for patient and family to ask questions and relay concerns by including 30 minutes for this every shift.
11. Incorporate care of other health team members to address collaborative needs, including:
    a. Pediatrician or subspecialist
    b. Clinical nurse specialist
    c. Physical therapist
    d. Occupational therapist
    e. Respiratory therapist
    f. Play therapist
    g. Family therapist
    h. Social service
    i. Public health nurse
    j. Child protective services

12. Devote appropriate attention to prevention of major complications such as shock, cardiac failure, tissue necrosis, infection, fluid and electrolyte imbalance, convulsions or loss of consciousness, respiratory failure, and renal failure.
13. Provide teaching to address unknown and necessary information for child and family in terms they can relate to (e.g., temperature measurement).
14. Administer medications as ordered. Monitor effects and record.
15. Anticipate safety needs according to patient's age and development status.
16. Monitor safe functioning of equipment used in thermoregulation.
17. Allow for appropriate attention to resolution of psychological trauma, especially in instances of severe exposure to cold.
18. Make appropriate arrangements for follow-up and discharge from hospital.
19. Identify support groups in the community to help foster resources for long-term management.

WOMEN'S HEALTH

(Note: This nursing diagnosis will pertain to the woman the same as to any other adult. The reader is referred to the other sections—Adult Health, Home Health, and Mental Health—for specific nursing orders and objectives pertaining to women and hypothermia).

Newborn

1. To prevent hypothermia in the newborn:
   a. Dry new infant thoroughly;
   b. Cover with blanket;
   c. Lay next to mother's body (cover mother and infant by placing blanket over them);
   d. Place infant under radiant heat source;
   e. Keep out of drafts.
2. Observe infant for hypoglycemia.
3. Check temperature every hour until stable, then every 4 hours for 24 hours. May be taken rectally, by axilla, or by skin (continuous probe).

MENTAL HEALTH

(Note: The objectives and nursing orders for the mental health client will be the same as those described for adult health. The following nursing orders are specific considerations of the mental health client.)

1. Monitor client's mental status every 2 hours (note times here); report alterations to physician.
2. If client is receiving antipsychotics or antidepressants report this to the physician when alteration is first noted.
3. Protect client from contact with uncontrolled hot objects such as space heaters and radiators by teaching clients and family to remove these from the environment.
4. Allow client to use heating pads and electric blankets *only* with supervision.
5. Teach client the potential for medications to affect body temperature regulation, especially in the elderly.
6. Teach client and family measures to decrease or eliminate the potential for hypothermia, to include:
   a. Wearing appropriate clothing when outdoors
   b. Maintaining room temperature at minimum of 65°F.
   c. Wearing clothing in layers
   d. Covering the head, hands, and feet when outdoors (especially the head)
   e. Removing wet clothing
7. Teach client about the kinds of behavior that increase the risk for hypothermia:
   a. Drug and alcohol abuse
   b. Working, living, or playing outdoors

   c. Poor nutrition, especially when body fat is reduced below normal levels as in anorexia nervosa

8. Teach client and family signs and symptoms of early hypothermia:
   a. Confusion, disorientation
   b. Slurred speech
   c. Low blood pressure
   d. Difficulty in awakening
   e. Weak pulse
   f. Cold stomach
   g. Impaired coordination
9. Consult with appropriate assistive resources as indicated:
   a. Energy audit by public service company to identify possible sources
   b. Social services to provide information on emergency shelters, clothing, and food banks
   c. Financial counseling if heating the home is difficult financially
   d. Clinical nurse specialist
   e. Physician

HOME HEALTH

1. Monitor for factors contributing to the potential for hypothermia.
2. Involve patient and family in planning, implementing, and promoting reduction or elimination of the potential for hypothermia.
3. Teach patient and family measures to decrease or eliminate potential for hypothermia:
   a. Wearing appropriate clothing when outdoors
   b. Keeping room temperature at a minimum of 65° F
   c. Wearing clothing in layers
   d. Covering hands, feet, and head
   e. Intervening early with gradual rewarming; removing wet clothing
4. Assist patient and family to identify life-style changes that may be required.
   a. Avoiding drug and alcohol abuse
   b. Learning survival techniques if client works or plays outdoors (e.g., camping, hiking, skiing, etc.)
   c. Keeping person dry
   d. Transporting to health care facility
   e. Using emergency transport system
5. Teach patient and family signs and symptoms of early hypothermia:
   a. Confusion, disorientation
   b. Slurred speech
   c. Low blood pressure
   d. Difficulty in awakening
   e. Weak pulse
   f. Cold stomach
   g. Impaired coordination
6. Consult with appropriate assistive resources as indicated:
   a. YMCA or YWCA for classes on outdoor recreation and survival
   b. Energy audit by public service company to identify possible sources of heat loss from the home
   c. Financial counseling if heating the home is difficult financially
   d. Nurse
   e. Physician

EVALUATION
OBJECTIVE 1

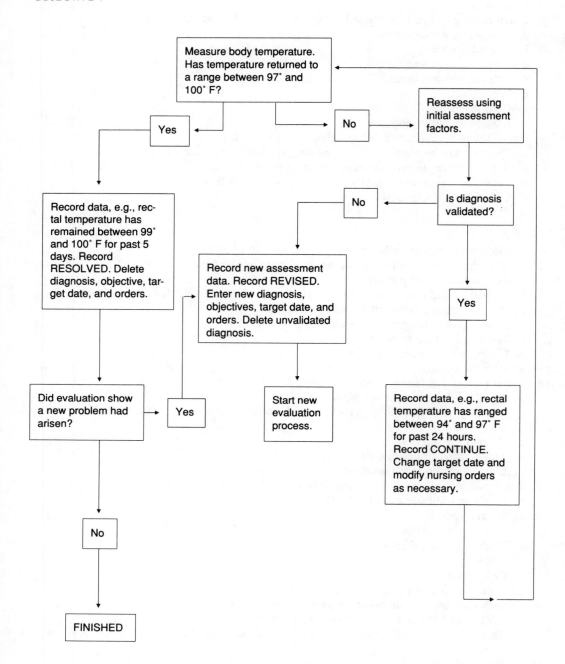

OBJECTIVE 2

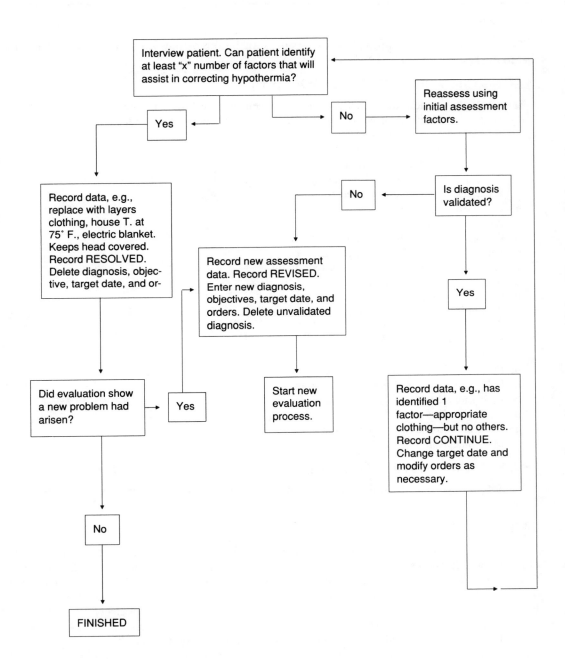

Nutrition, Altered: Less than Body Requirements

DEFINITION

The state in which an individual experiences an intake of nutrients insufficient to meet metabolic needs (NANDA, 1987, p. 15).

DEFINING CHARACTERISTICS (NANDA, 1987, p. 15)

The nurse will review the initial pattern assessment for the following defining characteristics to determine the diagnosis of Nutrition, Altered: Less Than Body Requirements.
1. Major defining characteristics
    a. Loss of weight with adequate food intake
    b. Body weight 20% or more under ideal
    c. Reported inadequate food intake less than RDA (recommended daily allowance)
    d. Weakness of muscles required for swallowing or mastication
    e. Reported or evidence of lack of food
    f. Aversion to eating
    g. Reported altered taste sensation
    e. Satiety immediately after ingesting food
    f. Abdominal pain with or without pathology
    g. Sore, inflamed buccal cavity
    h. Capillary fragility
    i. Abdominal cramping
    j. Diarrhea or steatorrhea
    k. Hyperactive bowel sounds
    l. Lack of interest in food
    m. Perceived inability to ingest food
    n. Pale conjuctival and mucous membranes
    o. Poor muscle tone
    p. Excessive loss of hair
    q. Lack of information, misinformation
    r. Misconception

RELATED FACTORS (NANDA, 1987, p. 15)

Inability to ingest or digest food or absorb nutrients due to biologic, psychologic, or economic factors.

DIFFERENTIATION

Nutrition, Altered: Less Than Body Requirements would need to be differentiated from several other nursing diagnoses. For example, the primary problem may not be nutritional but may be Oral Mucous Membranes, Altered. If the Oral Mucous Membranes, Altered is of such an extent that it interferes with the intake of food, then the person may have Nutrition, Altered: Less Than Body Requirements secondary to the Oral Mucous Membranes, Altered. Conversely, the Nutrition, Altered may be a result of what happens to the food once it is ingested. Bowel Elimination, Altered: Diarrhea could really be the primary problem. The body does not have time to absorb the necessary nutrients because the digested food material passes through the gastrointestinal tract too rapidly. Once the food has been ingested, digested, and absorbed, its components must get to the cells. If there is Tissue Perfusion, Altered, the nutrients may not be able to get to the cells in sufficient quantities to do any good. The results would be Nutrition, Altered: Less Than Body requirements. The person would literally be starving to death even though taking in enough nutrients.

Self-Care Deficit: Feeding; Sensory Perception, Altered: Visual, Olfactory, and/or Gustatory; Thought Process, Altered; or Health Maintenance, Altered may also be the primary problem. If the person does not sense hunger through the usual means—seeing, smelling, or tasting; or if the person thinks he or she has already eaten, then the desire to eat may not exist. Even if the person senses hunger, the inability to feed oneself or Health Maintenance, Altered may result in Nutrition, Altered: Less Than Body Requirements. Comfort, Altered: Pain may also be the primary problem. If the pain prevents the person from ingesting enough food, then the person may have Nutrition, Altered: Less Than Body Requirements secondary to the Pain. Fear, Dysfunctional Grieving, Social Isolation, Body Image Disturbance, Alteration in Self-Esteem, and Spiritual Distress are also psychosocial problems that may really be the primary nursing diagnosis. Each of these may create a decreased desire to eat or, even if food is eaten, the person may vomit because the stomach will not accept the food. Additionally, if the person eats, he or she may only pick at the food and not ingest enough to maintain the body's need for nutrients.

Nutrition, Altered: Less Than Body Requirements may really be secondary to a Knowledge Deficit. The person may not really know how much or what kind of food is more beneficial to his or her body. Teaching is of prime importance in this instance.

OBJECTIVES

1. Will gain (number) pounds by (date).

AND/OR

2. Will design and implement a personal nutritional improvement plan by (date) that is accurate, achievable, and realistic.

TARGET DATE

This diagnosis reflects a long-term care problem; therefore, a target date of 5 days or over, from the date of admission, would be acceptable.

NURSING ORDERS

ADULT HEALTH

1. Increase food and fluid intake at each meal or feeding via:
   a. Reducing noxious stimuli:
      (1) Open all food containers and release odors outside patient's room.
      (2) According to individual needs, either provide privacy for eating *or* provide communal dining.
      (3) Administer appropriate medications 30 minutes before meals (e.g., analgesics, antiemetics). Record effects of medications within 30 minutes of administration.
   b. Providing at least a 30-minute rest period prior to meal.
   c. Giving oral hygiene 30 minutes before meals and as required.
   d. Assisting patient to eat *or* feeding patient:
      (1) Raise head of bed
      (2) Help wash hands
      (3) Open cartons and packages
      (4) Cut food into small, bite-size pieces
      (5) Provide assistive devices (e.g., large-handled spoon or fork, all-in-one utensil, plate guard)
   e. Offering small, frequent feedings every 2–3 hours rather than just 3 meals per day. Allow patient to assist with food choices and feeding schedules.
   f. Focusing fluid intake between meals. Limit at meals. Offer wine at meals or immediately prior to meals to stimulate appetite.
   g. Encouraging patient to eat slowly.

    h. Having patient chew gum before meals to stimulate salivation, or having patient visualize lemons, sour pickles.

    i. Offering between-meal supplements. Focus on high-protein diet and liquids.

    j. Avoiding gas-producing foods and carbonated beverages.

    k. Avoiding very hot or very cold foods.

    l. Encouraging significant other to bring special food from home.

2. Measure and total intake and output every 8 hours. Total each 24 hours.

3. Weigh daily at (state time) and in same-weight clothing. Have patient empty bladder before weighing.

4. Monitor:

    a. Vital signs every 4 hours while awake and as required;

    b. Airway, sensorium, chest sounds, bowel sounds, skin turgor, mucous membranes, bowel function, urine specific gravity, and glucose level at least once per shift;

    c. Laboratory values (e.g., electrolyte levels, hematocrit, hemoglobin, blood glucose).

5. Teach patient and significant others:

    a. Balanced diet based on the basic four food groups;

    b. Role of diet in health (e.g., healing, energy, normal body functioning);

    c. How to keep food diary with calorie count;

    d. Adding spices to food to improve taste and aroma;

    e. Use of exchange lists;

    f. Relaxation techniques;

    g. How to weigh self properly (refer to Nursing Order 3).

6. Provide positive reinforcement as often as possible for:

    a. Weight gain;

    b. Increased intake;

    c. Ignoring weight loss;

    d. Using consistent approach.

7. Encourage exercise at least twice per shift to the extent possible without tiring. If exercise capacity is limited, do passive/active range of motion every 4 hours while awake.

8. Refer, as necessary, to other health care providers:

    a. Dietitian or nutritionist

    b. Psychiatric nurse clinician

    c. Social services

    d. Dentist

    e. Visiting nurse service

    f. Meals on Wheels

Additional Information

There will be situations in which the patient's nutritional condition has progressed to the point that tube feedings, intravenous therapy, or total parenteral nutrition will become necessary. In addition to the nursing orders for the overall nursing diagnosis of Nutrition, Altered: Less Than Body Requirements, the following orders should be added:

1. Tube feedings

    a. Check placement and patency prior to each feeding.

    b. Aspirate tube prior to each feeding. Measure amount of residual from previous feeding. If 150 ml or more, delay feeding and notify physician.

    c. Check temperature of feeding before administering. Temperature should be slightly below room temperature.

    d. Measure amount of feeding exactly. Flush tube with water immediately after feeding.

    e. Crush medications in water or dissolve in water before giving.

    f. Keep patient in semi-Fowler's position for at least 30 minutes following feeding.

g. Cleanse and lubricate nares after each feeding.

h. Check taping of tube for security and comfort following each feeding.

i. If feeding is to be administered by gravity method (preferred), make sure all air is out of tubing.

2. Intravenous

a. Check insertion site for warmth, redness, swelling, leakage, and pain at least every 4 hours (state times here).

b. Check flow rate at a maximum of every hour (state times here).

c. Check for signs and symptoms of circulatory overload at least every 2 hours (state times here) (e.g., headache, neck vein distention, tachycardia, increased blood pressure, respiratory changes).

3. Total parenteral nutrition

a. Do not administer without pump.

b. Change tubing and filter daily.

c. Change dressing every other day beginning (date):

(1) Use aseptic technique.

(2) Gently cleanse area around catheter with (state how here).

(3) Use a bacteriostatic, not antibiotic, ointment.

(4) Apply a dry, airtight dressing.

CHILD HEALTH

(Note: This diagnosis represents a long-term care issue. Therefore, a series of subgoals of smaller amounts of weight to be gained in a lesser period of time may be necessary. Long-term goals are still to be formulated and revised as the patient's status demands. Also, there will undoubtedly be instances in which overlap may exist for other nursing diagnoses. Specifically, as an example, in the instance of an alteration in nutrition related to actual failure to thrive, one must refer to appropriate role performance on the part of the mother with consideration for holistic nursing management. It would be most critical to include a few specific nursing process components to reflect the critical needs for the mother-infant dyad.)

Refer to aforementioned sections of Adult Health for guidelines for Nutrition, Altered: Less Than Body Requirements and select those aspects which apply, plus the following as applicable:

1. Feed the infant on a regular schedule which offers nutrients appropriate to metabolic needs. For example, an infant of less than 5 lb will eat more often, but in lesser amounts (2–3 oz every 2–3 hr) than an older infant of 15 lb (4–5 oz every 3–4 hr).

2. If patient requires suctioning, do so at least 15 minutes before mealtime. Keep suctioning equipment available but out of immediate eating site.

3. Assist or feed patient:

a. Elevate head of bed or place infant in infant seat, and older infant or toddler in high chair with safety belt in place. If necessary, hold infant. (This will be dictated in part by patient's status and presence of various tubes and equipment.)

b. Help patient wash hands. For infants and toddlers, administer diaper change as needed.

c. Warm foods and formula as needed and test on wrist before feeding infant or child.

d. Provide aids appropriate for age and physical capacity as needed, such as two-handled cups for toddlers, favorite spoon, or Velcro strap for utensils for child with cerebral palsy.

e. Offer small, age-appropriate feedings with input from family members regarding preferences when possible.

f. Encourage patient to eat slowly and to chew food thoroughly. For infant, bubble before, during, and after feeding.

4. Encourage favorite snacks or foods to be prepared at home and brought in by family.

5. Allow for rest periods after feeding without interruption to the degree possible and according to patient's status.

6. Provide role-modeling opportunities in a nonthreatening, nonjudgmental manner to assist parents in learning about feeding an infant or child.
7. Weigh patient on same scale (infants without clothes, older children in underwear).
8. Teach patient and family:
   a. Balanced diet appropriate for age using basic four food groups.
   b. Role of diet in health (e.g., healing, energy, normal body functioning). If infant is diagnosed as Failure to Thrive, offer appropriate support emotionally and allow time for exploring dyad relationships.
   c. How to use spices and child-oriented approach in encouraging child to eat (e.g., peach fruit salad, with peach as a face, garnished with cherries and raisins for eyes and nose, pineapple rounded for mouth).
   d. Monitoring for possible food allergies, especially in toddlers with history of allergies.
   e. How to weigh self appropriately if applicable, or for parents to weigh child.
9. Provide positive reinforcement as often as possible or appropriate for parents and child demonstrating critical behavior.

Additional Information

There will be situations in which the patient's nutritional status has deteriorated with the necessity of tube feedings, intravenous therapy, or total parenteral nutrition. In addition to the nursing orders for the nursing diagnosis Nutrition, Altered: Less Than Body Requirements, the following orders should be added:
1. Tube feedings
   a. Aspirate tube gently prior to each feeding. Measure amount of residual. If 50% or more of total feeding volume, notify physician for possible change in ordered amount.
   b. Suction patient before feedings as necessary.
   c. Administer feeding per gravity at approximately 1–2 ml/minute for total volumes of less than 30 ml. If feeding is to be infused continuously, use pump and maintain appropriate rate and function.
   d. Keep patient in semi-Fowler's position after feeding or allow infant to sit in infant seat for at least 30 minutes after feeding.
2. Intravenous
   a. Check insertion site for warmth, redness, swelling, leaking, and pain every hour on (odd/even) hour.
   b. Check flow rate every 15 minutes, (state times here).
   c. Check for signs and symptoms of circulatory overload at least every 2 hours (state times here) (gallop rhythm, tachycardia, jugular venous distention, elevated BP).
   d. Ensure proper labeling of solution for accuracy of content, including additives, flow rate, time hung, and other ordered specifics.
   e. Assess intravenous fluid solution for compatibility of additives and medications.
   f. Restrain patient judiciously if needed to ensure safety of intravenous administration.
3. Total parenteral nutrition
   a. Change dressing as ordered, (daily at least):
      (1) Assess site for redness, warmth, or irritation.
      (2) Report temperature elevation above 101° F to physician.
      (3) Restrain patient judiciously if needed to ensure safe administration of parenteral nutrition.

WOMEN'S HEALTH

(Note: Poverty and substance abuse are often associated with nutritional deficits. Remember that underweight women who are pregnant will exhibit a different pattern of weight gain [rapid weight

gain at the beginning of the 1st trimester of about 1 pound per week; by 20 weeks weight gain can be as much as 18 to 20 pounds]. Remember to teach the parents signs and symptoms of weight loss in the neonate.)

1. Collaborate with dietitian in planning and teaching diet.
   a. Emphasize high-quality calories (cottage cheese, lean meats, fish, tofu, whole grains, fruits, vegetables).
   b. Avoid excess intake of fats and sugar in a regular pattern through the day.
2. Assist client in identifying methods to keep caloric intake within the recommended limit.
3. Verify prepregnant weight.
4. Determine if weight loss during 1st trimester is due to nausea and vomiting.
5. Check activity level against daily dietary intake.
6. Check for food intolerances.
7. Check environmental influences.
   a. Hot weather
   b. Cultural practices
   c. Pica eating
   d. Economic situation
8. Assess economic status and ability to buy food.
9. Assess woman's emotional response to the pregnancy and to additional weight gain.

(Note: Dieting is never recommended during pregnancy because "it deprives mother and fetus of nutrients needed for tissue growth and because weight loss is accompanied by maternal ketosis, a direct threat to fetal well-being [Neeson & May, 1986; Olds, London & Ladewig, 1988].)

10. Identify additional caloric needs and sources of those calories for the nursing mother.
    a. Additional 500 calories per day above normal dietary intake is needed to produce adequate milk (depending on the individual, a total of 2500 to 3000 calories per day).
    b. Additional fluids are necessary to produce adequate milk.
    c. Collaborate with nutritionist to provide a healthy dietary pattern for the lactating mother.
11. Monitor mother's energy levels and health maintenance.
    a. Does she complain of fatigue?
    b. Does she have insufficient energy to complete her daily activities?
    c. Does a dietary assessment show irregular dietary intake?
    d. Is she more than 10% below the ideal weight for body stature?
12. For breast feeding the newborn or neonate during the first 6 months, teach mother:
    a. The major source of nourishment is human milk.
    b. Vitamin supplements can be used as recommended by physican.
       (1) Vitamin D
       (2) Flouride
       (3) If indicated, iron
    c. Infant should be taking in approximately 420 ml daily soon after birth and building to 1200 ml daily at the end of 3 months.
13. Monitor for fluid deficit at least daily.
    a. "Fussy baby," especially immediately after feeding.
    b. Constipation (remember breast-fed babies have less stools than formula-fed babies).
    c. Weight loss or slow weight gain.
       (1) Closely assess baby, mother, and nursing routine.
       (2) Is baby getting empty calories (e.g., a lot of water between feedings)?
       (3) Avoid nipple confusion—from switching baby from breast to bottle and vice versa many times.
       (4) Count number of diapers per day (should have 6–8 really wet diapers per day).
    d. Intolerance to mother's milk or bottle formula.
    e. Illness or lactose intolerance.

f. Infrequent nursing can cause slow weight gain.

MENTAL HEALTH

(Note: Due to long-term care requirements for these clients, target dates should be determined in weeks or months, not hours or days.)

1. Do not attempt teaching or long-term goal setting with client until concentration has improved (symptom of starvation).
2. Establish contract with client to remain on prescribed diet and not to perform maladaptive behavior (i.e., vomiting, use of laxatives). State specific behavior for client here.
3. Place client on 24-hour constant observation (this will be discontinued when client ends maladaptive behavior or at specific times that nursing staff assess are low risk).
4. Place client on constant observation during meals and at high-risk times for maladaptive behavior (such as 1 hour after meals or while using the bathroom). This order will take effect when the preceding one is discontinued.
5. Do not allow client to discuss weight or calories. Excessive discussion of food is also discouraged.
6. Require client to eat prescribed diet (all food on tray each meal except for those three or four foods client was allowed to omit in the admission contract). (List client's omitted food here.)
7. Sit with client during meals and provide positive support and encouragement for the feelings and concerns the client may have.
8. Do not threaten client with punishment (tube feeding or IVs).
9. Report all maladaptive behavior to the client's primary nurse or physician for confrontation in individual therapy sessions.
10. Spend (number) minutes with client every (number) minutes to establish relationship.
11. Respond to queries related to fears of being required to gain too much weight with reassurance that the goal of treatment is to return client to health and he or she will not be allowed to become overweight.
12. If client vomits, have him or her assist with the cleanup and require him or her to drink an equal amount of a nutritional replacement drink.
13. Encourage client to attend group therapy (specific encouraging behavior should be listed here, such as assisting client to complete morning care on time or other interventions that are useful for this client).
14. Encourage client's family by (list specific encouraging behaviors for this family) to attend family therapy sessions.
15. Assist client with clothing selection (clothes should not be too loose, hiding weight loss, or too tight, assisting client to feel overweight even though appropriate weight is achieved).
16. When maintenance weight is achieved assist client with selection of appropriate foods from hospital menu.
17. When maintenance weight is achieved refer to dietitian for teaching about balanced diet and home maintenance.
18. When maintenance weight is achieved refer to occupational therapist for practice with menu planning, trips to grocery stores to purchase food, and meal preparation.
19. When maintenance weight is achieved plan passes with client for trips to restaurants for meals.
20. Client will be allowed to do exercise (number) minutes (number) times per day while supervised (this will be altered as client reaches maintenance weight).
21. Client will be allowed to do the following exercises during the exercise period (these are graded to the client's physical condition; consultation with the occupational therapist is useful).
22. Client will be allowed (number) of (number) minute walks on hospital grounds with a staff member each day.
23. Refer client to appropriate assistive resources:
    a. Anorexia/bulimia support groups

b. Nutritionist

c. Dentist

d. Psychiatric nurse clinician

e. Occupational therapist

f. Stress reduction classes

HOME HEALTH

1. Reduce associated factors, for example:
   a. Minimize noxious odors by using foods that require minimal cooking; or if someone else is cooking for patient, arrange for patient to be away from cooking area.
   b. Provide social atmosphere desired by patient.
   c. Plan medications to decrease pain and nausea around mealtime.
   e. Plan meals away from area where treatments are performed.
   f. Maintain oral hygiene (e.g., before and after meals); instruct patient and family in proper brushing, flossing, and use of water pick.
2. Provide eating assistance as needed (e.g., operate devices, open pre-packaged items, cut food).
3. Teach patient and family to try small, frequent feedings every 2–3 hours.
4. Teach patient and family to add high-calorie, high-protein, and high-fat items to meal preparation activities (e.g., use milk in soups, add cheese to food, use butter or margarine in soups, vegetables, etc.).
5. Teach patient and family to try high-calorie, high-protein supplements between meals.
6. Teach patient or provide patient assistance to rest before meals. If patient is doing the meal preparation, teach patient to cook large quantities and freeze several meals at a time and to seek assistance in meal preparation when fatigued.
7. Encourage patient to prepare favorite foods.
8. Teach patient and family to avoid foods that contribute to noxious symptoms such as gas, nausea, or GI distress.
9. Discourage fasting.
10. Teach stress-reduction exercises.
11. Maintain exercise program as tolerated.
12. Refer to appropriate assistive resources as indicated:
    a. Anorexia/bulimia support groups
    b. Nutritionist
    c. Dentist
    d. Psychiatric nurse clinician
    e. Meals on Wheels
    f. Occupational therapist
    g. Stress reduction classes

EVALUATION
OBJECTIVE 1

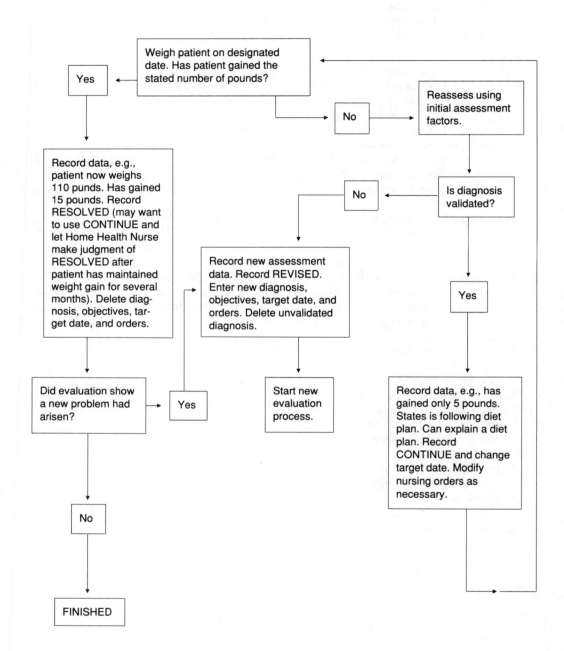

OBJECTIVE 2

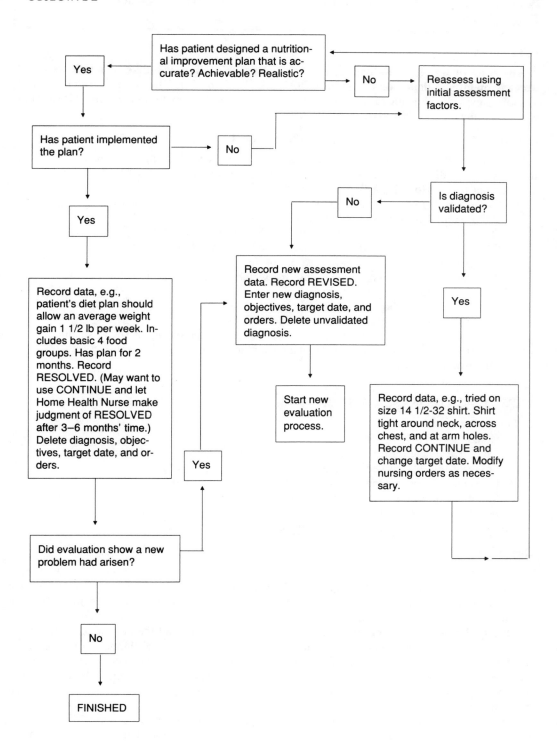

Has patient designed a nutritional improvement plan that is accurate? Achievable? Realistic?

Yes

No

Reassess using initial assessment factors.

Has patient implemented the plan?

No

Yes

Is diagnosis validated?

No

Yes

Record data, e.g., patient's diet plan should allow an average weight gain 1 1/2 lb per week. Includes basic 4 food groups. Has plan for 2 months. Record RESOLVED. (May want to use CONTINUE and let Home Health Nurse make judgment of RESOLVED after 3–6 months' time.) Delete diagnosis, objectives, target date, and orders.

Record new assessment data. Record REVISED. Enter new diagnosis, objectives, target date, and orders. Delete unvalidated diagnosis.

Start new evaluation process.

Record data, e.g., tried on size 14 1/2-32 shirt. Shirt tight around neck, across chest, and at arm holes. Record CONTINUE and change target date. Modify nursing orders as necessary.

Yes

Did evaluation show a new problem had arisen?

No

FINISHED

Nutrition, Altered: Potential for or More than Body Requirements

DEFINITION

The state in which an individual is at risk of experiencing an intake of nutrients which exceeds metabolic demands (Potential) (NANDA, 1987, p. 16). The state in which an individual is experiencing an intake of nutrients which exceeds metabolic needs (More Than Body Requirements) (NANDA, 1987, p. 14).

DEFINING CHARACTERISTICS (NANDA, 1987, pp. 14–16)

The nurse will review the initial pattern assessment for the following defining characteristics to determine the diagnosis of Nutrition, Altered: Potential for or More Than Body Requirements.
1. Potential for or More Than Body Requirements
   a. Major defining characteristics (risk factors)
      (1) Reported or observed obesity in one or both parents
      (2) Rapid transition across growth percentiles in infants or children.
      (3) Reported use of solid food as major food source before 5 months of age.
      (4) Observed use of food as reward or comfort measure
      (5) Reported or observed higher baseline weight at beginning of each pregnancy
      (6) Dysfunctional eating patterns:
          (a) Pairing food with other activities
          (b) Concentrating food intake at end of day
          (c) Eating in response to external cues such as time of day or social situation
          (d) Eating in response to internal cues other than hunger (e.g., anxiety)
   b. Minor defining characteristics
      None given.

RELATED FACTORS (NANDA, 1987, pp. 14–16)

1. Potential for
   a. Hereditary predisposition
   b. Excessive intake during late gestational life, early infancy, and adolescence
   c. Frequent, closely spaced pregnancies
   d. Dysfunctional psychological conditioning in relation to food
   e. Membership in lower socioeconomic group
2. More Than Body Requirements
   a. Excessive intake in relation to metabolic need

DIFFERENTIATION

Nutrition, Altered: Potential for or More Than Body Requirements may be confused with other nursing diagnoses which are the primary problems. Differentiation is based on assessment data related to usual eating patterns. Potential obesity may be only the result of another, more pressing problem. For example, Knowledge Deficit may be the primary problem. The patient, because of cultural background, may not know the appropriate food groups and the nutritional value of the foods. Additionally, the cultural beliefs held by a patient may not value thinness. Therefore, the people of a particular culture may actually promote obesity. Health Maintenance, Altered is another example of a primary nursing diagnosis that must be differentiated from potential obesity. Patients may be unable or unwilling to modify nutritional intake even though they have information about good nutritional patterns.

There are several nursing diagnoses from the psychosocial province that need to be differentiated from potential obesity. Powerlessness, Self-Esteem Disturbance, Social Isolation, Body Image

Disturbance, or Ineffective Individual Coping may be the primary problem. Potential obesity may only be the manifestation of psychosocial problems.

OBJECTIVES

1. Will lose (number) pounds by (date).

AND/OR

2. Will have (percentage) decrease in body fat by (date).
(Note:Goal is 22% fat for women and 15% fat for men [Bailey, 1978; Remington, Fisher, & Parent, 1983].)

TARGET DATE

Because this diagnosis reflects long-term care in terms of both cause and correction, a target date of 5 days or over would not be unreasonable.

NURSING ORDERS

ADULT HEALTH

1. Assist patient to identify dysfunctional eating habits by:
   a. Reviewing 1 week's dietary intake;
   b. Associating times of eating and types of food with corresponding events:
      (1) In response to internal cues;
      (2) In response to external cues;
   c. Reviewing 1 week's exercise pattern.
2. Assist patient to establish a food diary which should be maintained until weight has stabilized within normal limits:
   a. What eating—caloric intake.
   b. Where eating—all actual sites.
   c. When eating—time of day, length of time spent eating, circumstances leading to deciding to eat.
3. Collaborate with physical therapist in establishing an exercise program.
4. Teach patient principles of balanced diet or refer to clinical dietitian for instructions:
   a. Basic four food groups
   b. Recommended daily allowances
   c. Weighing and measuring foods
   d. Exchanges
5. Review pros and cons of alternate weight-loss options with patient:
   a. Fad diets
   b. Diet pills
   c. Liquid diet preparations
   d. Surgery
   e. Diuretics
   f. Laxatives
   g. Bingeing and purging
6. Weight patient daily at (state time). Teach patient to weigh self at the same time each morning in same clothing. Help patient to establish a graphic to allow visualization of progress (e.g., bar chart, chart with gold star for each weight-loss day).
7. Teach stress reduction techniques (e.g., progressive relaxation, scheduled quiet time, time management).
8. Demonstrate adaptations in eating that could promote weight loss:
   a. Smaller plate
   b. One-half of usual serving

   c. No second servings
   d. Laying fork down between bites
   e. Chewing each bite at least "X" number of times
9. Have patient design own weight loss plan:
   a. Caloric intake
   b. Activity
   c. Behavioral or life-style changes
10. Limit patient's intake to number of calories recommended by physician or nutritionist.
11. Consult with family and visitors regarding importance of patient's adhering to diet. Caution against bringing food, etc. from home.
12. Use appropriate behavior modification techniques to reinforce teaching. Refer patient and family to psychiatric nurse clinician for appropriate techniques to use at home as well as assistance with guilt, anxiety, etc. over being obese.
13. Provide good skin care and assess skin daily, especially skin folds and areas where skin meets skin.
14. Measure total intake and output every 8 hours. Encourage intake of low-calorie, caffeine-free drinks to help offset "hunger pains."
15. Refer to community resources for long-term support at least 3 days prior to discharge:
   a. Weight Watchers
   b. TOPS (Take Off Pounds Sensibly)
   c. Overeaters Anonymous
16. Suggest patient contract with a significant other or home health nurse for added reinforcement and support in weight loss.

CHILD HEALTH

Orders are the same as for the adult. Make orders specific to the child according to the child's developmental level.

WOMEN'S HEALTH

1. Verify the prepregnancy weight.
2. Obtain a 24-hour diet history.
3. Calculate the woman's calorie and protein intake.
4. Rule out excessive edema and hypertension.
5. Check activity level against her daily dietary intake.
6. Encourage client to increase her activity by:
   a. Walking up stairs instead of riding elevators at work;
   b. Taking walks in the evening before retiring;
   c. Joining exercise groups for pregnancy (usually found in childbirth classes or hospitals in communities);
   d. Joining swim exercise groups for pregnancy (usually found at YWCAs or community centers in communities).
7. If recommended intake is 2400 calories/day but 24-hour diet recall reveals a higher caloric intake:
   a. Recommend reduction of fat in diet (e.g., decrease amount of cooking oil used, use less salad dressing and margarine, cut excess fat off meat, and take skin off of chicken before preparing);
   b. Check out size of food portions;
   c. Stress appetite control with high-quality sources of energy and protein.
8. Use visual aids to increase effectiveness of diet teaching.
9. Schedule adequate time for teaching—convey positive attitude and reinforce information about food groups.

10. Assist mothers with cultural or economic restrictions to introduce more variety into their diets.
11. Stress that weight gain is the only way the fetus can be supplied with nourishment.
12. Point out that added body fat will be burned and will provide necessary energy during lactation (breast feeding).
13. Assist pregnant adolescents within 3 years of menarche to plan diets that have needed additional nutrients to meet their own growth needs as well as those of fetus.
14. Discourage any attempts at weight reduction or dieting.
(Note: Dieting during pregnancy, can result in the catabolization of fat and maternal ketosis which results in a poor outcome for the fetus [Neeson & May, 1986; Olds, London, & Ladewig, 1988]).
15. Refer to appropriate support groups for assistance in exercise programs for the pregnant woman (e.g., physical therapist, local groups who have swimming classes for pregnant women, and childbirth classes).
16. Encourage good skin care and assess skin daily, especially skin folds and areas where skin meets skin.

Additional Information

A satisfactory pattern of weight gain for the average woman as reported in Neeson and May (1986, p. 390) is shown below.

10 weeks of gestation	650 gm (approximately 1.5 lb)
20 weeks of gestation	4,000 gm (approximately 9.0 lb)
30 weeks of gestation	8,500 gm (approximately 19.0 lb)
40 weeks of gestation	12,500 gm (approximately 27.5 lb)

Over the course of the pregnancy, a total weight gain of 25–35 pounds is recommended for both nonobese and obese pregnant women. During the 2nd and 3rd trimesters, a gain of about 1 pound per week is considered desirable

MENTAL HEALTH

1. Discuss with client potential or real motivation for desiring to lose weight at this time. (This will assist in developing an understanding of the client's motivation and assist in developing rewards.)
2. Discuss with client past attempts at weight loss and factors that contributed to their success or failure.
3. Develop with client a diet plan (this would be listed here).
4. Provide client with a food diary to be kept for 1 week. This should include information about the food eaten, when it is eaten, where it is eaten, activity during this time, and feelings and emotions before, during, and after eating. Space should also be provided for the client to list all physical activity (i.e., walked 1½ blocks from car to office).
5. Review food diary with client and list those factors that will assist with a weight-loss plan and those that will hinder a weight-loss plan.
6. Develop with client alternative kinds of behavior that will replace those factors that will inhibit a weight-loss plan.
7. Develop a list of rewards for positive changes. These rewards should be ones the client will give himself or herself or that can be given by the health care team or client support system and should not be related to food. Many clients will have difficulty identifying nonfood rewards, and a great deal of support may be needed. Rewards should initially be scheduled on a daily basis for successful achievement of behavior related to weight loss and can then be gradually expanded to weekly or monthly rewards. The client's reward schedule should be listed here.
8. Teach client relaxation technique and practice technique 30 minutes a day at (time).

9. Instruct client to postpone desires to eat between meals by doing 5 minutes of slow deep breathing and reviewing three of the identified positive motivating factors for weight loss for this client. If the desire to eat remains, have the client drink a glass of water or cup of herb tea and spend 7 minutes engaged in an activity such as writing a letter, working on a hobby, reading, sewing, playing with children or spouse or significant other—anything but watching television (this activity generally contains too many food cues).
10. Instruct client to grocery shop from a list soon after eating.
11. Discuss with client and significant others necessary alterations in eating behavior, and develop a list of ways significant others can be supportive of these alterations.
12. Teach alternative food preparation habits that will reduce calories while increasing nutritional content of diet:
    a. Boil or broil instead of frying food.
    b. Use non-stick spray for pans instead of butter, margarine, or fat.
    c. Use fruits and vegetables.
    d. Increase use of fish or poultry over beef or pork.
    e. Drink water or herb tea for thirst, do not confuse thirst for hunger.
    f. Reduce or eliminate fat and sugar from recipes.
    g. Use fresh ingredients whenever possible for increased flavor.
    h. Use fresh fruit fruit canned in its own juice for sweetening instead of sugar.
    i. Use plain yogurt or blended and seasoned tofu as substitutes for sour cream.
13. Discuss with client those foods that provide the greatest risk of decreasing self-control and developing a plan for eliminating them from the diet.
14. Provide client with a calorie list of fast food items and plan for maintaining desired goals by:
    a. Developing a list of those fast food items that provide the best food value for the calories;
    b. Assisting the client with developing recipes to use at home that are calorie-wise and easily prepared to decrease the temptation to use fast food;
    c. Developing a list of those restaurants that provide options for reducing calorie intake as with salad bars or the option to eliminate certain items from a serving such as high-calorie condiments.
15. Assist client in selecting an exercise program (provide client with a broad range of options and select one the client will enjoy). This could include swimming, cycling, dancing, aerobic dance, jogging, walking.
16. Develop a schedule and goals for implementing the exercise plan. (Set goals that are achievable, usually this is 50% of what the client estimates is achievable).
17. Develop a reward schedule for achievement of exercise goals and record this plan here.
18. Spend 30 minutes two times a day with client reviewing the benefits of weight loss and the progress made to this point (record times here).
19. Do not focus on the concept of loss when talking with client, use terms such as reduction and gains in self-concept to provide positive frames.
20. Discuss with client the concept of set point and methods to alter this. List client's choices here.
21. Discuss with client other life achievements and strategies that assisted with these achievements. Focus on the concept of perseverance in achieving this goal or discuss with client the last long trip taken and apply the concept of persevering hazards in achieving this goal. Relate this to the task of weight loss.
22. Present the concept of approaching goals one day at a time rather than attempting or reflecting on all of the task.
23. Plan for times when client will indulge in high-calorie meals or snacks such as holidays by developing an attitude of nonfailure and regained control or coping. Time may be planned for the client to ''break''the diet.

24. If bingeing has been a problem and other techniques have not effectively eliminated it, then assist the client in planning the next binge to the final detail. If the client does not follow up, this will demonstrate client control over binges and remove feelings of powerlessness. If the client does the planned binge this also demonstrates control and the client regains power and can then proceed to schedule and plan binges altering the frequency and amount consumed gradually. Either option should be positively received by the nurse with appropriate follow-up.

25. Assist client in contacting support groups for long-term follow-up to include as appropriate:
    a. Weight Watchers
    b. TOPS
    c. Overeaters Anonymous
    d. Nutritionist
    e. YWCA/YMCA
    f. Exercise classes
    g. Stress reduction classes
    h. Special interest sports clubs such as jogging, walking or cycling groups
    i. Psychiatric nurse clinician

HOME HEALTH

1. Assist patient in identifying life-style changes that may be required:
   a. Regular exercise at least three times per week which includes stretching, flexibility, and aerobic activity (20 minutes) at target training rate.
   b. Nutritional habits should include decreasing fats and simple carbohydrates and increasing complex carbohydrates.

2. Teach those responsible for food preparation techniques for reducing fat and simple carbohydrates in meal preparation, for example:
   a. Boil and broil instead of frying foods.
   b. Use non-stick spray for pans instead of butter, margarine, or fat.
   c. Use fruits and vegetables.
   d. Identify recipes which provide balanced meals without added fats (e.g., Weight Watchers).
   e. Drink water for thirst, and do not confuse thirst with hunger. (Often excess food is consumed for water content when water would satisfy the need.)

3. Assist patient and family in identifying cues other than focus on weight and calories, such as feeling of well-being, percent of body fat, increased exercise endurance, better-fitting clothes, etc. (Excess focus on the weight as measured by the scale and on calorie counting may increase the probability of failure and encourage the pattern of repeated weight loss followed by weight gain. This pattern results in increased percentage of body fat.)

4. Have patient and family design personalized plan:
   a. Menu planning
   b. Decreased fats and simple carbohydrates and increase complex carbohydrates
   c. Regular, balanced exercise
   d. Life-style changes

EVALUATION
OBJECTIVE 1

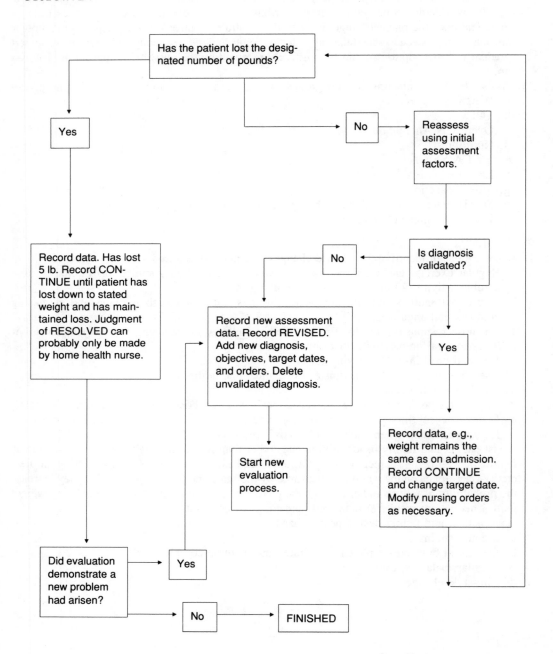

OBJECTIVE 2

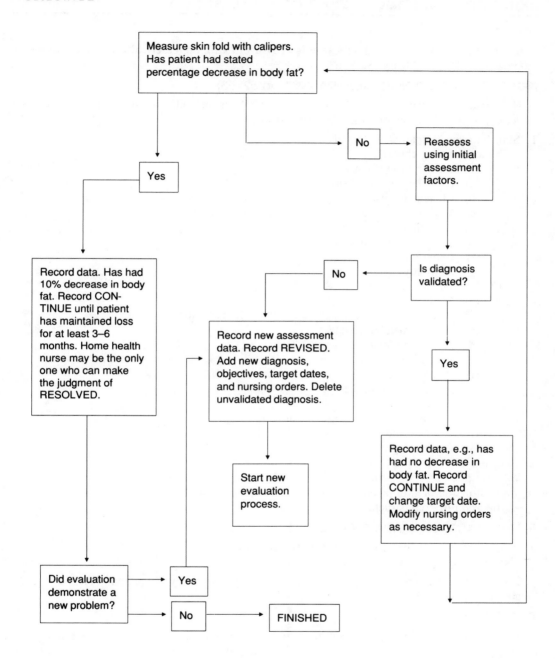

Skin Integrity, Impaired: Potential or Actual

DEFINITION

A state in which the individual's skin is at risk of being adversely altered or is adversely altered (NANDA, 1987, pp. 52,53).

DEFINING CHARACTERISTICS (NANDA, 1987, pp. 52–53)

The nurse will review the initial pattern assessment for the following defining characteristics to determine the diagnosis of Skin Integrity, Impaired.

1. Skin Integrity, Impaired: Potential
   a. Major defining characteristics
      (1) External (environmental)
         (a) Hypothermia or hyperthermia
         (b) Chemical substance
         (c) Mechanical factors (shearing forces, pressure, restraint)
         (d) Radiation
         (e) Physical immobilization
         (f) Excretions or secretions
         (g) Humidity
      (2) Internal (somatic)
         (a) Medication
         (b) Alterations in nutritional state (obesity, emaciation)
         (c) Altered metabolic state
         (d) Altered circulation
         (e) Altered sensation
         (f) Altered pigmentation
         (g) Skeletal prominence
         (h) Developmental factors
         (i) Alterations in skin turgor (change in elasticity)
         (j) Psychogenic
         (k) Immunologic
2. Skin Integrity, Impaired: Actual
   a. Disruption of skin surface
   b. Destruction of skin layers
   c. Invasion of body structure

RELATED FACTORS (NANDA, 1987, pp. 52, 53)

1. Skin Integrity, Impaired: Potential No related factors given.
2. Skin Integrity, Impaired: Actual

The major and minor defining characteristics of Skin Integrity, Impaired: Potential are the related factors for Skin Integrity, Impaired: Actual.

DIFFERENTIATION

Physical Mobility, Impaired means that the person is unable to adequately move his or her body. Compression of the skin, underlying tissue, and blood vessels occurs. Tissue perfusion is then compromised or altered and a breakdown in the skin may occur.

The by-products of digestion and metabolism can be very damaging to the skin if they are allowed to remain on the skin for any length of time. If the primary problem is Bowel or Urinary Elimination, Altered: Diarrhea or Incontinence, the skin loses its protective mechanisms and becomes prone to breakdown from the caustic substances in the products of elimination as well as simply from the constant state of wetness.

The skin needs adequate amounts of both food and fluid to remain healthy. When there is either Nutrition, Altered: Less Than Body Requirements or a Fluid Volume Deficit, the skin does not receive what it needs which predisposes it to a skin breakdown.

Sensory Deficit, Uncompensated means that the person lacks perception and interpretation of stimuli from one or more of the five senses. In case of Skin Integrity, Impaired, that sense is touch. The person does not perceive or appropriately interpret the stimuli and thus does not respond appropriately.

Verbal Communication, Impaired may be the primary problem. The person may accurately perceive and interpret touch stimuli but if he or she is unable to communicate to anyone that there is a problem, then intervention will not be done to resolve problems and Skin Integrity, Impaired may result.

OBJECTIVES

1. Will exhibit no signs or symptoms of increased skin integrity problems (e.g., increased size, infection) by (date).

AND/OR

2. Will demonstrate proper skin care measures by (date).

TARGET DATE

An appropriate target date will be every 2 days beginning 2 days following admission.

NURSING ORDERS

ADULT HEALTH

1. Cleanse area daily at (time) according to prescribed regimen. Collaborate with an enterstomal therapist and the physician regarding care specific to the patient:
   a. Protect open surface with such products as:
      (1) Karaya powder
      (2) Skin gel
      (3) Wafer barrier
      (4) Other commercial skin preparations
   b. Avoid use of adhesive tape.
   c. Avoid use of doughnut ring.
   d. Use mild soap (or soap substitute) and cool water.
   e. Avoid vigorous rubbing but do massage gently using a lanolin-based lotion.
   f. Pat area dry. Be sure area is thoroughly dry.
   g. Expose to air, sunlight, or heat lamp at least four times a day. Check patient at least every 5 minutes if using heat lamp.
2. Do active/passive range of motion at least every 4 hours on (odd/even) hours while awake.
   a. Ambulate to extent possible.
   b. Change position and teach patient to change position at least every 2 hours on (odd/even) hour. Do not position on affected area.
   c. If patient is unable to turn self, have several available to help lift, then turn.
   d. Gently massage pressure points and bony prominences following each position change.
3. Gently massage bony prominences and pressure points at least every 4 hours.
4. Assist patient to avoid shearing forces:
   a. Provide assistive devices for turning (e.g., trapeze bar, siderails kept up).
   b. Use soft, wrinkle-free linen only.
   c. Place cornstarch or powder on linens.
   d. Make sure footboard is in place for patient to use for bracing.
5. Reduce pressure on affected skin surface by using:
   a. Egg crate;

   b. Alternating air mattress;
   c. Sheepskin;
   d. Commercial wafer barriers;
   e. Thick dressing used as pad;
   f. Bed cradle.
 6. Collaborate with dietitian regarding nutrition—high protein, high carbohydrates, supplemental vitamins and minerals. Assist patient to eat and drink as necessary.
 7. Monitor:
   a. Skin surface and pressure areas at least every 4 hours at (state times here) for blanching, erythema, temperature difference (e.g., increased warmth), or moisture.
   b. Size and color of lesion at least every 4 hours at (state times here).
   c. Fluid and electrolyte balance. Particularly watch for signs or symptoms of edema:
      (1) Intake and output every 8 hours. Total each 4 hours.
      (2) Collaborate with physician regarding frequency of measurement of electrolyte levels.
 8. Caution patient and assist to avoid scratching irritated areas.
   a. Trim and file nails.
   b. Apply cool compresses.
   c. Collaborate with physician regarding medicated baths (e.g., oatmeal) and topical ointments.
   d. Keep room cool with low humidity level.
 9. Cleanse perineal area carefully after each urination or bowel movement. Monitor closely for any urinary or fecal incontinence.
10. Teach patient principles of good skin hygiene.
11. Administer medications as ordered (e.g., antihistamines, medicated lotions).

CHILD HEALTH

1. Handle infant gently; especially caution paramedical personnel regarding need for gentle handling.
2. Place patient on sheepskin or flotation pad, or if parents choose allow infant or child to be held frequently.
3. Caution patient and parents to avoid scratching irritated area:
   a. Trim nails with appropriate scissors; receive parental permission first if necessary.
   b. Make small mitts if necessary from cotton stockinette used for precasting.
   c. Keep room at cool temperature, approximately 72° F with low humidity.
4. Cleanse perineal area after each urination or bowel movement (monitor for possible allergy to diapers).
5. Cleanse area daily at (specific time).
   a. Use mild soap, unscented if possible, and lukewarm water.
   b. Avoid vigorous rubbing; gently massage using unscented lotion or ointment as ordered.
   c. Allow area to air dry.
6. Assist patient to avoid shearing forces:
   a. Assist in moving slowly.
   b. Avoid stiffly starched linens and clothes.
   c. Use tape of nonallergenic nature if any tape at all.
   d. Avoid use of rubber or plastic in direct contact with patient.
7. Assist patient to eat and drink as needed.
   a. Encourage fluids.
      (1) Infants—250–300 ml/24 hours
      (2) Toddler—1150–1300 ml/24 hours
      (3) Preschooler—1600 ml/24 hours.
      (These are approximate ranges, or as ordered according to weight and condition).
   b. Collaborate with physician and dietitian regarding possible need for high-protein diet.

WOMEN'S HEALTH

Childbirth

1. Monitor perineum and rectum after childbirth for injury or healing at least once per shift.
2. Collaborate with physician regarding:
   a. Applying ice packs or cold pads to perinium for the first 12 hours after delivery to reduce edema and increase comfort;
   b. Sitz baths twice a day or as needed after the first 24 hours;
   c. Analgesics and topical anesthetics as necessary for pain and discomfort.
3. Teach good perineal hygiene and self-care.
   a. Rinse perineal area with warm water after each voiding.
   b. Pat dry gently from front to back to prevent contamination.
   c. Apply perineal pad from front to back to prevent contamination.
   d. Change pads frequently to prevent infection and irritation.
4. Provide factual information on resumption of sexual activities after childbirth.
   a. First intercourse should be after adequate healing period (usually 3–4 weeks).
   b. Intercourse should be slow and easy (woman on top can better control angle, depth, and penetration).
5. Teach postmenopausal women the signs and symptoms of atrophic vaginitis.
   a. Watery discharge
   b. Burning and itching of vagina or vulva
6. Encourage examinations (Pap smears) for estrogen levels at least annually.
7. In collaboration with physician, encourage use as needed of:
   a. Estrogen replacement creams or vaginal suppositories;
   b. Extra lubrication during intercourse.
8. Teach breastfeeding mothers about breast care.
   a. Inspect for cracks or fissures in nipples.
   b. Wear supportive bra (breast binder to relieve engorgement).
   c. Shower daily, do not use soap on breasts, allow to air dry.
   d. Use lanolin-based cream (Vitamin E cream, Massé or A & D cream to prevent drying and cracking of nipples)
9. Enhance let-down reflex.
   a. Early, frequent feedings. Ten minutes on each side is easier on sore nipples than nursing less frequently.
   b. Nurse at both breasts each feeding. Switch sides to begin nursing each time (e.g., if baby nursed first on left side before, begin on right side this time. A safety pin or small ribbon on bra strap will remind mother which side she used first last time).
   c. Change positions from one feeding to next (distributes sucking pressure).
   d. Check baby's position on breast; be certain areola is in mouth, not just nipple.
   e. Begin nursing on least sore side first (if possible to encourage let-down reflex, then switch baby to other side).
   f. Apply ice to nipple just before nursing to decrease pain (fold squares, put them in the freezer and apply as needed).
10. Consult physician for pain medication if needed. Do not take over-the-counter pain medication, as some medications are passed to baby in breast milk.

MENTAL HEALTH

1. Refer to Chapter 8 for stress reduction measures and interventions for the stressors that produce psychogenic skin reactions.
2. Restraint care.
   a. Assess the integrity of skin under restraints every 15 minutes.

b. Apply lanolin-based lotion and cornstarch or powder to area under restraint as needed (at least every 2 hours).
c. Pad restraints with nonabrasive materials such as sheepskin.
d. Keep area of restraint next to the skin clean and dry.
e. Release restraints one at a time every 2 hours or as required. Remove restraints as soon as the client will tolerate one-to-one care without risk to self or others.
f. Maintain proper movement and alignment of affected body parts.
g. Change client's position every 2 hours on (odd/even) hours.
h. Offer client fluids every 15 minutes (list preferred fluids here).
i. While client is very agitated and physically active provide constant one-to-one observation.
3. Teach client to avoid excessive wind and sun exposure, especially with antipsychotic drugs.
4. If client is taking antipsychotic drugs suggest the use of a sunscreen containg PABA.
5. Refer to appropriate assistive resources as indicated:
   a. Visiting nurse
   b. Nutritionist
   c. Physical therapist
   d. Occupational therapist
   e. Physician

HOME HEALTH

1. Teach patient and family measures to promote skin integrity.
   a. Keep skin clean and dry (wash urine and feces off of skin immediately).
   b. Maintain adequate hydration (e.g., oral fluids, mild soap for bathing, place nonscented lotion or petroleum jelly on skin after bathing to moisturize).
   c. Maintain adequate protein intake.
   d. Use mild laundry detergent on clothes; double-rinse clothes, linens, and diapers if skin is sensitive.
   e. Change position at least every 2 hours; avoid prolonged sitting, standing, or lying in one position for extended periods.
   f. Use sunscreen to prevent sun damage.
   g. Avoid excessive wind and sun exposure.
   h. Wear properly fitting shoes.
   i. Avoid shearing force when moving in bed or chair.
2. Teach patient and family signs and symptoms of skin breakdown.
   a. Redness over bony prominences
   b. Pain or discomfort in localized area
   c. Skin lesions
   d. Itching
   e. Physical activity (active or passive) which develops full range of motion of all joints and relieves pressure on risk area
3. Teach patient and family self-monitoring techniques to prevent skin breakdown and initiate early treatment.
   a. Inspect the skin.
   b. Change positions at least every 2 hours.
   c. Massage pressure points and bony prominences gently.
   d. Avoid rubber or plastic mattress covers or sheets.
   e. Use proper body alignment and padding to reduce pressure on affected areas.
   f. Consult health care provider for treatment of actual skin lesions.
   g. Avoid scratching lesions.
4. Refer to appropriate assistive resources as indicated:
   a. Nutritionist
   b. Physical therapist
   c. Physician

EVALUATION
OBJECTIVE 1

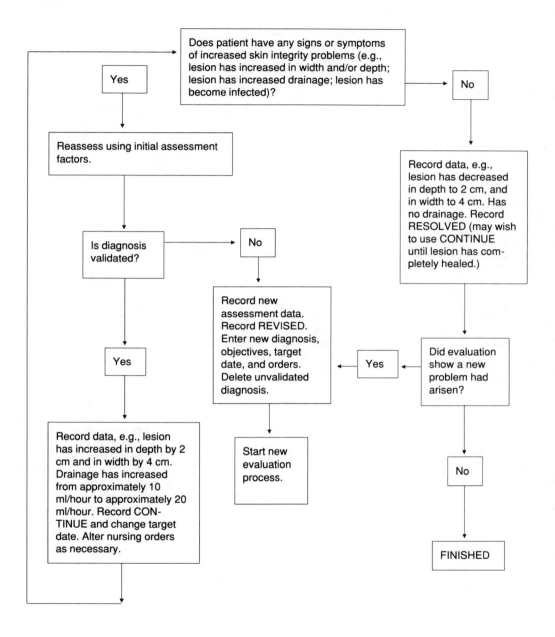

OBJECTIVE 2

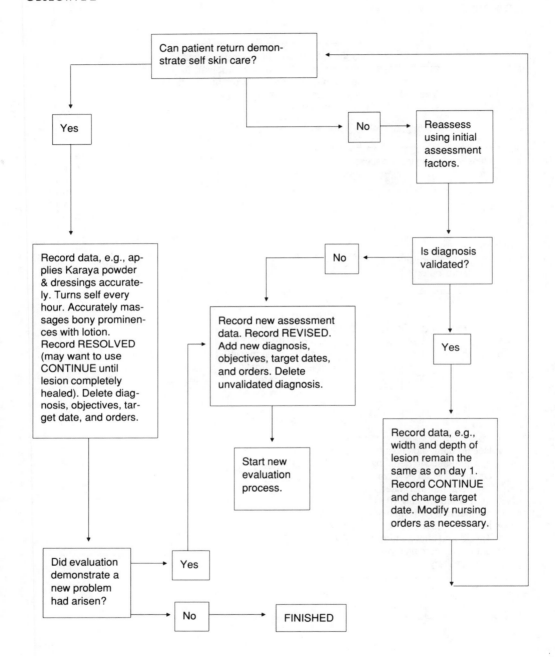

Swallowing, Impaired

DEFINITION

The state in which an individual has decreased ability to voluntarily pass fluids or solids from the mouth to the stomach. (NANDA, 1987, p. 88)

DEFINING CHARACTERISTICS (NANDA, 1987, p. 88)

The nurse will review the initial pattern assessment for the following defining characteristics to determine the diagnosis of Swallowing, Impaired.

1. Major defining characteristics
   a. Observed evidence of difficulty in swallowing (e.g., stasis of food in oral cavity, coughing, choking).
2. Minor defining characteristics
   a. Evidence of aspiration

RELATED FACTORS (NANDA, 1987, p. 88)

1. Neuromuscular impairment (e.g., decreased or absent gag reflex, decreased strength or excursion of muscles involved in mastication, perceptual impairment, facial paralysis).
2. Mechanical obstruction (e.g., edema, tracheostomy tube, tumor)
3. Fatigue
4. Limited awareness
5. Reddened, irritated oropharyngeal cavity

DIFFERENTIATION

Swallowing Impaired needs to be differentiated from Oral Mucous Membrane, Altered and Nutrition, Altered: Less Than Body Requirements.

Swallowing Impaired implies that there is a mechanical or physiological obstruction between the oropharynx and the esophagus. An Oral Mucous Membrane, Altered indicates that only the oral cavity is involved. Structures below the oral cavity, per se, are not affected. If liquids or solids are able to pass through the oral cavity, there will be nothing obstructing its passage through the esophagus to the stomach. Therefore, if solids or liquids are able to pass into the stomach without cawing coughing or choking, the appropriate nursing diagnosis is *not* Swallowing, Impaired.

Swallowing Impaired, might well be the primary reason someone has Nutrition, Altered: Less Than Body Requirements. However, in the case of the nursing diagnosis of Swallowing, Impaired, the Nutrition, Altered is a secondary problem. Additionally, Nutrition, Altered has several other related etiologic factors. Therefore, differentiation between these two nursing diagnoses needs to be done to appropriately prioritize nursing intervention.

OBJECTIVES

1. Will be able to freely swallow (solids) (fluids) by (date).

AND/OR

2. Will not have any aspiration problems by (date).

TARGET DATE

Since impaired swallowing can be so life-threatening the patient should be checked for progress daily. After the condition has improved, progress could be checked at 3-day intervals.

NURSING ORDERS

ADULT HEALTH

1. Stay with the patient while he or she tries to eat.
2. Be supportive, as it is very frustrating for the patient who has impaired swallowing.
3. Provide for rest periods, as coughing and choking can be very tiring.
4. Have a suction at hand in case of aspiration.
5. Have a tracheostomy tray at hand in case of respiratory obstruction.
6. Teach the patient who has had supraglottis surgery an alternate method of swallowing.
    a. Have the patient clear his or her throat by coughing and expectorating or suctioning the secretions.
    b. Have the patient inhale as he or she puts food in the mouth.
    c. Have the patient then perform a Valsalva maneuver as he or she swallows.
    d. Have the patient cough, swallow again, and exhale deeply.
    e. Start with soft, nonacidic, noncrumbly foods rather than liquids. Liquids are more difficult to control.
7. Support hydration and caloric intake as ordered (e.g., IVs, etc.).
8. Provide privacy for the patient as he or she learns alternate swallowing.
9. Include the family in the plan of care.

CHILD HEALTH

1. Monitor for contributory factors, especially palate formation, possible tracheolesophageal fistula, or other congential anomalies.
2. Monitor for lesions or infectious processes of the mouth and oropharynx.
3. Monitor, prior to every offering of food, fluid, etc., for presence of gag reflex.
4. Test swallowing capacity only with clear, sterile water and in presence of suctioning apparatus.
5. Maintain appropriate upright position during feeding to facilitate swallowing.
6. Warm fluids to assist in swallowing.
7. Advance diet as tolerated.
8. Maintain infant in upright position after feedings for at least 1½ hours.
9. Address anticipatory safety needs for possible choking:
    a. Have appropriate suctioning equipment available.
    b. Teach parents CPR.
    c. Provide parenting support for CPR and suctioning.
10. Assist family to identify ways to cope with swallowing disorder (e.g., extra help in feeding).
11. Administer medications as ordered. Avoid powder or pill forms. Use elixirs or mix as needed.
12. Include collaboration and referral as required for related health team members:
    a. Surgeon, pediatrician
    b. Clinical nurse specialist
    c. Speech therapist
    d. Occupational therapist
    e. Respiratory therapist
    f. Family therapist
    g. Social service
    h. Community health nurse
13. Assist parents in identifying support groups for long-term care.
14. Provide for follow-up appointments before dismissal from hospital.

WOMEN'S HEALTH

The nursing orders for a woman with the nursing diagnosis of Swallowing, Impaired are the same as those for adult health.

MENTAL HEALTH

(Note: The nursing orders for the mental health client will be the same as those described for adult health. The following nursing orders are specific considerations for the mental health client. These orders are directed to the client that has impairment that is caused or increased by anxiety. Refer to mental health nursing orders for the diagnosis of Anxiety for interventions related to decreasing and resolving the client's anxiety. If swallowing problems are related to an eating disorder, refer to mental health nursing orders for Nutrition, Altered: Less Than Body Requirements for additional nursing orders.)

1. Provide a quiet, relaxed environment during meals by discussing with client the situations that increase anxiety and excluding those factors from the situation. Provide things such as favorite music and friends or family that increase relaxation (note information provided by client here, especially those things that need to be provided by the nursing staff).
2. Provide medications in liquid or injectable form (note any special preference client may have in presentation of medications here).
3. Teach client deep muscle relaxation (refer to the mental health nursing orders for Anxiety for orders related to decreasing anxiety).
4. Discuss with client foods that are the easiest and the most difficult to swallow. Note information from this discussion here. (Note time and person responsible for this discussion here.)
5. Consult with nutritionist about client's preferred food list and about enhancing the nutritional value of those foods that are easier for the client to swallow (e.g., adding an egg to frozen milk drinks or products, adding vitamins to warm liquids).
6. Plan client's most nutritious meals for the time of day client is most relaxed and note that time here.
7. Provide client with high-energy snacks several times during the day (note snacks preferred by client and time it is to be offered here).
8. Maintain an intake and output record.
9. Weigh client each day at the same time (note time here).
10. Assign primary nurse to sit with client 30 minutes (this can be increased to an hour as client tolerates interaction time better) two times a day to discuss concerns related to swallowing (this can be included in the time described under the nursing orders for Anxiety). As the nurse-client relationship moves to a working phase, discussions can include those factors that precipitated client's focus on swallowing. These factors could be a trauma directly related to swallowing, such as an attack in which the client was choked or in which oral sex was forced, etc.
11. Teach client and client's support system nutrition facts that will improve swallowing and maintain adequate nutrition. Note here the names of those persons client would like included in this teaching. Note time arranged and person responsible for this teaching here.
12. Consult with appropriate assistive resources as indicated:
    a. Physician
    b. Dentist
    c. Community health nurse
    d. Occupational therapist
    e. Nutritionist
    f. Clinical nurse specialist

HOME HEALTH

1. Teach patient and family to monitor for factors contributing to impaired swallowing (e.g., fatigue, obstruction, neuromuscular impairment, irritated oropharyngeal cavity) on at least a daily basis.
2. Involve patient and family in planning, implementing, and promoting reduction or elimination of impaired swallowing by establishing regular family conferences to provide for mutual goal setting and to improve communication.

3. Teach patient and family measures to decrease or eliminate impaired swallowing:
   a. Principles of oral hygiene
   b. Small pieces of food or puréed food as necessary
   c. Aspiration precautions (e.g., eat and drink sitting up, do not force feed or fill mouth too full, CPR)
   d. Proper nutrition and hydration
   e. Use of adaptive equipment as required
4. Assist patient and family in life-style changes that may be required:
   a. Patient may need to be fed
   b. Meal times should be quiet,uninterrupted, and at consistent times on a daily basis
   c. Patient may require special diet and special utensils
5. Consult with appropriate assistive resources as indicated:
   a. Red Cross or American Heart Association for CPR training
   b. Physician
   c. Nurse
   d. Dentist
   e. Occupational therapist
   f. Home health aid
   g. Nutritionist

EVALUATION
OBJECTIVE 1

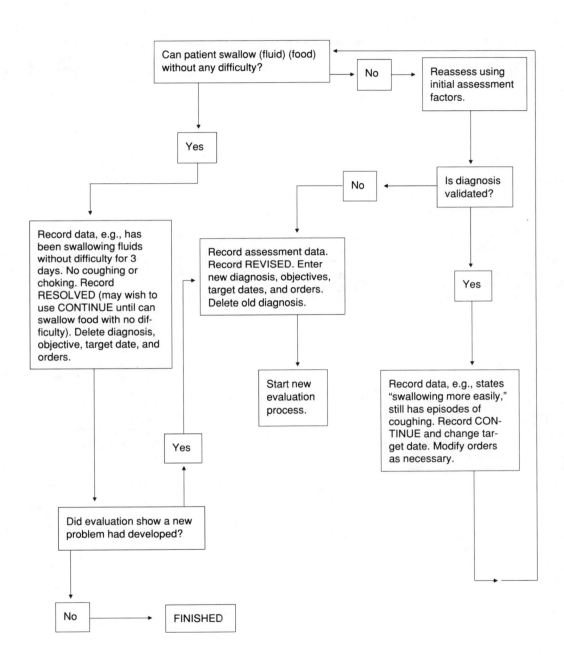

OBJECTIVE 2

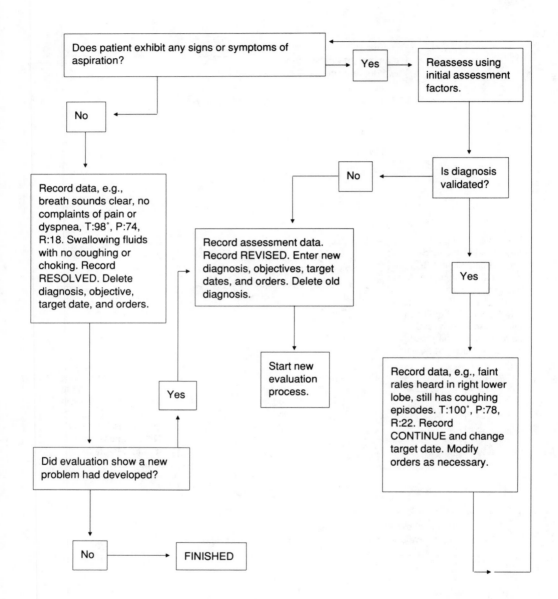

Thermoregulation, Ineffective

DEFINITION

The state in which the individual's temperature fluctuates between hypothermia and hyperthermia. (NANDA, 1987, p. 21)

DEFINING CHARACTERISTICS (NANDA, 1987, p. 21)

The nurse will review the initial pattern assessment for the following defining characteristics to determine the diagnosis of Thermoregulation, Ineffective

1. Fluctuation in body temperature above or below the normal range.
2. See also major and minor characteristics present in Hyperthermia and Hyperthermia.

RELATED FACTORS (NANDA, 1987, p. 21)

1. Trauma or illness
2. Immaturity
3. Aging
4. Fluctuating environmental temperature

DIFFERENTIATION

Thermoregulation, Ineffective needs to be differentiated from Hyperthermia, Hypothermia, and Body Temperature, Altered: Potential.

Hyperthermia means that a person maintains a body temperature greater than normal for himself on herself. By definition, Thermoregulation, Ineffective means that a person's temperature fluctuates or vacillates between being too high and being too low. Therefore, these two nursing diagnoses can be differentiated by time. If a person's temperature remains high rather than fluctuating, the person has Hyperthermia rather than Thermoregulation, Ineffective.

The same would hold true for Hypothermia. If the person's temperature remains low rather than fluctuating, the person has Hypothermia rather than Thermoregulation, Ineffective.

Body Temperature, Altered: Potential indicates that a person is potentially unable to regulate heat production and heat dissipation within a normal range. The potential for dysfunction of thermoregulation is there. However, in Thermoregulation, Ineffective, the potential is realized and the person is unable to regulate production and dissipation of heat.

OBJECTIVES

1. Will maintain a body temperature between 97° and 99° F by (date).

AND/OR

2. Will identify at least (number) measures to use in correcting ineffective thermoregulation by (date).

TARGET DATE

Initial target dates will be stated in terms of hours. After stabilization, an appropriate target date would be 3 days.

NURSING ORDERS

ADULT HEALTH

1. Maintain room temperature around 72° F.
2. If the patient is hypothermic:
   a. Warm the patient quickly. Use warm blankets, warm water (102°–105° F), extra clothing, warm drinks (if conscious). Do not use a heat lamp or hot water bottles.
   b. Prevent injury by gently massaging the body to stimulate circulation. Do *not* rub a body part if frostbite is evident, as rubbing may lead to tissue death and gangrene.

    c. As temperature and circulation increase, the patient may increase activity or exercise of body parts.

    d. Give fluids (salt and soda solution); have patient sip slowly; do *not* give alcohol.

    e. Monitor respiration rate and depth.

3. If the patient is hyperthermic:

    a. Reduce temperature quickly by sponging the patient with cool water *or* rubbing alcohol *or* by placing him or her in a tub of cool water until temperature is lowered. (Be careful not to overchill the patient.) Dry patient off.

    b. Use a fan or place patient in front of an air conditioner to promote cooling. Cool the environment.

    c. *Do not* give stimulants.

    d. Give sips of salt water if conscious and not vomiting. Up to 3000 ml of fluids in 24 hours may be given.

    e. Give antipyretic drugs as ordered.

    f. Give frequent skin, mouth, and nasal care.

CHILD HEALTH

1. Provide for other primary nursing needs, especially convulsions, fluid replacement, or related factors.
2. Monitor neurologic vital signs and temperature every 2 hours on (odd/even) hours. Notify physician if temperature falls below 97°F or goes above 100°F, or as ordered.
3. Provide warmth or cooling as needed to maintain temperature in desired range; avoid drafts and chilling for patient.
4. Administer medications as ordered and monitor for effects and possible untoward effects.
5. Protect child from excessive chilling during bathing or procedures.
6. Monitor for pattern of temperature on an ongoing basis.
7. Assist in answering parent's or child's questions regarding monitoring temperature procedures, or other educational needs such as administration of medications.
8. Assist parents in dealing with anxiety in times of unknown causes or prognosis by allowing 30 minutes per shift for venting anxiety.
9. Involve parents and family in child's care whenever appropriate, especially for comforting child.
10. Make referrals for appropriate follow-up before dismissal from hospital.

WOMEN'S HEALTH

1. Assist patient in identifying life-style adjustments that may be needed, due to physiologic function or needs during experiential phases of life (e.g., pregnancy, menopause).

    a. Keep room cooler.

    b. Layer blankets or covers that can be discarded or added as necessary.

    c. Have client drink cool fluids (i.e., iced tea, cold soda, etc.)

    d. Have client wear clothing that is layered, so that jackets can be discarded or added as necessary.

    e. In collaboration with physician, administer estrogen replacement therapy as required.

    f. Provide support and factual information to client about body heat fluctuations during menopause.

MENTAL HEALTH

(Note: The objectives and nursing orders for the mental health client will be the same as those described for adult health. The following nursing orders are specific considerations for the mental health client.)

1. Monitor client's mental status every 2 hours and report any alterations to the physician.
2. Assign client's care to a primary care nurse, and if client experiences alteration in mental status assign someone to be with that client at all times until thermoregulation is reestablished.
3. Monitor client's temperature every 2 hours on the (odd/even) hours and report alterations below 97° or above 100° F to physician.
4. Monitor for a pattern of temperature alteration over time.
5. Answer client's questions related to the alteration in temperature.
6. Place client in a quiet environment.
7. Reduce client's anxiety by:
   a. Providing a primary care nurse;
   b. Providing client with as much information as possible about procedures related to care;
   c. Talking with client about concerns related to alteration in physical status;
   d. Directing client through a deep muscle relaxation procedure if physical condition permits.
8. Consult with appropriate assistive resources as indicated:
   a. Clinical nurse specialist
   b. Physician
   c. Nutritionist
   d. Financial counselor
   e. Home energy audit
   f. Social services
   g. Emergency housing authority

HOME HEALTH

1. Monitor for factors contributing to ineffective thermoregulation (illness, trauma, immaturity, aging, fluctuating environmental temperature).
2. Involve patient and family in planning, implementing, and promoting reduction or elimination of ineffective thermoregulation.
3. Teach patient and family measures to decrease or eliminate ineffective thermoregulation (see Hyperthermia and Hypothermia).
4. Assist patient and family to identify life-style changes that may be required (see Hyperthermia and Hypothermia).
5. Teach patient and family early signs and symptoms of effective thermoregulation (see Hyperthermia and Hypothermia).
6. Consult with appropriate assistive resources as indicated:
   a. Nurse
   b. Physician
   c. Nutritionist
   d. Financial counselor
   e. Home energy audit
   f. YMCA/YWCA for classes on outdoor recreation and survival

EVALUATION
OBJECTIVE 1

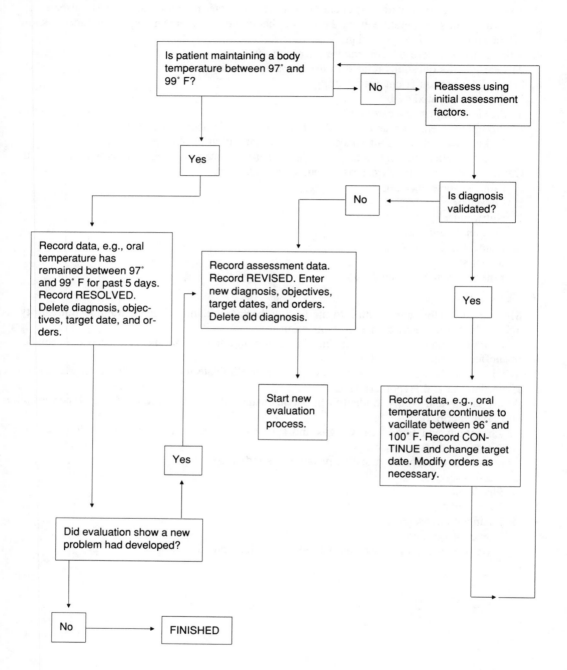

OBJECTIVE 2

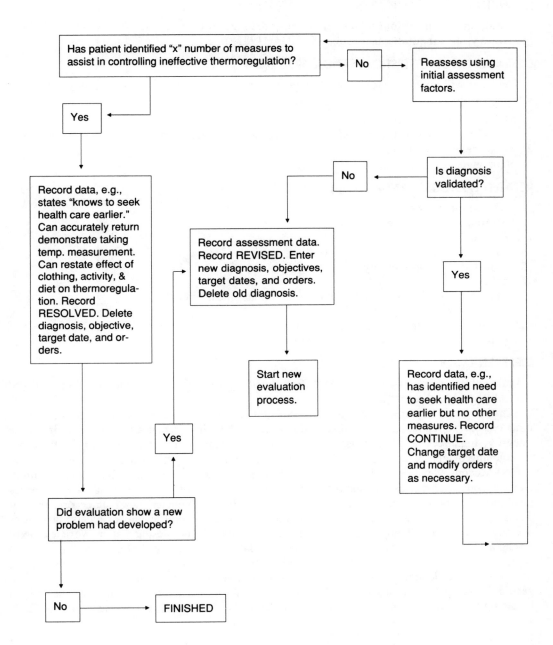

Tissue Integrity, Impaired

DEFINITION

A state in which an individual experiences damage to mucous membrane, corneal, integumentary, or subcutaneous tissue. (NANDA, 1987, p. 54).

DEFINING CHARACTERISTICS (NANDA, 1987, p. 54)

The nurse will review the following defining characteristics to determine the diagnosis of Tissue Integrity, Impaired.

1. Major defining characteristics
   a. Damaged or destroyed tissue (cornea, mucous membrane, integumentary, or subcutaneous).
2. Minor defining characteristics
   None given.

RELATED FACTORS (NANDA, 1987, p. 54)

1. Altered circulation
2. Nutritional deficit or excess
3. Fluid deficit or excess
4. Knowledge deficit
5. Impaired physical mobility
6. Irritants
7. Chemicals (including body excretions, secretions, medications)
8. Temperature extremes
9. Mechanical factors (pressure, sheer, friction)
10. Radiation (including therapeutic radiation)

DIFFERENTIATION

Impaired tissue integrity needs to be differentiated primarily from Skin Integrity, Impaired and Oral Mucous Membranes, Impaired.

Skin Integrity, Impaired means that the skin, the covering of the body, is not performing its functions of heat regulation, protection, and sensation. The skin covers underlying tissue. In Tissue Integrity, Impaired, it is this underlying tissue that is affected rather than the skin itself. These two nursing diagnoses are closely related but are differentiated by the depth of damage.

Oral Mucous Membranes, Impaired is a fifth-level diagnosis under Tissue Integrity, Impaired. Oral Mucous Membranes, Impaired is defined as the state in which an individual experiences disruptions in the tissue layers of the oral cavity. Defining characteristics include oral pain or discomfort, coated tongue, xerostomia (dry mouth), stomatitis, oral lesions or ulcers, lack of or decreased salivation, leukoplakia, edema, hyperemia, oral plaque, desquamation, vesicles, hemorrhage, gingivitis, carious teeth, and halitosis. Related factors are pathologic conditions—oral cavity (radiation to head or neck), dehydration, trauma (chemical, e.g., acidic foods, drugs, noxious agents, alcohol; mechanical, e.g., ill-fitting dentures, braces, tubes [endotracheal/nasogastric], surgery in oral cavity), NPO for more than 24 hours, ineffective oral hygiene, mouth breathing, malnutrition, infection, lack of or decreased salivation, and medication (NANDA, 1987, p. 56).

OBJECTIVES

1. Will have no signs or symptoms of impaired tissue integrity by (date).

AND/OR

2. Will implement plan to avoid future episodes of impaired tissue integrity by (date).

TARGET DATE

An appropriate target date would be 3 days from the date of diagnosis.

NURSING ORDERS

ADULT HEALTH

(Note: The specific nursing orders for Tissue Integrity, Impaired would depend on the specific tissue affected. In general, the following nursing orders would apply.)

1. Turn patient every 2 hours on (odd/even) hours.
2. Pad bony prominences.
3. Massage back and pressure areas at least every 4 hours while awake on (odd/even) hours.
4. Perform active and passive range of motion exercises at least once per shift at (state times here).
5. Feed patient well-balanced diet.
6. Monitor dietary intake and avoid irritant food and fluid intake.
7. Encourage fluid intake to at least 2000 ml per 24 hours.
8. Measure and total intake and output every 8 hours.
9. Keep skin around perineum clean and dry.
10. Have patient cough and deep breathe every 2 hours on (odd/even) hours.
11. Administer oral hygiene at least twice a day as well as required:
    a. Brush teeth, gums, and tongue with soft-bristled brush, sponge stick, or gauze-wrapped finger.
    b. Floss teeth.
    c. Rinse mouth thoroughly after brushing:
       (1) Avoid commercial mouthwashes, preparations with alcohol, lemon, or glycerine. Use normal saline or oxidizing agent (mild hydrogen peroxide solution, Gly-oxide, sodium bicarbonate solution).
       (2) If patient is unable to rinse, turn on side and do oral irrigation.
       (3) Teach patient use of water pick.
12. Teach patient and significant others proper oral hygiene.
13. If patient has dentures, cleanse with equal parts of hydrogen peroxide and water.
14. Apply lubricant to lips at least every 3 hours (e.g., petroleum jelly, glycerine).
15. Maintain good body hygiene.
16. Monitor for signs of infection daily.
17. Keep room temperature and humidity constant.
18. Darken room, if necessary, to protect eyes.
19. Encourage patient to chew sugar-free gum to stimulate salivation.
20. Administer medications as ordered and record response (e.g., topical oral antibiotics [note response daily such as decreased size, redness, etc.], analgesic mouthwash [note response within 15 minutes of administration]).
21. Encourage patient to avoid smoking.
22. Provide between-meal food or fluids that patient describes as soothing (e.g., warm, cool).
23. Refer to dental practitioner and dietitian.

CHILD HEALTH

1. Address primary nursing needs related to impaired tissue integrity (adult health nursing orders).
2. Provide protection such as bandage or dressing to tissue site involved.
3. Collaborate with health team members as appropriate, especially:
    a. Surgeon or subspecialist, especially cardiovascular
    b. Pediatrician
    c. Clinical nurse specialist
    d. Physical therapist

    e. Occupational therapist
    f. Respiratory therapist
    g. Dietitian
    h. Social worker
    i. Community health nurse
    j. Play therapist

4. Monitor and document in depth for circulation of tissue and limb involved via:
    a. Peripheral arterial pulses
    b. Blanching or capillary refill
    c. Color of tissue
    d. Sensation to touch, pain
    e. Condition of tissue or wound
    f. Drainage noted, odor, bleeding
    g. Range of motion of joint involved

5. Administer oral hygiene according to needs and status (glycerine and lemon swabs for NPO infant; special orders for postoperative cleft palate lip repair client).

6. Teach parents of need to limit length of time infant sucks bottle in reclining position to best limit possible "bottle syndrome" and decayed teeth.

7. Protect the altered tissue site as needed during movement with support of limb.

8. Provide range of motion or ambulation as permitted to encourage vascular return.

9. Position patient while in bed so that the head of the bed is elevated slightly and involved limb is elevated approximately 20°.

10. Address altered thermoregulation and especially protect patient from chilling or shock, as from dehydration or sepsis.

11. Provide appropriate skin care to involved site as needed or ordered.

12. Use restraints judiciously for involved limb or body site.

13. Monitor intravenous infusion and administration of medications cautiously; avoid use of sites in close proximity to area of altered tissue integrity.

14. Allow patient and family to express concerns related to the altered tissue integrity by alloting 15 minutes per shift for discussion and ventilation of fears.

15. Provide appropriate teaching for patient and family regarding:
    a. Bandage or dressing changes
    b. Medications: administration and side effects
    c. Need for future follow-up
    d. Signs and symptoms to be reported
        (1) Increased temperature (101°F or above)
        (2) Foul odor of drainage or tissue
        (3) Failure of healing to occur or increase in site area size
        (4) Loss of sensation or pulsation in limb or site
    e. Prosthetic device if indicated
    f. Aids in mobility, such as crutches, walker
    g. Need to avoid constrictive clothing
    h. Appropriate dietary restrictions or needs
    i. Other related metabolic needs, such as diabetic or cardiac related

WOMEN'S HEALTH

(Note: The specific nursing orders for Tissue Integrity, Impaired would depend on the specific tissue affected. For instance, in an episiotomy after childbirth, one would need to judge the depth (i.e., is there a 4th-degree tear into the rectum, or is it a mediolateral episiotomy involving layers of muscle?).

The same nursing orders would apply as found in Skin Integrity, Impaired with the following additions:

1. Monitor the episiotomy site frequently for redness, edema, hematomas:
   a. Each 15 minutes immediately after delivery for 1 hour;
   b. Each shift thereafter.
2. Administer ice packs for the first 2 hours.
3. Thereafter give warm sitz baths 3 4 times daily.
4. In collaboration with the physician, administer for pain relief;
   a. Analgesic sprays
   b. Oral analgesics
5. Teach postmenopausal women the signs and symptoms of atrophic vaginitis.
   a. Watery discharge
   b. Burning and itching of vagina and vulva
6. Relate necessity for Pap smears for estrogen levels at least annually.
7. In collaboration with physician, encourage use as needed of:
   a. Estrogen replacement creams or vaginal suppositories;
   b. Extra lubrication during intercourse.

(Note: Between the 3rd and 6th months of pregnancy the process of tooth calcification [hardening] begins in the fetus. What the mother consumes in her diet will affect the development of the unborn child's teeth. A well balanced diet will usually provide correct amounts of nutrients for both mother and child.)

8. Teach patient to practice good oral hygiene at least twice a day as well as required.
   a. Each time client eats and if nauseated and vomiting, after each attack of vomiting.
   b. If the smell of toothpaste or mouth rinse makes client nauseated, use baking soda.
9. Reduce the number of times sugar-rich foods are eaten between meals.
10. Teach client to snack on fruits, vegetables, cheese, cottage cheese, whole grains, or milk.
11. Have client increase daily calcium intake by at least 0.49 gm (total of 1.2 gm of calcium per day is needed during pregnancy).
12. Collaborate with obstetrician and dentist to plan needed dental care during pregnancy.
13. Assist in planning best time in pregnancy for dental visits.
    a. Not during the first 3 months if:
       (1) Previous obstetric history includes miscarriage;
       (2) Threatened miscarriage;
       (3) Other medical indications;
       (4) Hypersensitive to gagging (will increase nausea and vomiting).
    b. Not during the last 3 months if:
       (1) Not able to sit in dental chair for long periods of time;
       (2) Obstetric history of premature labor.
14. Emphasize having only *needed* x-rays.
    a. Provide a lead apron to prevent any exposure to fetus.

Additional Information

A care plan for newborn health immediately follows this care plan. The authors inserted this additional care plan in this one instance because the newborn's oral mucous membrane problem can easily be overlooked.

NEWBORN HEALTH

1. In collaboration with dentist, teach parents the oral and dental needs of the neonate.
   a. Use of fluoride
   b. Pacifying
      (1) Do not use homemade pacifiers

        (2) Use pacifiers recommended by dentist

        (3) Allow infant who is teething to chew on soft toothbrush

           (a) Hold on to brush

           (b) Give to infant only when adult is present

           (c) Allows infant to become use to toothbrush in mouth (will encourage later brushing of teeth)

    c. Oral hygiene

        (1) Massage and rub infant's gums with finger daily

           (a) Helps circulation in gums and promotes healthy tissue

           (b) Gets infant use to finger in mouth, lessens fear when child has to go to dentist

           (c) Allows adult to inspect oral cavity for hygiene and problems

    d. First dental visit

    e. Nursing

        (1) Dental caries (dental decay) as a result of prolonged nursing or delayed weaning

           (a) Infant permitted to nurse at breast or bottle beyond required feeding time

           (b) Allowed to sleep habitually at the breast or with a bottle

2. Encourage client not to give sweet liquids (soft drinks) or fruit juices in bottles to infant.
3. Encourage client not to allow infant to nurse on either the bottle or breast while sleeping.
    a. Liquids pool around teeth (sleeping infant does not swallow).
    b. If Infant needs bottle between meals, use unsweetened liquid or water in bottle.
4. Encourage client to wean child from bottle to cup soon after first birthday.
    (Note: This refers to infant who is bottle feeding only; but nursing mothers should nurse only at necessary mealtimes for nutritional purposes and follow good oral hygiene for their infants.).
5. Encourage client to arrange for dental examination as soon as possible.
    (Note: "Baby's first teeth need to remain sound and healthy for several years because they are very important to the normal growth and development of the jaws and permanent teeth. Nursing caries are very destructive and the destruction occurs so rapidly that the teeth must frequently be removed to eliminate pain and infection" [American Society of Dentistry for Children, 1986].)
6. Use good hand-washing techniques to prevent infection with or reinfection of thrush.
7. Do not place infant on sheets where mother has been sitting. Thrush is caused by *Candida albicans* and infection is usually caused by direct contact with an "infected birth canal, hands (mother's or others), feeding equipment, breast, or bedding" (Jensen & Bobak, 1985, p. 905).
8. Thoroughly clean feeding equipment.
    a. Clean and properly store bottles.
    b. Clean breasts before each feeding.
9. In collaboration with physician, administer medications and treatments as ordered.
    a. Chemotherapy (gentian violet).
    b. Antibiotics (Mycostatin).
    c. Rinse mouth with sterile water.

MENTAL HEALTH

(Note: The objectives and nursing orders for the mental health client will be the same as those described for adult health. The following orders are specific considerations for the mental health client.)

1. If client is placed in restraints, remove every 2 hours to monitor condition of the skin and underlying tissue. Remove restraints one limb at a time if client's behavior does not allow the removal of all restraints. Note schedule and order for restraint removal here.
2. While limb is out of restraint have client move limb through range of motion.

3. If client is in four-point restraints, place him or her on side or stomach and change this position every 2 hours. Monitor skin condition of pressure areas. Note schedule for position change here.
4. If client is in four-point restraint, provide one-on-one observation.
5. Continually remind client of reason for restraint and conditions for having the restraints removed.
6. Talk with client in calm, quiet voice.
7. Use client's name.
8. Use restraints that are wide and have padding. Make sure padding is kept clean and dry and free of wrinkles.
9. If impaired tissue integrity is the result of self-harm, place client on one-on-one observation until the risk of future harm has diminished.
10. Monitor self-inflicted injuries hourly for the first 24 hours for signs of infection and further damage. Note information on a flow sheet. After the first 24 hours, monitor as required (note frequency here).
11. Provide equipment and time for the client to practice oral hygiene twice a day or as required or ordered (list times here).
12. Discuss with client life-style changes to improve condition of mucous membranes, including:
    a. Nutritional habits;
    b. Use of tobacco products;
    c. Use of alcohol;
    d. Maintenance of proper hydration;
    e. Effects of frequent vomiting.
13. Discuss with client side effects of medications that contribute to alterations in oral mucous membranes, such as:
    a. Antibiotics
    b. Antihistamines
    c. Phenytoin
    d. Antidepressants
    e. Antipsychotics
14. Teach client to use lemon juice and glycerine mouth swabs, nonsucrose candy or gum to stimulate flow of saliva. Obtain these supplies as necessary.
15. Consult with health team members as appropriate.
    a. Physician
    b. Clinical nurse specialist
    c. Physical therapist
    d. Occupational therapist
    e. Social services
    f. Client's family
    g. Nutritionist

HOME HEALTH

The nursing orders for Tissue Integrity, Impaired are the same as those for Skin Integrity, Impaired, and the adult health orders.

EVALUATION
OBJECTIVE 1

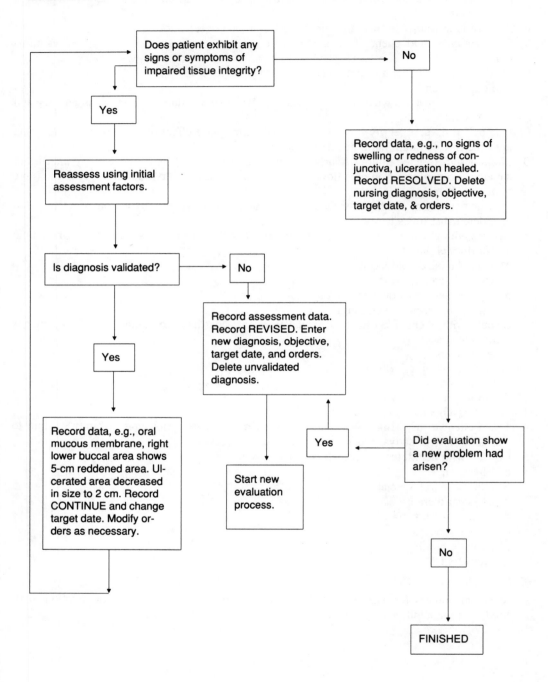

OBJECTIVE 2

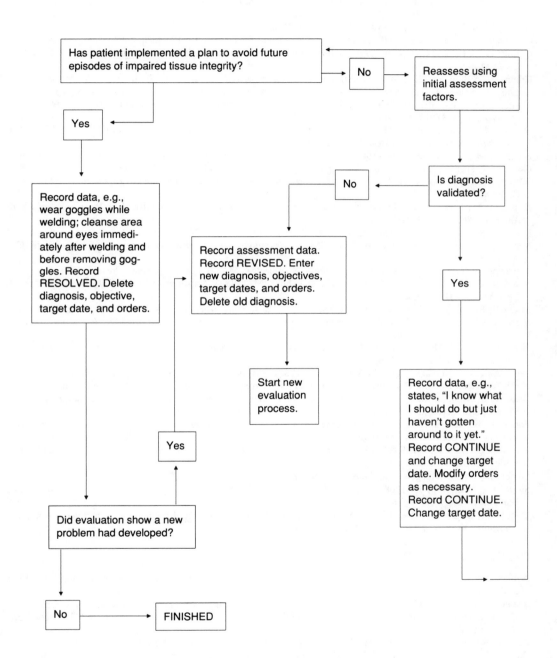

REFERENCES

American Society of Dentistry for Children. (1986). *Infant nursing: An important message to parents*. Chicago: Author.

Bailey, C. (1978). *Fit or fat?* Boston: Houghton Mifflin.

Carnevali, D., & Patrick, M. (1979). *Nursing management for the elderly*. Philadelphia: J. B. Lippincott.

Chinn, P., & Leitch, C. (1979). *Child health maintenance: A guide to clinical assessment* (2nd ed.). St. Louis: C. V. Mosby.

Chinn, P., & Leonard, K. (Eds.). (1980). *Current practice in pediatric nursing*. St. Louis: C. V. Mosby.

Cugini, P., Scavo, D., Halberg, F., Schramm, A., Pusch, H., & Franke, H. (1982). Methodologically critical interaction of circadian rhythm, sex and aging characterize serum aldosterone and female adenopause. *Journal of Gerontology,37* (4), 403–411.

Driscoll, J., & Heird, W. (1973). Maintenance fluid therapy during the neonatal period. In R. Winters (Ed.), *The body fluids in pediatrics*. Boston: Little, Brown.

Flynn, J. M., & Heffron, P. B. (1984). *Nursing: From concept to practice*. Bowie, MD: Brady Communication.

Guyton, A. (1981). *Textbook of medical physiology* (6th ed.). Philadelphia: W. B. Saunders.

Jensen, M. D., & Bobiak, I. M. (1985). *Maternity and gynecologic care: The nurse and the family*. St. Louis: C. V. Mosby.

Kopak, C. (1983). Sensory loss in the aged: The role of the nurse and the family. *Nursing Clinics of North America,18*(2), 373–384.

Korones, S. (1981). *High-risk newborn infants* (3rd ed.). St. Louis: C. V. Mosby.

Masiac, M., Naylor, M., & Hayman, L. (1985). *Fluids and electrolytes through the life cycle*. East Norwalk, CT: Appleton-Century-Crofts.

McCrory, W. (1972). *Developmental nephrology*. Cambridge, MA: Harvard University Press.

Mitchell, H., Rynbergen, H., Anderson, L., & Dibble, M. (1982). *Nutrition in health and disease* (17th ed.). New York: J. B. Lippincott.

Mitchell, P. H., & Loustau, A. (1981). *Concepts basic to nursing practice*. New York: McGraw-Hill.

Murray, R., & Zentner, J. (1985). *Nursing assessment and health promotion through the life span* (3rd ed.). Englewood Cliffs, NJ: Prentice-Hall.

Neeson, J. D., & May, K. A. (1986). *Comprehensive maternity nursing: Nursing process and the childbearing family*. Philadelphia: J. B. Lippincott.

North American Nursing Diagnosis Association. (1988). *Taxonomy I with complete diagnoses*. St. Louis: Author.

North American Nursing Diagnosis Association. (1988). *Proposed nursing diagnoses*. St. Louis: Author.

Olds, S. B., London, M. L., & Ladewig, P. A. (1988). *Maternal newborn nursing: A family-centered approach*. Menlo Park, CA: Addison-Wesley.

Potter, P. A., & Perry, A. G. (1985). *Instructors' manual for fundamentals of nursing: Concepts, process and practice*. St. Louis: C. V. Mosby.

Schuster, C., & Ashburn, S. (1986). *The process of human development: A holistic life-span approach*. Boston: Little, Brown.

Shafer, J. (1965). Dysageusia in the elderly. *Lancet, 1*, 35.

Stone, L., & Church, J. (1968). *Childhood and adolescence: A psychology of the growing person*. New York: Random House.

Young, C., Bogan, A., Roe, D., & Lutwak, L. (1968). Body composition of pre-adolescent and adolescent girls. *Journal of the American Diabetic Association, 53*(6),579–587.

SUGGESTED READINGS

Adams, C., & Macione, A. (Eds.) (1983). *Handbook of psychiatric mental health nursing*. New York: John Wiley & Sons.

Anderson, A., Morse, C., & Santmyer, K. (1985). Inpatient treatment for anorexia nervosa. In D. Garner & P. Garfinkel (Eds.), *Handbook of psychotherapy for Anorexia Nervosa and Bulimia* (pp. 311–343). New York: The Guilford Press.

Armstrong, M. E., et al. (1979). *McGraw-Hill handbook of clinical nursing*. New York: McGraw-Hill.

Bassuk, E., & Schoonover, S. (1977). *The practitioner's guide to psychoactive drugs*. New York: Plenum.

Bressler, R., & Conrad, K. (1983). Clinical pharmacology. In F. Steinberg (Ed.), *Care of the geriatric patient* (6th ed.). St. Louis: C. V. Mosby.

Bricklin, M. (1979). *Lose weight naturally*. Emmaus, PA: Rodale Press.

Carpenito, L. J. (1983). *Nursing diagnosis: Application to clinical practice*. Philadelphia: J. B. Lippincott.

Carpenito, L. J. (1984). *Handbook of nursing diagnosis*. Philadelphia: J. B. Lippincott.

Crittendon, R. (1983). *Discharge planning*. Bowie, MD: Robert J. Brady.

Eiger, M. S., & Olds, S. W. (1972). *The complete book of breast feeding*. New York: Doubleday.

Ewy, D., & Ewy, R. (1985). *Postpartum nursing: Health care of women*. New York: Doubleday.

Friebery, K. (1983). *Human development: A life span approach*. Monterey, CA: Wadsworth Health Sciences Division.

Frisch, R. E., & McArthur, J. (1974). Menstrual cycles: Fatness as a determinant of minimum weight for height necessary for their maintenance or onset. *Science,185*, 949–951.

Gettrust, K. V., Ryan, S. C. & Engleman, D. S. (1985). *Applied nursing diagnosis*. New York: John Wiley & Sons.

Gordon, M. (1985). *Manual of nursing diagnosis*. New York: McGraw-Hill.

Griffin, C., & Lockhart, J. (1987). Learning to swallow again. *American Journal of Nursing,87*(3),314–17.

Haber, J., Hoskins, P., Leach, A., & Sideleau, B. (Eds.) (1987). *Comprehensive psychiatric nursing* (3rd ed.). New York: McGraw-Hill.

Hadek, M. (1987). *Clinical judgment in community health nursing*. Boston: Little, Brown.

Haley, J. (1976). *Problem solving therapy*. San Francisco: Jossey-Bass.

Hawkins, J. W., & Gorvine, B. (1985). *Postpartum nursing: Health care of women*. New York: Springer.

Humphrey, C. (1986). *Home care nursing handbook*. East Norwalk, CT: Appleton-Century-Crofts.

Jaffe, M., & Skidmore-Roth, L. (1988). *Home health nursing care plans*. St. Louis: C. V. Mosby.

Kelly, M. A. (1985). *Nursing diagnosis source book*. East Norwalk, CT: Appleton-Century-Crofts.

Kneisl, C., & Wilson, H. (1984). *Handbook of psychosocial nursing care*. Menlo Park, CA: Addison-Wesley.

La Leche League International. (1981). *The womanly art of breast feeding*. New York: New American Library.

Lobel, S., Spratto, G., & Heckheimer, E. (1983). *The nurse's drug handbook* (3rd ed.). New York: John Wiley & Sons.

McClelland, E., Kelly, K., & Buckwalter, K. (1984). *Continuity of care: Advancing the concept of discharge planning*. Orlando, FL: Grune & Stratton.

McFarland, G., & Wasli, E. (1986). *Nursing diagnoses and process in psychiatric mental health nursing*. Philadelphia: J. B. Lippincott.

Murray, R. (1980). *The nursing process in later maturity*. Englewood Cliffs, NJ: Prentice-Hall.

National League for Nursing. (1986). *Policies and procedures*. New York: Accreditation Division for Home Care, National League for Nursing.

National League for Nursing. (1988). *Accreditation program for home care and community health: Criteria and standards*. New York: Author.

Parfett, A., & Kleenekiper, M. (1980). Clinical disorders of calcium, phosphorous and magnesium metabolism. In M. Maxwell & C. Kellman (Eds.), *Clinical disorders of fluid and electrolyte metabolism* (3rd ed.). New York: McGraw-Hill.

Pregnancy and Oral Health. (1981). Chicago: American Dental Association.

Remington, D., Fisher, G., & Parent, E. (1983). *How to lower your fat thermostat*. Provo, UT: Vitality House.

Rinke, L. (1988). *Outcome standards in home health*. New York: National League for Nursing.

Steffi, B, & Eide, I. (1978). *Discharge planning handbook*. New York: Charles B. Slack.

Steinberg, F. (1983). The aging of organs and organ systems. In F. Steinberg (Ed.), *Care of the geriatric patient*. (6th ed.). St. Louis: C. V. Mosby.

Stuart, G., & Sundeen, S. *Principles and practice of psychiatric nursing* (3rd ed.). St. Louis: C. V. Mosby.

Sykes, J., Kelly, P., & Kennedy, J. (1981). Black skin problems. *American Journal of Nursing, 81*(6),29–33.

Tonna, E. (1977). Aging of skeletal-dental systems and supporting tissue. In C. Finch & L. Hayflick (Eds.), *Handbook of the biology of aging*. New York: Van Nostrand, Reinhold.

Walsh, J., Persons, C., & Wieck L. (1987). *Manual of home health care nursing*. Philadelphia: J. B. Lippincott.

CHAPTER FOUR

Elimination Pattern

Pattern Description

The elimination pattern is a frequent focus for both the health care deliverer and the health care recipient. The elimination pattern may be the primary reason for seeking health care or may arise secondary to another health problem such as impaired mobility. There are very few of the other patterns or nursing diagnoses that will not have an ultimate impact on the elimination pattern from either a physiologic, psychologic, or sociologic direction.

The elimination pattern focuses on bowel and bladder excretions. The individual's habits in terms of excretory regularity, aids to maintaining habits, and perceived normality or abnormality are essential to planning the best care for the patient who has a problem in the elimination pattern.

Pattern Assessment

1. Patient's description of usual bowel elimination functioning:
    a. Regularity (e.g., once per day, once every 2 days, etc.)
    b. Color (e.g., brown, tarry, clay-colored)
    c. Amount
    d. Consistency (e.g., soft, well-formed, liquid, hard, dry, ribbon-shaped)
    e. Discomfort (e.g., pain, flatulence, distention)
    f. Control
    g. Any changes in usual functioning:
        (1) Onset
        (2) Duration
        (3) Measures taken to correct
        (4) Effect of corrective measures
2. Patient's description of usual bladder elimination functioning:
    a. Frequency
    b. Amount each voiding
    c. Color
    d. Odor
    e. Discomfort (e.g., pain, burning)
    f. Nocturia
    g. Control
    h. Any changes in usual functioning:
        (1) Onset
        (2) Duration
        (3) Measures taken to correct
        (4) Effect of corrective measures
3. Patient's current weight and any recent changes in weight.
4. Patient's description of activity level:
    a. Occupation

    b. Planned or recreational exercise
5. Patient's description of usual intake:
    a. Food:
        (1) Amount
        (2) Inclusion of basic four food groups
        (3) Times of day
        (4) Relationship to output:
            (a) Timing
            (b) Flatulence-producing
            (c) Diarrhea-producing
    b. Fluid:
        (1) Amount
        (2) Type
        (3) Caffeine-containing
        (4) Relationship to output
6. Patient's description of aids for excretion:
    a. Medications:
        (1) Physician recommended or prescribed.
        (2) Over-the-counter.
    b. Enemas
    c. Manual pressure over the bladder
    d. Self-catheterization
    e. Herbs or vitamins
    f. Massage
7. Other medications patient takes:
    a. Prescribed
    b. Over-the-counter
8. Signs and symptoms of fluid or electrolyte balance.
9. Vital signs.
10. Abdominal examination:
    a. Scars
    b. Distention
    c. Rigidity
    d. Bowel sounds
    e. Ascites
    f. Masses
    g. Presence of artificial orifices:
        (1) Type:
            (a) Colostomy
            (b) Ileostomy
            (c) Ureterostomy, etc.
        (2) Location
        (3) Stoma appearance
        (4) Tissue integrity around stoma
        (5) Type of appliance(s)
11. Perineal area examination:
    a. Presence of hemorrhoids
    b. Color
    c. Tissue integrity
    d. Odor

    e. Patient's description of perineal hygiene and any problems with discomfort, drainage, itching, etc.
12. Recent history of:
    a. Travel to foreign countries
    b. Surgery
    c. Trauma
    d. Stress
13. Results of routine screening:
    a. Occult blood
    b. Clinitest
    c. Acetest
    d. Urinalysis
14. Patient's description of perspiration:
    a. Amount
    b. Odor
15. Balance between intake and output.

Conceptual Information

Elimination, simply defined, refers to the excretion of waste and nondigested products of the metabolic process. Elimination is essential in maintaining fluid, electrolyte, and nutritional balance of the body. A disruption in an individual's usual elimination pattern can be life-threatening, since a person cannot live long without the ability to rid his or her body of waste products (Bruya, 1981; Long & Durham, 1983).

Elimination depends on the interrelated functioning of the gastrointestinal system, urinary system, nervous system, and skin. This chapter will only include the lower urinary tract and lower gastrointestinal tract since the skin and nervous system are related to nursing diagnoses in other chapters. Also, since the nursing diagnoses related to elimination refer only to elimination and not to the collection and formation of the waste materials, inclusion of other conceptual information would be confusing.

Our society has a rather dichotomous attitude toward elimination. A great deal of time, effort, and money is expended in designing and advertising bathrooms and aids to elimination, but to discuss elimination is considered rude (Bruya, 1981). Therefore, obtaining a reliable, complete elimination pattern assessment may be difficult. Added to this difficulty is the fact that each person has his or her own normal elimination habit.

Elimination is highly individualized and can be influenced by age, circadian rhythms, culture, diet, activity, stress, and a number of other factors. Elimination has elements of both involuntary and voluntary control. Involuntary control relates primarily to the production of waste materials and the neural signals that the bladder or bowel needs to be emptied. However, each person can usually control both the timing of bowel and bladder evacuation and the use of abdominal and perineal muscles to assist in evacuation.

Food and fluid intake are extremely important in elimination. A fluid intake of 2000 ml per day and a food intake of high-fiber foods would, in the majority of instances, ensure an adequate elimination pattern (Flynn, & Heffron 1984; Kelly, 1985). Alteration in elimination may cause psychosocial problems, such as social isolation due to embarrassment, as well as physiologic problems, such as fluid and electrolyte problems.

Bowel Elimination

The lower gastrointestinal tract includes the small and large intestines. The small bowel includes the duodenum, jejunum, and ileum and is about 20 feet in length and 1 inch in diameter. The large bowel includes the cecum, colon, and rectum and terminates at the anus. The large bowel is about 5 feet long and about 2½ inches in diameter. The small bowel and large bowel connect at the ileocecal valve (Long & Durham, 1983).

The intestines receive partially digested food from the stomach and move the food element through the lower tract thus assisting in proper absorption of water, nutrients, and electrolytes. The intestines also provide secretory and storage functions. They secrete mucus, potassium, bicarbonate, and enzymes.

The chyme (small intestine contents) is moved by peristalsis and the feces (large intestine contents) is propelled by mass movements which are stimulated by the gastrocolic reflex. The gastrocolic reflex occurs in response to food entering the stomach and causing distention, so mass movement occurs only a few times a day. The gastrocolic reflex occurs within 30 minutes after eating and is most predominant after the first meal of the day. Therefore, after the first meal of the day is the most frequent time for bowel elimination. Other reflexes involved in elimination are the duodenocolic reflex and the defecation reflex. The duodenocolic reflex is stimulated by the distention of the duodenum as food passes from the stomach to the duodenum. The gastrocolic and duodenocolic reflexes stimulate rectal contraction and, usually, a desire to defecate. The defecation reflex occurs in response to feces entering the rectum. This reflex promotes relaxation of the internal anal sphincter thus also promoting a desire to defecate. Extra fluids upon morning waking potentiate the gastrocolic reflex. If the fluids are warm or contain caffeine they will also stimulate peristalsis (Bruya, 1981; Long & Durham, 1983).

The secretions of the gastrointestinal tract assist with food passage and further digestion. The passage rate of the contents through the intestines helps determine the absorption amount. The small intestine is responsible for about 90% of the absorption of amino acids, sodium, calcium chloride, fatty acids, bile salts, and water. Potassium and bicarbonate are excreted. The usual amount of time for chyme to move from the stomach to the ileocecal valve varies from 3 to 10 hours. It takes about 12 hours for feces to travel from the ileocecal valve to the rectum. One bowel movement may be the result of meals eaten over the past 3–4 days, but most of the food residue from any particular meal will have been excreted within 4 days. Passage of contents is primarily influenced by the amount of residue and the motility rate. Feces is normally evacuated on a moderately regular schedule, but the schedule will vary from 3 times daily to once per week depending on the individual.

When proper absorption does not occur, necessary nutrients and electrolytes are lost for subsequent body use. Small bowel loss can cause metabolic acidosis and hypokalemia. Large bowel loss can lead to dehydration and hyponatremia.

The squatting, leaning forward position is the most supportive position for defecation because it increases intraabdominal pressure and promotes easier abdominal and perineal muscle contraction and relaxation. Beside positioning, diet, and fluid intake, other aids to elimination include enemas and laxatives.

Enemas assist in evacuation through either promotion of peristalsis, chemical irritation, or lubrication. Volume enemas, 500–1000 ml of fluid, cause distention which increases peristalsis. The addition of heat and soapsuds, for example, adds chemical irritation and increases peristalsis. Straight tap water enemas should be used cautiously since they are hypotonic and may disturb water balance. Electrolyte enemas are usually prepackaged and are hypertonic. Hypertonic enemas increase fluid amounts in the bowel through osmosis, thus slightly increasing distention and providing a relatively mild chemical irritation. Both the distention and irritation also result in increased peristalsis. Oil enemas are usually small volume enemas (100–200 ml) and provide lubrication as well as stool softening (Bruya, 1981; Gettrust, Ryan, & Engelman, 1985).

Laxatives assist elimination through producing bulk, providing lubrication, causing chemical irritation, or softening stool. The action of laxatives ranges from harsh to mild.

Both laxatives and enemas can be abused. Persistent use of either will diminish normal reflexes so that the individual will begin to require more and more aid. The individual then establishes an aid-dependent habit just as a drug abuser does.

While constipation and diarrhea are the two most common problems with bowel elimination, flatulence may be an associated problem. Flatus (intestinal gas) is normal. A problem arises when the individual cannot pass the gas or when abnormally large amounts of gas are produced. Flatus is produced by swallowed air, diffusion of gases from the bloodstream to the gastrointestinal tract, from carbon dioxide formed by the action of bicarbonate with hydrochloric acid or fatty acids, and from bacterial decomposition of food residue. Common causes of gas problems include gas-producing foods (beans, for example), highly irritating foods (pizza, for example), constipation, medications (codeine, for example), and inactivity. The problems relate directly to the amount of gas produced and decreased motility. Increased flatus causes distention which, in turn, can cause pain, respiratory difficulty, and further problems with intestinal motility (Bruya, 1981).

As previously mentioned, any bowel elimination problem can ultimately be life-threatening. Any bowel elimination problem, whether it be constipation, diarrhea, or flatulence, that lasts over 1–2 weeks in an adult or over 2–3 days for an infant or elderly person requires immediate health care intervention.

Urinary Elimination

The lower urinary tract is composed of the ureters, bladder, and urethra. These anatomical structures serve as storage and excretory passageways for the waste secreted by the kidneys. The ureters extend from the kidney pelvis to the trigone area in the bladder. The ureters are small tubes composed of smooth muscle which propels urine by peristalsis from the kidney to the bladder. The bladder stores the urine until it is excreted through the urethra. Between the base of the bladder and the top of the urethra is the urethral sphincter. The sphincter opens under learned voluntary control. Opening the urethral sphincter allows the urine to pass through the urethra and meatus for elimination. The female urethra is about 3–5 cm long and the male urethra is about 20 cm long (Miller, 1983).

The desire to void occurs when the bladder (adult) has reached a capacity of 250–450 ml of urine. As urine collects to the bladder capacity, the stretch receptors in the bladder muscle are activated. This stretching stimulates the voiding reflex center in the spinal cord (sacral levels 2, 3, and 4) which sends signals to the midbrain and the pons. These stimuli result in inhibition of the spinal reflex center and pudendal nerve which allows relaxation of the external sphincter and contraction of the bladder, and voiding occurs. The bladder is under parasympathetic control with the learned voluntary control being guided by the cortex, midbrain, and medulla (Bruya, 1981; Miller, 1983).

The anatomically correct positions for voiding are sitting for the female and standing for the male. An individual generally voids 200–450 ml each avoiding time and it is within normal limits to void 5–10 times per day. Common times for urination are upon arising and before retiring. Other times will vary with habits and correspond with work breaks and availability of toilet facilities (Bruya, 1981; Miller, 1983).

Urine volume will vary according to the individual. Urine volume depends on normal kidney functioning, amount of fluid and food intake, environmental temperature, fluid requirements of other organs, presence of open wounds, output by other areas (skin, bowel, respiration) and medications such as diuretics. The amount of solutes in the urine, an intact neuromuscular system, and the action of the antidiuretic hormone also influence output. A significant impact on urinary output is the opportunity to void at socially acceptable times in private (Bruya, 1981).

Inadequate urinary output may arise from either the kidney not producing urine (suppression) or blockage of urine flow (retention) somewhere between the kidney and external urinary meatus. Suppression may result from diseases of the kidneys or other body structures and inadequate fluid intake. Retention may be either mechanical or functional in nature. Mechanical retention is due to anatomic blockage such as a stricture or a calculus. Functional retention actually refers to any retention that is not mechanical and includes such areas as neurogenic problems (Miller, 1983).

Urinary control relates to the integrity and strength of the urinary sphincters and perineal musculature. Inability to control urinary output will soon lead to social isolation due to embarrassment over control and odor.

Urine is a waste product formed as a part of body metabolism. Urine is normally produced at a rate of 30–50 ml per hour. Under normal circumstances output will balance with intake about every 72 hours. An hourly output under 30 ml, a 24-hour output 500 ml or under, or an intake-output imbalance lasting over 72 hours requires immediate intervention (Bruya, 1981; Kelly, 1985).

Developmental Considerations

Elimination depends on the interrelatedness of fluid intake, muscle tone, regularity of habits, culture, state of health, and adequate nutrition (Murray & Zentner, 1985).

Infant

Kidney function does not reach adult levels until 6 months to 1 year of life. However, nervous system control is inadequate and renal function does not reach a mature status until approximately 1 year of life (Murray & Zentner, 1985). Voiding is stimulated by cold air. The infant usually voids 15–60 ml at each voiding during the first 24 hours of life. By the 3rd day, the infant may void 8–10 times during each 24 hours, equaling about 100–400 ml.

Uric acid crystals may be found in concentrated urine causing a rusty discoloration to the diaper (Schuster & Ashburn, 1986).

Urinary output is affected by the amount of fluid consumed, the amount of activity (increased activity, less urine) and the environmental temperature (increased temperature, less urine) (Schuster & Ashburn, 1986).

The muscles and elastic tissues of the infant's intestines are poorly developed and nervous system control is inadequate. Water and electrolyte absorption is functional but immature. The intestines are proportionately longer than in the adult. While some digestive enzymes are present, they can only break down simple foods. These digestive enzymes are unable to break down complex carbohydrates or protein.

Meconium is the first waste material that is eliminated by the bowel. This usually occurs during the first 24 hours. After 24 hours, the characteristics of the bowel movement change as it mixes with milk. The characteristics of the stool will depend on whether the infant is breast fed or bottle fed. The breast-fed infant will have soft, semiliquid stools that are yellow or golden in color. The bottle-fed infant will have a more formed stool which is light yellow to brown in color.

The infant may have 4–8 soft bowel movements a day during the first 4 weeks of life. Flatus often accompanies the passage of stool and there may be a sour odor to the bowel movement. By the 4th week of life, the number of bowel movements has decreased to 2–4 a day. By 4 months, there is a predictable interval between bowel movements.

It is common for the infant to push or strain at stool. However, if the stools are very hard or dry, the infant should be assessed for constipation. The bottle-fed infant is more prone to constipation than the breast-fed infant.

Infants sometimes suffer from what is known as colic. Colic is described as daily periods of distress caused by rapid, violent peristaltic waves and increased gas pressure in the rectum (Murray & Zentner, 1985). The cause is unknown but may have to do with the simple (rather than the complex) digestive enzymes of the infant or a decreased amount of vitamin A, K, or E. Most authorities agree that colic disappears as digestive enzymes become more complex and when normal bacterial flora accumulate (Murray & Zentner, 1985). Yogurt has been found to alleviate some of the colic symptoms.

Toddler and Preschooler

By 2 years of age, the kidneys are able to conserve water and to concentrate urine almost on an adult level, except under stress. The bladder increases in size and is able to hold about 88 ml of urine.

Nervous system and gastrointestinal maturation has occurred during infancy and the beginning of the toddler years. By the time children are 2–3 years of age, they are ready to control bowel and bladder functioning. Bowel elimination control is usually attained first; daytime bladder control is second and nighttime bladder control is third. The child must be able to walk a few steps, control the sphincter, recognize and interpret that the bladder is full, and be able to indicate that he or she wants to go to the bathroom. The child must also value dryness. He or she must recognize that it is more socially acceptable to be dry than to be wet.

Parents should not attempt toilet training, even if the child is ready, if there are family or environmental stressors. Regression is normal during toilet training and, coupled with undue stress, could cause physical or psychosocial problems.

Bladder training takes time to accomplish. Both the parent and the child must have patience and not get unduly upset when accidents occur. In fact, nighttime bladder control may not be attained until 5–8 years of life. Doctors and researchers disagree on the age at which nighttime bedwetting (enuresis) becomes a problem (Schuster & Ashburn, 1986). Parents should limit fluids at night, have the child void before going to bed and get the child up at least once during the night to assist in attaining nighttime control.

In order to toilet train, the parent should watch for patterns of defecation. Eating stimulates peristaltic activity and evacuation. The child can then be taken to the potty at the expected time after eating. The child should be told what is expected while on the potty. Give the child enough time to evacuate the bowel but do not have the child sit on the potty too long. The child (and the parent) may then become frustrated.

Children at this age like to give and to please their parents. Evacuation of the bowel is a natural process and should not be approached as if it is a dirty or unnatural process. The children should be rewarded when able to defecate, but should not be punished if unable to have a bowel movement. Children should feel a pride in accomplishment but may feel shame or doubt if punished for not giving what is expected.

Children usually do not need enemas or laxatives to make them regular. In fact, those artificial aids may be dangerous. Lack of parental understanding of the elimination process and of the developmental aspects of children coupled with harsh punishment for "accidents" may lead a child to an obsessive, meticulous, and rigid personality.

Accidents can and do occur even after a child has been completely toilet trained. These accidents usually occur because the child ignores the defecation urge. Usually this occurs because the child is engrossed in another activity and does not want to take the time to go to the bathroom or because other stressors have a higher priority at the moment.

School-Age Child

The urinary system is functioning maturely by this age. The normal output is 500 ml/day. Urinary tract infections are normal because of careless hygiene practices.

The gastrointestinal system attains adult functional maturity during the school years.

Adolescent

There are no noticeable differences in patterns of urinary elimination in this age group. The intestines grow in length and width. The muscles of the intestines become thicker and stronger.

This developmental stage is important in developing bowel habits. The teenager is engaged in developing sexuality. This group may ignore warning signals for elimination because they do not want to leave their activities or because of the close association of the anus to the teenager's developing sexual organs. Additionally, if a problem arises with elimination, adolescents are reluctant to talk about it with either their peers or an adult.

Young Adult

There is no noticeable difference in patterns of elimination during this developmental period. Total urinary output for 24 hours is 1000–2000 ml. The rate of passage of feces is influenced by the nature of the foods consumed and the physical health of the individual. Hemorrhoids are possible in this developmental group, especially females.

Adult

Adequate daily fluid intake helps to maintain proper elimination functions. There is a gradual decrease in the number of nephrons (the functional unit of the kidney) and therefore decreased renal functioning with age.

Digestive enzymes (gastric acid, pepsin, ptyalin, pancreatic enzymes) begin to decrease. This may lead to an increasing incidence of intestinal disorders, cancer, and gastrointestinal complaints.

Older Adult

Renal function is slowed by both the structural and functional changes of aging. This is mainly due to the decrease in the number of nephrons. However, the heart also pumps less blood to the kidney, leading to a decrease in the glomerular filtration rate and a decrease in the concentrating and diluting ability of the kidneys. Wastes can be effectively processed by the kidney but it takes longer.

The older male adult may have an enlarged prostate gland. An enlarged prostate gland can lead to urethritis, incomplete emptying of the bladder, and difficulty in initiating stream. Both male and female older adults have an increased incidence of urinary tract infections.

The female may, as a result of decreased muscle tone in the peritoneal area, have stress incontinence and uterine prolapse. This situation leads to embarrassment and self-imposed social isolation.

There are many changes in routines in the older adult. Activity is slowed; diet habits are erratic; and there is physical, social, and environmental immobility. There are also neurologic changes or alterations in the interpretation of neurologic signs that may then alter elimination. The older adult tends to pass urine more frequently because of decreased bladder capacity and will have a degree of urgency in urination (Carnevali & Patrick, 1979).

There is a continued decrease in digestive enzymes. There is also a decreased absorption rate which leads to a decreased absorption of nutrients and drugs. Intestinal muscle tone is decreased but the muscles are thicker. This leads to slower peristalsis and slower elimination.

Constipation is a usual factor of aging based not only on the above factors but also on the changes in dietary habits, routine, activity, and mobility (physical, social, environmental) of the elderly.

Applicable Nursing Diagnoses

Bowel Elimination, Altered: Constipation or Intermittent Constipation

DEFINITION

A state in which an individual experiences a change in normal bowel habits characterized by a decrease in frequency or passage of hard, dry stools (North American Nursing Diagnosis Association [NANDA], 1987, p. 22).

DEFINING CHARACTERISTICS (NANDA, 1987, p. 22)

The nurse will review the initial pattern assessment for the following defining characteristics to determine the diagnosis of Bowel Elimination, Altered: Constipation or Intermittent Constipation Pattern.

1. Major defining characteristics
   a. Decreased activity level
   b. Frequency less than usual pattern
   c. Hard form stools
   d. Palpable mass
   e. Reported feeling of pressure in rectum
   f. Reported feeling of rectal fullness
   g. Straining at stool
2. Minor defining characteristics
   a. Abdominal pain
   b. Appetite impairment
   c. Back pain
   d. Headache
   e. Interference with daily living
   f. Use of laxatives

RELATED FACTORS

None given.

DIFFERENTIATION

Bowel Elimination, Altered: Constipation or Intermittent Constipation Pattern would need to be differentiated from several other nursing diagnoses.

For example, Nutrition, Altered: Less or More Than Body Requirements may be the primary nursing diagnosis. Either of these diagnoses influences the amount and consistency of the feces. Fluid Volume Deficit may also be the primary problem. The feces needs adequate lubrication to pass through the gastrointestinal tract. If there is a Fluid Volume Deficit, the feces is harder, more solid, and unable to move through the system.

Bowel Elimination, Altered: Constipation also needs to be differentiated from diarrhea or incontinence. Diarrhea or incontinence may be a secondary condition to constipation, as semiliquid feces may pass around the area of constipation.

Physical Mobility, Altered could be the underlying cause for constipation. Decrease in physical mobility affects every body system. In the GI tract, peristalsis is slowed, which may lead to a backlog of feces and to constipation. Self-Care Deficit: Toileting may also be the primary cause.

Coping, Ineffective and Anxiety are two psychosocial nursing diagnoses from which Bowel Elimination, Altered: Constipation needs to be differentiated. Both of these psychosocial diagnoses initiate stress as an autonomic response, and the parasympathetic system stimuli (which controls motility of the GI tract) is reduced. This reduced motility may lead to constipation.

Other diagnoses which are included in the taxonomy under the heading of Constipation are Colonic Constipation and Perceived Constipation. Colonic constipation is defined as a state in which an individual's pattern of elimination is characterized by hard, dry stool which results from a delay in passage of food residue. Colonic constipation includes the major defining characteristics of decreased frequency; hard, dry stool; straining at stool; painful defecating; abdominal distention; and palpable mass.

Minor defining characteristics include rectal pressure, headache, appetite impairment, and abdominal pain. Related factors include less-than-adequate fluid intake, less-than-adequate dietary intake, less-than-adequate fiber, less-than-adequate physical activity, immobility, lack of privacy, emotional disturbances, chronic use of medication and enemas, stress, change in daily routine, metabolic problems (e.g., hypothyrodism, hypocalcemia, hypokalemia) (NANDA, 1988).

Perceived constipation is defined as a state in which an individual makes a self-diagnosis of constipation and ensures a daily bowel movement through use of laxatives, enemas, and suppositories. Major defining characteristics are expectation of a daily bowel movement with the resulting overuse of laxatives, enemas, and suppositories and expected passage of stool at same time every day. No minor defining characteristics have been given. Related factors include cultural or family health beliefs, faulty appraisal, and impaired thought processes (NANDA, 1988).

OBJECTIVES

1. Will return, as nearly as possible, to usual bowel elimination habits by (date).

AND/OR

2. Will design and carry out a plan to avoid constipation by (date).

TARGET DATE

Target dates should be based on the individual's usual bowel elimination habits. A target date 3–5 days from admission would be reasonable for the majority of patients.

NURSING ORDERS

ADULT HEALTH

1. Collaborate with dietitian regarding a high-fiber, high-roughage diet.
2. Force fluids, of patient's choice, to at least 2000 ml daily. Encourage 8 ounces of fluid every 2 hours on the (odd/even) hour beginning at awakening each morning.
3. Increase patient's activity to extent possible through ambulation at least three times per shift while awake.
4. Collaborate with physical therapist regarding exercise program.
5. Help patient assume anatomically correct position for bowel movements.
6. Collaborate with physician regarding mild analgesics and ointments for control of pain associated with bowel movements.
7. Provide privacy and sufficient time for bowel elimination.
8. Use rectal tube, heat, activity, and frequent change of position for problems with flatulence.
9. Measure and total intake and output every shift. Be sure to include estimation of loss by perspiration.
10. Monitor anal skin integrity at least once per shift.
11. Assist patient with exercises, every 4 hours while awake, to strengthen pelvic floor and abdominal muscles:
    a. Bent-knee situps.
    b. Straight- or bent-leg lifts.
    c. Alternating contraction and relaxation of perineal muscles while sitting in a chair and with feet placed apart on floor. Have patient repeat each exercise at least 5 times.
12. Assist patient with implementation of stress reduction techniques at least once per shift.
13. Teach patient:

    a. To understand importance of a daily routine;
    b. To stimulate gastrocolic reflex through drinking prune juice or hot liquid upon arising;
    c. To allow sufficient time for bowel movement;
    d. To include high-fiber foods and extra liquid in daily diet;
    e. To avoid prolonged use of elimination aids such as laxatives and enemas;
    f. To avoid straining;
    g. To use proper perineal hygiene;
    h. To understand the relationship of diet and activity to bowel elimination.
14. Record amount, color, and consistency of bowel movement following each bowel movement. Question patient regarding bowel movements at least once per shift. Also record if no bowel movement on each shift.
15. Provide a room deodorizer for patient.
16. If fecal impaction:
    a. Attempt digital removal using gloves and lubrication.
    b. Administer oil retention enema of small volume. Have patient retain for at least 1 hour.
    c. Use small volume saline enema if oil retention does not relieve impaction.
    d. Collaborate with physician regarding use of glycerine or other types of suppositories.
17. Collaborate with physician regarding use of stool softeners, laxatives, suppositories, and enemas.
18. Digitally stimulate anal sphincter and defecation reflex.
19. Use cool compresses to alleviate anal itching.
20. Collaborate with enterstomal therapist regarding ostomy care (i.e., irrigations, stoma and skin care, appliances).

CHILD HEALTH

1. Monitor and record symptoms associated with passage of bowel movement:
    a. Any straining, pain, or headache
    b. Any rectal bleeding or fissures
2. Encourage daily intake of fluids, including juices, according to child's requisites and preferences.
3. Collaborate with physician and other health personnel regarding:
    a. Dietary teaching and considerations for increased fiber;
    b. Use of stool softeners or laxatives and precautions;
    c. Counseling for child and family regarding possible underlying emotional components;
    d. Physical therapy, exercise, or diversion;
    e. Specific plan to ensure privacy, comfort, and consistency in dealing with elimination patterns;
    f. Enterostomal therapy for specific stomal care;
    g. Follow-up planning for home and usual daily activities of living with emphasis on stress, etc.

WOMEN'S HEALTH

1. Assist patient in identifying life-style adjustments that may be needed due to changes in physiologic function or needs during experiential phases of life (e.g., pregnancy, postpartum, and after gynecologic surgery).
    a. Establishing regular bowel habits
    b. Establishing exercise program
2. Teach client changes that occur during pregnancy which contribute to decreased gastric motility.
3. Describe anatomic shifting of abdominal contents due to fetal growth.
4. Describe hormonal influences (e.g., increased progesterone) on bodily functions:

    a. Decreased stomach emptying time

    b. Decreased peristalsis

    c. Increase in water reabsorption

    d. Decrease in exercise

    e. Relaxation of abdominal muscles

    f. Increase in flatulence

5. Describe the effects of the increase in oral iron or calcium supplements on the gastrointestinal tract.

6. Assist patient in planning diet which increases bulk, fiber, and fluid intake.

7. Review daily schedule with patient and assist patient in planning an exercise program.

8. Describe the physical changes present in the immediate postpartum period that affect the gastrointestinal tract.

    a. Lax abdominal muscles

    b. Fluid loss (perspiration, urine, lochia, dehydration during labor and delivery)

    c. Hunger

9. Assist patient in planning diet which will promote healing, replace lost fluids, and help with return to normal bowel evacuation.

10. Instruct in the use of ointments, anesthetic sprays, sitz baths, and witch hazel compresses to relieve episiotomy pain and reduce hemorrhoids.

11. Collaborate with physician regarding use of stool softeners, laxatives, suppositories, and enemas.

12. Instruct in pelvic floor exercises (Kegel exercises) to assist healing and reduce pain.

13. Teach nursing mothers alternate methods of assistance with bowel evacuation other than cathartics (cathartics are expressed in breast milk).

    a. Prune juice

    b. Hot liquids

    c. High-fiber, high-roughage diet

    d. Daily exercise

14. Describe the physical changes present in the immediate postoperative period that affect the gastrointestinal tract.

    a. Fluid loss (blood loss or dehydration as a result of being NPO and surgery)

    b. Decreased peristalsis

        (1) Bowel manipulation during surgery

        (2) Increased use of analgesics and anesthesia

MENTAL HEALTH

The nursing orders for this diagnosis in mental health application are the same as those for adult health or child health. Please refer to those orders.

HOME HEALTH

1. Teach patient and family the definition of constipation. Determine if problem is perceived by patient due to incorrect definition or is based on physiologic dysfuntion.

2. Teach patient and family measures to ensure adequate bowel elimination.

    a. High-fiber, high-roughage diet

    b. Fluids to at least 2000 ml daily

    c. Regular exercise and activity

    d. Warm fluids ½ hour prior to scheduled elimination to stimulate evacuation

    e. Exercises to strengthen pelvic floor and abdominal muscles:

        (1) Bent-leg situps

        (2) Isometric contraction of perineal muscles while sitting in chair with feet on floor

            (a) Correct position for elimination

        (b) Perineal hygiene

        (c) Avoidance of straining

3. Assist patient and family in identifying life-style changes that may be required:
   a. Food, fluids, and exercise as above
   b. Avoidance of laxative and enema abuse
   c. Establishment of a regular elimination routine based on cultural and individual variations
   d. Stress management techniques
   e. Decrease in concentrated, refined foods
   f. Need for privacy
   g. Identification of any food intolerances or allergies and avoidance of those foods
   h. Environmental conditions conducive to proper elimination:
      (1) Privacy
      (2) Sufficient time
      (3) Room deodorizer
      (4) Reading material if desired
4. Monitor and teach importance of appropriate medications as ordered by physician.
5. Teach patient and family appropriate use and frequency of use of over-the-counter medications.
6. Teach patient and family to monitor color, frequency, consistency, and pattern of symptoms.
7. Refer to appropriate assistive resources as indicated:
   a. Visiting nurse
   b. Physician
   c. Physical therapist
   d. Nutritionist

EVALUATION
OBJECTIVE 1

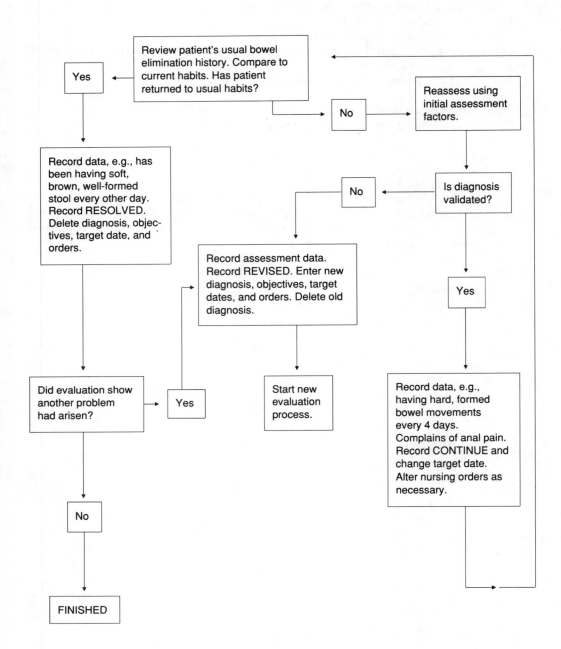

OBJECTIVE 2

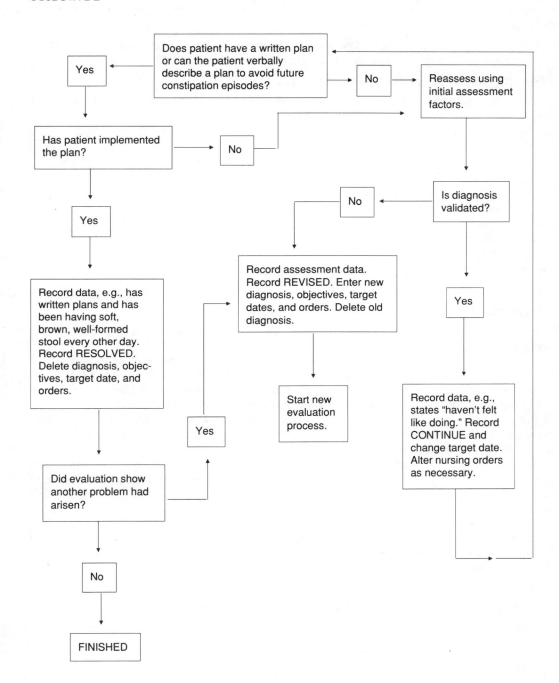

Bowel Elimination, Altered: Diarrhea

DEFINITION

A state in which an individual experiences a change in normal bowel habits characterized by the frequent passage of loose, fluid, unformed stools (NANDA, 1987, p. 23).

DEFINING CHARACTERISTICS (NANDA, 1987, p. 23)

The nurse will review the initial pattern assessment for the following defining characteristics to determine the diagnosis of Bowel Elimination, Altered: Diarrhea.

1. Major defining characteristics
   a. Abdominal pain
   b. Cramping
   c. Increased frequency
   d. Increased frequency of bowel sounds
   e. Loose, liquid stools
   f. Urgency
2. Minor defining characteristics
   a. Change in color

RELATED FACTORS

None given.

DIFFERENTIATION

Bowel Elimination, Altered: Diarrhea would need to be differentiated from several other nursing diagnoses.

For example, with Bowel Elimination, Altered: Constipation, diarrhea may be secondary to a primary problem of constipation if semiliquid feces is leaking around the constipated feces.

Nutrition, Altered: Less Than Body Requirements could be the primary problem. The individual is not ingesting enough food or sufficient bulk to allow feces to be well formed. Fluid Volume Deficit and Fluid Volume Excess are also nursing diagnoses that need to be differentiated from Bowel Elimination, Altered: Diarrhea. The amount of fluid ingested or absorbed by the body can affect the consistency of the fecal material.

Anxiety, Self-Esteem Disturbance, or Ineffective Coping may also be confused with Bowel Elimination, Altered: Diarrhea. Any of these diagnoses precipitates a stress response. Indices of stress include gastrointestinal signs and symptoms, including diarrhea, vomiting, and "butterflies" in the stomach.

A Sleep Pattern Disturbance may be the primary diagnosis and should be differentiated from Bowel Elimination, Altered: Diarrhea. If a person's biologic clock is changed because of altered sleep-wake patterns, body responses attuned to the biologic clock will also be altered. This includes usual elimination patterns. Diarrhea may result.

OBJECTIVES

1. Will have no more than one soft, formed bowel movement per day by (date).

AND/OR

2. Will return to usual bowel elimination habits by (date).

TARGET DATE

Target dates should be based on the individual's usual bowel elimination habits. Thus, a target date 3 days from the day of admission would be reasonable for the majority of patients. Since diarrhea can be particularly life-threatening for infants and older adults, a target date of 2 days would not be too soon.

NURSING ORDERS

ADULT HEALTH

1. Make sure bathroom facilities are readily available.
2. Increase fluid intake to at least 2500 ml per day. Offer fluids high in potassium and sodium at least once per hour. Serve fluids at tepid temperatures. Avoid hot or cold fluids.
3. Collaborate with dietitian regarding low-fiber, low-residue, soft diet. Avoid irritant foods described by patient.
4. Monitor anal skin integrity at least once per shift.
5. Provide room deodorizer and chlorophyll tablets for patient.
6. Record amount, color, consistency, and odor following each bowel movement.
7. Provide perineal skin care after each bowel movement.
8. Measure and total intake and output each shift.
9. Monitor weight and electrolytes at least every 2 days while diarrhea persists.
10. Assist patient with stress reduction techniques at least once per shift; provide quiet, restful atmosphere.
11. Administer antidiarrheal medications as ordered.
12. If tube feedings are causal factor, collaborate with physician regarding:
    a. Infusion rate
    b. Temperature of feeding
    c. Dilution of feeding
    d. Following feeding with water.
13. Teach patient:
    a. Diet—avoid irritating foods, include basic four food groups, influence of fiber.
    b. Fluids—maintain good fluid balance.
    c. Medications—those that are antidiarrheal, those that promote diarrhea.

CHILD HEALTH

1. Monitor intake and output accurately.
   a. Weigh diapers for urine and stools, assess specific gravity every voiding.
   b. Note consistency of stool and presence of reducing substances, and document same.
   c. Ensure proper administration of fluids as ordered.
   d. Monitor for signs and symptoms of dehydration to include:
      (1) Depressed anterior fontanel in infants
      (2) Poor skin turgor
      (3) Decreased urinary output
2. Monitor signs and symptoms associated with bowel movements, including cramping, flatus, crying.
3. Monitor bowel movements every shift and for 24-hour period.
4. Weigh patient daily at same time, on same scale.
5. Collaborate with physician regarding:
   a. Frequent stooling (more than three times per shift);
   b. Excessive vomiting;
   c. Possible dietary consultation for specific formula or diet;
   d. Monitoring electrolytes and renal function;
   e. Maintenance of IV fluids;
   f. Antidiarrheal medications;
   g. Possible relationship to tube feedings.
6. Provide prompt and gentle cleansing after each diaper change. For older children offer warm soaks after diarrhea episodes.
7. Provide air freshener for room as needed.

8. Exercise appropriate care in disposal of stool, and follow appropriate guidelines for infection control and enteric precautions if applicable.

WOMEN'S HEALTH

(Note: Some women experience diarrhea 1 or 2 days before labor begins. It is not certain why this occurs but is thought to be due to the irritation of the bowel by the contracting uterus and the decrease in hormonal levels [estrogen and progestrone] in late pregnancy. See Adult Health. Nursing orders 1–12 listed there apply to women's health. For diarrhea which is a preceptor to labor the following nursing orders apply.)

1. Offer oral electrolyte solutions such as:
    a. Gatorade
    b. Coca-Cola (Classic)
    c. Jello
    d. "New runner's drink" from Coca-Cola Company
    e. Pedialyte

MENTAL HEALTH

1. Maintain fluid intake to at least 2500 ml per day. Provide fluids that are high in potassium and sodium. Serve fluids at room temperature. (List client's preferred fluids here so they can be provided.)
2. Ask client about those foods that are irritating and list them here so they can be eliminated from the diet.
3. Teach client the importance of diet in diarrhea and inform client about:
    a. Increasing intake of fluids high in sodium and potassium during diarrhea;
    b. Limiting intake of caffeine, high-fiber foods, milk, fruits, and those foods that are personally irritating.
4. Discuss with client the role stress and anxiety play in this problem.
5. Develop with client stress reduction plan and practice specific interventions three times a day at (list times here).
6. Refer to Chapter 8 for specific interventions related to the diagnosis of Anxiety.
7. Provide room deodorizer, chlorophyll tablets, and fresh parsley for client.

HOME HEALTH

1. Teach patient and family measures to decrease diarrhea.
    a. Avoid foods known to be irritants to the individual.
    b. Make diet low in fiber, low in fruits, low in roughage, and soft.
    c. Decrease or avoid caffeine.
    d. Administer antidiarrheal medications as directed by physician.
    e. Avoid hot or cold fluids (tepid only).
2. Teach family and patient principles of maintaining fluid and electrolyte balance. (2500 ml fluid daily; foods high in potassium and sodium).
3. Teach family and patient techniques of perianal hygiene.
4. Teach family and patient techniques for monitoring perianal skin integrity.
5. Assist patient and family in identifying life-style changes that may be required.
    a. Avoid drinking local water when traveling in areas where water supply may be contaminated (foreign countries, streams and lakes when camping).
    b. Practice stress management.
    c. Avoid laxative or enema abuse.
    d. Avoid foods which cause symptoms.
    e. Avoid bingeing behavior.
6. Monitor and teach importance of appropriate medications as ordered by physician.

7. Teach patient and family appropriate use and frequency of use of over-the-counter medications.
8. Assist patient and family to set criteria to help them to determine when a physician or other intervention is required.
9. Refer to appropriate assistive resources as indicated:
    a. Nutritionist
    b. Physician

EVALUATION
OBJECTIVE 1

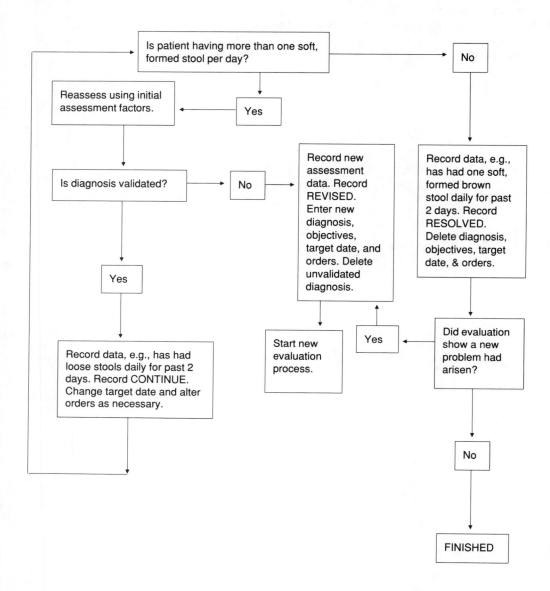

OBJECTIVE 2

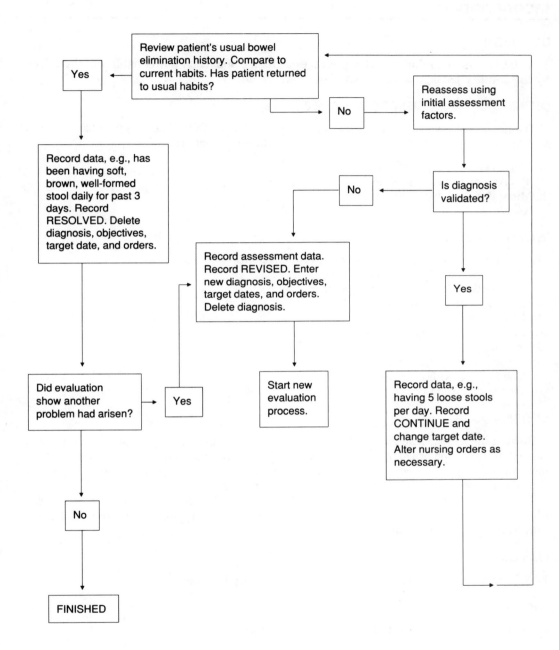

Bowel Elimination, Altered: Incontinence or Bowel Incontinence

DEFINITION

A state in which an individual experiences a change in normal bowel habits characterized by involuntary passage of stool (NANDA, 1987, p. 24).

DEFINING CHARACTERISTICS (NANDA, 1987, p. 24)

The nurse will review the initial pattern assessment for the following defining characteristics to determine the diagnosis of Bowel Elimination, Altered: Incontinence.

1. Major defining characteristics
   a. Involuntary passage of stool
2. Minor defining characteristics
   None given.

RELATED FACTORS

1. Organic changes in neural innervation of the rectum.
2. Decreased sensation of rectal filling.
3. Increased excitability of rectal sphincter.
4. Decreased anal muscle tone.
5. Loss of cortical control.
6. Inflammation or cancer of the rectum.
7. Rectal prolapse.
8. Quality of fecal material.
9. Constipation with impaction and overflow.
10. Mental confusion.

DIFFERENTIATION

Bowel Elimination, Altered: Incontinence needs to be differentiated from Bowel Elimination, Altered: Constipation or Diarrhea. The problem may really be due to constipation with impaction. Incontinence may occur because some feces is leaking around the impaction site and the individual is unable to control its passage and thus appears incontinent.

The nursing diagnosis of Self-Care Deficit: Toileting may be one that is confused with Bowel Elimination, Altered: Incontinence. If the individual is unable to appropriately care for his or her evacuation needs, incontinence may result.

OBJECTIVES

1. Will have no more than one soft, formed stool per day by (date).

AND/OR

2. Will return to usual bowel elimination habits by (date).

TARGET DATE

Target dates should be based on the individual's usual bowel elimination pattern. Incontinence may require additional retraining time and effort. Therefore, a target date 5 days from admission may be tried. Also, remember that there must be a realistic potential that bowel continence can be regained by the patient.

NURSING ORDERS

ADULT HEALTH

1. Record timing of each incontinent episode and the amount, color, and consistency of each stool.
2. Record events associated with incontinent episode, including events both before and after the episode (i.e., activity, stress, etc.).
3. Check for fecal impaction and implement nursing orders from Bowel Elimination, Altered: Constipation.
4. Initiate bowel training:
   a. Suppository ½ hour after eating
   b. Toilet ½ hour after suppository insertion
   c. Toilet prior to activity
   d. Stimulate defecation reflex with circular movement in rectum using gloved, lubricated finger
5. Monitor anal skin integrity at least once per shift.
6. Keep anal area clean and dry.
7. Provide room deodorizer and chlorophyll tablets for patient.
8. Provide emotional support for patient through teaching, providing time for listening, etc. Refer to psychiatric nurse clinician as necessary.
9. Teach patient:
   a. Pelvic floor strengthening exercises (See Bowel Elimination, Altered: Constipation);
   b. Diet—Role of fiber and fluids;
   c. Use of assistive devices—Velcro closings on clothes, pads;
   d. Perineal hygiene;
   e. Appropriate use of suppositories, antidiarrheal medications.
10. Refer for home health care assistance.

CHILD HEALTH

Nursing orders for Bowel Elimination, Altered: Incontinence for the child are the same as for adult health. Modifications would be made for developmental levels such as medications.

WOMEN'S HEALTH

Bowel incontinence in women caused by uterine prolapse and pelvic relaxation with displacement of pelvic organs (particularly the rectum) is relieved only by surgical repair (Fogel & Woods, 1981). Otherwise, nursing orders for incontinence in women's health are the same as in adult health.

MENTAL HEALTH

(Note: The nursing orders for the mental health client will be the same as those described for adult health. The following orders are specific considerations that should be added for the mental health client.)

1. Record events associated with incontinent episode, including events both before and after the episode (i.e., activity, stress, location, persons present, etc.).
2. If a pattern forms around specific events, develop plan to:
   a. Encourage person to use bathroom before the event;
   b. Alter the manner in which specific task is performed to prevent stress;
   c. Discuss with client alternative ways of coping with stress;
   d. If assessment suggests secondary gains associated with episodes, decrease these by:
      (1) Withdrawing social contact after an episode;
      (2) Having client clean himself or herself;

(3) Providing social contact or interactions with the client at times when no incontinence is experienced.
3. If not related to secondary gain spend (number) minutes with client after each episode to allow expression of feelings.
4. Discuss with client effects this problem has on life-style.
5. Refer to appropriate assistive resources to include:
   a. Visiting nurse
   b. Nutritionist
   c. Occupational therapist
   d. Physical therapist

HOME HEALTH

1. Teach patient and family to monitor and maintain skin integrity.
2. Keep bed linens and clothing clean and dry.
3. Monitor and teach importance of appropriate medication as ordered by physician.
4. Teach patient and family appropriate use and frequency of use of over-the-counter medications.
5. Teach patient and family to monitor color, frequency, consistency, and pattern of symptoms.
6. Teach patient and family measures to ensure adequate bowel elimination.
   a. Proper diet
   b. Fluid and electrolyte balance
   c. Pelvic floor and abdominal exercises
7. Refer to appropriate assistive resources as indicated:
   a. Psychiatric clinical specialist
   b. Nutritionist
   c. Physical therapist
   d. Rehabilitation specialist

EVALUATION
OBJECTIVE 1

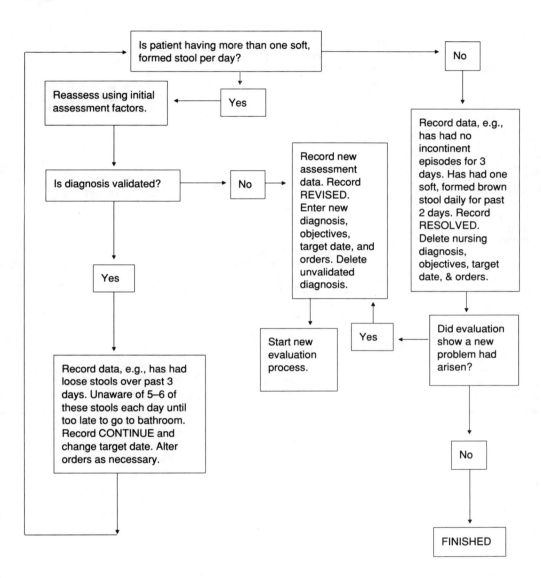

Is patient having more than one soft, formed stool per day?

No

Yes

Reassess using initial assessment factors.

Is diagnosis validated?

No

Record new assessment data. Record REVISED. Enter new diagnosis, objectives, target date, and orders. Delete unvalidated diagnosis.

Record data, e.g., has had no incontinent episodes for 3 days. Has had one soft, formed brown stool daily for past 2 days. Record RESOLVED. Delete nursing diagnosis, objectives, target date, & orders.

Yes

Start new evaluation process.

Yes

Did evaluation show a new problem had arisen?

Record data, e.g., has had loose stools over past 3 days. Unaware of 5–6 of these stools each day until too late to go to bathroom. Record CONTINUE and change target date. Alter orders as necessary.

No

FINISHED

OBJECTIVE 2

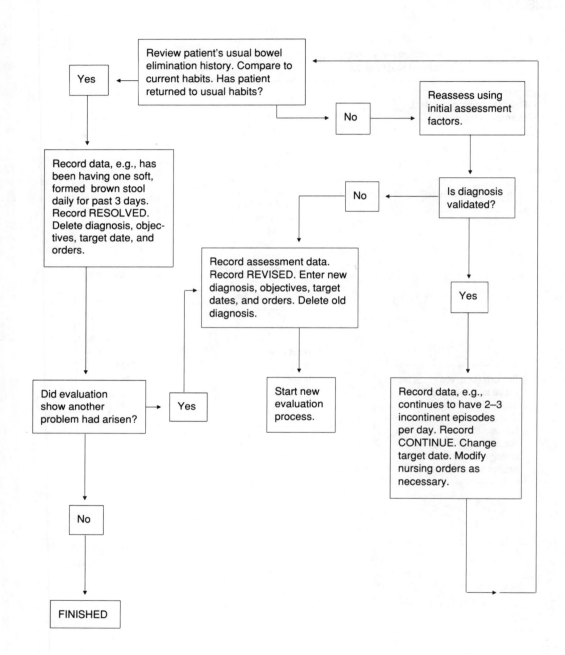

Urinary Elimination Patterns, Altered: Incontinence

DEFINITION

The state in which an individual experiences an involuntary loss of urine (NANDA, 1987, pp. 27–32).

DEFINING CHARACTERISTICS (NANDA, 1987, pp. 27–32)

The nurse will review the initial pattern assessment for the following defining characteristics to determine the diagnosis of Urinary Elimination Patterns, Altered: Incontinence.

1. Stress Incontinence—the state in which an individual experiences a loss of urine of less than 50 ml occurring with increased abdominal pressure (NANDA, 1987, p. 26).
   a. Major defining characteristics (NANDA, 1987, p. 26)
      (1) Reported or observed dribbling with increased abdominal pressure
   b. Minor defining characteristics (NANDA, 1987, p. 26)
      (1) Urinary urgency
      (2) Urinary frequency (more often than every 2 hours)
2. Reflex Incontinence—the state in which an individual experiences an involuntary loss of urine, occurring at somewhat predictable intervals when a specific volume is reached (NANDA, 1987, p. 28).
   a. Major defining characteristics (NANDA, 1987, p. 28)
      (1) No awareness of bladder filling
      (2) No urge to void or feelings of bladder fullness
      (3) Uninhibited bladder contraction or spasms at regular intervals
   b. Minor defining characteristics
      None given.
3. Urge Incontinence—the state in which an individual experiences involuntary passage of urine occurring soon after a strong sense to void (NANDA, 1987, p.29).
   a. Major defining characteristics (NANDA, 1987, p. 29)
      (1) Urinary urgency
      (2) Frequency (voiding more often than every 2 hours)
      (3) Bladder contraction or spasm
   b. Minor defining characteristics (NANDA, 1987, p. 29).
      (1) Nocturia (more than 2 times per night)
      (2) Voiding in small amounts (less than 100 ml)
      (3) Voiding in large amounts (more than 550 ml)
4. Functional Incontinence—the state in which an individual experiences an involuntary, unpredictable passage of urine (NANDA, 1987, p. 31).
   a. Major defining characteristics (NANDA, 1987, p. 31)
      (1) Urge to void or bladder contraction sufficiently strong to result in loss of urine before reaching an appropriate receptacle.
   b. Minor defining characteristics
      None given.
5. Total Incontinence—the state in which an individual experiences a continuous and unpredictable loss of urine (NANDA, 1987, p. 32).
   a. Major defining characteristics (NANDA, 1987, p. 32)
      (1) Constant flow of urine occurs at unpredictable times without distention or uninhibited bladder contraction or spasm.
   b. Minor defining characteristics (NANDA, 1987, p. 32)
      (1) Lack of perineal or bladder filling awareness

   (2) Unawareness of incontinence

RELATED FACTORS (NANDA, 1987, pp.26–32)

1. Degenerative changes in pelvic muscles and structural supports associated with increased age.
2. High intraabdominal pressure (e.g., obesity, gravid uterus).
3. Incompetent bladder outlet.
4. Overdistention of bladder between voidings.
5. Weak pelvic muscles and structural supports.
6. Neurologic impairment (e.g., spinal cord lesion which interferes with conduction of cerebral messages above the level of the reflex arc).
7. Decreased bladder capacity (e.g., history of pelvic inflammatory disease, abdominal surgeries, indwelling urinary catheter).
8. Irritation of bladder stretch receptors causing spasm (e.g., bladder infection).
9. Alcohol.
10. Caffeine
11. Increased fluids.
12. Increased urine concentration.
13. Altered environment.
14. Sensory, cognitive, or mobility deficits.
15. Neuropathy preventing transmission of reflex indicating bladder fullness.
16. Neurologic dysfunction causing triggering of micturition at unpredictable times.
17. Independent contraction of detrusor reflex due to surgery.
18. Trauma or disease affecting spinal cord nerves.
19. Anatomic (fistula).

DIFFERENTIATION

   Urinary Elimination Patterns, Altered: Incontinence needs to be differentiated from Bowel Elimination, Altered: Constipation; Fluid Volume, Altered: Deficit or Excess; Urinary Retention; Sensory-Perceptual Alterations; Input Deficit; Self-Esteem or Body Image Disturbance; Verbal Communication, Impaired; and Physical Mobility; Impaired.

   Anything in the body that creates additional pressure on the bladder or bladder sphincter may precipitate voiding. Bowel Elimination, Altered: Constipation can create this additional pressure because of the increased amount of fecal material in the sigmoid colon and rectum. Incontinence may then be a direct result of constipation or fecal impaction.

   Since urination depends on input of the stimulus that the bladder is full and since one of the ways the body responds to excess fluid volume is by increasing urinary output, the very fact that there is excess fluid volume may result in the bladder's inability to keep up with the kidney's production of urine. Thus incontinence may occur. Conversely, Fluid Volume Deficit can result in incontinence by eliminating the sensation of a full bladder and by decreasing the person's awareness of the sensation. Additionally, the perception and interpretation by the brain of the sensation that the bladder is full may be diminished. Thus a Sensory-Perceptual Deficit may occur with resultant incontinence.

   As previously stated, the person must be able to control the sphincter, walk a few steps, recognize and interpret that the bladder is full, and be able to indicate that he or she wants to go to the bathroom. Even if the person has some control of the sphincter and has correctly recognized and interpreted the cues of a full bladder, if he or she is unable to get to the bathroom or get there in time because of Physical Mobility, Impaired, the person may become incontinent. This may happen especially in a hospital. The ability to verbally communicate the need to urinate is important. If the person is unable to tell someone or have someone understand that he or she wants to go to the bathroom, incontinence may occur.

Sometimes the person may have an accident of incontinence. That person knows that control of urination is necessary for social acceptance. The person may then become very embarrassed and afraid that the accident may occur again, thus experiencing a Body Image Disturbance and an Alteration in Self-Esteem. In some ways this may become a self-fulfilling prophecy in that the greater the alteration in body image or self-esteem, the greater the incidence of incontinence and further alteration in body image and self-esteem.

OBJECTIVES

1. Will remain continent at least 90% of the time by (date).

AND/OR

2. Will design and carry out personal continence plan by (date).

TARGET DATE

Incontinence will require training time and effort; therefore, a target date 5 days from the date of admission would be reasonable to evaluate the patient's progress toward meeting the objectives. Additionally, there must be a realistic potential that urinary continence may be regained by the patient. For this reason, it would need to be qualified for use with handicapped or neurologically deficient clients according to exact level of continence hoped for.

NURSING ORDERS

ADULT HEALTH

1. Record:
    a. Time and amounts of each voiding;
    b. Whether voiding was continent or incontinent;
    c. Patient's activity before and after incontinent incidence.
2. Monitor, at least every 2 hours on (odd/even) hour, for continence.
3. Schedule toileting.
    a. Schedule at least 30 minutes before recorded incontinence times.
    b. Awaken patient once during night for voiding.
    c. Encourage patient to consciously hold urine to stretch bladder.
    d. Stimulate voiding at scheduled time by:
        (1) Assisting patient to maintain normal anatomic position for voiding;
        (2) Having patient lightly brush inner thighs or lower abdomen;
        (3) Running warm water over perineum (measure amount first);
        (4) Having patient listen to dripping water;
        (5) Placing patient's hands in warm water;
        (6) Using Crede's or Valsalva maneuver. (see Additional Information at end of chapter);
        (7) Gently tapping over bladder;
        (8) Drinking water while trying to void;
        (9) Providing privacy;
        (10) Providing night light and clear path to bathroom;
        (11) Sitting on firm towel roll when incontinence threatens;
        (12) Gradually increasing length of time, by 15 minutes, between voidings.
4. Establish a bladder retraining program (see Additional Information at end of chapter).
5. Respond immediately to patient's request for toileting.
6. Teach patient exercises to strengthen pelvic floor muscles (10 times each at least 4 times per day):
    a. Contracting posterior perineal muscles as if trying to stop a bowel movement.
    b. Contracting anterior perineal muscles as if trying to stop voiding.
    c. Starting and stopping urinary stream.
    d. Bent-knee situps.

e. Straight leg lifts.
7. Teach patient the importance of maintaining a daily routine:
   a. Voiding upon arising
   b. Awakening self once during the night
   c. Voiding immediately before retiring
   d. Not postponing voiding unnecessarily
8. Schedule fluid intake:
   a. Avoid fluids containing caffeine and other fluids that produce a diuretic effect (e.g., grapefruit juice, alcohol).
   b. Encourage 8 ounces every 2 hours during day.
   c. Limit fluids after 6 PM.
9. Maintain bowel elimination. Monitor bowel movements and record at least once each shift.
10. Monitor:
    a. Weight at least every 3 days;
    b. Lab values (e.g., electrolytes, WBC, urinanalysis);
    c. Perineal skin integrity at least once per shift:
       (1) Cleanse after each voiding.
       (2) Apply medicated ointments as ordered.
       (3) Use heat lamp as needed.
       (4) Consult with enterostomal therapist regarding any stoma care.
       (5) Give sitz baths.
    d. Intake and output each shift;
    e. For bladder distention at least every 2 hours.
11. Teach perineal skin care.
12. Collaborate with physician regarding:
    a. Intermittent catheterization;
    b. Medications (e.g., urinary antiseptics, analgesics, etc.).
13. Collaborate with dietitian regarding food and fluids to acidify urine (e.g., cranberry juice, citrus fruits).
14. Guard, and teach patient to guard, against nosocomial infection.
15. Encourage patient that he or she can be continent again and encourage to avoid social isolation:
    a. Wearing street clothes with protective pads in undergarments.
    b. Maintaining bladder retraining program
    c. Responding as soon as possible to voiding urge
    d. Taking oral chlorophyll tablets
    e. Losing weight if necessary
16. Assist patient with stress reduction and relaxation techniques at least once per shift.
17. Refer to home health care agency for follow-up.

CHILD HEALTH

Child health nursing orders for this diagnosis are the same as for adult health with appropriate modifications for developmental level.

WOMEN'S HEALTH

1. Assist client in identifying life-style adjustments that may be needed to accommodate changing bladder capacity due to anatomic changes of pregnancy.
   a. Illustrate reduction of bladder capacity due to enlarging uterus and anatomic changes of pregnancy.
2. Assist client in understanding the necessity for frequent voidings to avoid bladder distension.
   a. Voiding upon arising
   b. Voiding when urge is present during the day

   c. Voiding immediately before retiring

   d. Awakening self once during night

3. Teach and encourage client to do Kegel exercises to strengthen perineal muscles.

   a. Starting and stopping stream

   b. Contracting and relaxing perineal, vaginal, and anal muscles

   c. Straight leg lifts *should not be done* during pregnancy

4. Maintenance of fluid intake.

   a. Drink at least 2500 ml per 24 hours.

   b. Limit fluids after 8 PM.

5. Assist client in learning to recognize signs and symptoms of urinary tract infections.

   a. Urgency

   b. Burning

   c. Dysuria

6. Teach clients how to assess for temperature elevation (make certain they know how to read thermometer).

7. Instruct client to seek immediate medical care if symptoms of urinary tract infections appear.

MENTAL HEALTH

(Note: clients receiving the following drugs are at risk for this nursing diagnosis: hypnotics, antidepressants, and antipsychotics.)

If alteration is related to psychosocial issues and has no physiologic component, initiate the following plan (refer to Adult Health for physiologically produced problems):

1. Monitor times, places, persons present, and emotional climate around inappropriate voiding episodes.

2. Remind client to void before a high-risk situation or remove secondary gain process from situation.

3. Inform client of acceptable times and places for voiding and of consequences for inappropriate voiding.

4. Provide the client with supplies necessary to facilitate appropriate voiding behavior (e.g., urinal for client in locked seclusion area).

5. Have client assist with cleaning up any voiding that has occurred in an inappropriate place.

6. Provide as little interaction with client as possible during cleanup.

7. Provide client with positive reinforcement for voiding in appropriate place and time (list specific reinforcers for this client here).

8. Spend (number) minutes with client every hour in an activity the client has identified as enjoyable; do not provide this time or discontinue time if client inappropriately voids during the specified time (list identified activities here).

9. If client voids inappropriately (number) times during a shift he or she will spend (number) minutes (no more than 30) in time out. Each inappropriate voiding in time out adds 5 minutes to this time.

10. As behavior improves add rewards for accumulated times of appropriate voiding (e.g., one 2-hour pass for 1 day of appropriate voiding). Record those rewards here.

11. Refer to Chapter 8 for interventions related to the specific alterations that would promote this coping pattern.

HOME HEALTH

(Note: If this nursing diagnosis is made it is imperative that a physician referral be made. Vigorous intervention is required to prevent damage to the urinary tract or systemic infection. If referred to home care under physician's care, it is important to maintain and evaluate response to prescribed treatments.)

1. Assist patient and family in identifying life-style changes that may be required:
   a. Using proper perineal hygiene.
   b. Taking showers instead of tub baths.
   c. Drinking fluids to cause voiding every 2–3 hours to flush out bacteria; scheduling fluid intake.
   d. Voiding after intercourse.
   e. Avoiding perfumed soaps, toilet paper, feminine hygiene sprays.
   f. Wearing cotton underwear.
   g. Using proper handwashing techniques.
   h. Following a daily routine of voiding—scheduling (see Adult Health care plan).
   i. Establishing a bladder retraining program (see Additional Information at end of chapter).
   j. Doing exercises to strengthen pelvic floor muscles.
   k. Providing an environment conducive to continence—street clothes and protective undergarments, air purifier, activities as tolerated, unobstructed access to bathroom.
2. Teach patient and family to dilute and acidify the urine:
   a. Increase fluids.
   b. Introduce cranberry juice, poultry, etc. to increase acid ash.
   c. Avoid fluids that produce diuretic effect (e.g., caffeine, alcohol, teas).
3. Teach patient and family to monitor and maintain skin integrity.
   a. Keep skin clean and dry.
   b. Keep bed linens and clothing clean and dry.
   c. Use proper perineal hygiene.
4. Assist patient and family to set criteria to help them to determine when a physician or other intervention is required.
5. Monitor and teach importance of appropriate medications and treatments ordered by physician.
6. Teach patient and family signs and symptoms of increasing problem:
   a. Urgency
   b. Frequency
   c. Hematuria
   d. Dysuria
7. Refer to appropriate assistive resources as indicated:
   a. Nutritionist
   b. Physical therapist
   c. Physician
   d. Visiting nurse
   e. Rehabilitation specialist

EVALUATION
OBJECTIVE 1

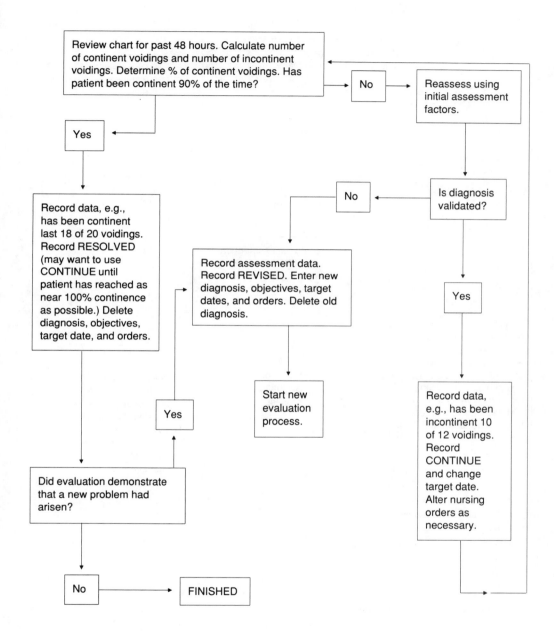

Review chart for past 48 hours. Calculate number of continent voidings and number of incontinent voidings. Determine % of continent voidings. Has patient been continent 90% of the time?

No

Reassess using initial assessment factors.

Yes

Is diagnosis validated?

No

Yes

Record data, e.g., has been continent last 18 of 20 voidings. Record RESOLVED (may want to use CONTINUE until patient has reached as near 100% continence as possible.) Delete diagnosis, objectives, target date, and orders.

Record assessment data. Record REVISED. Enter new diagnosis, objectives, target dates, and orders. Delete old diagnosis.

Record data, e.g., has been incontinent 10 of 12 voidings. Record CONTINUE and change target date. Alter nursing orders as necessary.

Yes

Start new evaluation process.

Did evaluation demonstrate that a new problem had arisen?

No → FINISHED

OBJECTIVE 2

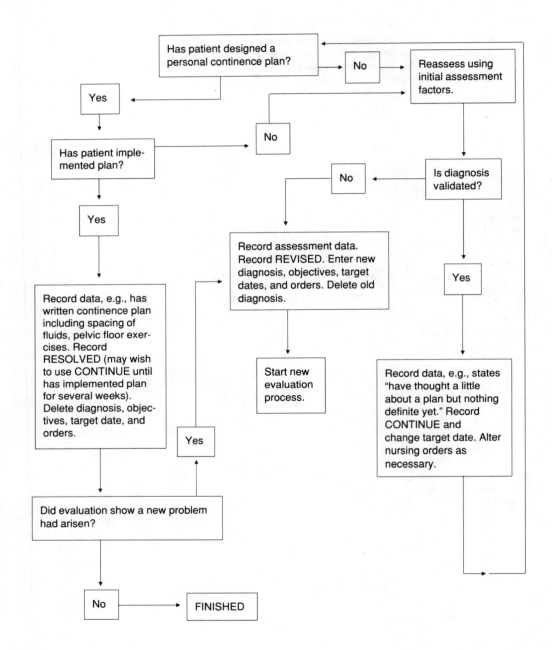

Urinary Retention

DEFINITION

The state in which the individual experiences incomplete emptying of the bladder (NANDA, 1987, p. 34).

DEFINING CHARACTERISTICS (NANDA, 1987, p. 34)

The nurse will review the initial pattern assessment for the following defining characteristics to determine the diagnosis of Urinary Retention.

1. Major defining characteristics (NANDA, 1987, p. 34)
   a. Bladder distention
   b. Small, frequent voiding
   c. Absence of urine output
2. Minor defining characteristics (NANDA, 1987, p. 34)
   a. Sensation of bladder fullness
   b. Dribbling
   c. Residual urine
   d. Dysuria
   e. Overflow incontinence

RELATED FACTORS (NANDA, 1987, p. 34)

1. High urethral pressure caused by weak detrusor urinae
2. Inhibition of reflex arc
3. Strong sphincter
4. Blockage

DIFFERENTIATION

Urinary Retention needs to be differentiated from Urinary Elimination Patterns, Altered: Incontinence. Overflow incontinence frequently occurs in patients whose primary problem is really retention. The bladder is overdistended in retention and some urine is passed involuntarily because of the pressure of the retained urine on the bladder sphincter.

Urinary Retention also needs to be differentiated from a Self-Care Deficit in Toileting, especially related to neurogenic bladder conditions. The bladder is chronically overdistended, resulting in Urinary Retention.

OBJECTIVES

1. Will void under voluntary control and emptying bladder at least every 4 hours by (date).

AND/OR

2. Will not demonstrate signs or symptoms of urinary retention by (date).

TARGET DATE

Urinary retention poses many dangers to the patient. An acceptable target date to evaluate for lessening of retention would be within 24–48 hours after admission.

NURSING ORDERS

ADULT HEALTH

1. Monitor bladder for distention at least every 2 hours on (odd/even) hour.
2. Measure and record intake and output each shift.
3. Collaborate with physician regarding:
   a. Intermittent catheterization;
   b. Medications (e.g., urinary antiseptics, analgesics, etc.);

    c. Teaching of Credé's and Valsalva maneuvers (see Additional Information at end of chapter);

    d. Daily fluid amounts.

4. Stimulate micturition reflex:

    a. Assist patient to assume anatomically correct position for voiding.

    b. Remind patient to consciously be aware of need-to-void sensations.

    c. Teach patient to assist bladder contraction:

       (1) Credé's maneuver

       (2) Valsalva maneuver

       (3) Abdominal muscle contraction

    d. Provide privacy.

    e. Awaken at least once during night to void.

5. Initiate bladder training program (see Additional Information at end of chapter).

6. Teach patient exercises to strengthen pelvic floor muscles:

    a. Bent-knee situps

    b. Straight or bent leg lifts

    c. Contracting posterior perineal muscles as if trying to stop a bowel movement

    d. Contracting anterior perineal muscles as if trying to stop voiding

    e. Starting and stopping voiding

7. Maintain fluid intake:

    a. Encourage fluids to at least 2000 ml per day.

    b. Limit fluids after 6 PM.

8. Monitor:

    a. Bowel elimination at least once per shift;

    b. Urinanalysis, electrolytes, and weight at least every 3 days.

9. Increase patient activity:

    a. Frequent ambulation

    b. Collaboration with physical therapist regarding an exercise program

10. Refer to home health agency for continued monitoring.

CHILD HEALTH

(Note: For young infants and children less than 20 lb, it would be necessary to calculate exact intake and output requisites and consider the etiologic factors present. A note to also address voluntary control would also need to reflect potential as it relates to physiologic and developmental factors.)

1. Monitor patient for bladder distention every 1–2 hours by gentle palpation or measurement of abdominal girth if necessary.

2. Monitor parental (patient as applicable) knowledge of preventive health care for patient regarding as appropriate:

    a. Teaching and observation of urinary catheterization;

    b. Maintenance of catheters and supplies;

    c. How to obtain supplies;

    d. How to obtain a sterile culture specimen;

    e. Appropriate restraint of infant;

    f. Potential regarding urinary control.

3. Provide opportunities for parental participation in the care of the infant or child.

    a. Feedings

    b. Bathing

    c. Monitoring intake and output

    d. Planning for care to include individual preferences when possible

    e. Assisting with procedures when appropriate

    f. Provision of anticipatory safety

    g. Cautious handwashing to prevent infection

    h. Appropriate emotional support

    i. Appropriate diversional activity and relaxation

    j. Need for pain medication

4. Provide opportunities for child and parents to verbalize concerns or views related to body image disturbances related to urinary control and retention.

5. Collaborate with paraprofessionals as needed to resolve any related issues of urinary retention to include:

    a. Physicians and subspecialists

    b. Clinical nurse specialist

    c. Occupational therapist

    d. Physical therapist

    e. Play therapist

    f. Teachers or tutors

6. Assist family to identify support groups represented in the community for future needs.

7. Reassure patients they are not being judged for loss of control.

WOMEN'S HEALTH

1. Collaborate with physician regarding intermittent catheterization. (It is not easy to catheterize a woman postpartum nor is it desirable to introduce an added risk of infection, so every effort and support should be directed toward helping the woman to void on her own. If, however, she is unable to void or to empty her bladder, an indwelling catheter may be placed for 24–48 hours to rest the bladder and allow it to heal, edema to subside, and bladder and urethral tone to return [Hawkins & Gorvine, 1985, p. 41].)

2. Stimulate micturition reflex:

    a. Use warm water to stimulate urge to void.

        (1) Hearing water run

        (2) Warm water poured over vulva

    b. Teach relaxation techniques.

    c. Use pelvic floor (Kegel) exercises before and after delivery.

MENTAL HEALTH

(Note: Clients receiving antipsychotic and antidepressant drugs are at increased risk for this diagnosis. Refer to Adult Health for general orders related to this diagnosis.)

1. Place clients receiving antipsychotic or antidepressant medications on daily assessment for this diagnosis. Elderly clients should be evaluated more frequently if their physical status indicates.

2. Monitor bladder for distention at least every 4 hours if verbal reports are unreliable or if they indicate a voiding frequency greater than every 4 hours.

3. Increase client's activity by:

    a. Walking with client (number) minutes three times a day (list times here);

    b. Collaborating with physical therapist regarding an exercise program;

    c. Placing client in a room distant from the day area, nursing station, and other areas of activity if condition does not contraindicate this;

    d. Providing physical activities that client indicates are of interest (list these here with the time for each).

4. Teach deep muscle relaxation and spend 30 minutes twice a day at (list times here) practicing this with client. Associate relaxation with breathing so that client can eventually relax with deep breathing while attempting to void.

5. Teach client the importance of relaxation while voiding, and teach the use of deep breathing as a method of promoting this state.

6. Refer to appropriate community agencies as indicated:

   a. Visiting nurse
   b. Occupational therapist
   c. Nutritionist
   d. Physical therapist
   e. Psychiatric nurse clinical specialist

HOME HEALTH

(Note: If this nursing diagnosis is made it is imperative that physician referral be made. If referred to home care under physician's care, it is important to maintain and evaluate response to prescribed treatments.)

1. Assist patient and family in life-style changes that may be required:
   a. Monitor bladder for distention.
   b. Record intake and output.
   c. Stimulate micturition reflex (see Adult Health).
   d. Institute bladder training program (see Additional Information).
   e. Perform exercises to strengthen pelvic floor muscles.
   f. Use proper position for voiding.
   g. Maintain fluid intake.
   h. Maintain physical activity as tolerated.
   i. Use straight catheterization.
2. Assist patient and family to set criteria to help them to determine when a physician or other intervention is required.
3. Monitor and teach importance of appropriate medications and treatments ordered by physician.
4. Refer to appropriate assistive resources as indicated.
   a. Nutritionist
   b. Physician
   c. Rehabilitation specialist
   d. Home health aid

EVALUATION
OBJECTIVE 1

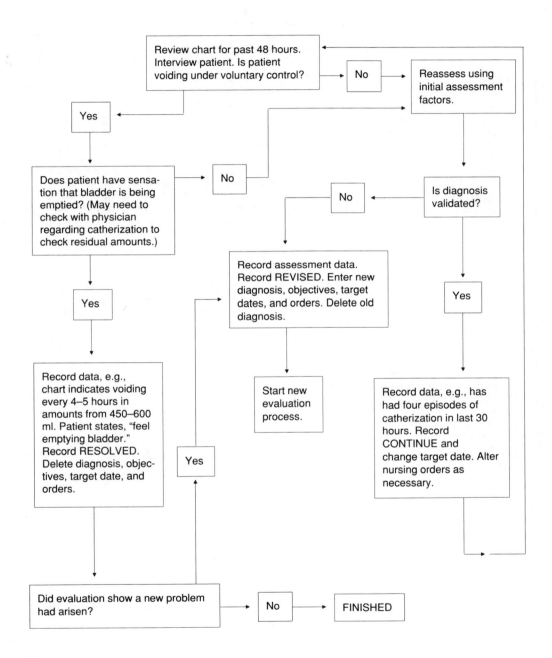

OBJECTIVE 2

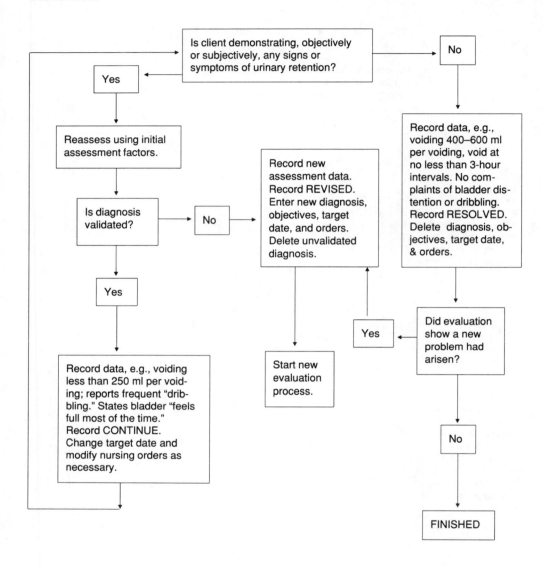

ADDITIONAL INFORMATION

Bladder retraining programs may vary according to individual hospitals and physicians. Consultation with a rehabilitation nurse clinician will provide the most current and reliable information regarding a quality bladder retraining program. The following article by Clay describes one such program:

Clay, E. (1980). Urinary continence/incontinence. Habit retraining: A tested method to regain urinary control. *Geriatric Nursing,* November-December *1* (4), 252–254.

Crede's maneuver involves placing the fingertips together at the midline of the pelvic crest then massaging deeply and smoothly down to the pubic bone. Check with the physician first, since there are contraindications such as ureteral reflux (Gettrust et al., 1985).

The Valsalva maneuver involves asking the patient to simulate having a bowel movement. Have the patient take a deep breath, hold it and then bear down as if expelling a bowel movement. Check with the physician first, since there are contraindications such as impaired circulation (Gettrust et al., 1985).

REFERENCES

Bruya, M. A. (1981). Elimination status. In P. Mitchell & A. Loustau (Eds.), *Concepts basic to nursing.* New York: McGraw-Hill.

Carnevali, D., & Patrick, M. (1979). *Nursing management for the elderly.* Philadelphia: J. B. Lippincott.

Flynn, J., & Heffron, P. (1984). *Nursing: From concept to practice.* Bowie, MD: Brady Communication.

Fogel, C. I., & Woods, N. F. (1981). *Health care of women: A nursing perspective.* St. Louis: C. V. Mosby.

Gettrust, K., Ryan, S., & Engleman, D. (1985). *Applied nursing diagnosis: Guides for comprehensive care planning.* New York: John Wiley & Sons.

Hawkins, J. W., & Gorvine, B. (1985). *Postpartum nursing: Health care of women.* New York: Springer.

Kelly, M. A. (1985). *Nursing diagnosis source book.* East Norwalk, CT: Appleton-Century-Crofts.

Long, B., & Durham, N. (1983). Assessment of lower gastrointestinal tract function. In W. Phipps, B. Long, & N. Woods (Eds.), *Medical-surgical nursing: Concepts and clinical practice.* St. Louis: C. V. Mosby.

Miller, P. (1983). Assessment of urinary function. In W. Phipps, B. Long, & N. Woods (Eds.), *Medical-surgical nursing: Concepts and clinical practice.* St. Louis: C. V. Mosby.

Murray, R., & Zentner, J. (1985). *Nursing assessment and promotion through the life span.* Englewood Cliffs, NJ: Prentice-Hall.

North American Nursing Diagnosis Association. (1987). *Taxonomy I with complete diagnoses.* St. Louis: Author.

North American Nursing Diagnosis Association. (1988). *Proposed nursing diagnoses.* St. Louis: Author.

Schuster, C., & Ashburn, S. (1986). *The process of human development* (2nd ed.). Boston: Little, Brown.

SUGGESTED READINGS

Aukamp, V. (1984). *Nursing care plans for the childbearing family.* East Norwalk, CT: Appleton-Century-Crofts.

Carpenito, L. J. (1983). *Nursing diagnosis: Application to clinical practice.* Philadelphia: J. B. Lippincott.

Crittendon, R. (1983). *Discharge planning.* Bowie, MD: Robert J. Brady.

Gilbert, E. S., & Harmon J. S. (1986). *High-risk pregnancy and delivery: Nursing perspectives.* St. Louis: C. V. Mosby.

Gordon, M. (1985a). *Manual of nursing diagnosis.* New York: McGraw-Hill.

Gordon, M. (1985b). *Nursing diagnosis: Process and application.* New York: McGraw-Hill.

Hadeka, M. (1987). *Clinical judgment in community health nursing.* Boston: Little, Brown.

Humphrey, C. (1986). *Home nursing care handbook.* East Norwalk, CT: Appleton-Century-Crofts.

Jaffe, M., & Skidmore-Roth, L. (1988). *Home health nursing care plans.* St. Louis: C. V. Mosby.

Kneisl, C., & Wilson, H. (1984). *Handbook of psychosocial nursing care.* Menlo Park, CA: Addison-Wesley.

Martin, L. L. (1978). *Health care of women.* Philadelphia: J. B. Lippincott.

McClelland, E., Kelly, K., & Buckwalter, K. (1984). *Continuity of care: Advancing the concept of discharge planning.* Orlando, FL: Grune & Stratton.

National League for Nursing. (1986). *Policies and procedures.* New York: Accreditation Division for Home Care, National League for Nursing.

National League for Nursing. (1988). *Accreditation program for home care and community health: Criteria and standards.* New York: Author.

Neeson, J. D., & May, K. A. (1986). *Comprehensive maternity nursing: Nursing process and the childbearing family*. St. Louis: J. B. Lippincott.

Potter, P., & Perry, A. (1985). *Instructor's manual for use with fundamentals of nursing: Concepts, process, and practice*. St. Louis: C. V. Mosby.

Raffensperger, E., Zusy, M., & Marchesseault, L. (1986). *Clinical nursing handbook*. Philadelphia: J. B. Lippincott.

Rinke, L. (1988). *Outcome standards in home health*. New York: National League for Nursing.

Steffi, B., & Eide, I. (1978). *Discharge planning handbook*. New York: Charles B. Slack.

Walsh, J., Persons, C., & Wieck, L. (1987). *Manual of home health care nursing*. Philadelphia: J. B. Lippincott.

CHAPTER FIVE

Activity-Exercise Pattern

Pattern Description

This pattern focuses on the activities of daily living (ADL) and the amount of energy the individual has available to support these activities. The ADL include all aspects of maintaining self-care and incorporates leisure time as well. Because the individual's energy level and mobility for ADL are affected by the proper functioning of the neuromuscular, cardiovascular, and respiratory systems, nursing diagnoses related to dysfunctions in these systems are included.

As with the other patterns, a problem in the activity-exercise pattern may be the primary reason for the patient entering the health care system or may arise secondary to problems in another functional pattern. Any admission to a hospital may promote the development of problems in this area because of the therapeutics required for the medical diagnosis (e.g., bed rest) or because of agency rules and regulations (e.g., limited visiting hours).

Pattern Assessment

1. Review the patient's activities of daily living:
   a. Have patient describe usual activities for at least 1 weekday and 1 weekend day.
   b. Question patient regarding any difficulties with ADL:
      (1) Self-care (e.g., feeding, bathing, home maintenance)
      (2) Energy level (e.g., fatigue, weakness, vertigo)
      (3) Mobility (e.g., pain, stiffness, paralysis)
      (4) Bowel and bladder function, etc., constipation, need for rectal stimulation, urinary retention, presence of urinary catheter
2. Review patient's exercise program:
   a. Frequency (e.g., daily for 30 minutes; three times a week for one hour)
   b. Type (e.g., jogging, walking, aerobics)
3. Review patient's leisure time activities:
   a. Type (e.g., sport, reading, traveling, gardening, hobbies)
   b. Frequency (e.g., daily, only when on vacation)
4. Complete physical assessment of:
   a. Cardiovascular system
      (1) Heart
      (2) Circulatory
   b. Respiratory system
      (1) Lungs
      (2) Ear, nose, and throat
   c. Neuromuscular system
      (1) Neuro examination

          (a) Mental status
          (b) Cranial nerves
          (c) Reflexes, particularly gag reflex
          (d) Sensory and motor nerve functioning
      (2) Skeletal system
          (a) Range of motion
          (b) Joint size
          (c) Posture
      (3) Muscular pattern and functioning
          (a) Gait
          (b) Coordination
          (c) Strength
          (d) Size and tone of muscles
   d. Integumentary system
      (1) Integrity
      (2) Lesions
   e. Compare and contrast findings with normals for age (normal growth and development guidelines)
5. Question patient regarding pain (e.g., chest, upon movement).
6. Assess for use of any prosthetic or assistive devices.
7. Check vital signs.

Conceptual Information

There are several nursing diagnoses included in this pattern that, at first glance, seem to have little relationship with each other. However, closer investigation demonstrates that there is one concept common to all of the diagnoses—immobility. Immobility can contribute to the development of any of these diagnoses, or any of these diagnoses can ultimately lead to the development of immobility.

Mobility and immobility are end points on a continuum with many degrees of impaired mobility or partial immobility between the two points (Potter & Perry, 1985). Immobility is usually distinguished from impaired mobility by the permanence of the limitation. A person who is quadriplegic has immobility because it is permanent; a person with a long cast on the left leg has impaired mobility because it is temporary (Kelly, 1985).

Mobility is defined as the ability to move freely and is one of the major means by which we define and express ourselves. A problem with mobility can be a measure of the degree of illness or health problem an individual has (Mitchell, 1981).

Patients with self-care deficits are most often those who are experiencing some type of mobility problem (Kelly, 1985). The problem with mobility requires greater energy expenditure which leads to activity intolerance, diversional activity deficit, and impaired home maintenance simply due to the lack of energy to engage in these activities.

Problems with mobility also lead to physical problems. When a person has impaired mobility or immobility, bed rest is quite often prescribed or is voluntarily sought in an effort to conserve energy. Mitchell (1981), Lentz (1981), and Pardue (1984) provide the best description of these problems according to each system:

1. Respiratory—Decreased chest and lung expansion causes slower and more shallow respiration. Pooling of secretions occurs secondary to decreased respiratory effort and the effects of gravity. The cough reflex is decreased due to decreased respiratory effort, gravity, and decreased muscle strength.
2. Cardiovascular—Circulatory stasis is caused by vasodilation and impaired venous return. Muscular inactivity leads to vein dilation in dependent parts. Gravity effects also occur. Decreased

respiratory effort and gravity lead to decreased changes in thoracic and abdominal pressures which usually assist in promoting blood return to the heart. Quite often patients have increased use of the Valsalva maneuver, which leads to increases in preload and afterload of cardiac output and ultimately a decreased cardiac output. Continued limitation of activity leads to decreased cardiac rate, circulatory volume, and arterial pressure due to redistribution of body fluids. Venous stasis contributes to the potential for deep venous thrombosis and pulmonary embolus. After prolonged bed rest the normal mechanism of the cardiovascular system that prevents large shifts in blood volume does not adequately function. When the individual who has experienced extended bed rest attempts to assume an upright position, gravity pulls an excessive amount of blood volume to the feet and legs, depriving the brain of adequate oxygen. As a result, the individual experiences orthostatic hypotension (Lentz, 1981).

3. Musculoskeletal—Inactivity causes decreased bone stress and decreased muscle tension. Osteoblastic and osteoclastic activities become imbalanced, leading to calcium and phosphorus loss. Decreased muscle use leads to decreased muscle mass and strength due to infrequent muscle contractions and protein loss.

4. Metabolic—Basal metabolic rate and oxygen consumption decrease, leading to decreased efficiency in using nutrients to build new tissues. Normally, body tissues break down nitrogen, but apparently muscle mass loss with accompanying protein loss leads to nitrogen loss and a negative nitrogen balance. Changes in tissue metabolism lead to increased potassium and calcium excretion. Decreased energy use and decreased basal metabolic rate (BMR) lead to appetite loss, which leads to decreased nutrient intake necessary to offset losses.

5. Skin—The negative nitrogen balance previously discussed, coupled with continuous pressure on bony prominences, leads to a greatly increased potential for skin breakdown.

Immobility is not the sole causative factor of the nursing diagnoses in this pattern. Many of the diagnoses can be related to specific medical diagnoses such as congestive heart failure. However, the concept of immobility does not serve to point out the interrelatedness of the diagnoses.

Since fatigue plays a major role in determining the quality and amount of musculoskeletal activity undertaken, consideration of the factors that influence fatigue is an essential part of nursing assessment for the sleep-rest pattern. It is likely that the activity-exercise pattern and nutritional-metabolic pattern will also be considered as key concepts related to sleep-rest needs.

Fatigue might be considered in two general categories—experiential and muscular.

The degree to which the individual participates in activity is significant in determining the fatigue experienced. Activities which the individual enjoys are less likely to produce fatigue than are those not enjoyed. Preferences should be considered within the framework of capacity and needs. Obviously other factors that must be considered include the physical and medical condition of the person and his or her emotional state, level of growth and development, and state of health in general. Oxygenation needs would also need to be addressed. Factors extrinsic to the person must also be considered. A most critical extrinsic factor is the immediate environment. If there is overstimulation as with noise, extremes of temperature, or interruption of routines, a greater amount of fatigue can be expected. Sensory understimulation with resultant boredom can also contribute to fatigue.

Fatigue can develop as a result of too much waste material accumulating and too little nourishment going to the muscles. Muscle fatigue usually is attributed to the accumulation of too much lactic acid in the muscles. Certain metabolic conditions, such as congestive heart failure, place a person at greater risk for fatigue.

Developmental Considerations

Activity is influenced by diet, musculoskeletal factors, and respiratory and cardiovascular mechanism. Developmental considerations for diet are addressed in Chapter 3. The developmental considerations discussed below specifically relate to musculoskeletal, respiratory, and cardiovascular factors.

Infant

Physical and motor abilities are influenced by many things, including genetic, biologic, and cultural factors. Nutrition, maturation of the central nervous system, skeletal formation, overall physical health status, amount of stimulation, environmental conditions, and consistent loving care also play a part in physical and motor abilities (Murray & Zentner, 1985). Girls usually develop more rapidly than boys, although the activity level is higher in boys (Murray & Zentner, 1985).

All muscular tissue is formed at birth but growth occurs as the infant uses the various muscle groups. This use stimulates increased strength and function.

The infant engages in various types of play activity at various times in infancy because of developing skills and changing needs. The infant needs the stimulation of parents in this play activity to fully develop. However, parents should be aware of the dangers in overstimulation. Fatigue, inattention, and injury to the infant may result (Murray & Zentner, 1985).

Interruptions in the normal developmental sequence of play activities due to illness or hospitalization, for example, can have a detrimental effect on the future development of the infant or child. An understanding of the normal sequence of play development is important to have so that therapeutic interventions can be designed to approximate the developmental needs of the individual.

The structural description of play development focuses on the Piagetian concepts of the increasing cognitive complexity of play activities. Elementary sensorimotor-based games emerge first, with the gradual development of advanced social games in adulthood (Schuster & Ashburn, 1985).

Play activities assist in the child's development of psychomotor skills and cognitive development. Socialization skills are learned and practiced via the interaction with others during play. As the child begins to learn more about his or her body during play, he or she will incorporate more complicated gross and fine motor skills. Play is extremely valuable in the development of language and other communication skills. Play helps the individual to establish control over self and a sense of accomplishment. Through play activities, the infant learns to trust the environment. Play also affords the child the opportunity to express emotions which would be unacceptable in other normal social situations.

Practice games begin during the sensorimotor level of cognitive development at 1–4 months of age and continues with increasing complexity throughout childhood. These games include skills that are performed for the pleasure of functioning, that is, for the pleasure of practice.

Symbolic games appear later during the sensorimotor period than do practice games—about age 12–18 months. Make-believe is now added to the practice game. Elements of absent objects or persons are represented by other objects.

The air conducting passages (the nose, pharynx, larynx, trachea, bronchi, bronchioles, and alveoli) and lungs of the infant are small, delicate, and immature. The air that enters the nose is cool, dry, and unfiltered. The nose is unable to filter the air and the mucous membranes of the upper respiratory tract, being immature, are unable to produce enough mucus to humidify or warm the inhaled air. Therefore, the infant is more susceptible to respiratory tract infections.

Additionally, the infant is a nose breather. When upper respiratory tract infections do occur, the infant is unable to appropriately clear the airways and may get into some difficulty until he or she learns to breathe through his or her mouth (at about 3–4 months of age). The cough of the infant is not very effective and the infant quickly becomes tired with the effort.

In the lungs, the alveoli are functioning, but not all alveoli may be expanded. Therefore, there is a large amount of dead space in the lungs. The infant has to work harder to exchange enough oxygen and carbon dioxide to meet body demands. The elevated respiratory rate of the infant (30–60 per minute) reflects this increased work. Additionally, arterial blood gases of the infant may show an acid-base imbalance. The rate and rhythm of respiration in the infant is somewhat irregular and it is not unusual for the infant to use accessory muscles of respiration. Retractions with respiration are common.

The alveoli of the infant increase in number and complexity very rapidly. By 1 year of age, the alveoli and the lining of the air passages have matured considerably.

Respiratory tract obstructions are common in this age group because of the short trachea and the almost straight-line position of the right main stem bronchus. Additionally, the epiglottis does not effectively close over the trachea during swallowing. Thus, foreign objects are aspirated into the lungs.

In terms of cardiovascular development, the foramen ovale closes during the first 24 hours and the ductus arteriosus closes after several days. The neonate can survive mild oxygen deprivation longer than an adult. The Apgar scoring system is used to measure the physical status of the newborn and includes heart rate, color, and respiration. There is no day-night rhythm to the neonate's heart rate, but from the 6th week on the rate will be lower at night than during the day. Axilliary temperature and age-sized blood pressure cuffs should be used to assess vital signs. The vital signs will not be stable in the neonate of infant. Temperature ranges from 97° to 100° F.; pulse is 120–150 beats minute; respiration ranges from 35 to 50/minute; and BP ranges from 40 to 90 mm Hg systolic and 6 to 20 mm Hg diastolic. Vital signs becomes more stable over the 1st year. Listening for murmurs should be done over the base of the heart rather than at the apex. Breath sounds are bronchovesicular. The neonate has limited ability to respond to environmental temperature changes and will lose heat rapidly. This leads to an increased BMR and an increased workload on the heart. Until age 7, the apex is palpated at the fourth interspace just to the left of the midclavicular line.

Toddler and Preschooler

By this age, the child is walking, running, climbing, and jumping. The toddler is very active and very curious. He or she gets into everything. This helps the toddler organize his or her world and develop spatial and sensory perception (Murray & Zentner, 1985).

The toddler is fairly clumsy, but gross and fine motor coordination is improving. Neuromuscular maturation and repetition of movements help the child further develop skills (Murray & Zentner, 1985). Muscles grow faster than bones during these years.

Bathing and Hygiene. By the age of 3, the child can wash and dry hands with some wetting of clothes; can brush teeth, but requires assistance to perform adequately. By the 4th birthday the child may bathe himself or herself with assistance. The child will be able to bathe himself or herself without assistance by the age of 5.

(Note: The nurse must always keep in mind the safety issues involved in bathing: the child requires supervision in selection of water temperature and in the prevention of drowning.)

Dressing and Grooming. At age 18–20 months the child has the fine motor skills required to unzip a large zipper. By 24–28 months the child can unbutton large buttons. The child can put on a coat with assistance by age 2; the child can undress himself or herself in most situations and can put on his or her own coat without assistance by age 3. At 3½ years the child can unbutton small buttons and by 4 years can button a small button. Dressing without assistance and beginning ability to lace shoes are accomplishments of the 5-year-old.

(Note: The development of fine motor skills is required for most of the tasks of dressing. It is important that the child's clothing have fasteners that are appropriate for the motor skill development. The child will require assistance with deciding the appropriateness of clothing selected; seasonal variations in weather and culturally accepted norms regarding dressing and grooming are learned by the child with assistance.)

Feeding. The child can drink from a cup without much spilling by 18 months. The child will have frequent spills while trying to get the contents of a spoon into his or her mouth at this age.

By 2 years the child can drink from a cup; use of the spoon has improved at this age, but the child will still spill liquids (soup) from a spoon when eating. The child can eat from a spoon without spilling by 3½ years. Accomplished use of the fork occurs at 5 years.

Toileting. By age 3 the child can go to the toilet without assistance; the child can pull pants up and down for toileting without assistance at this stage as well.

(Note: The development of food preferences, preferred eating schedules and environment, and toileting behavior are imparted to the child by learning. Toileting, food, and the eating experience may also include pleasures, control issues, and learning tasks in addition to the development of the motor skills required to accomplish the task. Delays or regressions in the tasks of self-feeding may reflect issues other than a self-care deficit, e.g., discipline, family coping, role-relationships, etc.)

During the preschool years, the child seems to have an unlimited supply of energy. However, he or she does not know when to stop and may continue activities past the point of exhaustion.

Parents should provide a variety of activities for the age group, as the attention span is short.

The lung size and volume of the toddler have now increased and thus the oxygen capacity of the toddler has increased. The toddler is still susceptible to respiratory tract infections but not to the extent of the infant. The rate and rhythm of respiration has decreased and respirations average 25–35 per minute. Accessory muscles of respiration are infrequently used now and respirations are primarily diaphragmatic.

The respiratory structures (trachea and bronchi) are positioned farther down in the chest now and the epiglottis is effective in closing off the trachea during swallowing. Thus, aspiration and airway obstruction are reduced in this age group.

The respiratory rate of the preschooler is about 30 per minute. The preschooler is still susceptible to upper respiratory tract infections. The lymphatic tissues of the tonsils and adenoids are involved in these respiratory tract infections. Tonsillectomies and adenoidectomies are not performed "routinely" any more. These tissues serve to protect the respiratory tract and valid reasons must be presented to warrant their removal.

The temperature of the toddler ranges around 99° F ± 1°; pulse ranges around 105 beats/minute ± 35; respirations range from 20 to 35/minute; and blood pressure ranges from 80 to 100 mm Hg systolic and 60 to 64 mm Hg diastolic. The size of the vascular bed increases in the toddler, thus reducing resistance to flow. Lung volume increases. The capillary bed has increased ability to respond to environmental temperature changes. Breath sounds are more intense and more bronchial, and expiration is more pronounced. The toddler's chest should be examined with the child in an erect position, then recumbent, and then turned to the left position. Arrhythmias and extrasystoles are not uncommon but should be recorded.

The temperature of the preschooler is 98.6° F ± 1°; pulse ranges from 80 to 100 beats per minute; respiration is 30/minute ± 5; and BP is 90/60 mm Hg ± 15. There is continued increase of the vascular bed, lung volume, etc. in keeping with physical growth.

School-Age Child

The skeletal system is growing rapidly during these years—faster than the muscles are growing. Children may experience "growing pains" because of the stretching of muscles with the growth of the long bones.

There is a gradual increase in muscle mass and strength, and the body takes on a leaner appearance. The child loses his or her baby fat. Muscle tone increases. Loose movements disappear.

Adequate exercise is needed to maintain strength, flexibility, and balance and to encourage muscular development (Schuster & Ashburn, 1986). Males have a greater number of muscle cells than females.

Poor posture may be reflective of fatigue as well as skeletal defects (Schuster & Ashburn, 1986). Fatigue may be exhibited by quarrelsomeness, crying, or lack of interest in eating.

Neuromuscular coordination is sufficient to permit the school child to learn most skills (Murray & Zentner, 1985). Hands and fingers manipulate things well.

Children age 7 have a lower activity level but have an increased attention span and cognitive skills. Therefore, they tend to engage in quiet games as well as active ones.

Games with rules develop as the child engages in more social contacts. These games characteristically emerge during the operational phase of cognitive development in the school-age child. These rule games may also be practice or symbolic in nature, but now the child attaches social significance and order to the play by imposing the structure of rules.

Eight-year-olds have grace and balance. Nine-year-olds move with less restlessness; strength and endurance increase; and the 9-year-old has good hand-eye coordination (Murray & Zentner, 1985). The 10–12-year-olds have energetic, active, restless movements with tension release through finger drumming, foot tapping, or leg swinging.

The respiratory rate of the school-age child slows to 18–22 minute. The respiratory tissues reach adult maturity, and the lung capacity is proportionate to body size.

The school-age child is still susceptible to respiratory tract infections. The frontal sinuses are fairly well developed by this age and all the mucous membranes are very vulnerable to congestion and inflammation.

The temperature, pulse, and respiration of the school-age child are gradually approaching adult norms, with temperature ranging from 98° to 98.6° F, pulse (resting) 60 to 70 beats/minute, and respiration from 18 to 21/minute. Systolic BP ranges from 94 to 112 mm Hg and diastolic from 56 to 60 mm Hg. The heart grows more slowly during this period and is smaller in relation to the rest of the body. But it must continue to supply the metabolic needs, so the child should be advised against sustained physical activity. After age 7 the apex of the heart lies at the interspace of the fifth rib at the midclavicle line. Circulatory functions reach adult capacity. The child will still have some vasomotor instability with rapid vasodilation. A third heart sound and sinus arrhythmias are fairly common but, again, should be recorded.

Adolescent

Growth in skeletal size, muscle mass, adipose tissue, and skin are significant in adolescence. The skeletal system grows faster than the muscles; the large muscles grow faster than the smaller muscles. Poor posture and decreased coordination result. Males are more clumsy than females. Muscle growth continues in males during late adolescence because of androgen production (Murray & Zentner, 1985).

Adolescents participate in physical activities that are socially determined. Males participate in activities that require physical abilities to demonstrate their manliness. Females participate in social functions and domestic skills as well as such activities as swimming, gymnastics, and dancing. Physical activities provide a way for adolescents to enjoy the stimulation of conflict in a socially acceptable way. Some form of physical activity should be encouraged to promote physical development, prevent overweight, formulate a realistic body image, and promote peer acceptance.

More rest and sleep are needed now than earlier. The teenager is expending large amounts of energy and functioning with an inadequate oxygen supply; both of these factors contribute to fatigue and cause the need for additional rest. Parents may need to set limits. Rest does not necessarily mean sleep and can also include quiet activites (Murray & Zentner, 1985).

There is a correlation between the maturation of the skeletal system and the reproductive system.

Because of the very rapid growth during this period, the adolescent may not have sufficient energy left for strenuous activities. He or she tires easily and may frequently complain of needing to sit down. Gradually the child is able to increase both speed and stamina during exercise. An increase in muscular and skeletal strength, as well as the increased ability of the lungs and heart to provide adequate oxygen to the tissues, facilitates maintenance of homeostasis and rate of recovery after exercise. The body reaches its peak of physiologic resilience during late adolescence and early adulthood. Both strength and tolerance to strenuous activity can be increased by regular physical training and an individualized conditioning program.

Faulty nutrition is another major cause of fatigue in the adolescent. Poor eating habits established during the school-age years, combined with the typical quick-service, quick-energy food consumption patterns of adolescents frequently lead to anemia, which in itself can lead to activity intolerance (Schuster & Ashburn, 1986).

The adolescent may be given responsibility for assisting with the maintenance of the family home, or may be responsible for his or her own home if he or she is living independent from the family of origin. The role exploration characteristic of adolescence may lead to temporary changes in hygiene practices.

Recreational activities in adolescence often take the form of organized sports and other competitive activities. Social relationships are developed and enhanced, specific motor and cognitive skills related to the specific sport are refined, and a sense of mastery can be developed. Group activities and peer approval and acceptance are important.

The adolescent responds to peer activities and experiments with different roles and life-styles. The nurse must distinguish self-care practices that are acceptable to the peer group from those that indicate a self-care deficit.

The respiratory rate of the adolescent is 16–20/minute. The body is growing at various rates but the respiratory system does not grow proportionately. Therefore, the adolescent may have inadequate oxygenation and become more fatigued. The lung capacity correlates with the adolescent's structural form. Males have a larger lung capacity than females due to greater shoulder width and chest size. Males have greater respiratory volume, greater vital capacity, and increased respiratory rate. The male's lung capacity matures later than the female's. The female's lungs mature at age 17 or 18.

The heart continues to grow during adolescence but more slowly than the rest of the body, so inadequate oxygen and fatigue are common. The heart continues to enlarge until age 17 or 18. Systolic pulse pressure increases and the temperature is the same as an adult level. The pulse ranges from 60 to 68 beats/minute; respiration ranges from 18 to 20/minute and BP is 100–120/50–70 mm Hg. Females have slightly higher pulse rates and basal body temperatures, and lower systolic pressures than males. Hypertension incidence increases. Athletes have slower pulse rates than peers. Heart sounds are heard readily at the fifth left intercostal space. Functional murmurs should be outgrown. Chest pain may arise from musculosketal changes, but cardiovascular pain should always be investigated. Cardiovascular problems are the fifth leading cause of death in adolescents. Essential hypertension incidence is approximately equal between races for this age group.

Young Adult

Growth of the skeletal system is essentially complete by age 25. Muscular efficiency is at its peak between 20 and 30. Energy level and control of energy are high. Thereafter, muscular strength declines with the rate of muscle aging depending on the specific muscle group and the activity of the person and the adequacy of his or her diet.

Regular exercise is helpful in controlling weight and maintaining a state of high-level wellness. Muscle tone, strength, and circulation are enhanced by exercise. Problems arise especially when sedentary life-styles decrease the amount of exercise available with daily activities.

The general concern in this generation is with physical fitness. Calorie intake and exercise should be balanced.

Adequate sleep is important for good physical and mental health. Lack of sleep results in progressive sluggishness of both physical and cognitive functions.

This age group gets the majority of its activity from work and leisure activities. The young adult should learn to balance his or her work with leisure time activities. Getting started in a career can be very stressful and can lead to burnout if an appropriate balance is not found. "Physical fitness reflects ability to work for a sustained period with vigor and pleasure, without undue fatigue, with energy left over for enjoying hobbies and recreational activities and for meeting emergencies" (Murray & Zentner, 1985).

Basic to fitness are regular physical exercise, proper nutrition, adequate rest and relaxation, conscientious health practices, and good medical and dental care. Regular physical fitness is a natural tranquilizer releasing the body's own endorphins which reduce anxiety and muscular tension.

The respiratory system of the young adult has completely matured. Oxygen demand is based on exercise and activity now but gradually decreases between ages 20 and 40. The body's ability to use oxygen efficiently is dependent on the cardiovascular system and the needs of the skeletal muscles.

Respiratory system, heart, and circulatory systems change gradually with age but the rate of change is highly dependent on the individual's diet and exercise pattern. Generally, contraction of the myocardium decreases. The maximum cardiac output is reached between the ages of 20 and 30. The arteries become less elastic. The maximum breathing capacity decreases between ages 20 and 40. Cardiac and respiratory function can be improved with regular exercise. Hypertension (BP $^{140}/90$ mm Hg or higher) and mitral valve prolapse syndrome are the most common cardiovascular medical diagnoses of the young adult.

Adult

Basal metabolism rate gradually decreases. Although there is a general and gradual decline in quickness and level of activity, people who were most active among their age group during adolescence and young adulthood tend to be the most active during middle and old age. In women, there is frequently a menopausal rise in energy and activity (Noble, 1982). Less time and energy go into childrearing; she may feel more self-confident and satisfied and she is less competitive. There is less physical and mental energy used on the worrisome details of everyday life. Judicious exercise balanced with rest and sleep may modify and retard the aging process. Exercise stimulates circulation to all parts of the body, thereby improving body functions. Exercise can also be an outlet for emotional tension. If the person is beginning exercises after being sedentary, certain precautions should be taken: gradually increase exercise to a moderate level; exercise consistently; and avoid overexertion.

The adult is beginning to have a decrease in bone mass and a loss of skeletal height. Muscle strength and mass are directly related to active muscle use. The adult needs to maintain the patterns of activity and exercise of young adulthood and not become sedentary. Otherwise, muscles lose mass structure and strength more rapidly.

The normal adult should be able to perform activities of daily living without assistance.

The needs for close relationships and intimacy of adulthood can be initiated by leisure activities with identified partners or a small group of close friends (e.g., hiking, tennis, golf, attending concerts, theatres, etc.). The middle-aged adult is often interested in the personal satisfaction of diversional activities.

The adult will most likely be responsible for home maintenance as well as outside employment. Role strain or over-taxation of the adult is possible. Illness or injury to the adults in the household will significantly affect the ability of the family unit to maintain the home.

The lung tissue becomes thicker and less elastic with age. The lungs cannot expand as they once did, and breathing capacity is reduced. The respiratory rate may increase to compensate for the reduced breathing capacity.

Temperature for the adult ranges from 97° to 99.6° F; pulse ranges from 50 to 100 beats/minute; respiration ranges from 16 to 20/minute; and BP $^{120}/80$ mm Hg ± 15. Decreasing elasticity of the blood vessels causes more susceptibility to hypertension and cardiovascular diseases. Females become as prone to coronary disease after menopause as males, so estrogen appears to be a protective agent. Cardiac output gradually decreases. BMR generally decreases. Essential and secondary hypertension and angina occur more frequently in this age group.

Older Adult

A decrease in skeletal mass affects all the bones of the skeleton. Decrease in skeletal mass leads to decreased strength. The tissues of the joints and bones stiffen; thus, movement and range of motion markedly decrease. The oxygen supply to the muscles may also be decreased as a result of the reduced cardiac output. Mobility is lessened and the older adult moves more slowly. The older adult should be encouraged to maintain optimum range of motion through planned exercise and activity.

There is a decline in exercise tolerance and work capacity as one ages. Cardiovascular changes, decreased pulmonary function, disuse of muscle groups, poor nutrition, and debilitating diseases may all contribute to less-than-optimum functioning and decreased mobility. Oxygen supply to muscles is decreased. Muscles may function but cardiac output may be so poor that normal activity is impossible.

There is decreased physical reserve and muscle strength. The older adult should view exercise and activity as a means of promoting and maintaining health and well-being. Activity and exercise can help keep an individual in shape and to maintain an optimal functioning level. The older adult should pace exercise and activity and recognize that it will take longer to do things than it once did.

Time available for leisure activities may dramatically increase for the individual at retirement or for the couple who have accomplished child-rearing or career-establishing tasks. Diversional activities provide physical activity as well as reestablish social contacts and form new friendships.

The older adult is more likely to experience the impairments discussed in the physiological section, thereby altering their ability to maintain their own homes. Impaired elderly may live with their adult children, thereby placing additional responsibilities on the adult children for adequate home maintenance.

Decreased sensory and motor abilities and muscle weakness may occur more frequently in the elderly.

Lung tissue continues to lose elasticity and becomes thicker. Alveolar sacs collapse and thus there are fewer functional units exposed to gas exchange. Additionally, the muscles of respiration have become rigid so lung expansion is not as great. The blood flow through the lungs is decreased because of reduced cardiac output. All these changes of aging result in a reduced breathing capacity, a decreased amount of oxygen in the blood (decreased pO_2), an increase in air trapped in the lungs (increased pCO_2), and changes in respiratory rate, rhythm, and depth. The work of breathing is increased but adequate functioning is decreased.

The ability and effectiveness of the cough is also decreased due to diminished muscle tone and decreased sensitivity to stimuli (Murray & Zentner, 1985).

Cardiovascular diseases are the highest cause of death in the older adult group, with the most common medical diagnosis being atherosclerosis. Physiologic cell and tissue changes (increased connective and collagen tissues, disappearance of some cellular elements, reduction in the number of normally functioning cells, increased amount of fat, decreased oxygen utilization, decreased cardiac output, decreased muscle strength) require the heart to work harder to provide adequate oxygenation. Exercise or stress raises heart rate and BP more in the older adult than in younger adults, and it takes longer for these rates to return to normal. Heart valves become more rigid and thick. This may give rise to the development of murmurs. Inelasticity of vessels, loss of cell integrity, and decrease in cardiac output and stroke volume combine to produce hypoxia. Blood flow through the coronary arteries decreases. Maximum breathing capacity, vital capacity, and inspiratory reserve volume decrease. The area of alveolar contact decreases as does the diffusing capacity; hence, there is a decrease in the oxygen content of the blood. Congestive heart failure, chronic occlusive arterial disease and stasis ulcers rise in incidence with this age group. The BP usually measures $^{140}/_{80}$ to $^{150}/_{90}$ mm Hg, but the rest of the vital signs remain in the same range as for the middle-aged adult. Downward dislocation of the cardiac apex and increased kyphosis may alter isolation of the apical pulse and usual chest landmarks.

Applicable Nursing Diagnoses

Activity Intolerance: Potential or Actual

DEFINITION

A state in which an individual is at risk of experiencing or has insufficient physiologic or psychologic energy to endure or complete required or desired daily activities (North American Nursing Diagnosis Association [NANDA], 1987, pp. 81–82).

(Note: When this diagnosis is made, the nurse should specify the level of the activity intolerance [Gordon, 1985, p. 126].)

Level I: The patient walks at his or her usual pace on a flat surface indefinitely; the patient can also walk up one or more flights of stairs without stopping but becomes more short of breath than usual.

Level II: The patient can walk approximately 500 feet on a flat surface; the patient can also walk up one flight of stairs without stopping but does have to walk slowly and does have some shortness of breath.

Level III: The patient can only walk approximately 50 feet on a flat surface; the patient must stop while walking up one flight of stairs.

Level IV: The patient has shortness of breath and fatigue even when he or she is not performing any activity.

DEFINING CHARACTERISTICS (NANDA, 1987, p. 81–82)

The nurse will review the initial pattern assessment for the following defining characteristics to determine the diagnosis of Activity Intolerance: Potential or Actual:

1. Activity Intolerance Potential:
   a. Major defining characteristics (risk factors)
      (1) History of previous intolerance
      (2) Deconditioned status
      (3) Presence of circulatory or respiratory problems
      (4) Inexperience with the activity
   b. Minor defining characteristics (risk factors)
      None given.
2. Activity Intolerance: Actual.
   a. Major defining characteristics
      (1) Verbal report of fatigue or weakness
      (2) Abnormal heart rate or blood pressure response to activity
      (3) Exertional discomfort or dyspnea
      (4) Electrocardiographic changes reflecting arrythmias or ischemia
   b. Minor defining characteristics None given.

RELATED FACTORS (NANDA, 1987, p. 81)

1. Activity Intolerance, Potential:
   The risk factors (defining characteristics) serve as the related factors.
2. Activity Intolerance, Actual:
   a. Bedrest or immobility
   b. Generalized weakness
   c. Sedentary life-style
   d. Imbalance between oxygen supply and demand

DIFFERENTIATION

Activity Intolerance: Actual or Potential needs to be differentiated from Physical Mobility, Impaired. Physical Mobility, Impaired implies that an individual would be able to move independently if something were not limiting the motion. Activity Intolerance, on the other hand, implies that the individual is freely able to move but cannot endure or adapt to the increased energy or oxygen demands made by the movement or activity.

Activity Intolerance: Actual or Potential also needs to be differentiated from Self-Care Deficits. Self-Care Deficits imply that the patient has some dependence on another person. Activity Intolerance implies that the patient is independent but is unable to perform activities because the body is unable to endure or adapt to the increased energy or oxygen demands made by the movement or activity. A person may have a Self-Care Deficit because of Activity Intolerance, but these two nursing diagnoses need to be differentiated.

Individual Coping, Ineffective is another nursing diagnosis that needs to be differentiated from Activity Intolerance: Actual or Potential. Persons with the nursing diagnosis of Individual Coping, Ineffective may be unable to participate in their usual roles or in their usual self-care because they feel they lack control or the motivation to do so. Activity Intolerance, on the other hand, implies that the person is willing and able to participate in activities but is unable to endure or adapt to the increased energy or oxygen demands made by the movement or activity.

OBJECTIVES

1. Will verbalize less fatigue and weakness by (date).

AND/OR

2. Will participate in increased self-care activities by (date). Specify which self-care activity (i.e., bathing, feeding, dressing, ambulation).

TARGET DATE

Appropriate target dates will have to be very individualized according to the degree of activity intolerance. An appropriate range would be 3–5 days.

NURSING ORDERS

ADULT HEALTH

1. Encourage rest as needed between activities. Assist client in planning a balanced rest-activity program.
2. Provide for a quiet, nonstimulating environment.
3. Limit number of visitors and length of their stay.
4. Assist patient with self-care activities as needed. Let patient determine how much assistance is needed.
5. Instruct patient in energy-saving techniques of daily care (e.g., prepare meals sitting on a high stool rather than standing).
6. Encourage oxygen therapy as needed.
7. Encourage progressive activity and increased self-care as tolerated. Schedule moderate increase in activities on a daily basis (e.g., will walk 10 feet farther each day).
8. Monitor blood pressure, pulse, and respiration before and after activities.
9. Determine motivators for activities.
10. Assist the patient in weight reduction, if needed.
11. Encourage adequate dietary input.
12. Teach relaxation and alternate pain relief measures.

CHILD HEALTH

1. Monitor current potential for desired activities, including:
   a. Physical limitations related to illness or surgery.
   b. Factors which relate to desired activities.
   c. Realistic expectations for actualizing potential for desired activities.

   d. Objective criteria by which specific progress may be measured (e.g., distance, time, observable signs or symptoms such as apical pulse, respiration).
   e. Previous level of activities patient enjoyed (this may be difficult to address if ambulation was impossible due to casting or congenital anomalies).
2. Provide collaboration in appropriate planning for desired or prescribed activity regimen to include:
   a. Aids to desired activity (e.g., walker, crutches, wheelchair).
   b. Pediatrician or subspecialists
   c. Physical therapist
   d. Occupational therapist
   e. Play therapist
   f. Clinical nurse specialist
   g. Psychiatrist or psychologist
   h. Support group role model
3. Provide opportunities of 15–30 minutes per shift for allowing patient and family to verbalize concerns regarding activity.
4. Provide patient and family opportunities to contribute to plans for activity as appropriate.
5. Allow for individual preference and suggestions on an ongoing basis.
6. Provide opportunities for success in meeting expected goals by using subgoals or increments which lead to desired activity.
7. Introduce necessary teaching according to the readiness of patient and family with appropriate modifications to best meet patient's needs.
8. Provide learning modules and practice sessions with materials suitable for child's age and developmental capacity (e.g., dolls, videos, pictures).
9. Provide for continuity in care by assigning same nurses for care during critical times for teaching and implementation.
10. Modify expected behavior to incorporate appropriate developmental needs (e.g., allow for shared cards, messages, or visitors to lobby if possible for adolescent patients).
11. Reinforce adherence to regimen with stickers or other appropriate measures to document progress.

WOMEN'S HEALTH

Postpartum (Cesarean Section or Vaginal Delivery)

1. Encourage client to limit number of visitors and their length of stay.
2. Encourage progressive activity and increased self-care as tolerated:
   a. Ambulation
   b. Bathing
   c. Care of infant
3. Provide quiet, supportive atmosphere for interaction with infant:
   a. Attachment
   b. Care-taking activities
   c. Feeding
      (1) Breast
      (2) Bottle
4. Instruct client in energy-saving activities of daily care.
   a. Take care of self and baby only.
   b. Let significant others take care of the housework and other children.
   c. Let significant others take care of baby for a prearranged time during the day, so mother can spend quality time with other children.
   d. Learn to sleep when the baby sleeps.
   e. Have specific set times for visiting of friends or relatives.

   f. If breastfeeding, significant other can bring infant to mother at night (mother does not always have to get up every time for infant).

Sexual Activity During Pregnancy and Postpartum Periods

5. Provide client with factual information about sexual changes during pregnancy.
   a. Answer questions promptly and factually.
   b. Meet people who have had similar experiences.
   c. Discuss fears about sexual changes.
   d. Discuss aspects of sexuality and intercourse during pregnancy.
      (1) Positions for intercourse during different stages of pregnancy
      (2) Frequency of intercourse
      (3) Effect of intercourse on pregnancy or fetus
   e. Describe healing process postpartum and timing of resumption of intercourse.

MENTAL HEALTH

1. Discuss with client his or her perceptions of activity appropriate to his or her current capabilities.
   a. If the client estimates a routine that far exceeds current capabilities (as with eating disorder clients or clients experiencing elated mood):
      (1) Establish appropriate limits on exercise (The limits and consequences for not maintaining limits established should be listed here. If the excessive exercise pattern is related to an elated mood, set limits in a manner that allows client some activity while not greatly exceeding metabolic needs until psychologic status is improved.);
      (2) Begin client slowly (i.e., with stretching exercise for 15 minutes twice a day);
      (3) As physical condition improves, gradually increase exercise to 30 minutes of aerobic exercise once per day;
      (4) Discuss with client the hazards of overexercise;
      (5) Discuss with client appropriate levels of exercise considering his or her age and metabolic pattern;
      (6) Establish a reward system for clients who maintain the established exercise schedule (the schedule for the client should be listed here with those reinforcers that are to be used);
      (7) Stay with client while he or she is engaged in appropriate exercise;
      (8) Develop a schedule for the client to be involved in an occupational therapy program to assist client in identifying alternative forms of activity other than aerobic exercise;
      (9) Limit number of walks off the unit to accommodate client's weight, level of exercise on the unit, and physiology (the frequency and length of the walk should be listed here);
      (10) For further information related to eating disorder clients see Nutrition Altered: Less Than Body Requirements.
   b. If client's expectations are much less than current capabilities (as with depressed or poorly motivated client), implement the following orders:
      (1) Establish very limited goals that client can accomplish (i.e., a 5-minute walk in a hallway once a day or walking in the client's room for 5 minutes) (the goal established should be listed here).
      (2) Establish a reward system for achievement of goals (the reward program should be listed here with a list of items the *client* finds rewarding).
      (3) Develop a schedule for the client to be involved in an occupational therapy program (note schedule here).
      (4) Establish limits on the amount of time the client can spend in bed or in his or her room during waking hours (establish limits the client can achieve, and note limits here).

    (5)   Stay with client during exercise periods and time out of the room until the client is performing these tasks without prompting.

    (6)   Provide the client with firm support for initiating the activity.

    (7)   Place a record of goal achievement where client can see it and mark each step toward the goal with a reward marker.

    (8)   Provide positive verbal reinforcement for goal achievement and progress.

    (9)   For further information about clients with depressed mood refer to Individual Coping, Ineffective (Chapter 11).

2. Collaborate with a physical therapist in establishing an appropriate exercise plan.
3. Collaborate with an occupational therapist for appropriate diversional activity schedule.
4. Teach client appropriate exercise methods to prevent injury (i.e., no straight-leg sit ups; proper muscle stretching and warmup before aerobic exercise; reaching target heart rate; stopping exercise if experiencing pain, excessive fatigue, nausea, breathlessness, etc.).
5. Teach client relationship between nutrition and exercise tolerance, and assist in developing a diet that is appropriate for nutritional and metabolic needs (see Chapter 3 for further information).
6. Assist client in acquiring equipment to perform desired exercise (list needed equipment here; this could include proper shoes, eyeglasses, weights, etc.).
7. Monitor effect current medications may have on activity tolerance and teach client necessary adjustments (e.g.,psychotropic medications may cause postural hypotension and client should be instructed to change position slowly).
8. Schedule time to discuss plans and special concerns with client and client's support system. This could include teaching and answering questions. Schedule daily during initial days of hospitalization and one longer time just before discharge. Note scheduled times and person responsible for this here.
9. Refer to appropriate community agencies for follow-up.
   These could include:
   a. Visiting nurse
   b. Physical therapist
   c. Occupational therapist
   d. Physician
   e. Social services
   f. Psychiatric nurse clinician

HOME HEALTH

1. Teach patient and family appropriate monitoring of causes, signs, and symptoms of potential or actual activity intolerance:
   a. Prolonged bed rest
   b. Circulatory or respiratory problems
   c. New activity
   d. Fatigue
   e. Dyspnea
   f. Pain
   g. Vital signs (before and after activity)
   h. Malnutrition
   i. Previous inactivity
   j. Weakness
   k. Confusion
2. Assist patient and family in identifying life-style changes that may be required.
   a. Progressive exercise to increase endurance
   b. Range of motion and flexibility exercises

   c. Treatments for underlying conditions (cardiac, respiratory, musculoskeletal, circulatory, etc.)
   d. Motivation
   e. Assistive devices as required (walkers, canes, crutches, wheelchairs, etc.)
   f. Adequate nutrition
   g. Adequate fluids
   h. Stress management
   i. Pain relief
   j. Prevention of hazards of immobility
   k. Changes in occupation, family, or social roles
   l. Changes in living conditions
   m. Economic concerns
3. Teach patient and family purposes and side effects of medications and proper administration techniques.
4. Assist patient and family to set criteria to help them to determine when physician or other intervention is required.
5. Consult with or refer to appropriate assistive resources as indicated.
   a. Visiting nurse
   b. Occupational therapist
   c. Rehabilitation
   d. Physical therapist
   e. Social service
   f. Psychiatric nurse clinician
   g. Nutritionist
   h. Physician

EVALUATION
OBJECTIVE 1

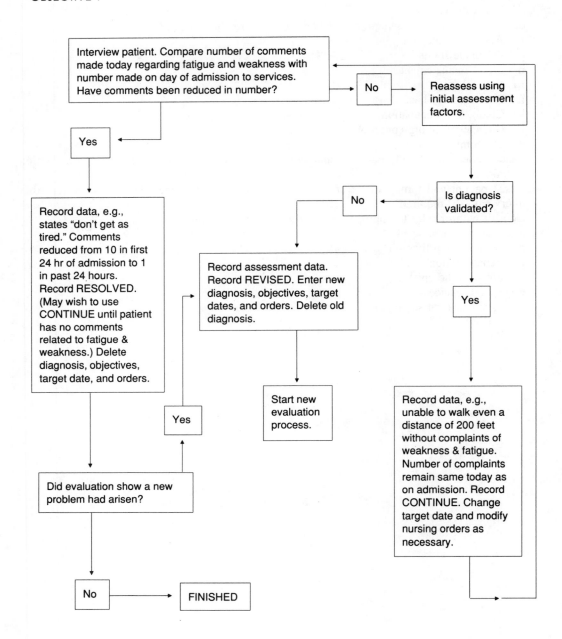

OBJECTIVE 2

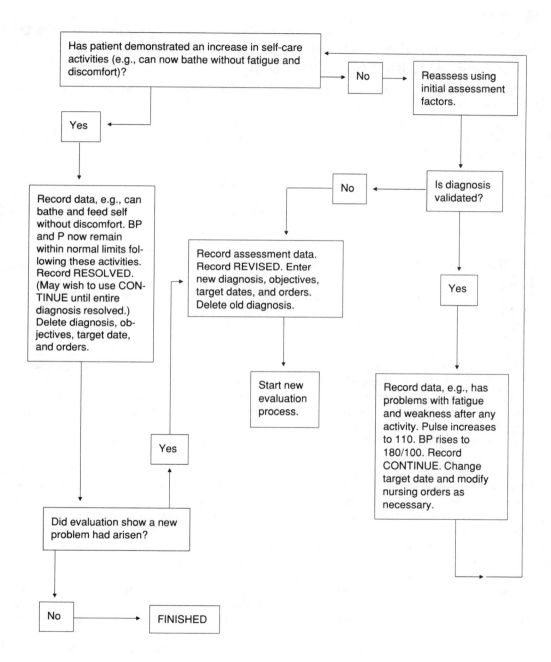

Airway Clearance, Ineffective

DEFINITION

A state in which an individual is unable to clear secretions or obstructions from the respiratory tract to maintain airway patency (NANDA, 1987, p. 43)

DEFINING CHARACTERISTICS (NANDA, 1987, p. 43)

The nurse will review the initial pattern assessment for the following defining characteristics to determine the diagnosis of Airway Clearance, Ineffective.

1. Major defining characteristics
   a. Abnormal breath sounds: rales (crackles), rhonchi (wheezes)
   b. Changes in rate or depth of respiration
   c. Tachypnea
   d. Cough (effective or ineffective, with or without sputum)
   e. Cyanosis
   f. Dyspnea
2. Minor defining characteristics
   None given.

RELATED FACTORS (NANDA, 1987, p. 43)

1. Decreased energy; fatigue
2. Tracheobronchial infection, obstruction, secretion
3. Perceptual or cognitive impairment
4. Trauma

DIFFERENTIATION

Airway Clearance, Ineffective needs to be differentiated from Breathing Pattern, Ineffective; Gas Exchange, Impaired; Knowledge Deficit; Fluid Volume Deficit; and Comfort, Altered: Pain.

Breathing Pattern, Ineffective implies an alteration in the rate, rhythm, depth, or type of respiration such as hyperventilation or hypoventilation. These patterns are not effective in supplying oxygen to the cells of the body or in removing the products of respiration. However, air is able to move freely through the air passages. In ineffective airway clearance, the air passages are obstructed in some way.

Gas Exchange, Impaired is another nursing diagnosis that should be differentiated from ineffective airway clearance. Impaired gas exchange means that air has been inhaled through the air passages but that oxygen and carbon dioxide are not appropriately exchanged at the alveolar-capillary level. Air has been able to pass through clear air passages but a problem arises at the cellular level.

Knowledge Deficit would be an appropriate primary nursing diagnosis if the patient does not know the most efficient and effective methods to cough or to clear the airway. Ineffective airway clearance is then secondary to the knowledge deficit.

Fluid Volume Deficit may be the differential diagnosis when the decreased fluid volume is sufficient to make the secretions of the respiratory tract thick and tenacious. Then the patient would be unable to effectively expel the secretions no matter how hard he or she tried, and ineffective airway clearance would result.

Comfort, Altered: Pain is another nursing diagnosis that should be differentiated from ineffective airway clearance. If the pain is sufficient to prevent the patient from coughing to clear the airway then ineffective airway clearance will result secondary to the pain.

OBJECTIVES

1. Will have an open, clear airway by (date).

AND/OR

2. Will easily expectorate secretions from airway by (date).

TARGET DATE

Ineffective airway clearance is life-threatening; therefore, progress toward meeting the objective should be evaluated at least on a daily basis.

ADDITIONAL INFORMATION

The various ways of measuring lung capacity are summarized and defined in Table 5.1.

NURSING ORDERS

ADULT HEALTH

1. Monitor effects of medications used to open patient's airways (bronchodilators, corticosteroids). Document effect within 30 minutes after administration.
2. Maintain adequate fluid intake to liquefy secretions. Encourage intake up to 3000 ml per day. Measure output each 8 hours.
3. Assist patient in coughing efforts to make them more productive:
   a. Sitting up
   b. Placing hands on upper abdomen and exerting inward, upward pressure during cough
   c. Humidifying inspired air
4. Assist with cupping and clapping activities. Teach family these procedures.
5. Suction as needed. Provide oxygen as needed.
6. Instruct patient to avoid irritating substances, large crowds, and persons with upper respiratory infections.
7. Give mucolytic agents via nebulizer or intermittent positive-pressure breathing (IPPB) treatments as ordered.
8. Collaborate with physician regarding frequency of blood gas measurements.

Table 5.1.
Lung Capacities and Volumes

Measurement	Average Value, Adult Male	Definition
Tidal volume (TV)	500 ml (resting)	Amount of air inhaled or exhaled with each breath
Inspiratory reserve volume (IRV)	3100	Amount of air that can be forcefully inhaled after a normal tidal volume inhalation
Expiratory reserve volume (ERV)	1200	Amount of air that can be forcefully exhaled after a normal tidal volume exhalation
Residual volume (RV)	1200	Amount of air left in the lungs after a forced exhalation
Total lung capacity (TLC)	6000	Maximum amount of air that can be contained in the lungs after a maximum inspiratory effort: $TLC = TV + IRV + ERV + RV$
Vital capacity (VC)	4800	Maximum amount of air that can be expired after a maximum inspiration: $VC = TV + IRV + ERV$ (should be 80% of TLC)
Inspiratory capacity (IC)	3600	Maximum amount of air that can be inspired after a normal expiration: $IC = TV + IRV$
Functional residual capacity (FRC)	2400	Volume of air remaining in the lungs after a normal tidal volume expiration: $FRC = ERV + RV$

9. Monitor respiratory rate, depth, and breath sounds at least every 4 hours.
10. Administer oral hygiene at least every 4 hours while awake.

CHILD HEALTH

1. Monitor patient factors which relate to ineffective airway clearance, including:
   a. Feeding tolerance or intolerance
   b. Allergens
   c. Emotional aspects
   d. Stressors of recent or past activities
   e. Congenital anomalies
   f. Parental anxieties
   g. Infant or child temperament
   h. Abdominal distention
   i. Related vital signs, especially heart rate
   j. Diaphragmatic excursion
   k. Retraction in respiratory effort
   l. Choking, coughing
   m. Flaring of nares
   n. Appropriate functioning of respiratory equipment
2. Provide appropriate attention to suctioning and related respiratory maintenance:
   a. Appropriate size for catheter as needed
   b. Appropriate administration of humidified oxygen as ordered per physician if applicable
   c. Appropriate follow-up of blood gases if applicable (to be specified for limits to report to physician)
   d. Documentation of oxygen administration, characteristics of secretions obtained by suctioning, vital signs during suctioning, reporting apical pulse below 70 or above 149 beats/minute for infant, below 90 or above 120 beats/minute for young child.
3. Encourage parental input in planning care for patient with attention to individual preferences when possible.
4. Promote rest and relaxation by scheduling treatments and activities with appropriate rest periods.
5. Administer medications as ordered and monitor for specific side effects (Example—Aminophylline IV drip: Ensure appropriate dilution, note incompatibility factor. Monitor for nausea, increased heart rate, irritability, etc.).
6. Provide health teaching as needed based on assessment and child's situation.
7. Plan for appropriate follow-up with health team members to include:
   a. Pediatric nurse specialist
   b. Respiratory therapist
   c. Play therapist
   d. Pediatric subspecialist (e.g., allergist or pulmonologist)
   e. Social service
   f. Support groups such as Cystic Fibrosis Society
   g. Community health nurse
   h. Dietitian
8. Reduce apprehension by providing comforting behavior and meeting developmental needs of patient and family.
9. Allow for diversional activities to approximate tolerance of child.
10. Encourage family members to assist in care of patient with use of return-demonstration opportunities for teaching required skills.
11. Provide for appropriate safety maintenance, especially with oxygen administration (no smoking) and appropriate precautions for age and developmental level.

12. Maintain appropriate emergency equipment as dictated by situation (e.g., tracheostomy sterile setup, suctioning apparatus).
13. Provide for appropriate follow-up by scheduling appointments before dismissal.
14. Allow ample time for parental mastery of skills identified in care of child.

WOMEN'S HEALTH

(Note: The following nursing orders pertain to the newborn infant in the delivery room, immediately following delivery. See Adult Health or Home Health for orders related to the mother.)

1. Evaluate and record the respiratory status of the newborn infant:
    a. Suction mouth and pharynx with bulb syringe.
        (1) Clear mouth and oropharynx with bulb syringe.
        (2) Avoid deep suctioning if possible.
2. Continue to evaluate infant's respiratory status and to act if necessary to resuscitate. Depending on infant's response, the following nursing measures can be taken.
    a. Administer warm, humid oxygen with face mask
    b. If no improvement, administer oxygen with bag and mask
    c. If no improvement, be prepared for:
        (1) Endotracheal intubation
        (2) Ventilation with positive pressure
        (3) Cardiac massage
        (4) Transport to neonatal intensive care unit

MENTAL HEALTH

1. Discuss with client factors contributing to ineffective clearance.
2. Discuss with client importance of maintaining proper position to include:
    a. Side-lying position while in bed
    b. Sitting or standing position with shoulders back and back as straight as possible to facilitate expansion of the diaphragm
3. Remind client of proper positioning as required.
4. Maintain or have client maintain oral hygiene.
5. Lubricate lips with a moisturizing agent.
6. Do not allow the use of oil-based products around the nose.
7. Remind client to chew food well, and sit with him or her during mealtime if cognitive functioning indicates a need for close observation. Note any special adaptations here (i.e., soft foods, observation during meals, etc.).
8. Assist client with clearing secretions from mouth or nose by:
    a. Providing tissues;
    b. Using gentle suctioning if necessary.
9. Encourage intake of 2–4 quarts of fluid per day, if this is not contraindicated by medical condition, by:
    a. Having client's favorite fluids available;
    b. Reminding client to drink fluids at least every hour (note schedule here);
    c. Provide warm or hot drinks instead of cold fluids.
10. Teach client appropriate breathing and coughing techniques to include:
    a. Sitting in an upright position
    b. Taking a deep, slow breath while expanding abdomen, allowing diaphragm to expand
    c. Holding breath for 3–5 seconds
    d. Exhaling the breath slowly through the mouth while abdomen moves inward
    e. Pausing briefly before next breath in
    f. Coughing with the second breath inward, coughing forcefully from the chest (these should be two short, forceful coughs)

11. Observe client practicing proper breathing techniques 30 minutes twice a day (note time of practice sessions here).
12. Maintain adequate humidity in environment.
13. Collaborate with physician for possible use of saline gargles or anesthetic lozenge for sore throats (report all sore throats to physician, especially if client is receiving antipsychotic drugs and in the absence of other flu or cold symptoms).
14. Refer for appropriate consultations. These could include:
    a. Respiratory therapy
    b. Physical therapy
15. Discuss with client the role smoking plays in ineffective airway clearance and refer to a stop smoking program at a community agency such as:
    a. American Cancer Society
    b. American Heart Association
    c. American Lung Association

HOME HEALTH

1. Teach patient and family appropriate monitoring of signs and symptoms of ineffective airway clearance.
    a. Cough (effective or ineffective)
    b. Sputum
    c. Respiratory status (cyanosis, dyspnea, rate)
    d. Abnormal breath sounds (noisy respirations)
    e. Nasal flaring
    f. Intercostal, substernal retraction
    g. Choking, gagging
    h. Diaphoresis
    i. Restlessness, anxiety
    j. Impaired speech
    k. Collection of mucus in mouth
2. Assist patient and family in identifying life-style changes that may be required:
    a. Eliminating smoking
    b. Treating fear or anxiety
    c. Treating pain
    d. Performing pulmonary hygiene: clearing the bronchial tree by controlled coughing, decreasing viscosity of secretions via humidity and fluid balance, postural drainage
    e. Learning stress management
    f. Ensuring adequate nutritional intake
    g. Learning diaphragmatic breathing
    h. Administering pain relief
    i. Beginning progressive ambulation (avoid fatigue)
    j. Maintaining position so that danger of aspiration is decreased
    k. Maintaining body position to minimize work of breathing and clearing airway
    l. Ensuring adequate oral hygiene
    m. Clearing secretions from throat
    n. Suctioning as needed
    o. Keeping area free of dust and potential allergens or irritants
    p. Ensuring adequate hydration (monitor intake and output)
3. Teach patient and family purposes, side effects, and proper administration techniques of medications.
4. Assist patient and family to set criteria to help them to determine when physician or other intervention is required.

5. Teach family basic CPR.
6. Consult with or refer to appropriate assistive resources as indicated:
    a. American Lung Association
    b. Cystic Fibrosis Foundation
    c. American Cancer Society
    d. Visiting nurse
    e. Homemaker
    f. Occupational therapist
    g. Physical therapist
    h. Nutritionist
    i. Psychiatric nurse clinician
    j. Social service
    k. American Red Cross
    l. Respiratory therapist

EVALUATION
OBJECTIVE 1

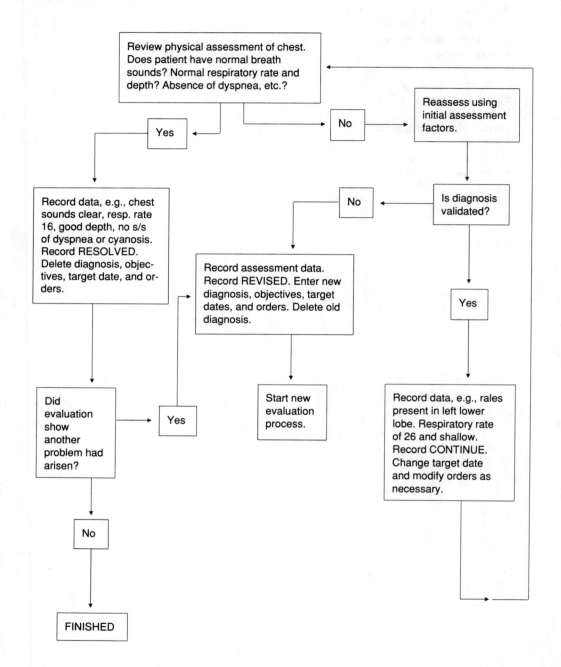

OBJECTIVE 2

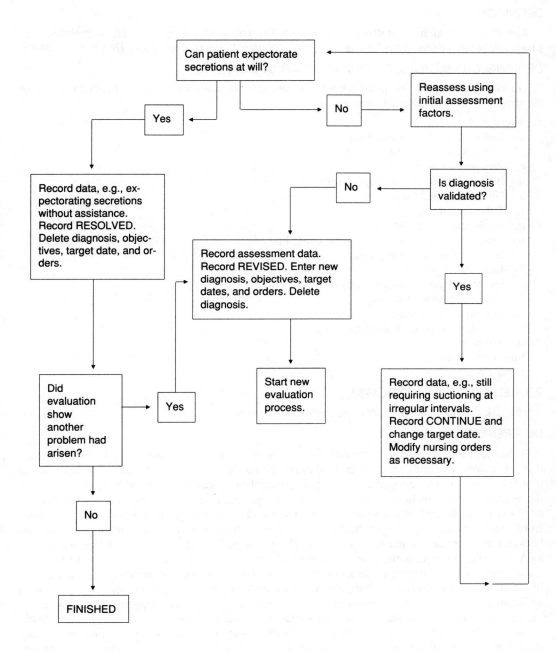

Aspiration, Potential

DEFINITION

The state in which an individual is at risk for entry of gastrointestinal secretions, oropharyngeal secretions, or solids or foods into tracheobronchial passages (NANDA, 1988).

DEFINING CHARACTERISTICS (RISK FACTORS) (NANDA, 1988)

The nurse will review the initial pattern assessment for the following characteristics to determine the diagnosis of Aspiration, Potential.

1. Major risk factors
   a. Reduced level of consciousness
   b. Depressed cough and gag reflexes
   c. Presence of tracheostomy or endotracheal tube
   d. Incomplete lower esophageal sphincter
   e. Gastrointestinal tubes
   f. Tube feedings
   g. Medication administration
   h. Situations hindering elevation of upper body
   i. Increased intragastric pressure
   j. Increased gastric residual
   k. Decreased gastrointestinal motility
   l. Delayed gastric emptying
   m. Impaired swallowing
   n. Facial, oral, or neck surgery or trauma
   o. Wired jaws
2. Minor risk factors
   None given.

RELATED FACTORS (NANDA, 1988)

The risk factors listed also serve as the related factors.

DIFFERENTIATION

Aspiration, Potential needs to be differentiated from Swallowing, Impaired. Swallowing means that when food or fluids are present in the mouth, the brain signals both the epiglottis and the true vocal cords to move together to close off the trachea so that the food and fluids can pass into the esophagus and thus into the stomach. Swallowing, Impaired implies that there is a mechanical or physiologic obstruction between the oropharynx and the esophagus that prevents food or fluids from passing into the esophagus. In Aspiration, Potential, there may or may not be an obstruction between the oropharynx and the esophagus. The major pathophysiologic dysfunction that occurs in Aspiration, Potential is the inability of the epiglottis and true vocal cords to move to close off the trachea. This inability to close off the trachea may occur because of pathophysiologic changes in the structures themselves; or because messages to the brain are absent, decreased, or impaired; or because messages from the brain to the structures are absent, misinterpreted, or impaired.

Aspiration, Potential should also be differentiated from Airway Clearance, Ineffective. In Airway Clearance, Ineffective, the patient is unable to effectively clear secretions from the respiratory tract due to some of the same related factors as are found with Aspiration, Potential. However, in Airway Clearance, Ineffective, the defining characteristics (abnormal breath sounds, cough, change in rate or depth of respirations, etc.) are associated directly with respiratory function, whereas the defining characteristics of Aspiration, Potential are directly or indirectly related to the oropharyngeal mechanisms that protect the tracheobronchial passages from the entrance of foreign substances.

OBJECTIVES

1. Will demonstrate no risk factors of aspiration by (date).

AND/OR

2. Will implement plan to offset potential for aspiration by (date).

TARGET DATE

Aspiration is life-threatening. Initial target dates should be stated in hours. After the number of risk factors have been reduced, the target date can be moved to 2–4 day intervals.

NURSING ORDERS

ADULT HEALTH

1. Sit patient up or elevate head of bed if there are no contradictory orders.
2. Feed slowly.
3. Cut food into small bites.
4. Instruct patient to chew thoroughly.
5. Teach patient to be cognizant of closing off trachea before attempting to swallow.
6. Offer small, more frequent feedings rather than 3 large meals/day.
7. Delay fluids associated with meals for at least 30 minutes after the meal.
8. Have suction equipment available.
9. Have patient cough and clear secretions prior to offering any food or fluid.
10. Teach patient to limit conversation while either eating or drinking.

CHILD HEALTH

1. Determine best position for client as determined by underlying risk factors (e.g., head of bed elevated 30° with infant propped on right side after feeding).
2. Monitor patient's status on an ongoing basis with specific attention to possibility of aspiration:
   a. Every 30 minutes check for breath sounds bilaterally (or as needed) or any change in respiratory status.
   b. Assess amount of residual in nasogastric tube and report excess of 10–20 ml of volume of feeding or as ordered.
   c. Note the presence of facial trauma or surgery of face, head, or neck-associated drainage.
   d. Assess the potential for increased intracranial pressure or condition which may cause vomiting such as Reye's syndrome.
   e. Check for nausea secondary to medications, especially post-operatively.
   f. Determine if patient has a history of cerebral palsy or neurologic damage which predisposes child to possible difficulty in swallowing or aspirations.
3. Assist patient and family to identify factors which will help prevent aspiration.
4. Provide opportunities for patient and family to ask questions or ventilate regarding potential for aspiration.
5. Assess patient and family perception of need and worth of learning CPR and first aid to deal with potential for aspiration.
6. Provide teaching for patient and family on CPR and first aid for choking.
7. Teach patient and family suctioning technique as needed, including appropriate ordering of supplies.
8. Begin discharge planning soon after admission to best afford discharge follow-up.
9. Assist family in identification of resources in the community, including available funding for equipment for suctioning, etc.
10. Collaborate with other health team members as applicable:
    a. Pediatrician or subspecialist
    b. Clinical nurse specialist, especially pediatric

c. Respiratory therapist
d. Public health nurse
e. Social workers
f. Dietitian
g. Occupational therapist

WOMEN'S HEALTH

(Note: The following nursing orders pertain to the newborn infant in the presence of meconium in amniotic fluid.)

1. Alert obstetrician and pediatrician of the presence of meconium in amniotic fluid.
2. Assemble equipment and be prepared for resuscitation of the newborn at the time of delivery.
3. Be prepared to suction infant's nasopharynx and oropharynx while head of infant is still on the perineum.
4. Evaluate and record the respiratory status of the newborn infant.
5. Assist pediatrician in viewing the vocal cords of infant (have various sizes of pediatric laryngoscopes available); if meconium is present, be prepared to insert endotracheal tube for further suctioning.
6. Continue to evaluate and record infant's respiratory status.
7. Reassure parents (mother) by keeping them informed of actions.
8. Allow opportunities for mother and significant others to verbalize fears and ask questions.

MENTAL HEALTH

(Note: Clients receiving electroconvulsive therapy (ECT) are at risk for this diagnosis, in addition to those clients experiencing any of the symptoms mentioned under Defining Characteristics. Refer to the adult health care plan. The interventions listed here are to be used in addition to those in the adult health care plan.)

1. Discuss with client the purpose for any alterations in care necessitated by this diagnosis.
2. Remind client to chew food well, and sit with him or her during mealtime if cognitive functioning indicates a need for close observation. Note any special adaptations here (i.e., soft foods, observation during meals, etc.).
3. Provide calm, relaxed atmosphere during mealtime and assist client with relaxation exercises as needed (see Anxiety, Chapter 8, for information on relaxation training).
4. Remain with client who has had ECT until gag reflex and swallowing have returned to normal.
5. Place client who has had ECT on side until reactive.
6. Clients in four-point restraint should be placed on side or stomach. Elevate client's head to eat and remove restraints one at a time to facilitate eating.
7. Request that oral medications be provided in liquid form.
8. Observe clients receiving antipsychotic agents for possible suppression of cough reflex.

HOME HEALTH

The nursing orders for home health care of this diagnosis are the same as the orders enumerated in the adult health care plan. Please refer to the adult health nursing orders.

EVALUATION
OBJECTIVE 1

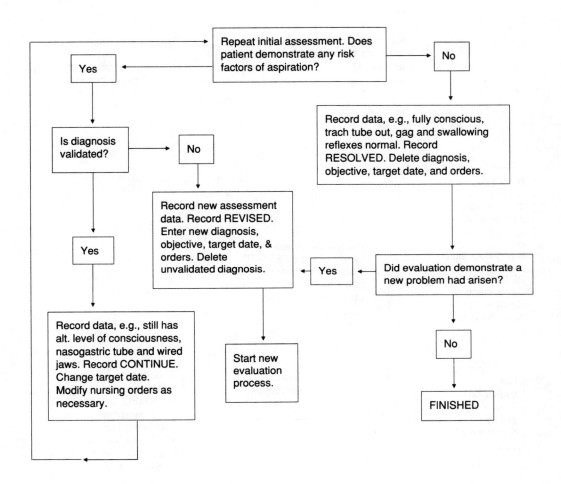

OBJECTIVE 2

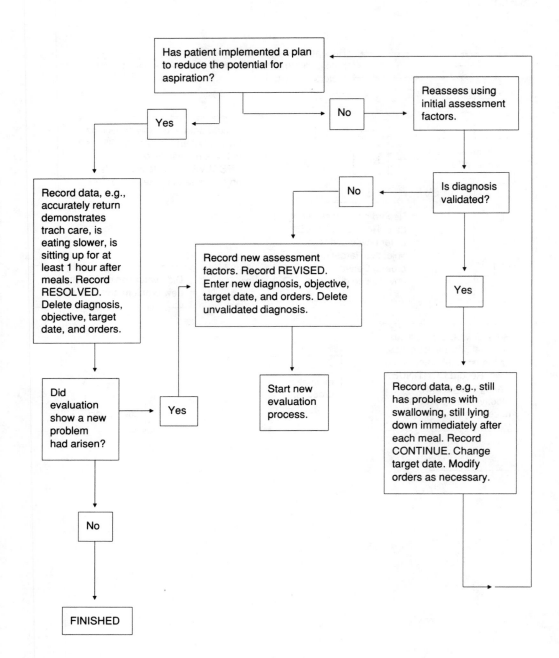

Breathing Pattern, Ineffective

DEFINITION

The state in which an individual's inhalation or exhalation pattern does not enable adequate pulmonary inflation or emptying (NANDA, 1987, p. 44).

DEFINING CHARACTERISTICS (NANDA, 1987, p. 44)

The nurse will review the initial pattern assessment for the following defining characteristics to determine the diagnosis Breathing Pattern, Ineffective.

1. Major defining characteristics
   a. Dyspnea
   b. Shortness of breath
   c. Tachypnea
   d. Fremitus
   e. Abnormal arterial blood gas
   f. Cyanosis
   g. Cough
   h. Nasal flaring
   i. Respiratory depth changes
   j. Assumption of 3-point position
   k. Pursed-lip breathing or prolonged expiratory phase
   l. Increased anteroposterior diameter
   m. Use of accessory muscles
   n. Altered chest excursion
2. Minor defining characteristics
   None given.

RELATED FACTORS (NANDA, 1987, p. 44)

1. Neuromuscular impairment
2. Pain
3. Muscloskeletal impairment
4. Perception or cognitive impaired
5. Anxiety
6. Decreased energy fatigue

DIFFERENTIATION

Breathing Pattern, Ineffective needs to be differentiated from Airway Clearance, Ineffective and Gas Exchange, Impaired.

Airway Clearance, Ineffective means that something is blocking the air passage, but when air gets to the alveoli there is adequate gas exchange. In Breathing Pattern, Ineffective, the ventilatory effort is insufficient to bring in enough oxygen or to get rid of sufficient amounts of carbon dioxide. However, air is able to freely move through the air passages.

Gas Exchange, Impaired indicates that enough oxygen is brought into the respiratory system and the carbon dioxide that is produced is exhaled, but there is insufficient exchange of oxygen and carbon dioxide at the alveolar-capillary level. There is no problem with either the ventilatory effort or the air passageways. The problem exists at the cellular level.

OBJECTIVES

1. Will demonstrate an effective breathing pattern by (date) as evidenced by (specify criteria here; e.g., normal breath sounds, arterial blood gases within normal limits, no evidence of cyanosis.)

AND/OR

2. Will demonstrate methods necessary to improve breathing pattern by (date).

TARGET DATE

Evaluation should be made on a daily basis, since this diagnosis has the potential to be life-threatening.

NURSING ORDERS

ADULT HEALTH

1. Collaborate with physician on monitoring of blood gases; report abnormal results immediately.
2. Reduce fear and anxiety by spending at least 15 minutes every 2 hours with patient.
3. Reduce chest pain using noninvasive techniques and analgesics.
4. Perform nursing orders to maintain effective airway clearance (see Airway Clearance, Ineffective; enter those orders here).
5. Raise head of bed 30° or more if not contraindicated.
6. Administer or assist with IPPB as ordered. Remain with patient during treatment.
7. Encourage patient's mobility as tolerated (see Physical Mobility, Impaired).
8. Instruct in diaphragmatic deep breathing and pursed-lip breathing.
9. Administer oxygen as ordered.
10. Turn every 2 hours.

CHILD HEALTH

1. Monitor baseline respiratory data with regard for:
   a. Respiratory rate and pattern;
   b. Use of intercostal and accessory muscles;
   c. Position of comfort;
   d. Nares for flaring;
   e. Grunting or related noises such as stridor;
   f. Coughing, nature of secretions;
   g. Breath sounds;
   h. Related vital signs, especially apical pulse and blood pressure;
   i. Aids required for respiration and airway maintenance;
   j. Skin color, hydration, and elimination;
   k. Arterial blood gases as ordered;
   l. Appropriate related equipment such as arterial line, IV;
   m. Oxygen administration per order;
   n. Documentation of all the above.
2. Determine perception of illness by patient and parents.
3. Provide teaching based on needs of patient and family regarding:
   a. Illness;
   b. Procedures, related nursing care;
   c. Implications for rest, relief of anxiety secondary to respiratory failure;
   d. Advocacy role.
4. Collaborate with appropriate related health team members as needed, considering:
   a. Respiratory therapist
   b. Pediatrician and subspecialist such as pulmonologist, neonatalogist, or pediatric cardiologist
   c. Pediatric clinical nurse specialist
   d. Play therapist
   e. Occupational therapist
   f. Dietitian
   g. Community health nurse

    h. Social worker
    i. Community resource groups
5. Include parents in care of child as appropriate, to include comfort measures, assisting with feeding, and the like.
6. Allow at least 5–15 minutes per shift for parents and child to verbalize concerns related to illness.
7. Maintain appropriate emergency equipment in an accessible place. (Specify actual size of endotracheal tube for infant, child, or adolescent, trach set size, and suctioning catheters or chest tube for size of patient.)
8. Maintain appropriate attention to relief of pain and anxiety via positioning, suctioning, and administration of medications as ordered.
9. Maintain appropriate caution for possible side effects of respiratory depression for specific medication such as morphine or Valium.

WOMEN'S HEALTH

(Note: The nursing orders found in Adult Health and Home Health apply to women. The following relates to pregnancy).

1. Assist client and significant other in identifying life-style changes that may be required to prevent ineffective breathing pattern.
2. Carefully monitor maternal respiration during the laboring process.
    a. Amount and type of analgesia and anesthesia given to client during labor can cause maternal hypoxia and reduce fetal oxygen.
    b. Administer pure oxygen (10–12 liters/minute) to mother before delivery and until cessation of pulsation in cord.
3. Develop exercise plan for cardiovascular fitness during pregnancy.
4. Avoid wearing constrictive clothing.
5. Teach and encourage client to practice correct breathing techniques for labor to prevent hyperventilation.
6. During the latter stages of pregnancy, when the chest cavity has less room to expand because of the enlarging uterus, encourage patient to:
    a. Walk up stairs slowly;
    b. Lie on left side, to get more oxygen to fetus;
    c. Position herself in bed with pillows for optimum comfort and adequate air exchange;
    d. Take frequent rest breaks during the work day.

Newborn

7. Evaluate and record the respiratory status of the newborn infant:
    a. Determine the 1-minute Apgar score.
    b. Suction mouth and pharynx with bulb syringe.
        (1) Clear mouth and oropharynx with bulb syringe.
        (2) Avoid deep suctioning if possible.
    c. Dry excess moisture off infant with towel or blanket.
        (1) Helps stimulate infant
        (2) Prevents evaporative heat loss
    d. Stimulate (if necessary), using firm but *gentle* tactile stimulation:
        (1) Slapping sole of foot
        (2) Rubbing up and down spine
        (3) Flicking heel
    e. Place in warm environment:
        (1) Under radiant heat warmer

(2) Next to mother's skin
    (a) Cover infant's head with stocking cap
    (b) Cover both mother and infant with warm blanket
  f. Determine and record the 5-minute Apgar score.
8. Continue to evaluate infant's respiratory status and to act if necessary to resuscitate. Depending on infant's response, the following nursing measures can be taken:
  a. Administer warm, humid oxygen with face mask.
  b. If no improvement, administer oxygen with bag and mask.
  c. If no improvement, be prepared for:
    (1) Endotracheal intubation;
    (2) Ventilation with positive pressure;
    (3) Cardiac massage;
    (4) Transport to neonatal intensive care unit.

MENTAL HEALTH

1. Monitor causative factors.
2. Place client in calm, supportive environment.
3. Maintain a calm, supportive attitude, reassuring client that you will assist him or her in maintaining control.
4. Give client clear, concise directions.
5. Have client maintain direct eye contact with nurse.
6. Instruct client to take slow, deep breaths, demonstrating them to the client.
7. Breathe with the client, providing him or her with constant, positive reinforcement for appropriate breathing patterns.
8. Remain with the client until the episode is resolved.
9. If client does not respond to the attempts to control breathing, have client breathe into a paper bag to rebreathe air with a higher CO_2 content that will slow the respiratory rate.
10. Distract client from focus on breathing by beginning a deep muscle relaxation exercise that begins at the client's feet.
11. Use successful resolution of a problematic breathing episode as an opportunity to teach client that he or she can gain conscious control over breathing and that these episodes are not out of his or her control.
12. Discuss with client the role smoking plays in ineffective breathing patterns.
13. Teach client and significant others proper breathing techniques to include:
  a. Maintaining proper body alignment
  b. Using diaphragmatic breathing (see Airway Clearance, Ineffective for information on technique)
  c. Use of deep muscle relaxation before the onset of an ineffective breathing pattern begins
14. Practice with client diaphragmatic breathing twice a day for 30 minutes. Note practice times here.
15. Develop a plan with client for initiating slow, deep breathing when an ineffective breathing pattern begins.
16. Identify with client those situations that are most frequently associated with the development of ineffective breathing patterns and assist him or her in practicing relaxation in response to these situations one time a day for 30 minutes. Note time of practice session here.
17. Refer for appropriate consultations as needed to include:
  a. Respiratory therapy
  b. Physical therapy
  c. Psychiatric nurse clinician
  d. Stop smoking program in a community agency

HOME HEALTH

(Note: If this diagnosis is suspected when caring for a patient in the home, it is imperative that a physician referral be obtained immediately. If the patient has been referred to home health care by a physician, the nurse will collaborate with the physician in the treatment of the patient.)

1. Teach patient and family appropriate monitoring of signs and symptoms of ineffective breathing pattern:
   a. Cough
   b. Sputum production
   c. Fatigue
   d. Respiratory status: cyanosis, dyspnea, rate
   e. Lack of diaphragmatic breathing
   f. Nasal flaring
   g. Anxiety or restlessness
   h. Impaired speech
2. Assist patient and family in identifying life-style changes that may be required in assisting to prevent ineffective breathing pattern:
   a. Stopping smoking
   b. Prevention and early treatment of lung infections
   c. Avoidance of known irritants and allergens
   d. Pulmonary hygiene: clearing bronchial tree by controlled coughing, decreasing vicosity of secretions via humidity and fluid balance, postural drainage
   e. Treatment of fear, anxiety, anger, depression, thorax trauma, or narcotic overdoses
   f. Adequate nutritional intake
   g. Stress management
   h. Adequate hydration
   i. Breathing techniques (diaphragmatic, pursed lips)
   j. Progressive ambulation
   k. Pain relief
   l. Preventing hazards of immobility
   m. Appropriate use of oxygen (dosage, route, safety factors)
3. Teach patient and family purposes, side effects, and proper administration techniques of medication.
4. Assist patient and family to set criteria to help them to determine when physician or other intervention is required.
5. Teach family basic CPR.
6. Consult with or refer to appropriate assistive resources as indicated:
   a. American Red Cross
   b. American Lung Association
   c. Cystic Fibrosis Foundation
   d. American Cancer Society
   e. American Heart Association
   f. Visiting nurse
   g. Psychiatric nurse clinician
   h. Homemaker assistance
   i. Occupational therapist
   j. Physical therapist
   k. Group support
   l. Nutritionist
   m. Stop-smoking program

n. Psychiatric nurse clinician
o. Social service
p. Occupational counseling
q. Physician
r. Respiratory therapist

EVALUATION
OBJECTIVE 1

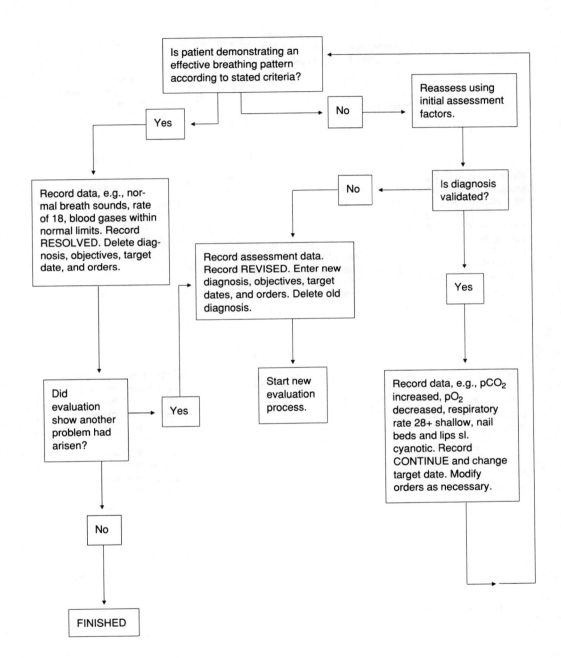

OBJECTIVE 2

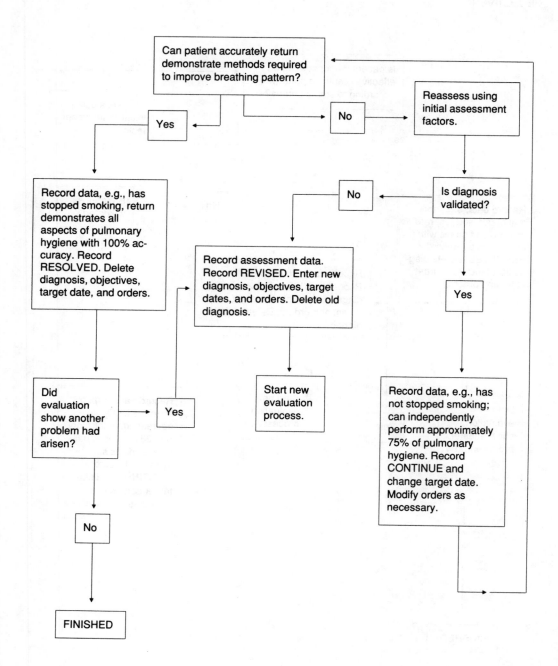

Cardiac Output, Altered: Decreased

DEFINITION

A state in which the blood pumped by an individual's heart is sufficiently reduced that it is inadequate to meet the needs of the body's tissues (NANDA, 1987, p. 41).

DEFINING CHARACTERISTICS (NANDA, 1987, p. 41)

The nurse will review the intial pattern assessment to determine the diagnosis of Cardiac Output, Altered: Decreased.

1. Major defining characteristics
   a. Variations in blood pressure readings
   b. Arrhythmias
   c. Fatigue
   d. Jugular vein distention
   e. Color changes (skin and mucous membranes)
   f. Oliguria
   g. Decreased peripheral pulses
   h. Cold, clammy skin
   i. Rales
   j. Dyspnea, orthopnea
   k. Restlessness
2. Minor defining characteristics
   a. Change in mental status
   b. Shortness of breath
   c. Syncope
   d. Vertigo
   e. Edema
   f. Cough
   g. Frothy sputum
   h. Gallop rhythm
   i. Weakness

RELATED FACTORS (NANDA, 1987, p. 41)

None given.

DIFFERENTIATION

Cardiac Output, Altered: Decreased has to be differentiated from Tissue Perfusion, Altered. Cardiac Output, Altered: Decreased relates specifically to a heart malfunction while Tissue Perfusion, Altered relates to deficits in the peripheral circulation which will have cellular-level impact. Tissue perfusion problems may develop secondary to decreased cardiac output, but can also exist without cardiac output problems (Doenges & Moorhouse, 1985).

In either diagnosis, close collaboration will be needed with medical practitioners to ensure the best possible interventions for the patient.

OBJECTIVES

1. Will exhibit no signs or symptoms of decreased cardiac output by (date).

AND/OR

2. Will implement a self-designed plan to decrease the likelihood of future decreased cardiac output episodes by (date).

TARGET DATE

Because the nursing diagnosis Cardiac Output, Altered: Decreased is so life-threatening, process toward meeting the objective should be evaluated daily for 3–5 days. If significant progress is demonstrated, then the target date can be increased to 3-day intervals. Patients who develop this diagnosis should be referred to a medical practitioner immediately and transferred to a critical care unit.

NURSING ORDERS

ADULT HEALTH

1. Place on cardiac monitor and monitor cardiac rhythm and rate continuously.
2. Monitor, at least every 2 hours:
   a. Vital signs
   b. Chest sounds
   c. Apical-radial pulse deficit
   d. Pulse pressure
   e. Other hemodynamic readings possible (e.g., wedge pressures, central venous pressure [CVP])
   f. Neck vein filling
3. Collaborate with physician regarding frequency of measurement of the following and closely monitor results:
   a. Arterial blood gases
   b. Electrolytes
   c. Cardiac enzymes
   d. Complete blood cell count
4. Explain reasons for tests and monitoring to patient as well as the role he or she plays in ensuring accurate results.
5. Measure urine output hourly. Total each 8 hours.
6. Measure intake and total at least every 8 hours. Collaborate with physician regarding limitation of intake.
7. Monitor pain and institute immediate relief measures.
8. Administer oxygen and medications as ordered and monitor effects.
9. Provide adequate rest periods:
   a. Schedule at least 5-minute rest after any activity.
   b. Schedule 30-to 60-minute rest period after each meal.
   c. Limit visitors and visiting time. Explain need for restriction to patient and significant others.
10. Keep siderails up and bed in low position for patient safety, particularly during periods of altered mental status.
11. Weigh daily at 7:30 AM.
12. Provide skin care at least every 2 hours:
    a. Change position and support in anatomical alignment.
    b. Elevate edematous extremities and use measures such as a bed cradle to keep pressure off of edematous parts.
    c. Use sheepskin, egg crate mattress, or alternating air mattress under patient.
    d. Keep linens free of wrinkles.
    e. Keep skin clean and dry. Avoid shearing forces in patient movement.
13. Position patient carefully to:
    a. Assist breathing;
    b. Avoid pressure;
    c. Maintain anatomical alignment.

14. Do range of motion exercises at least once per shift.
15. Monitor bowel elimination closely at least once per shift during waking hours. Collaborate with physician regarding stool softener to avoid straining and Valsalva maneuver.
16. Collaborate with dietitian regarding dietary restrictions (e.g., sodium, fluids, calories, cholesterol).
17. Collaborate with occupational therapist and family regarding diversional activities.
18. Assist patient with stress management and relaxation techniques every 4 hours while awake.
19. Plan to spend at least 15 minutes every 4 hours providing emotional support to patient and significant others.
20. Monitor intravenous therapy:
    a. Flow rate
    b. Insertion site
21. Teach patient and significant others:
    a. Risk factors (e.g., smoking, hypertension, obesity)
    b. Medication regiment (e.g., effects, toxicity)
    c. Need to balance rest and activity
    d. Monitoring of:
       (1) Weight—daily
       (2) Vital signs
       (3) Intake and output
    e. When to contact health care professional:
       (1) Chest pain
       (2) Dyspnea
       (3) Sudden weight gain
       (4) Decreased urine output
       (5) Increased fatigue
    f. Dietary adaptations, as necessary:
       (1) Low sodium
       (2) Low cholesterol
       (3) Caloric restriction
       (4) Soft
22. Refer to:
    a. Physical therapist for home exercise program
    b. Visiting nurse service

Additional Information (Kavanagh & Riegger, 1983)

Cardiac output refers to the amount of blood ejected from the left ventricle into the aorta per minute. Cardiac output (CO) is equivalent to the stroke volume (SV), the amount of blood ejected from the left ventricle with each contraction times the heart rate (HR) or the number of beats per minute.

$$CO = SV \times HR$$

The average amount of cardiac output is 5.6 liters per minute. This amount will vary according to the individual's amount of exercise and body size.

Cardiac output is dependent on the relationship between stroke volume and the heart rate. Cardiac output is maintained by compensatory adjustment of these two variables. If the rate slows, the time for ventricular filling (diastole) increases. This allows for an increase in the preload and a subsequent increase in stroke volume. If the stroke volume falls, the heart rate increases to compensate. Stroke volume is affected by preload, contractility, and afterload.

Preload is related to the amount of stretching of the myocardial fibers. The fibers stretch due to the increase in the volume of blood delivered to the ventricles during diastole. The degree of myocardial stretch before contraction is preload. Preload is determined by the venous return and ejection fraction (amount of blood left in the ventricle at the end of systole). Prolonged excessive stretching will lead to a decrease in cardiac output.

Contractility is a function of the intensity of the actinmyocin linkages. Increased contractility increases ventricular emptying and results in increased stroke volume. Contractility can be increased by sympathetic stimulation or by administration of such aids as calcium and epinephrine. Afterload is the amount of tension developed by the ventricle during contraction. The amount of peripheral resistence will predominantly determine the amount of tension. Excessive increases in the afterload will reduce stroke volume and cardiac output.

The heart rate is predominantly influenced by the autonomic nervous system through both the sympathetic and parasympathetic nervous systems. The sympathetic fibers can increase both rate and force, while the parasympathetic fibers act in an opposite direction. Other factors such as the central nervous system, pressoreceptor reflexes, cerebral cortex impulses, body temperature, electrolytes, and hormones also affect the heart rate, but the autonomic nervous system keeps the entire system in balance.

CHILD HEALTH

1. Provide in-depth monitoring and documentation related to:
   a. Cardiac monitoring, rate, rhythm, and regularity;
   b. Vital signs, including BP, every 1 hour or as ordered;
   c. Apical and peripheral pulses, especially pedal;
   d. Arterial and central venous pressure line maintenance and monitoring;
   e. Blood drawing (maintain an ongoing record for transfusion and replacement calculation);
   f. Liver position;
   g. Jugular venous filling and distention;
   h. Heart sounds for changes, presence of murmurs;
   i. Breath sounds for changes, presence of adventitious sounds;
   j. Oxygen administration, per (route), flow (as ordered);
   k. Ventilator if applicable:
      (1) If continuous positive airway pressure (CPAP) is on order, what setting
      (2) Peak pressure ordered
      (3) O_2 percentage desired as ordered
   l. Intake and output hourly and as ordered;
   m. Fluid and electrolyte balance;
   n. Urinary output (notify physician if below 10 ml/hour or as specified for size of infant or child);
   o. Excessive bleeding (if in postop status, notify physician if above 50 ml/hour or as specified);
   p. Tolerance of feedings if applicable;
   q. Abdominal distention and bowel sounds;
   r. Bowel movements;
   s. Level of consciousness;
   t. Notify physician for:
      (1) Premature ventricular contractions (PVCs) or other arrhythmias
      (2) Limits of pulse, respiratory rate, output criteria as specified for individual patient.
   u. Position of comfort, maintenance of neutral thermal environment;
   v. Activity tolerance;
   w. Cautious administration of medications as ordered, especially digoxin
      (1) Have another RN check dose and medication order.
      (2) Validate heart rate to be greater than specified lower limit parameter (e.g.,100 for infant before administering) and documentation of same, when to hold medication.
      (3) Apply knowledge regarding possible toxicity such as vomiting.

  (4) Ensure potassium maintenance.
  (5) Maintain digitalizing protocol.
  x. Evaluation for peripheral edema, as in extremities, eyelids, sacral area, and daily weight;
  y. Parental understanding of patient's status and treatment;
  z. Patient's response to suctioning, x-ray, or other procedures.
2. Collaborate with health team to include:
  a. Pediatrician, pediatric cardiologist, or cardiovascular surgeon
  b. Pediatric cardiac clinical nurse specialist
  c. Respiratory therapist
  d. Occupational therapist
  e. Play therapist
  f. Radiology technician
  g. Dietitian
  h. Social service worker
  i. Clergyman
  j. State crippled children services
3. Allow for parents to voice concern on a regular basis; set aside 10–15 minutes per shift for this purpose.
4. Encourage parental input in care, such as with feeding, positioning, monitoring intake and output as appropriate.
5. Encourage patient as applicable to participate in care.
6. Allow for sensitivity to time and understanding of diagnosis and seemingly abstract nature of underlying cardiac physiology, especially in noncyanotic heart disease.
7. Support parents in usual coping methodologies.
8. Maintain appropriate technique in dressing change (asepsis and cautious handwashing).
9. Limit visitors in immediate postoperative status as applicable.
10. Help reduce patient parental anxiety by touching and allowing patient to be held and comforted, especially in infant population.
11. Provide teaching with sensitivity to patient and parental needs regarding equipment, procedures, or routines (for example, use a doll for demonstration with toddler).
12. Encourage parents to meet parents of similarly involved cardiac patients.
13. Address need for parents to continue with activities of daily living with confidence regarding knowledge of restrictions in child's status.
14. Deal appropriately with related health conditions or issues.
15. Ensure availability of crash cart and emergency equipment as needed to include:
  a. Cardiac or emergency drugs
  b. Defibrillator
  c. Ambu bag (pedi or infant size)
  d. Endotracheal tube, according to size of patient
  e. Appropriate suctioning equipment

WOMEN'S HEALTH

(Note: Women will have the same nursing orders as applied to adult health, mental health, and home health in all those various situations and settings. The following nursing orders relate directly to pregnancy, labor, and delivery.)

1. Assist client with relaxation techniques.
2. Assist in developing an exercise plan for cardiovascular fitness during pregnancy. *(Note: Caution the client never to begin a new vigorous exercise plan while pregnant. Teach the client to exercise slowly, in moderation, and according to the individual's ability. A good rule of thumb is to use moderation and with the consent of the physician continue with the pre-pregnant established exercise plan. Most professionals discourage aerobics and hot tubs or*

spas because of the heat. It is not known at this time if overheating by the mother is harmful to the fetus.) Some good exercises are:

    a. Swimming

    b. Walking

    c. Bicycling

    d. Jogging (if patient has done this before and is used to it) (*But* remember that during pregnancy joints and muscles are more susceptible to strain; if patient feels pain, fatigue, or overheating, should slow down or stop exercise.)

3. Refer client to support groups that understand that physiology of pregnancy and have developed exercise programs based on this physiology, such as swimming classes for pregnant women at the local YWCA, childbirth education classes, or the exercise videotapes produced by the American College of Obstetricians and Gynecologists (available through ASPO/Lamaze, P. O. Box 952, McLean, VA 22101).

4. Teach patient and significant others how to avoid "supine hypotension" during pregnancy (particularly the later stages).

    a. Lying on left side to reduce pressure on vena cava

    b. Taking frequent rest breaks during the day

    c. Wearing support hose (not knee-high) to reduce venous pooling in lower extremities

    d. Propping feet up while sitting or resting

5. During the 2nd stage of labor avoid straining and Valsalva maneuver by:

    a. Encouraging patient to attend childbirth education classes to learn how to work with her body during labor;

    b. Allowing client to assume whatever position aids her in the 2nd stage of labor (i.e., upright, squatting, kneeling position, etc.)

    c. Providing client with proper physical support during the 2nd stage of labor (*including* allowing the partner or support person to sit or stand beside her and support her head or shoulders; or behind her supporting her with his or her body; or in front of her allowing her to lean on his or her shoulders with her arms about his or her neck; as well as the use of a birthing bed or chair, pillows, over-the-bed table, or bars);

    d. Not urging the woman to "push, push" or to hold breath during the 2nd stage of labor. Allow the woman to bear down with her contractions at her own pace:

        (1) Keeping pelvic floor muscles relaxed

        (2) Keeping shoulders rounded forward

        (3) Keeping chin tucked against chest

        (4) Pressing and rounding (rocking pelvis) lower back

        (5) Encouraging spontaneous, even breathing patterns that flow with the contractions and allow pushing with the diaphragm while relaxing abdominal muscles (Kitzinger, 1984).

MENTAL HEALTH

1. Monitor risk factors: medications, past history of cardiac problems, age, current condition of the cardiovascular system, weight, exercise patterns, nutritional patterns, psychosocial stressors.

2. Monitor every (number) hours (depends on level of risk, can be anywhere from 2 to 8 hours) client's cardiac functioning (list times to observe here).

    a. Vital signs

    b. Chest sounds

    c. Apical-radial pulse deficit

    d. Mental status

3. Closely monitor results of:

    a. Arterial blood gases

    b. Electrolytes

    c. Cardiac enzymes
    d. Complete blood cell count
4. Report alterations to medical practitioner.
5. Weigh client daily at same time with same-weight clothing.
6. If acute situation develops, notify medical practitioner and implement the following plan:
    a. Place on cardiac monitor and monitor cardiac rhythm and rate continuously.
    b. Collaborate with physician regarding frequency of measurement of the following and closely monitor results:
        (1) Arterial blood gases
        (2) Electrolytes
        (3) Cardiac enzymes
        (4) Complete blood cell count
    c. Monitor vital signs every 15 minutes to 2 hours dependent on client's condition (list times here).
    d. Measure intake and output hourly.
    e. Restrict fluids as indicated.
    f. Administer O_2 as indicated.
    g. Provide a calm, restful environment by decreasing stimuli and scheduling tests in a manner that provides for adequate rest periods.
    h. Administer medications as ordered.
    i. Answer questions from the client and the client's support system in an honest manner.
    j. Do not use physical restraints, as client may become more agitated and increase physical activity.
    k. Keep siderails on bed elevated to prevent injury when client is confused. If the unit has no beds with siderails, client may be placed on mattress on the floor until one can be obtained.
    l. Position client in a manner that:
        (1) Facilitates breathing (may need head elevated);
        (2) Maintains cardiac flow (horizontal trunk with legs slightly raised);
        (3) Avoids pressure;
        (4) Maintains anatomical alignment.
7. If client's condition or other factors necessitate client remaining in the mental health area beyond the acute stage, refer to Adult Health care plan for care on an ongoing basis. This is not recommended due to the lack of equipment and properly trained staff to care for this situation on most specialized care units.
8. If client is placed on unit while in the rehabilitation stage of this diagnosis, implement the following care plan:
    a. Discuss with client current rehabilitation schedule and record special considerations here.
    b. Provide appropriate rest periods following activity. This varies according to the client's stage in rehabilitation. Most common times of needed rest are after meals and after any activity.
    c. Assist client with implementation of exercise program. List types of activity, time spent in activity, and times of activity here. Also list special motivators the client may need, such as a companion to walk for 30 minutes three times a day.
    d. Provide diet restrictions (i.e., low sodium, low calorie, low fat, low cholesterol, fluid restrictions).
    e. Monitor intake and output each shift.
    f. Assess for and teach client to assess for:
        (1) Potassium loss (muscle cramps)
        (2) Chest pain
        (3) Dyspnea
        (4) Sudden weight gain

(5) Decreased urine output

(6) Increased fatigue

g. Assess increased risk factors and assist client in developing a plan to reduce these (i.e., smoking, obesity, stress) (refer to appropriate nursing diagnosis for assistance in developing interventions).

h. Spend 30 minutes twice a day teaching client deep muscle relaxation and practicing this process (list times here).

i. Discuss with support system the life-style alterations.

j. Develop stress reduction program with client and provide necessary environment for implementation. This could include massage therapy, meditation, aerobic exercise as tolerated, hobbies, music, etc.

9. Refer to appropriate community supports to include:

a. Visiting nurse

b. Physical therapist

c. Occupational therapist

d. Nutritionist

e. Weight loss support groups

f. Anorexia support groups

g. Stop-smoking groups

h. Psychiatric mental health nurse clinical specialist

HOME HEALTH

(Note: If this diagnosis is suspected when caring for a client in the home, it is imperative that a physician referral be obtained immediately. If the client has been referred to home health care by a physician, the nurse will collaborate with the physician in the treatment of the client.)

1. Teach patient and family appropriate monitoring of signs and symptoms of decreased cardiac output:

a. Pulse

b. Blood pressure

c. Edema

d. Urinary output

e. Fatigue

f. Weight fluctuation

g. Chest pain

h. Respiratory status (dyspnea, cyanosis, rate)

i. Physiologic responses to physical activity

2. Assist patient and family in identifying life-style changes that may be required.

a. Eliminating smoking

b. Cardiac rehabilitation program

c. Stress management

d. Weight control

e. Dietary restrictions

f. Decreased alcohol

g. Relaxation techniques

h. Bowel regime to avoid straining and constipation

i. Maintenance of fluid and electrolyte balance

j. Changes in role functions in family

k. Concerns regarding sexual activity

l. Monitoring activity and responses to activity

m. Providing diversional activities when physical activity is restricted (see Diversional Activity, Deficit)

    n. Pain control
3. Teach family basic CPR.
4. Teach patient and family purposes and side effects of medications and proper administration techniques.
5. Teach patient and family to refrain from activities which increase the demands on the heart.
6. Assist patient and family to set criteria to help them to determine when a physician or other intervention is required.
7. Consult with or refer to appropriate assistive resources as indicated:
    a. American Red Cross
    b. Visiting nurse
    c. Homemaker
    d. American Heart Association
    e. Stop-smoking group
    f. Cardiac rehabilitation
    g. Physical therapist
    h. Occupational therapist
    i. Nutritionist
    j. Physician
    k. Social services
    l. Occupational counseling
    m. Psychiatric nurse clinician
    n. Pharmacist

EVALUATION
OBJECTIVE 1

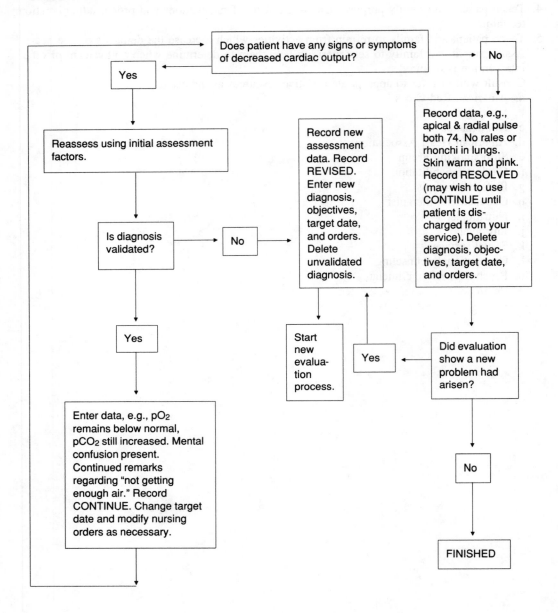

OBJECTIVE 2

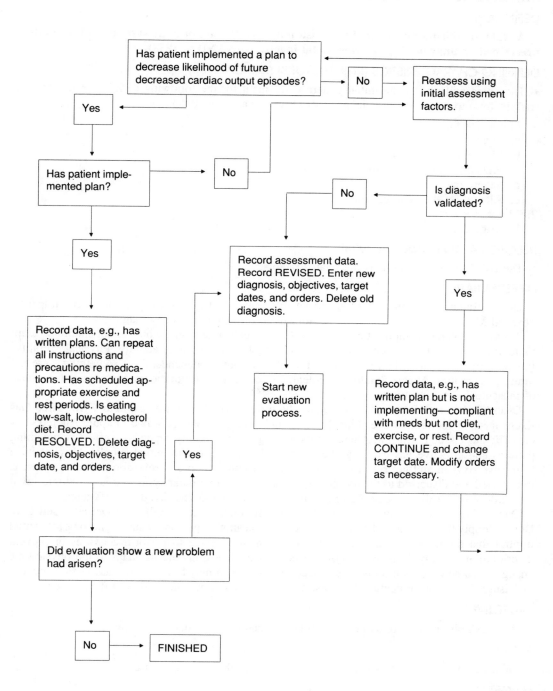

Disuse Syndrome, Potential

DEFINITION

A state in which an individual is at risk for deterioration of body systems as the result of prescribed or unavoidable muscloskeletal inactivity (NANDA, 1988).

DEFINING CHARACTERISTICS (RISK FACTORS) (NANDA, 1988)

The nurse will review the initial pattern assessment for the following defining characteristics (risk factors) to determine the diagnosis of Disuse Syndrome, Potential.

1. Major risk factors
   a. Paralysis
   b. Mechanical immobilization
   c. Prescribed immobilization
   d. Severe pain
   e. Altered level of consciousness
2. Minor risk factors
   None given.

RELATED FACTORS (NANDA, 1988)

The risk factors also serve as the related factors.

DIFFERENTIATION

Disuse Syndrome, Potential needs to be differentiated from Activity Intolerance, Impaired Physical Mobility, and any of the respiratory or cardiovascular nursing diagnoses.

Activity Intolerance implies that the individual is freely able to move but cannot endure or adapt to the increased energy or oxygen demands made by the movement or activity. Physical Mobility, Impaired implies that an individual would be able to move independently if something were not limiting the motion. Disuse Syndrome, Potential refers to the deterioration of body systems because of musculoskeletal inactivity

Disuse Syndrome, Potential also needs to be differentiated from the respiratory (Impaired Gas Exchange and Ineffective Breathing Pattern) and cardiovascular (Cardiac Output, Altered: Decreased; and Tissue Perfusion, Altered) nursing diagnoses. Mobility depends on effective breathing patterns and effective gas exchange between the lungs and arterial blood supply. Muscles have to receive oxygen and get rid of carbon dioxide for contraction and relaxation. Since oxygen is transported and dispersed to the muscle tissue via the cardiovascular system, it is only logical that the cardiovascular diagnoses need to be differentiated from Disuse Syndrome, Potential

Disuse Syndrome, Potential also needs to be differentiated from Self-Care Deficits. Self-Care Deficits imply that the clients has some dependence on another person. Disuse Syndrome, Potential implies that the client is independent but is potentially unable to perform activities or prevent deterioration of body systems because the body is unable to endure or adapt to the physiologic changes created by the muscloskeletal inactivity. A person may have a Self-Care Deficit because of Disuse Syndrome, Potential, but these two nursing diagnoses need to be differentiated.

OBJECTIVES

1. Will exhibit no signs or symptoms of disuse syndrome by (date).

AND/OR

2. Will demonstrate (specify activities) to prevent development of disuse syndrome by (date).

TARGET DATE

Disuse Syndrome can develop rapidly after the onset of immobilization. The initial target date, therefore, should be 2 days.

NURSING ORDERS

ADULT HEALTH

1. Perform active and passive range of motion exercises to all joints at least once per shift.
2. Instruct patient to perform isotonic exercises at least every 4 hours.
3. Instruct patient on relaxation and pain-reducing methods.
4. Maintain adequate nutrition and fluid balance.
5. Orient patient to environment as necessary.
6. Turn and anatomically position patient every 2 hours on the (odd/even) hours.

(Note: Refer to Physical Mobility, Impaired for more detailed orders.)

CHILD HEALTH

1. Monitor for contributing factors to pattern of disuse.
2. According to patient's status, determine realistic potential and actual levels of functioning with regard to general physical condition.
   a. Cognition
   b. Mobility, head control, positioning
   c. Communication, receptive and expressive, verbal or non-verbal
   d. Augmentive aids for daily living
3. Assist family in development of an individualized plan of care to best meet child's potential.
4. Assist family in identification of factors that will facilitate progress as well as those factors that may hinder progress in meeting child's potentials.
5. Encourage patient and family to ventilate feelings which may relate to disuse—offer time of 15–20 minutes for each nursing shift or as needed.
6. Arrange daily activities with appropriate regard for rest as needed.
7. Assist family in identification of support system for best possible follow-up, to include:
   a. Possible support groups (post–motor vehicle accident organization)
   b. Peer support group
   c. Homebound teacher
   d. Therapists, both physical and occupational
   e. Public health nurse
   f. Home health nurse
   g. Social worker
   h. Clinical nurse specialist
   i. Mental health specialist
   j. Environmental advisor regarding least restrictive environment
   k. Pediatrician or subspecialist
8. Monitor patient and family for perceived and actual health teaching needs, including:
   a. Patient's status
   b. Patient's daily care
   c. Equipment required for patient's care
   d. Signs or symptoms to be reported to physician
   e. Medications, administration, instructions, side effects
   f. Plans for follow-up
   g. Troubleshooting

WOMEN'S HEALTH

This nursing diagnosis will pertain to women the same as to any other adult. The reader is referred to the other sections (Adult Health, Home Health, and Mental Health) for specific nursing orders and objectives pertaining to women and Disuse Syndrome, Potential.

MENTAL HEALTH

(Note: The interventions in this section reflect the potential for disuse syndrome related to mental health. This would include use of restraints and seclusion. If the inactivity is related to a physiologic or physical problem, refer to the appropriate care plan under Adult Health.)

1. Attempt all other interventions before considering immobilizing the client. (See Violence, Potential for, Chapter 9, for appropriate interventions.)
2. Carefully monitor client for appropriate level of restraint necessary. Immobilize the client as little as possible while still protecting the client and others.
3. Obtain necessary medical orders to initiate methods that limit the client's physical mobility.
4. Carefully explain to client in brief, concise language, reasons for initiating this intervention and what behavior must be present for the intervention to be terminated.
5. Attempt to gain client's voluntary compliance with the intervention by explaining to client what is needed and with a "show of force" (having the necessary number of staff available to force compliance if the client does not respond to the request).
6. Initiate forced compliance only if there is an adequate number of staff to complete the action safely (see Violence, Potential for for a detailed description of intervention with forced compliance).
7. Secure the environment the client will be in by removing harmful objects such as accessible light bulbs, sharp objects, glass objects, tight clothing, metal objects, shower curtain rods, etc.
8. If client is placed in four-point restraints, maintain one-to-one supervision.
9. If client is in seclusion or in bilateral restraints, observe client at least every 15 minutes, more frequently if agitated. (List observation schedule here.)
10. Leave urinal in room with client or offer toileting every hour.
11. Offer client fluids every 15 minutes while awake.
12. Discuss with client his or her feelings about the initiation of immobility and review at least twice a day the kinds of behavior necessary to have immobility discontinued.
13. When checking client, let him or her know you are checking by calling him or her by name and orienting him or her to day and time. Inquire about client's feelings and implement necessary reality orientation.
14. Provide meals at regular intervals on paper containers, providing necessary assistance (amount and type of assistance required should be listed here).
15. If client is in restraints, remove restraints at least every 2 hours one limb at a time. Have client move limb through a full range of motion and inspect for signs of injury. Apply lubricants such as lotion to area under restraint to protect from injury.
16. Pad the area of the restraint that is next to the skin with sheepskin or other nonirritating material.
17. Check circulation in restrained limbs in the area below the restraint by observing skin color, warmth, and swelling. Restraint should not interfere with circulation.
18. Change client's position in the bed every 2 hours. Have client cough and deep breathe during this time (list schedule for change here).
19. Place body in proper alignment to prevent complications and injury. Use pillows for support if client's condition allows.
20. If client is in four-point restraints, place on stomach or side to prevent aspiration or choking.
21. Place client on intake and output monitoring to ensure adequate fluid balance is maintained.
22. Have client in seclusion move around the room at least every 2 hours, during this time initiate active range of motion and have client cough and take deep breaths (note schedule of this activity here).
23. Administer medications as ordered for agitation.
24. Monitor blood pressure before administering antipsychotic medications.

25. Have client change position slowly, especially from lying to standing.
26. Assist client with daily personal hygiene (record time for this here).
27. Have environment cleaned on a daily basis.
28. Remove client from seclusion as soon as the contracted behavior is observed for the required amount of time (both of these should be very specific and listed here). (See Violence, Potential for, Chapter 9, for detailed information on behavior change and contracting specifics.)
29. Schedule time to discuss this intervention with client and his or her support system. Inform support system of the need for the intervention and about special considerations related to visiting with the client. This information must be provided with consideration of the support system before and after each visit.
30. Arrange consultations with appropriate resources after client is released from mobility limitations to assist client with developing alternate coping behaviors. This could include:
    a. Physical therapist
    b. Occupational therapist
    c. Psychiatric nurse clinician
    d. Social worker

HOME HEALTH

1. Teach patient and family appropriate monitoring of causes, signs, and symptoms of Disuse Syndrome, Potential.
    a. Prolonged bed rest
    b. Circulatory or respiratory problems
    c. New activity
    d. Fatigue
    e. Dyspnea
    f. Pain
    g. Vital signs (before and after activity)
    h. Malnutrition
    i. Previous inactivity
    j. Weakness
    k. Confusion
    l. Fracture
    m. Paralysis
2. Assist patient and family in identifying life-styles changes that may be required.
    a. Progressive exercise to increase endurance
    b. Range of motion and flexibility exercise
    c. Treatments for underlying conditions (cardiac, respiratory, musculoskeletal, circulatory, neurologic, etc.)
    d. Motivation
    e. Assistive devices as required (walkers, canes, crutches, wheelchairs, ramps, wheelchair access, etc.).
    f. Adequate nutrition
    g. Adequate fluids
    h. Stress management
    i. Pain relief
    j. Prevention of hazards of immobility (e.g., antiembolism stockings, range of motion exercises, position changes)
    k. Changes in occupation, family, or social roles
    l. Changes in living conditions
    m. Economic concerns
    n. Proper transfer techniques

    o. Bowel and bladder regulation
3. Teach patient and family purposes and side effects of medications and proper administration techniques (e.g., anticoagulants, analgesics).
4. Assist patient and family to set criteria to help them to determine when physician or other intervention is required.
5. Consult with or refer to appropriate resources as indicated.
    a. Visiting nurse
    b. Occupational therapist
    c. Rehabilitation
    d. Physical therapist
    e. Social service
    f. Psychiatric nurse clinician
    g. Nutritionist
    h. Physician
    i. Rehabilitation specialist
    j. Community government and other groups developing a barrier-free environment
    k. National Spinal Cord Injury Foundation
    l. National Wheelchair Association
    m. National Paraplegic Foundation

EVALUATION
OBJECTIVE 1

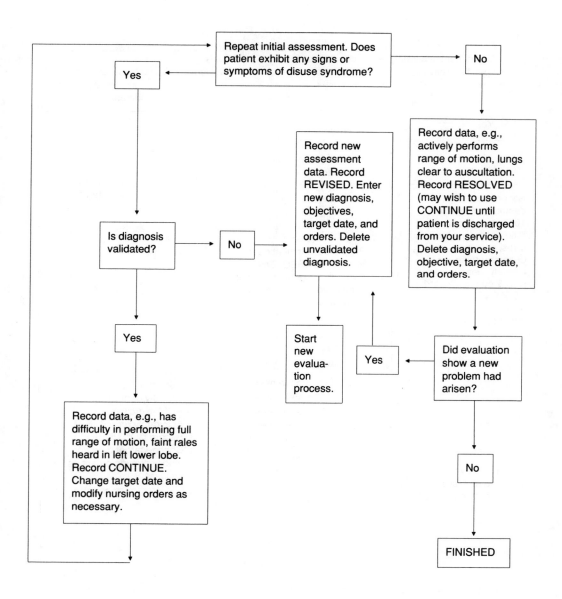

OBJECTIVE 2

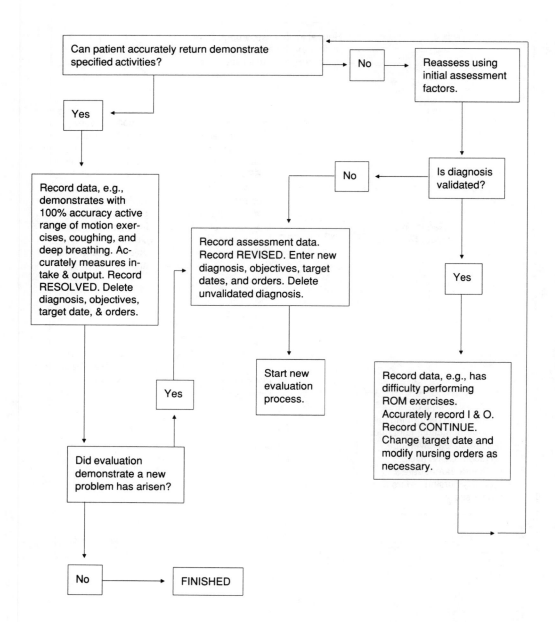

Diversional Activity Deficit

DEFINITION

The state in which an individual experiences a decreased stimulation from or interest or engagement in recreational or leisure activities (NANDA, 1987, p. 84).

DEFINING CHARACTERISTICS (NANDA, 1987, p. 84)

The nurse will review the initial pattern assessment for the following defining characteristics to determine the diagnosis of Diversional Activity Deficit.

1. Major defining characteristics
   Patient's statements regarding:
   a. Boredom (wish there was something to do, to read, etc.);
   b. Usual hobbies cannot be undertaken in hospital.
2. Minor defining characteristics
   None given.

RELATED FACTORS (NANDA, 1987, p. 84)

1. Environmental lack of diversional activity, as in:
   a. Long-term hospitalization;
   b. Frequent, lengthly treatments.

DIFFERENTIATION

Several other nursing diagnoses may need to be considered in the differential.

Activity Intolerance should be considered if the nurse observes or validates reports of the patient's inability to complete required tasks because of insufficient energy. Physical Mobility, Impaired is appropriate if the patient has difficulty with coordination, range of motion, muscle strength and control, or activity restrictions related to treatment.

Social Isolation should be considered if the patient demonstrates limited contact with community, peers, and significant others.

Uncompensated Sensory Deficit is of concern when a loss of acuity in vision, touch, smell, hearing, or balance is assessed.

The nursing diagnosis of Self-Care Deficit should be considered if the nurse observes or validates reports of inability to complete the tasks required because of inability to feed, bathe, toilet, dress, and groom self.

Self-Concept Disturbance is suggested when the patient refuses to accept rehabilitation efforts, denies the existence of a deformity or disfigurement, withdraws from social contact, and increases dependence on others.

Individual Coping, Ineffective should be suspected with verbalizations of inability to cope, with decreased problem solving, and with anxiety, fear, anger, and irritability.

Questions regarding the meaning of suffering, anger toward God, and verbalizations about conflicts with beliefs suggest the nursing diagnosis of Spiritual Distress.

OBJECTIVES

1. Will have decreased number of complaints regarding boredom by (date).

AND/OR

2. Will assist in designing and implementing a plan to overcome diversional activity deficit by (date).

TARGET DATE

Planning and accessing resources will require a moderate amount of time. A reasonable target date would be within 3–5 days.

NURSING ORDERS

ADULT HEALTH

1. Assist patient to review activity likes and dislikes.
2. Move patient to semi private room if possible and patient is amenable to move.
3. Encourage patient to discuss feelings regarding deficit and causes.
4. Alter daily routine (e.g., bathe at different times, increase ambulation).
5. Encourage significant others to assist in decreasing deficit:
   a. Bringing books, games, hobby materials.
   b. Visiting more frequently.
   c. Encouraging other visitors.
   d. Bringing a box of wrapped small items, one to be opened each day (e.g., paperback book, crossword puzzles, small jigsaw puzzle, small hand-held games).
6. Rearrange environment to facilitate activity:
   a. Provide ample light.
   b. Place bed near window.
   c. Provide radio as well as television set.
   d. Place books, games, etc. within easy reach.
   e. Provide clear pathway for wheelchair, ambulation, etc. Move furniture.
7. Involve patient, to extent possible, in more self-care activities.
8. Provide change of environment (e.g., out of room to sun deck or outside building, add posters to room decor).
9. Refer to:
   a. Occupational therapist
   b. Hospital volunteers
   c. Recreational therapist
   d. Librarian

CHILD HEALTH

1. Monitor patient's potential for activity or diversion according to:
   a. Attention span,
   b. Physical limitations and tolerance;
   c. Cognitive, sensory, and perceptual deficits;
   d. Preferences for gender, age, and interests;
   e. Available resources;
   f. Safety needs;
   g. Pain.
2. Encourage parental input in planning and implementing desired diversional activity plan.
3. Allow for peer interaction when appropriate through diversional activity.
4. Entertain use of appropriate specialists to best address holistic needs of child and family, including:
   a. Play therapist
   b. Social worker
   c. Pediatric or clinical nurse specialist
   d. Occupational therapist
   e. Physical therapist
   f. Community resource groups
5. Provide for appropriate adaptations in equipment or positioning to facilitate desired diversional activity.
6. Provide for scheduling of diversional activity at a time when patient is rested and without multiple interruptions.

WOMEN'S HEALTH

(Note: The following refers to those women placed on restrictive activities because of threatened abortions, premature labor, multiple pregnancy, or pregnancy-induced hypertension.)

1. Encourage family and significant others to participate in plan of care for client.
2. Encourage client to list life-style adjustments that need to be made.
3. Teach client relaxation skills and coping mechanisms.
4. Maintain proper body alignment with use of positioning and pillows.
5. Provide diversional activities:
   a. Hobbies such as:
      (1) Needlework
      (2) Reading
      (3) Painting
      (4) Television
   b. Job-related activities as tolerated (that can be done in bed).
      (1) Reading
      (2) Writing
      (3) Telephone conferences
   c. Activities with children.
      (1) Reading to child
      (2) Painting or coloring with child
      (3) Allowing child to "help" mother
         (a) Bringing water to mother
         (b) Assisting in fixing meals for mother
   d. Encourage help and visits from friends and relatives.
      (1) Visit in person
      (2) Telephone visit
      (3) Help with child care
      (4) Help with housework

MENTAL HEALTH

1. Assess source of diversional activity deficit. Is the nursing unit appropriately stimulating for the level or type of clients or is the problem the client's perceptions?

Nursing Unit Related Problems

2. Develop milieu therapy program.
   a. Include seasonal activities for clients such as parties, special meals, outings, games.
   b. Alter unit environment by changing pictures, adding appropriate seasonal decorations, updating bulletin boards, cleaning and updating furniture.
   c. Alter mood of unit with bright colors, seasonal flowers, appropriate music.
   d. Develop group activities for clients such as team sports, ping pong, bingo games, activity planning groups, meal planning groups, meal preparation groups, current events discussion groups, book discussion groups, exercise groups, crafts groups, etc.
   e. Decrease emphasis on television as primary unit activity.
   f. Provide books, newspapers, records, tapes, and craft materials.
   g. Use community service organizations to provide programs for clients.
   h. Collaborate with occupational therapist for ideas regarding activities and supplies.
   i. Collaborate with physical therapist regarding physical exercise programs.

Client Perception Related Problems

3. Discuss with client past activities, reviewing those that have been enjoyed and those that have been tried and not enjoyed.
4. List those activities that the client has enjoyed in the past with information about what keeps client from doing them at this time.

5. Monitor client's energy level and develop activity that corresponds to client's energy level and physiologic needs (i.e., manic client may be bored with playing cards and yet physiologic needs require less physical activity than the client may desire, so an appropriate activity would address both of these needs). Note assessment decisions here.

6. Develop with client a plan for reinitiating a previously enjoyed activity. Note that plan here.

7. Develop time in the daily schedule for that activity and note that time here.

8. Relate activity to enjoyable time such as a time for interaction with the nurse alone or interaction with other clients in a group area.

9. Provide positive verbal feedback to client about his or her efforts at the activity.

10. Assist client in obtaining necessary items to implement activity, and list necessary items here.

11. Develop plan with client to attempt one new activity—one that has been interesting for him or her but which he or she has not had time or direction to pursue.

12. Have client set realistic goals for activity involvement (i.e., one cannot paint like a professional in the beginning).

13. Discuss feelings of frustration, anger, and discomfort that may occur as client attempts a new activity.

14. Frame mistakes as positive tools of learning new behavior.

15. Refer to appropriate community agencies or groups:
    a. Special activity clubs
    b. Physical therapy
    c. Occupational therapy
    d. Sports clubs
    e. Community service organizations

HOME HEALTH

1. Monitor factors contributing to diversional activity deficit.

2. Involve patient and family in planning, implementing, and promoting reduction in diversional activity deficit:
    a. Family conference
    b. Mutual goal setting
    c. Communication

3. Assist patient and family in life-style adjustments that may be required:
    a. Time management
    b. Work, family, social, and personal goals and priorities
    c. Rehabilitation
    d. Learning new skills or games
    e. Development of support systems
    f. Stress management techniques
    g. Drug and alcohol use

4. Refer to appropriate assistive resources as indicated:
   a. Physician
   b. Social services
   c. Occupational therapist
   d. Rehabilitation specialist
   e. Job or education counselor
   f. Recreational therapist
   g. City and county recreation
   h. Community college or university
   i. YMCA/YWCA
   j. Financial counselor
   k. Psychiatric nurse clinician.
   l. Physical therapist
   m. Visiting nurse
   n. Play therapist
   o. Public library

EVALUATION
OBJECTIVE 1

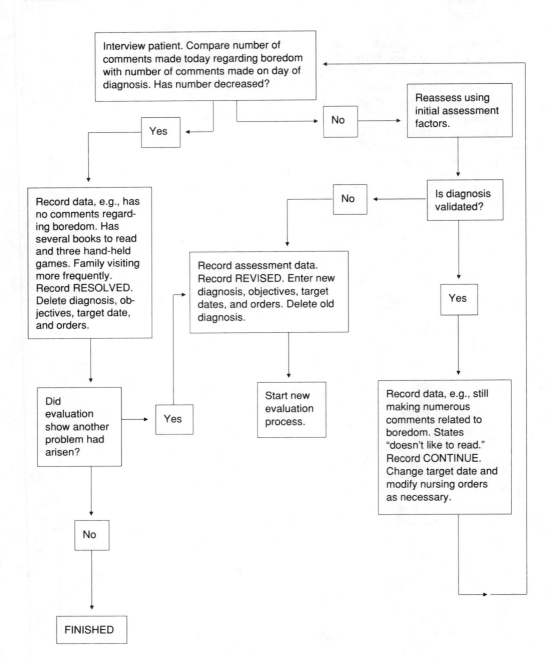

OBJECTIVE 2

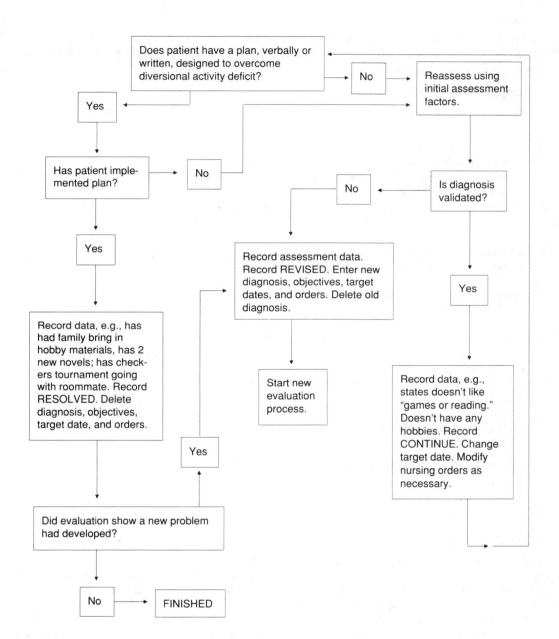

Dysreflexia

DEFINITION

The state in which an individual with a spinal cord injury at T7 or above experiences or is at risk to experience a life-threatening uninhibited sympathetic response of the nervous system to a noxious stimulus (NANDA, 1988).

DEFINING CHARACTERISTICS (NANDA, 1988)

The nurse will review the initial pattern assessment for the following defining characteristics to determine the diagnosis of Dysreflexia.

1. Major defining characteristics
   Individual with spinal cord injury (T7 or above) with:
   a. Paroxysmal hypertension (sudden, periodic elevated blood pressure with systolic pressure over 140 mm Hg and diastolic above 90 mm Hg)
   b. Bradycardia or tachycardia (pulse rate of less than 60 or over 100 beats/minute)
   c. Diaphoresis (above the injury)
   d. Red splotches on skin (above the injury)
   e. Pallor (below the injury)
   f. Headache (a diffuse pain in different portions of the head and not confined to any nerve distribution area)
2. Minor defining characteristics
   a. Chilling
   b. Conjunctival congestion
   c. Horner's syndrome (contraction of the pupil, partial ptosis of the eyelid, enophthalmos, and sometimes loss of sweating over the affected side of the face)
   d. Paresthesia
   e. Pilomotor reflex (gooseflesh formation when skin is cooled)
   f. Blurred vision
   g. Chest pain
   h. Metallic taste in mouth
   i. Nasal congestion

RELATED FACTORS (NANDA, 1988)

1. Bladder distention
2. Bowel distention
3. Skin irritation

DIFFERENTIATION

Dysreflexia occurs only in spinal cord injured patients and represents an emergency situation that requires immediate intervention. Cardiac Output, Altered may be suspected because of the changes in blood pressure. Skin Integrity, Impaired may be diagnosed because of skin blotchiness or concomitant lesions, and the presence of a headache may lead to the diagnosis of Comfort, Altered: Pain. Dysreflexia should be suspected in people with spinal cord injuries above T7 who experience bladder spasms, bladder distention, or untoward responses to urinary catheter insertion or irrigation. Bowel distention or rectal stimulation may also lead to Dysreflexia. Occasionally, symptoms are precipitated by skin lesions such as pressure sores and ingrown or infected nails (Lindan et al., 1980).

OBJECTIVES

1. Will have no signs or symptoms of dysreflexia by (date).

AND/OR

2. Will actively cooperate in care plan to prevent development of dysreflexia by (date).

TARGET DATE

Dysreflexia is a life-threatening response. For this reason, the target date should be expressed in hours on a daily basis.

NURSING ORDERS

ADULT HEALTH

1. Keep patient warm; avoid chilling.
2. Monitor fluid balance at least every 2 hours.
3. Monitor electrolyte balance at least daily.
4. Turn, cough, deep breathe patient every 2 hours on (odd/even) hour; keep in anatomic position.
5. Pad bony prominences.
6. Perform range of motion (active and/or passive).
7. At least every 4 hours, instruct patient on isotonic exercises. Encourage patient to perform isotonic exercises at least every 2 hours on (odd/even) hour.
8. Instruct on bladder and bowel conditioning.
9. Catheterize as necessary; use rectal tube if not contra indicated.
10. Provide appropriate skin care. Monitor skin integrity daily.
11. Maintain adequate food and fluid balance so that constipation is avoided.
12. Assist patient to repeat developmental stages as needed.
13. Involve family in plan of care such as positioning, feeding, exercising, etc.
14. Identify and encourage family to use community resources.
15. Be consistent and supportive in your approach.
16. Use abdominal binders and antiembolic stockings as needed.
17. Elevate head of bed if not contraindicated.

CHILD HEALTH

1. Administer medications as required to help control the blood pressure at appropriate levels for age and weight and thus prevent seizure activity.
2. Monitor the pulse as needed and blood pressure every 15 minutes until stable. Determine parameters for client per norms for age, site, and condition.
3. Assess family's understanding and perception of the problem.
4. Assess for appropriate related needs for family support during acute phase of problem, including emotional needs.
5. Develop a plan of care that reflects individual's needs and potentials.
6. Assist in appropriate referrals for long-term care to include:
   a. Rehabilitation nurse specialist
   b. Prevention of infection, especially urinary and integumentary

WOMEN'S HEALTH

(Note: This nursing diagnosis will pertain to women the same as to any other adult. The reader is referred to the other sections (Adult Health and Home Health) for specific nursing orders and objectives to women and dysreflexia. The following precautions should be taken when the victim is pregnant.)

1. Position the patient to prevent supine hypotension by:
   a. Placing the patient on her left side if possible;
   b. Using a pillow or folded towel under the right hip to tip to left;
   c. If neck injury is suspected, placing the patient on back board and then tipping the board to the left, thus keeping the weight of the uterus off the inferior vena cava.

2. Start an intravenous line for replacement of lost fluid volume (remember the pregnant woman has 50% more blood volume), as her vital signs may not change until a 30% reduction in mother's circulating blood volume has occurred.
3. Monitor the fetal status.
4. Monitor for uterine contractions.

MENTAL HEALTH

The objectives and nursing orders for the mental health client are the same as those for adult health. Refer to this section for the care of this client in the mental health setting.

HOME HEALTH

1. Teach patient and family measures to prevent dysreflexia.
   a. Bowel and bladder routines
   b. Prevention of skin breakdown (e.g., turning, transfer, prevention of incontinence)
   c. Use and care of indwelling urinary catheter
   d. Prevention of infection
2. Assist patient and family in identifying signs and symptoms of Dysreflexia.
   a. Teach family how to monitor vital signs and recognize tachycardia, bradycardia, and paroxysmal hypertension
3. Assist patient and family in identifying emergency referrals.
   a. Physician
   b. Emergency room
   c. Emergency medical system
4. Teach patient and family appropriate uses and side effects of medications and proper administration.
5. Consult with or refer to appropriate assistive resources as needed.
   a. Clinical specialist neuroscience nurse
   b. Rehabilitation specialist
   c. Physician

EVALUATION
OBJECTIVE 1

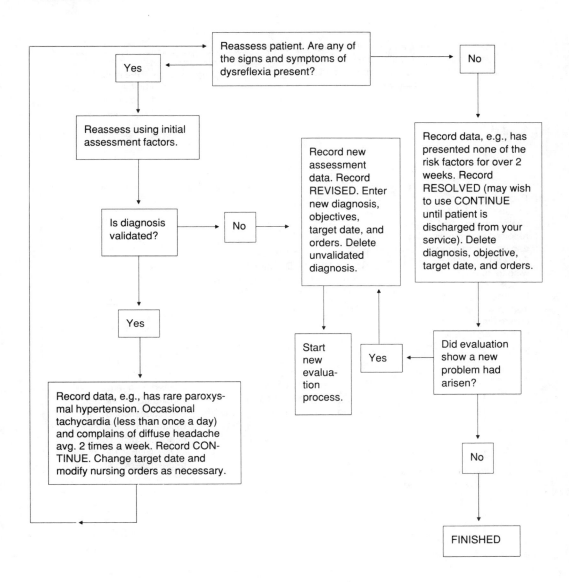

OBJECTIVE 2

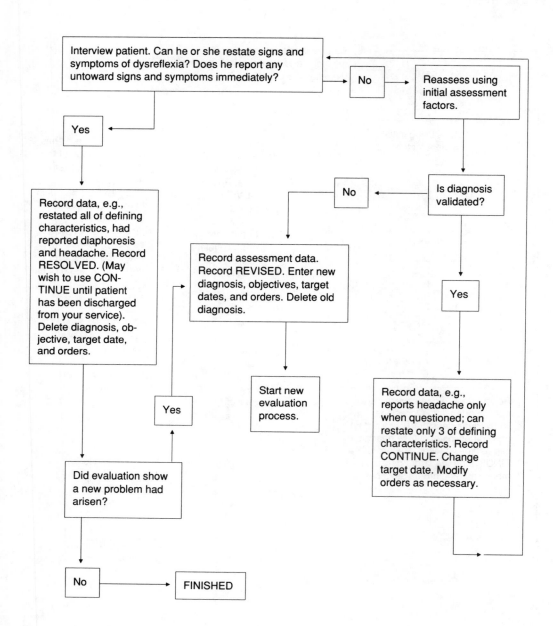

Interview patient. Can he or she restate signs and symptoms of dysreflexia? Does he report any untoward signs and symptoms immediately?

No

Reassess using initial assessment factors.

Yes

Record data, e.g., restated all of defining characteristics, had reported diaphoresis and headache. Record RESOLVED. (May wish to use CONTINUE until patient has been discharged from your service). Delete diagnosis, objective, target date, and orders.

No

Is diagnosis validated?

Record assessment data. Record REVISED. Enter new diagnosis, objectives, target dates, and orders. Delete old diagnosis.

Yes

Start new evaluation process.

Yes

Record data, e.g., reports headache only when questioned; can restate only 3 of defining characteristics. Record CONTINUE. Change target date. Modify orders as necessary.

Did evaluation show a new problem had arisen?

No

FINISHED

Fatigue

DEFINITION

An overwhelming sense of exhaustion and decreased capacity for physical and mental work (NANDA, 1988).

DEFINING CHARACTERISTIC (NANDA), 1988)

The nurse will review the initial pattern assessment for the following defining characteristics to determine the diagnosis of Fatigue.

1. Major defining characteristics
   a. Verbalization of an unremitting and overwhelming lack of energy.
   b. Inability to maintain usual routines.
2. Minor defining characteristics
   a. Perceived need for additional energy to accomplish tasks.
   b. Increase in physical complaints.
   c. Emotional lability or irritability.
   d. Impaired ability to concentrate.
   e. Decreased performance.
   f. Lethargy or listnessness.
   g. Disinterest in surroundings; intrajection.
   h. Decreased libido.
   i. Accident prone.

RELATED FACTORS (NANDA, 1988)

1. Decreased or increased metabolic energy production.
2. Overwhelming psychological or emotional demands.
3. Increased energy requirement to perform activities of daily living (ADL).
4. Excessive social or role demands.
5. States of discomfort.
6. Altered body chemistry (e.g., medications, drug withdrawal, chemotherapy).

DIFFERENTIATION

Fatigue is defined as a sense of exhaustion and decreased capacity for mental work regardless of adequate sleep. In this sense fatigue may be considered an alteration in quality of sleep and is subjective. Sleep Pattern Disturbance otherwise may be qualified according to the quantity of sleep or the expressed quality of the sleep.

Several alterations in nutritional-metabolic pattern might be considered according to the specific consequences resulting from the altered oxygenation needs.

The nurse must be responsible for differentiating between fatigue as a primary problem and fatigue as a consequence of any of the other primary diagnoses. Fatigue is uniquely qualified by a subjective component.

OBJECTIVES

1. Will have decreased complaints of fatigue by (date).

AND/OR

2. Will have implemented plan to offset fatigue by (date).

TARGET DATE

Fatigue can have far-reaching impact. For this reason the initial target date should be set at no more than 4 days.

NURSING ORDERS

ADULT HEALTH

1. Carefully plan activities of daily living and exercise schedules with detailed input from patient.
2. Provide frequent rest periods. Schedule at least 30 minutes' rest after any strenuous activity.
3. Avoid overstimulation—either cognitive or sensory—and understimulation.
4. Maintain adequate food and fluid balance.
5. Collaborate with nutritionist for in-depth dietary assessment and planning.
6. Instruct in stress reduction techniques. Have patient return demonstrate on a daily basis.
7. Encourage frequent deep breathing.
8. Assist patient to realistically appraise life short-and long-term goals.
9. Refer to exercise center for assistance with regular exercise plan.
10. Assist patient to schedule at least one recreational night per week and one rest evening per week.

CHILD HEALTH

1. Monitor for contributory factors on a daily basis.
2. Determine a plan to best address contributory factors as determined by verbalized perceptions of fatigue. (May be related to mother's or father's perceptions).
3. Provide adequate input about usual sleep pattern versus current pattern associated with fatigue.
4. Develop consistency by limiting staff to those who can best facilitate the plan to lessen fatigue.
5. Provide daily feedback regarding progress and reassess child and family perception of fatigue.
6. Determine how to best foster future patterns which will maintain optimal sleep-rest patterns without fatigue through planning ADL with patient and family.
7. If special conditions exist such as with apnea or the like, which may be perceived as fatigue-related, provide appropriate follow-up for family (e.g., support group for premature infants).
8. Consider medical status and condition as to chronic fatigue needs.
9. Determine to what extent any other patterns may potentially be interacting with fatigue component.
10. Ensure safety needs according to child's or infant's age and developmental capacity.

WOMEN'S HEALTH

1. Identify a support system that can assist patient in alleviating fatigue.
2. During pregnancy, schedule rest periods during day.
   a. Find restful area, one time in the morning and one time in the afternoon, to get away from work area and rest 5 minutes with feet propped above the abdomen.
   b. During lunch, leave work area to rest 10–15 minutes with feet propped above the abdomen or lying on left side.
3. Research the possibility of split time or job sharing at work during pregnancy.
4. Use relaxation techniques to induce a restful state.
5. Use music of preference to assist with relaxation during rest periods.
6. Plan for at least 6–8 hours of sleep during night (see Sleep Pattern Disturbance, Chapter 6, for nursing orders).
7. Involve significant others in discussion and problem-solving activities regarding life-style changes needed to reduce fatigue.
8. After delivery identify a support system that can assist patient with infant care and household duties to assist in alleviating fatigue.
9. Learn to rest and sleep when the infant sleeps.
10. Plan daily activities to alleviate unnecessary steps and to allow for frequent rest periods.
    a. If bottle feeding, prepare formula for 24 hours at a time.
    b. If breastfeeding, let spouse get up at night and bring baby to you.

    c. Prepare extra when cooking meals for family and freeze extra for future meals (i.e., prepare big batch of stew or spaghetti on one day and freeze portions for future meals).
11. Return to work slowly (i.e., work part-time for the first 2 weeks, gradually increasing time at work until full-time by end of 4 weeks).

MENTAL HEALTH

(Note: All goals established for the orders should be achievable and adjusted as client's condition changes.)

1. Client must be out of bed and dressed by (note time here). Initially this goal may be limited to client getting out of bed without dressing.
2. Assist client with the following grooming activities: (note here the degree of assistance needed as well as any special items needed).
3. While assisting client with grooming activities, teach performance of tasks in energy-efficient ways such as placing all necessary items in one place before grooming is begun.
4. Provide client with appropriate rewards for accomplishing established goals (note specific goals here with the reward for achievement of goal). Establish rewards with client input.
5. Establish time for client to rest during the day. Initially this will be more frequent and diminish as client's condition changes. Note times and duration of rest periods here.
6. Walk with client on unit (number) minutes (number) times a day.
7. Have client identify pleasurable activities that cannot be performed because of fatigue.
8. Identify one pleasurable activity and develop a gradually escalating plan for client involvement in this activity. Provide rewards for accomplishment of each step in this plan.
9. Provide client with foods that are high in nutritional value and are easy to consume.
10. Talk with client 30 minutes twice a day. Topics for this discussion should include:
    a. Client's perception of the problem.
    b. Identification of thoughts that support the feeling of fatigue.
    c. Identification of thoughts that decrease feelings of fatigue.
    d. Identification of unrealistic goals.
    e. Client's evaluation of and attitudes toward self.
    f. Identification of circumstances in the client's environment that support continuing feelings of fatigue (e.g., family stressors or secondary gain from fatigue).
    g. Identification of client's accomplishments.
11. After client has verbalized the effects negative thoughts have on feelings and behavior, teach client how to stop negative thoughts and replace them with positive thoughts.
12. Reward client for positive self-statements.
13. Assign client tasks on the unit and provide positive reinforcement for task accomplishment. Note task assigned and reward established here.
14. Involve client in group activity with other clients for (number) minutes (number) times a day.
15. Meet with client and client's family to evaluate interaction patterns and provide information that would assist them in assisting the client.
16. Have client identify those factors that will maintain feeling of well-being after discharge and develop a specific behavioral plan for implementing them.

HOME HEALTH

1. Teach patient and family measures to promote capacity for physical and mental work.
    a. Use of assistive devices as appropriate (wheelchairs, crutches, canes, walkers, adaptive eating utensils, etc.).
    b. Maintain sufficient pain control (analgesics, imagery, meditation, etc.).
    c. Provide a safe environment to reduce barriers to activity and decrease potential for accidents (throw rugs, stairs, blocked pathways, etc.).
    d. Provide balance of work and recreational activities.

   e. Provide housekeeping assistance as appropriate (e.g., homemaker, meals on wheels, etc.).

   f. Provide diversional activity as appropriate (visiting friends or family, doing hobbies on school work, etc.).

2. Assist patient and family in identifying risk factors pertinent to the situation.
   a. Chronic disease (e.g., arthritis, cancer, heart disease)
   b. Medications
   c. Pain
   d. Role strain

3. Consult with or refer to appropriate resources as indicated.
   a. Arthritis Foundation
   b. American Cancer Society
   c. American Heart Association
   d. Multiple Sclerosis Society
   e. Social service
   f. Psychiatric nurse clinician
   g. Occupational therapist
   h. Physical therapist
   i. Support group
   j. Medical equipment supplier
   k. Visiting nurse
   l. Homemaker
   m. Physician
   n. Occupational counselor
   o. Financial counselor
   p. YMCA/YWCA

EVALUATION
OBJECTIVE 1

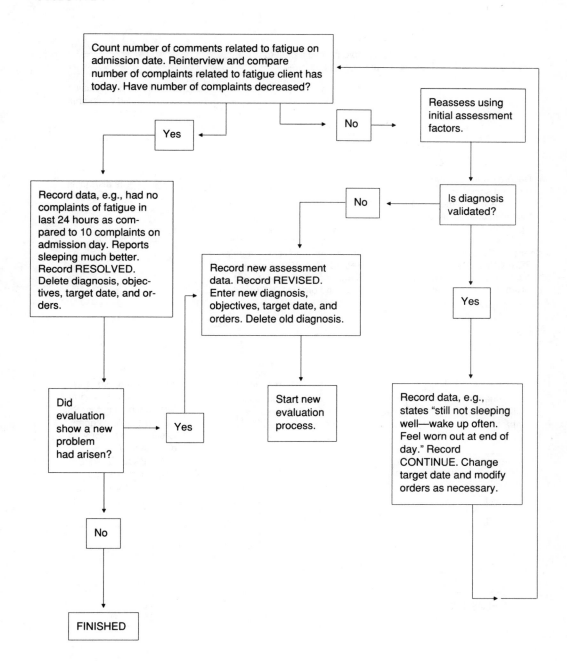

Count number of comments related to fatigue on admission date. Reinterview and compare number of complaints related to fatigue client has today. Have number of complaints decreased?

Yes

No

Reassess using initial assessment factors.

Record data, e.g., had no complaints of fatigue in last 24 hours as compared to 10 complaints on admission day. Reports sleeping much better. Record RESOLVED. Delete diagnosis, objectives, target date, and orders.

No

Is diagnosis validated?

Record new assessment data. Record REVISED. Enter new diagnosis, objectives, target date, and orders. Delete old diagnosis.

Yes

Did evaluation show a new problem had arisen?

Yes

Start new evaluation process.

Record data, e.g., states "still not sleeping well—wake up often. Feel worn out at end of day." Record CONTINUE. Change target date and modify orders as necessary.

No

FINISHED

OBJECTIVE 2

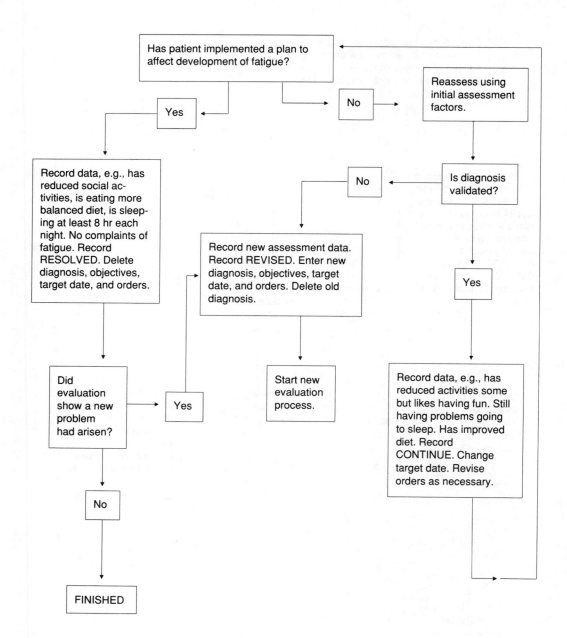

Has patient implemented a plan to affect development of fatigue?

Yes

No

Reassess using initial assessment factors.

Record data, e.g., has reduced social activities, is eating more balanced diet, is sleeping at least 8 hr each night. No complaints of fatigue. Record RESOLVED. Delete diagnosis, objectives, target date, and orders.

Is diagnosis validated?

No

Yes

Record new assessment data. Record REVISED. Enter new diagnosis, objectives, target date, and orders. Delete old diagnosis.

Did evaluation show a new problem had arisen?

Yes

Start new evaluation process.

Record data, e.g., has reduced activities some but likes having fun. Still having problems going to sleep. Has improved diet. Record CONTINUE. Change target date. Revise orders as necessary.

No

FINISHED

Gas Exchange, Impaired

DEFINITION

The state in which an individual experiences a decreased passage of oxygen or carbon dioxide between the alveoli of the lungs and the vascular system (NANDA, 1987, p. 42).

DEFINING CHARACTERISTICS (NANDA, 1987, p. 42)

The nurse will review the initial pattern assessment for the following defining characteristics to determine the diagnosis of Gas Exchange, Impaired.

1. Major defining characteristics
   a. Confusion
   b. Somnolence
   c. Restlessness
   d. Irritability
   e. Inability to move secretions
   f. Hypercapnea
   g. Hypoxia
2. Minor defining characteristics
   None given.

RELATED FACTORS (NANDA, 1987, p. 42)

1. Ventilation-perfusion imbalance

DIFFERENTIATION

Gas Exchange, Impaired, needs to be differentiated primarily from Airway Clearance, Ineffective; Breathing Patterns, Ineffective; and Cardiac Output, Altered: Decreased.

Airway Clearance, Ineffective means that something is blocking the air passages but that when and if air gets to the alveoli, there is adequate gas exchange. In Gas Exchange, Impaired, the air (oxygen) that reaches the alveoli is not sufficiently diffused across the alveoli-circulatory membrane.

Breathing Patterns, Ineffective suggests that the rate, rhythm, depth, and type of ventilatory effort is insufficient to bring in enough oxygen or get rid of sufficient amounts of carbon dioxide. These gases are sufficiently exchanged at the alveoli-circulatory membrane but the pattern of ventilation makes breathing ineffective.

Cardiac Output, Altered: Decreased implies that the heart is not pumping a sufficient amount of blood through the lungs to take up enough oxygen or release enough carbon dioxide to meet the body requirements. There is no impairment in the gas exchange, but there is not enough circulating blood to combine with sufficient amounts of oxygen to supply the body needs.

OBJECTIVES

1. Will have no signs or symptoms of impaired gas exchange by (date).

AND/OR

2. Will demonstrate improved blood gases and vital signs by (date). Note initial blood gases and vital signs here.

TARGET DATE

Because of the extreme danger of Gas Exchange, Impaired, progress should be evaluated daily until the client has stabilized. Thereafter, target dates at 3–5 days would be acceptable.

NURSING ORDERS

ADULT HEALTH

1. Collaborate with physician regarding monitoring of blood gases; report abnormal results immediately.
2. Reduce fear and anxiety by spending 15 minutes with patient every 2 hours.
3. Reduce chest pain by using noninvasive techniques and analgesic.
4. Perform nursing orders to maintain effective airway clearance. (See Airway Clearance, Ineffective; enter those orders here).
5. Raise head of bed 30° or more if not contraindicated.
6. Administer or assist with intermittent positive-pressure breathing (IPPB) as ordered. Stay with patient during treatment.
7. Encourage patient's mobility as tolerated.
8. Instruct in diaphragmatic deep breathing and pursed-lip breathing.
9. Administer oxygen as ordered.
10. Turn every 2 hours.
11. Provide teaching regarding bronchial hygiene:
    a. Breathe deeply and slowly while sitting up.
    b. Use diaphragmatic breathing.
    c. Hold the breath for 3–5 seconds and then slowly exhale through the mouth as much of the breath as possible.
    d. Take another deep breath, hold, and cough forcefully from deep in the chest, two times.
    e. Rest 15–20 minutes after coughing session.
    f. Assist with postural drainage and cupping and clapping exercises.
    g. Administer bronchodilators and mucolytic agents as ordered.
12. Provide teaching regarding respiratory exercises:
    a. Conscious, controlled deep breathing techniques.
    b. Breathe in deeply through the nose, hold for 2–3 seconds, breathe out slowly through pursed lips.
    c. Do the above several times every hour.

CHILD HEALTH

1. Monitor and document the following respiratory-related factors:
    a. Respiratory pattern, rate, and depth
    b. Symptoms noted with respiration, such as pain, difficulty in breathing, retraction of sternum or flaring of nares, allergies
    c. Equipment used in ventilation, including ventilator settings for:
       (1) Rate
       (2) Oxygen (FiO_2)
       (3) Peak pressure (PP)
       (4) If continuous positive airway pressure (CPAP) is needed
    d. Arterial blood gas values (notify physician of results, especially decreased pO_2, increased pCO_2, pH increased or decreased)
    e. Maintenance of a neutral thermal environment
    f. Auscultation of breath sounds every 1 hour or as needed, with follow-up chest x-ray as needed
    g. Tolerance of chest physiotherapy
    h. Suctioning tolerance, especially pluse rate
    i. Nature of secretions obtained via suctioning
    j. Observations of skin and mucous membranes for cyanosis
    k. Maintenance of fluid and electrolyte balance:

      (1) Administer appropriate fluids and electrolytes as ordered.

      (2) Monitor hourly intake and output.

      (3) Administer potassium only after voiding is noted.

      (4) Monitor specific gravity four times a day.

  l. Maintenance of appropriate and available emergency equipment to include:

      (1) Ambu bag

      (2) Endotracheal tube appropriate for age and size of infant (3.5)

      (3) Suctioning unit and catheters: infants,5 or 8 Fr; child, 8 or 10 Fr.

      (4) Crash cart with appropriate drugs

      (5) Defibrillation unit with guidelines

      (6) O_2tank (check amount of O_2 left)

      (7) Trachestomy sterile set

      (8) Chest tube tray, sterile

  m. Appropriate holistic assessment for related health needs

2. Provide for parental input in planning and implementing care as with comfort measures, assisting with feedings, and daily hygienic measures.

3. Allow at least 10–15 minutes per shift to allow family to verbalize concerns regarding child's status and changes.

4. Encourage parents to ask questions as needed by affording sensitivity to individual needs and possible clarification of issues.

5. Collaborate with related health team members as needed to include:

  a. Pediatrician, subspecialists such as neonatologist

  b. Radiologist

  c. Respiratory therapist

  d. Dietitian

  e. Pediatric clinical nurse specialist

  f. Play therapist

  g. Community health nurse

  h. Community support group

  i. Genetic counselor

6. Provide opportunities for parents and child to master essential skills necessary for long-term care, such as suctioning, while in hospital.

7. Allow for continuity in nursing care via Kardex, care plans, and same staff to the degree possible.

8. Ensure parents and family receive CPR training well before dismissal from hospital.

9. Provide long-term follow-up through appointments and appropriate referral to community nurses.

10. Encourage parents to use support system to aid in coping with illness and hospitalization.

11. Allow for sibling visitation as applicable within institution or specific situation.

WOMEN'S HEALTH

(Note: This nursing diagnosis will pertain to women the same as to any other adult. The reader is referred to the other sections (Adult Health, Home Health, and Mental Health) for specific nursing orders and objectives pertaining to women and impaired gas exchange. The following nursing orders will only focus on the fetal-placental unit during pregnancy.)

    Placental function is totally dependent on maternal circulation; therefore, any disease process which interferes with maternal circulation will affect the oxygen consumption of the placenta and therefore affect the fetus.

1. Assist client in developing an exercise plan for cardiovascular fitness during pregnancy.

2. Teach patient and significant others how to avoid ''supine hypotension'' during pregnancy (particularly during the later stages).

    a. Lying on left side to reduce pressure on vena cava.

    b. Taking frequent rest breaks during the day.

3. Assist patient in identifying life-style adjustments that may be needed due to changes in physiologic function or needs during pregnancy.

    a. Stop smoking.

    b. Avoid lying in supine position (see Nursing Order 2 above).

    c. Take no drugs unless so advised by physician.

4. Identify underlying maternal diseases that will affect the gas exchange of the fetal-placental unit during pregnancy.

Maternal Origin:

    a. Maternal hypertension (of any origin)

    b. Drug addiction

    c. Diabetes mellitus with vascular involvement

    d. Sickle cell anemia

    e. Maternal infections

    f. Maternal smoking

    g. Hemorrhage (abruptio placenta or placenta previa)

Fetal Origin:

    a. Premature or prolonged rupture of membranes

    b. Intrauterine infection

    c. RH disease

    d. Multiple pregnancy

MENTAL HEALTH

1. If client is demonstrating alterations in mental status, assess for increased hypoxia.

2. Observe client for signs of respiratory infection.

3. Protect client from respiratory infection by:

    a. Maintaining proper humidity in environment;

    b. Placing him or her in private room or monitoring roommate closely for signs and symptoms of respiratory infection and, if present, moving client to another room;

    c. Assigning staff members to client who are free of infection;

    d. Keeping client away from crowds;

    e. Assisting client in obtaining appropriate immunizations against influenza;

    f. Having client inform staff of signs of symptoms of respiratory infection when the earliest symptoms appear;

    g. Keeping environment as free of respiratory irritants as possible (i.e., dust, allergens, pollution, etc.).

4. Give client information in clear, concise manner, providing written notes if necessary. This is especially true for the client who has altered mental status as a result of hypoxia.

5. Discuss with client the effects smoking has on the respiratory system and refer to a stop smoking group if client wants this; if not, instruct client not to smoke 15 minutes before meals and physical activity.

6. Interact with client in a calm, supportive manner, especially during times of increased respiratory distress.

7. Decrease client's anxiety during periods of increased distress by:

    a. Talking in a calm, slow voice;

    b. Reassuring client that you can provide the necessary assistance;

    c. Having client take slow, deep breaths and follow proper breathing techniques;

    d. Staying with client until episode resolves.

8. Teach client proper breathing technique.

    a. Assume a sitting posture with back straight and shoulders relaxed.

    b. Take a slow, deep breath, expanding diaphragm downward (abdomen should rise).

    c. Hold breath 3–5 seconds.

    d. Exhale slowly through the mouth with pursed lips.

    e. Abdomen will sink down with the exhalation.

9. Have client practice proper breathing once every hour while awake. These sessions should be supervised by the nurse until the client masters the technique. Note schedule for practice session here.

10. Discuss with client the effects of alcohol and other depressant drugs on the respiratory system. Refer to a drug abuse recovery program as necessary.

11. Teach client appropriate hygiene of respiratory system to include:

    a. Use of daily coughing routine to clear lungs (this should be a deep, controlled cough that follows a deep breath);

    b. Maintenance of proper humidity in the environment;

    c. Instruction in postural drainage and chest clapping before coughing session (refer to physical or respiratory therapy if necessary).

12. Encourage drinking 2–3 liters of fluids per day unless contraindicated by other medical problems (i.e., alcohol withdrawal) by:

    a. Having favorite fluids available (list those here);

    b. Reminding client to drink 8 ounces every hour while awake;

    c. Providing fluids that are warm or at room temperature.

13. Maintain adequate nutrition (see Nutrition, Altered: Less than Body Requirements, Chapter 3).

14. Collaborate with physician regarding supplemental vitamins, especially thiamine if this is secondary to alcohol abuse.

15. Develop a schedule for activity and rest that provides client with the greatest amount of activity with the least fatigue (e.g., have chair in bathroom for being seated while doing daily hygiene). Note schedule here.

16. Spend 30 minutes twice a day with client discussing feelings and reactions to current situation. As feelings are expressed, begin to explore life-style changes with client. Refer to Individual Coping, Ineffective (Chapter 11) and Powerlessness (Chapter 8) for specific care plans related to coping styles.

17. Develop with client a plan for gradually increasing physical activity (see Activity Intolerance for specific behavioral interventions).

18. Practice with client the use of diaphragmatic breathing during exercise. This should be done with client during each exercise period until it can be accomplished without the nurse's coaching on a consistent basis.

19. Refer to appropriate community groups for ongoing support. These could include:

    a. Visiting nurse

    b. Physical therapist

    c. Occupational therapist

    d. Social services

    e. Disease-related support groups (e.g., American Lung Association)

    f. Alcoholics Anonymous, stop smoking programs

HOME HEALTH

(Note: If this diagnosis is suspected when caring for a patient in the home, it is imperative that a physician referral be obtained immediately. If the patient has been referred to home health care by a physician, the nurse will collaborate with the physician in the treatment of the patient.)

1. Teach patient and family appropriate monitoring of signs and symptoms of impaired gas exchange:

    a. Pursed-lip breathing

    b. Respiratory status: cyanosis, rate, dyspnea, orthopnea

    c. Fatigue

    d. Use of accessory muscles

    e. Cough

    f. Sputum production or change in sputum production

    g. Edema

    h. Decreased urinary output

    i. Gasping

2. Assist patient and family in identifying life-style changes that may be required.

    a. Prevention of impaired gas exchange: stopping smoking, prevention or early treatment of lung infections, avoidance of known irritants and allergens, influenza and pneumonia immunizations

    b. Pulmonary hygiene: clearing bronchial tree by controlled coughing, decreasing viscosity of secretions via humidity and fluid balance, postural drainage

    c. Daily activity as tolerated (remove barriers to activity)

    d. Breathing techniques to decrease work of breathing (diaphragmatic, pursed lips, sitting forward)

    e. Adequate nutritional intake

    f. Appropriate use of oxygen (dosage, route of administration, safety factors)

    g. Stress management

    h. Limiting exposure to upper respiratory infections

    i. Avoiding extreme hot or cold temperatures

    j. Keeping area free of animal hair and dander or dust

    k. Assistive devices required (oxygen, nasal cannula, suction, ventilator, etc.)

    l. Adequate hydration (monitor intake and output)

3. Teach patient and family purposes, side effects, and proper administration technique of medications.

4. Assist patient and family to set criteria to help them to determine when physician or other intervention is required.

5. Teach family basic CPR.

6. Consult with:

    a. American Red Cross

    b. American Lung Association

    c. Cystic Fibrosis Foundation

    d. American Cancer Society

    e. American Heart Association

    f. Visiting nurse

    g. Homemaker

    h. Occupational therapist

    i. Nutritionist

    j. Stop smoking program

    k. Group support

    l. Psychiatric nurse clinician

    m. Social service

    n. Occupational counselor

    o. Respiratory therapist

EVALUATION
OBJECTIVE 1

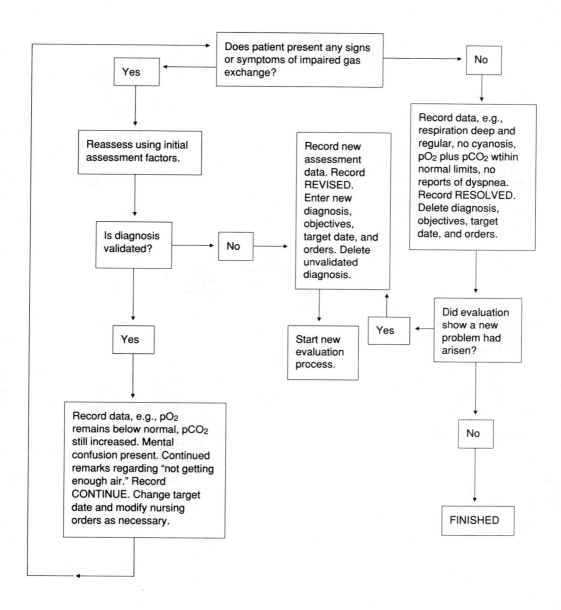

Does patient present any signs or symptoms of impaired gas exchange?

Yes

No

Reassess using initial assessment factors.

Record new assessment data. Record REVISED. Enter new diagnosis, objectives, target date, and orders. Delete unvalidated diagnosis.

Record data, e.g., respiration deep and regular, no cyanosis, pO_2 plus pCO_2 wtihin normal limits, no reports of dyspnea. Record RESOLVED. Delete diagnosis, objectives, target date, and orders.

Is diagnosis validated?

No

Yes

Start new evaluation process.

Yes

Did evaluation show a new problem had arisen?

Record data, e.g., pO_2 remains below normal, pCO_2 still increased. Mental confusion present. Continued remarks regarding "not getting enough air." Record CONTINUE. Change target date and modify nursing orders as necessary.

No

FINISHED

OBJECTIVE 2

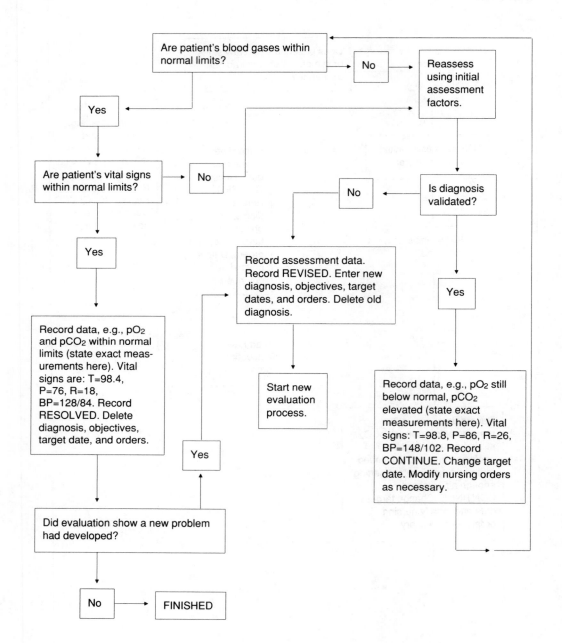

Growth and Development, Altered

DEFINITION

The state in which an individual demonstrates deviations in norms from his or her age group (NANDA, 1987, p. 92).

DEFINING CHARACTERISTICS (NANDA, 1987, p. 92)

The nurse will review the initial pattern assessment for the following defining characteristics to determine the diagnosis of Growth and Development, Altered.

1. Major defining characteristics
   a. Delay or difficulty in performing skills (motor, social, or expressive) typical of age group
   b. Altered physical growth
   c. Inability to perform self-care or self-control activities appropriate for age
2. Minor defining characteristics
   a. Flat affect
   b. Listlessness, decreased responses

RELATED FACTORS (NANDA, 1987, p. 92)

1. Inadequate caretaking
2. Indifference, inconsistent responsiveness, multiple caretakers
3. Separation from significant other
4. Environmental and stimulation deficiencies
5. Effects of physical disability
6. Prescribed dependence

DIFFERENTIATION

Several other nursing diagnoses may need to be considered in the differential, depending on what related factors are operating with the developmental alteration:

Sensory Deficit, Uncompensated should be considered when blindness, deafness, or neurologic impairment coexist.

Physical Mobility, Impaired may be indicated in situations in which physical disabilities are present.

Nutritional Deficit is possible when malnutrition is a factor.

Health Maintenance, Altered is a possible diagnosis when the person has difficulty maintaining normal growth and development, especially if the deviation is related to poor health.

Unilateral Neglect may be contributing to the alteration of growth and development if a neurologic deficit is a contributing factor.

Delayed development may also be a related factor in Thought Process, Altered.

The nursing diagnoses grouped under Gordon's (1987) Self-Perception and Self Concept Pattern, Role-Relationship Pattern, and Coping–Stress Tolerance Pattern should also be considered when alterations in growth and development are present.

OBJECTIVES

1. Will implement plan to offset, as much as possible, altered growth and development factors by (date).

AND/OR

2. Will return, as nearly as possible, to expected growth and development parameter for (specify exact parameter) by (date).

TARGET DATE

Assisting to modify altered growth and development factors will require a significant time; therefore, an initial target date of 7–10 days would be reasonable.

NURSING ORDERS

ADULT HEALTH

(Note: Nursing orders are varied and complex and incorporate nursing orders associated with other nursing diagnoses. For example, the patient may have either a total self-care deficit or a subdeficit in hygiene, grooming, feeding, or toileting. For an adult, any of these would be an alteration in growth and development. Therefore it would be appropriate to include the nursing orders associated with these nursing diagnoses in the nursing orders for the altered growth and development care plan.

Other nursing diagnoses that might indicate altered growth and development are Diversional Activity Deficit or Social Isolation.

An adult is generally able to find or initiate diversional and social activities. However, if the adult did not participate in diversional or social activities, it could indicate altered growth and development. Therefore, the nursing orders associated with Diversional Activity Deficit and Social Isolation would be appropriate to be included in the nursing orders for the altered growth and development care plan.)

In general, the nurse should:

1. Work collaboratively with other health care professionals and with the patient and family to develop and implement a plan that everyone can consistently use;
2. Provide adequate opportunities for the patient to be successful in whatever task he or she is attempting;
3. Reward and reinforce success, however minor;
4. Downplay relapses;
5. Have consistent, caring people in the care-giving role;
6. Allow patient to be as independent as possible.

CHILD HEALTH

1. Monitor child's growth and development status and determine what alterations there are (i.e., delays or precocity).
2. Determine what other primary health care needs exist, especially brain damage or residual of same.
3. Identify, with child or parents, realistic goals for growth and development.
4. Assist in collaboration with related health team members to include:
   a. Pediatrician
   b. Subspecialist
   c. Dietitician
   d. Occupational therapist
   e. Physical therapist
   f. Clinical nurse specialist
   g. School teacher
   h. Psychologist
   i. Speech therapist
5. Identify anticipatory safety for child related to altered growth and development.
6. In case of special diet, provide appropriate health teaching for parents.
7. Identify appropriate community resources to assist in fostering growth and development, such as the Early Childhood Intervention Services.

8. Provide for learning needs related to future development, including identification of schools for developmentally delayed children.
9. Identify state and national support groups, such as National Cerebral Palsy Association.
10. Provide for long-term follow-up with appointments before discharge.

WOMEN'S HEALTH

(Note: This nursing diagnosis will pertain to women the same as to any other adult. The reader is referred to the other sections (Adult Health, Home Health, and Mental Health) for specific nursing orders; the following nursing orders pertain only to women with reproductive anatomic abnormalities.)

1. Obtain a thorough sexual and obstetric history, especially noting any recurrent miscarriages in the first 3 months of pregnancy.
2. Assess for infertility.
3. Refer for further testing if primary amneorrhea is present.
4. Encourage client to verbalize her concerns and fears.
5. Encourage communication with significant others to identify concerns and explore options available.

MENTAL HEALTH

1. Provide a quiet, nonstimulating environment or an environment that does not add additional stress to an already overwhelmed coping ability.
2. Sit with client (number) minutes (number) times per day at (list specific times) to discuss current concerns and feelings.
3. Provide client with familiar or needed objects. These should be noted here.
4. Discuss with client perceptions of self, others, and the current situation. This should include client's perceptions of harm, loss, or threat. Assist client in altering perception of these situations so they can be seen as challenges or opportunities for growth rather than threats.
5. Provide client with an environment that will optimize sensory input. This could include hearing aids, eyeglasses, pencil and paper, decreased noise in conversation areas, appropriate lighting (these interventions should indicate an awareness of sensory deficit as well as sensory overload and the specific interventions for this client should be noted here, e.g., place hearing aid in when client awakens and remove before bedtime.)
6. Provide client with achievable tasks, activities, goals (these should be listed here). These activities should be provided with increasing complexity to give client an increasing sense of accomplishment and mastery.
7. Communicate to client an understanding that all coping behavior to this point has been his or her best effort and asking for assistance at this time is not failure; a complex problem often requires some outside assistance in resolution. (This will assist client in maintaining self-esteem and diminish feelings of failure.)
8. Provide client with opportunities to make appropriate decisions related to care at his or her level of ability. This may begin as a choice between two options and then evolve into more complex decision making. It is important that this be at the client's level of functioning so confidence can be built with successful decision-making experiences.
9. Provide constructive confrontation for client about problematic coping behavior. (See Kneisl & Wilson, 1984 for guidelines on constructive confrontation.) The kinds of behavior identified by the treatment team as problematic should be listed here.
10. Provide client with opportunities to practice new kinds of behavior either with role play or by applying them to graded real-life experiences.
11. Provide positive social reinforcement and other behavioral rewards for demonstration of adaptive behavior (those things that the client finds rewarding should be listed here with a schedule for use. The kinds of behavior that are to be rewarded should also be listed).

12. Assist client in identifying support systems and in developing a plan for their use.
13. Assist client with setting appropriate limits on aggressive behavior by (see Violence, Potential For, Chapter 9, for a detailed care plan if this is an appropriate diagnosis):
    a. Decreasing environmental stimulation as appropriate (this might include a secluded environment).
    b. Providing client with appropriate alternative outlets for physical tension. (This should be stated specifically and could include walking, running, talking with a staff member, using a punching bag, listening to music, doing a deep muscle relaxation sequence. These outlets should be selected with the client's input.)
14. Meet with client and support system to provide information on the client's situation and to develop a plan that will involve the support system in making changes that will facilitate the client's movement to age-appropriate behavior. Note this plan here.
15. Refer to appropriate assistive resources as indicated:
    a. Visiting nurse
    b. Social services
    c. Psychiatric nurse clinician
    d. Occupational therapist
    e. Physical therapist

HOME HEALTH

1. Monitor for factors contributing to the alteration in growth and development.
2. Involve patient and family in planning, implementing, and promoting reduction or correction of the alteration in growth and development:
    a. Family conference
    b. Mutual goal setting
    c. Communication
3. Teach patient and family measures to prevent or decrease alterations in growth and development.
    a. Expected norms of growth and development with anticipatory guidance. If the caretakers realize, for example, that the newborn begins to roll over by 2–4 months or that the 2-year-old can follow simple directions, then appropriate environmental and learning conditions can be provided to protect the child and to promote optimal development.
    b. Signs and symptoms of alterations in growth and development which may require professional evaluation.
    c. Parenting skills.
    d. Developmentally appropriate nutrition.
4. Assist patient and family to identify life-style changes that may be required.
    a. Care for handicaps (e.g., blindness, deafness, musculoskeletal or cognitive deficit)
    b. Proper use of assistive equipment
    c. Adapting to need for assistance or assistive equipment
    d. Determining criteria for monitoring patient's ability to function unassisted
    e. Time management
    f. Stress management
    g. Development of support systems
    h. Learning new skills
    i. Work, family, social, and personal goals and priorities
    j. Coping with disability or dependency
    k. Development of consistent routine
    l. Mechanism for alerting need for assistance
    m. Providing appropriate balance of dependence and independence

5. Assist patient and family to obtain assistive equipment as required (depending on alteration present and its severity).
   a. Adaptive equipment for eating utensils, combs, brushes, etc.
   b. Straw and straw holder
   c. Wheelchair, walker, motorized cart, cane
   d. Bedside commode, incontinence undergarments
   e. Hearing aid
   f. Corrective lenses
   g. Dressing aids: dressing stick, zipper pull, button hook, long-handled shoehorn, shoe fasteners, Velcro closures
   h. Bars and attachments and benches for shower or tub
   i. Hand-held shower device
   j. Medication organizers, magnifying glass
   k. Raised toilet seat
6. Consult with appropriate assistive resources as indicated:
   a. Occupational therapist
   b. Rehabilitation therapist
   c. Nutritionist
   d. Medical supplies manufacturer
   e. Meals on Wheels
   f. Crippled Children's Services
   g. Community transportation
   h. Psychiatric nurse clinician
   i. Respite care or delivery
   j. Special education teacher
   k. Job or education counselor
   l. Physical therapist
   m. Social service
   n. Visiting nurse
   o. Respiratory therapist
   p. Speech therapist
   q. Support groups
   r. Physician
   s. Home aid
   t. Pharmacist
   u. Psychologist

EVALUATION
OBJECTIVE 1

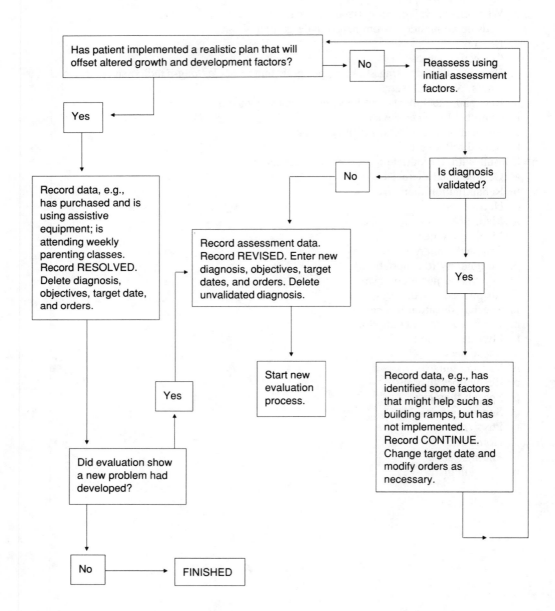

OBJECTIVE 2

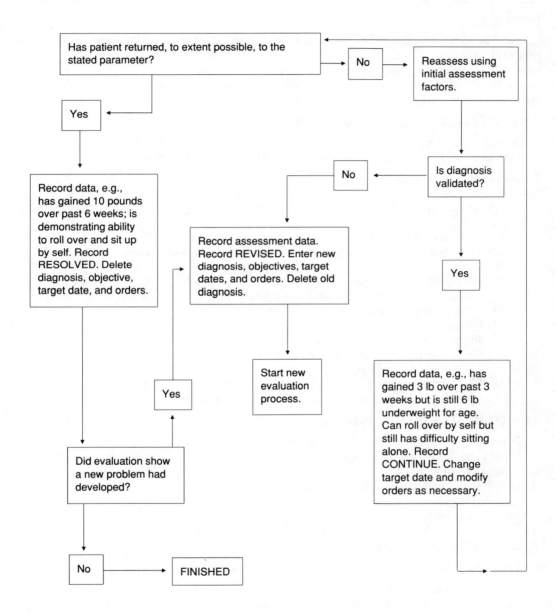

Home Maintenance Management, Impaired (Mild, Moderate, Severe, Potential, or Chronic)

DEFINITION

Inability to independently maintain a safe, growth-promoting immediate environment (NANDA, 1987, p. 88).

(Note: Different levels of this impairment may exist. The nurse must first assess the situation to determine if a potential exists. If Home Maintenance Management, Impaired is found to exist, then the nurse will assess for degree of severity.)

DEFINING CHARACTERISTICS (NANDA, 1987, p. 85)

The nurse will review the initial pattern assessment for the following defining characteristics to determine the diagnosis of Home Maintenance Management, Impaired.

1. Major defining characteristics
   a. Subjective:
      (1) Household members express difficulty in maintaining their home in a comfortable fashion.
      (2) Household requests assistance with home maintenance.
      (3) Household members describe outstanding debts or financial crisis.
   b. Objective:
      (1) Disorderly surroundings.
      (2) Unwashed or unavailable cooking equipment, clothes, or linen.
      (3) Accumulation of dirt, food wastes, or hygiene wastes.
      (4) Offensive odors.
      (5) Inappropriate household temperature.
      (6) Overtaxed family members (e.g., exhausted, anxious).
      (7) Lack of necessary equipment or aid.
      (8) Presence of vermin or rodents.
      (9) Repeated hygienic disorders, infestations, or infections.

RELATED FACTORS (NANDA, 1987, p. 85)

1. Individual or family member disease or injury.
2. Insufficient family organization or planning.
3. Insufficient finances.
4. Unfamiliarity with neighborhood resources.
5. Impaired cognitive or emotional functioning.
6. Lack of knowledge.
7. Lack of role modeling.
8. Inadequate support systems.

DIFFERENTIATION

Activity Intolerance should be considered if the nurse observes or validates reports of the patient's inability to complete required tasks because of insufficient energy. Physical Mobility, Impaired is appropriate if the patient has difficulty with coordination, range of motion, muscle strength and control, or activity restrictions related to treatment.

Uncompensated Sensory Deficit is of concern when a loss of acuity in vision, touch, smell, hearing, or balance is assessed.

Knowledge Deficit may exist if the client or family verbalizes less-than-adequate understanding of home maintenance.

Injury, Potential for exists if the patient is at risk for bodily harm.

The nursing diagnosis of Health Maintenance, Altered should be considered when a client or family fails to adhere to a therapeutic plan.

If the client exhibits impaired attention span; impaired ability to recall information; impaired perception, judgment, and decision making; or impaired conceptual and reasoning abilities, the nursing diagnosis of Thought Process, Altered should be made.

The nursing diagnosis of Self-Care Deficit should be considered if the nurse observes or validates reports of inability to complete the tasks required because of inability to feed, bathe, toilet, dress, and groom self.

Individual Coping, Ineffective, or Family Coping, Ineffective is suspected if there are major differences between reports by the patient and the family of health status, health perception, and health care behavior. Verbalizations by the client or family regarding inability to cope also indicate this differential nursing diagnosis. Through observing family interactions and communication, the nurse may assess that Family Process, Altered is a consideration. Poorly communicated messages, rigidity of family functions and roles, and failure to accomplish expected family developmental tasks are a few observations to alert the nurse to this possible diagnosis.

OBJECTIVES

1. Will identify factors contributing to impaired home maintenance management by (date).

AND/OR

2. Will demonstrate alteration necessary to reduce (potential or actual) impaired home maintenance management by (date).

TARGET DATE

Target dates will depend on the severity of impaired home maintenance management (mild, moderate, severe, etc.). Acceptable target dates for the first evaluation of progress toward meeting the objective would be 5–7 days.

NURSING ORDERS

ADULT HEALTH

A nurse in an acute care facility might very well receive enough information, while the patient is hospitalized, to make this nursing diagnosis. However, nursing orders specific for this diagnosis will require implementation in the home environment; therefore, the reader is referred to the Home Health care plan for this diagnosis.

CHILD HEALTH

1. Monitor risk factors or contributory etiologic factors of home maintenance management, to include:
   a. Addition of family member, birth
   b. Increased burden of care due to child's illness or hospitalization
   c. Lack of sufficient finances
   d. Loss of family member, death
   e. Hygienic practices
   f. History of repeated infections or poor health management
   g. Offensive odors
2. Identify ways to deal with home maintenance management alterations with assistance of applicable health team members, such as:
   a. Social service worker
   b. Clinical nurse specialist
   c. Community health nurse specialist
   d. Community resource groups
   e. Local and state agencies as applicable

   f. Women's Protective Services

   g. Legal counsel

3. Allow for individual patient and parental input in plan for addressing home maintenance management issues.

4. Monitor educational needs related to illness and the demands of the situation.

5. Provide health teaching with sensitivity to patient and family situation.

6. Provide 10–15 minutes each 8-hour shift as a time for discussion of patient and family feelings and concerns of management-related issues.

7. Encourage patient and family to identify support groups in the community to enhance coping.

8. If infant is at risk for sudden infant death by nature of prematurity or history of previous death in family, assist parents in learning about alarms and monitoring respiration, and institute CPR teaching.

9. Provide for appropriate follow-up after dismissal from hospital.

WOMEN'S HEALTH

1. Assist the client to describe her perception or understanding of home maintenance as it relates to her life-style and life-style decisions. Include areas related to:

   a. Stress-related problems and effects of environment

     (1) Allow client time to describe work situation

     (2) Allow client time to describe home situation

     (3) Encourage client to describe how she manages her responsibilities as a mother and a working woman

     (4) Encourage client to describe her assets and deficits as she perceives them

     (5) Encourage client to list life-style adjustments that need to be made

     (6) Monitor identified possible solutions, modifications, etc. designed to cope with each adjustment

     (7) Teach client relaxation skills and coping mechanisms

   b. Social network and significant others

     (1) Identify significant others in client's social network

     (2) Involve significant others if so desired by client in discussion and problem-solving activities regarding life-style adjustments

2. Encourage client to get adequate rest.

   a. Take care of self and baby only.

   b. Let significant others take care of the housework and other children.

   c. Learn to sleep when the baby sleeps.

   d. Have specific, set times for visiting friends or relatives.

   e. If breastfeeding, significant other can change infant and bring infant to mother at night (mother does not always have to get up every time for infant).

   f. Cook several meals at one time for family and freeze them.

   g. Prepare baby formula for a 24-hour period and refrigerate until use.

   h. Freeze breast milk, emptying breasts after baby eats; significant other can then feed infant one time at night so mother can get adequate, uninterrupted sleep.

     (1) Put breast milk into bottle and directly into freezer.

       (a) Can add milk each time breasts are pumped until needed amount is obtained.

       (b) Can freeze for 6 weeks if needed.

       (c) To use, remove from freezer and let thaw to room temperature

       (d) Once thawed must be used within a 12-to 24-hour period. DO NOT REFREEZE.

MENTAL HEALTH

1. Discuss with client concerns about returning home.

2. Develop with client and significant others list of potential home maintenance problems.

3. Teach client and family those tasks that are necessary for home care. Note tasks and teaching plan here.

4. Provide time to practice home maintenance skills as much as possible. This should be a minimum of 30 minutes once a day. Medication administration could be evaluated with each dose by allowing client to administer own medications. The times and types of skills to be practiced should be listed here.

5. If financial difficulties prevent home maintenance, refer to social services or a financial counselor.

6. If client has not learned skills necessary to cook or clean home, arrange time with occupational therapist to assess for ability and to teach these skills. Support this learning on unit by: (check all that apply)
   a. Having client maintain own living area;
   b. Having client assist with the maintenance of the unit (state specifically those chores client is responsible for);
   c. Having client assist with the planning and preparation of unit meals when this a milieu activity;
   d. Having client clean and iron own clothing.

7. If special aids are necessary for client to maintain self successfully, refer to social services for assistance in obtaining these items.

8. If client needs periodic assistance in organizing self to maintain home, refer to homemaker service or other community agency.

9. If meal preparation is a problem, refer to community agency for meals on wheels, or assist family with preparation of several meals ahead of time or exploring nutritious, easy ways to prepare meals.

10. Determine with client a list of rewards for meeting the established goals for achievement of home maintenance and then develop a schedule for the rewards. Note the reward schedule here.

11. Assess environment for impairments to home maintenance and develop with client and family a plan for resolving these difficulties (i.e., recipes that are simplified and written in large print are easier to follow).

12. Provide appropriate positive verbal reinforcers for accomplishment of goals or steps toward the goals.

13. Utilize group therapy once a day to provide:
    a. Positive role models;
    b. Peer support;
    c. Reality assessment of goals;
    d. Exposure to a variety of problem solutions;
    e. Socialization and learning of social skills;

14. Refer to appropriate community agencies for ongoing care at home. These could include:
    a. Social services
    b. Visiting nurse
    c. Homemaker services
    d. Meals on wheels
    e. Financial counseling
    f. Family therapy
    g. Adult day care
    h. Sheltered workshops
    i. Occupational therapy
    j. Psychiatric nurse clinician
    k. Family therapy

l. Group home

HOME HEALTH

1. Monitor factors contributing to impaired home maintenance management (items listed under etiologies section).
2. Involve patient and family in planning, implementing, and promoting reduction in the impaired home maintenance management:
   a. Family conference
   b. Mutual goal setting
   c. Communication
   d. Family members given specified tasks as appropriate to reduce the impaired home maintenance management (shopping, washing clothes, disposing of garbage and trash, yard work, washing dishes, meal preparation, etc.)
3. Assist patient and family in life-style adjustments that may be required.
   a. Hygiene practices
   b. Drug and alcohol use
   c. Stress management techniques
   d. Family and community support systems
   e. Removal of hazardous environmental conditions such as improper storage of hazardous substances, open heaters and flames, breeding areas for mosquitos or mice, congested walkways, etc.
   f. Proper food preparation and storage
4. Refer to appropriate assistive resources as indicated:
   a. Physician
   b. Social services
   c. Nutritionist
   d. Community home extension service
   e. Financial counseling
   f. Physical therapist
   g. Family counseling
   h. Stress reduction classes
   i. Job or education counseling
   j. Visiting nurse
   k. Homemaker assistance

EVALUATION
OBJECTIVE 1

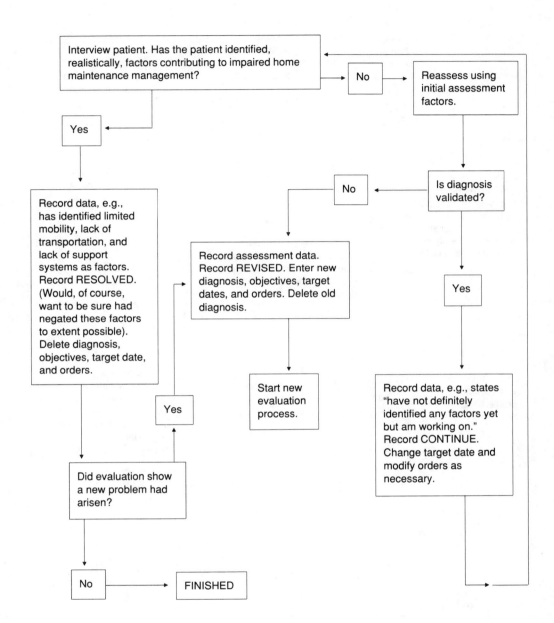

OBJECTIVE 2

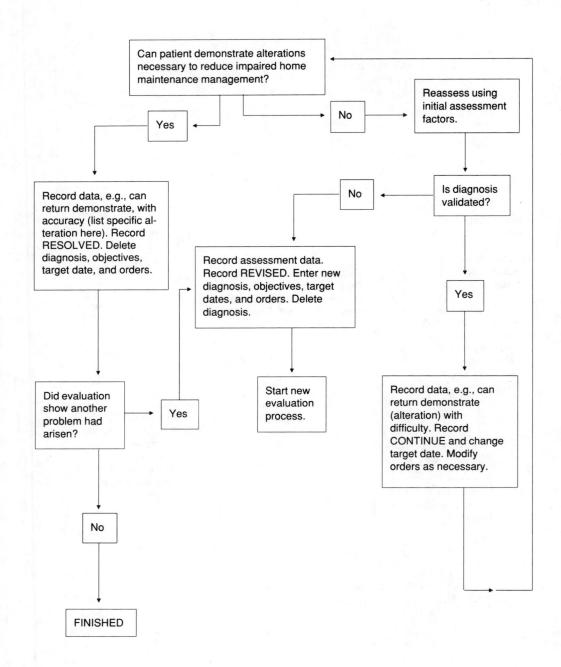

Physical Mobility, Impaired

DEFINITION

A state in which the individual experiences a limitation of ability for independent physical movement (NANDA, 1987, p. 80):

(Note: When this diagnosis is made the nurse should specify the level of the limitation.)

The suggested code for functional level classification are as follows (NANDA, 1987, p. 80):

0 = Completely independent
1 = Requires use of equipment or device
2 = Requires help from another person for assistance, supervision, or teaching
3 = Requires help from another person and equipment or device
4 = Dependent, does not participate in activity

DEFINING CHARACTERISTICS (NANDA, 1987, p. 80)

The nurse will review the initial pattern assessment for the following defining characteristics to determine the diagnosis of Physical Mobility, Impaired.

Major defining characteristics
a. Inability to purposefully move within the physical environment, including bed mobility, transfer, and ambulation
b. Reluctance to attempt movement
c. Limited range of motion
d. Decreased muscle strength, contact, and mass
e. Imposed restrictions of movement, including mechanical, medical protocol
f. Impaired coordination

RELATED FACTORS (NANDA, 1987, p. 81)

1. Intolerance to activity, decreased strength and endurance
2. Pain, discomfort
3. Perceptual or cognitive impairment
4. Neuromuscular impairment
5. Muscloskeletal impairment
6. Depression, severe anxiety

DIFFERENTIATION

Physical Mobility, Impaired needs to be differentiated from Activity Intolerance; any of the respiratory or cardiovascular nursing diagnoses; Nutrition, Altered: More or Less than Body Requirements, and Uncompensated Sensory Deficit.

Activity Intolerance implies that the individual is freely able to move but cannot endure or adapt to the increased energy or oxygen demands made by the movement or activity. Physical Mobility, Impaired, on the other hand, implies that an individual would be able to move independently if something were not limiting the motion.

Physical Mobility, Impaired also needs to be differentiated from the respiratory (Gas Exchange, Impaired, and Breathing Pattern, Ineffective) and cardiovascular (Cardiac Output, Altered: Decreased and Tissue Perfusion, Altered) nursing diagnoses. Mobility depends on effective breathing patterns and effective gas exchange between the lungs and arterial blood supply. Muscles have to receive oxygen and get rid of carbon dioxide for contraction and relaxation. Since oxygen is transported and dispersed to the muscle tissue via the cardiovascular system, it is only logical that the cardiovascular diagnoses need to be differentiated from primary Physical Mobility, Impaired.Nutrition, Altered: More or Less than Body Requirements should also be differentiated from Physical Mobility, Impaired. Nutritional deficits would indicate that the body is not receiving enough nutrients for its metabolic needs. Without adequate nutrition, the body (muscles) cannot function appropriately. Nutrition, Altered: More than Body Requirements or Exogenous Obesity may impair mobility simply because of the excess weight. In someone who is grossly obese, range of motion is limited, gait is altered, and coordination and tone are greatly reduced.

Uncompensated Sensory Deficit is another nursing diagnosis that should be differentiated from Impaired Physical Mobility. Uncompensated means that nothing has been done to help with problems of vision, hearing, touch, smell, or kinesthesia. Therefore, if these sensory inputs are uncompensated, the person will be unable to independently successfully navigate the environment. Physical Mobility, Impaired, as the definition states, is limited independent physical movement within the environment, but the assumption is that sensory functions are unimpaired.

OBJECTIVES

1. Will demonstrate measures (identify specifics) to increase mobility by (date).

AND/OR

2. Will demonstrate increased strength and endurance by (date).

TARGET DATE

These dates may be short-term or long-term based on the etiology of the diagnosis. An acceptable first target date would be 5 days.

NURSING ORDERS

ADULT HEALTH

1. Perform range of motion exercises (passive, active, and functional) as tolerated every 2 hours on the (odd/even) hour.
2. Turn, cough, and deep breathe every 1–2 hours. Massage pressure points after turning.
3. Maintain proper body alignment; support extremities with pillows, blanket, towel rolls, or sandbags.
4. Apply heat or cold as ordered.
5. Medicate for pain as needed and as ordered, especially before activity. Document effectiveness of medication within 30 minutes after administering medication.
6. Collaborate with physical therapist regarding exercise program.
7. Include patient and family or significant other in carrying out plan of care.
8. Use foot board, firm mattress, bed board, etc.
9. Monitor skin over pressure areas every 4 hours while awake.
10. Implement nursing orders specific to traction, casts, braces, prostheses, slings, and bandages.
11. Provide progressive mobilization as tolerated. Schedule increased mobilization on a daily basis (e.g., increase ambulation length by 25 feet each day).
12. Provide health teaching.
    a. Transfer methods
    b. Use of assistive devices
    c. Safety precautions
    d. Positioning, body mechanics
    e. Prescribed exercise
    f. Self-care activities
13. Maintain adequate nutrition.
14. Observe for complications of immobility (e.g., negative nitrogen balance, constipation, etc.).

CHILD HEALTH

1. Monitor alteration in mobility each 8-hour shift according to:
    a. Actual movement noted and tolerance for same;
    b. Factors related to movement;
    c. Situational factors;

    d. Pain;

    e. Circulation check to affected limb;

    f. Change in appearance of affected limb or joint.

2. Include related health team members in care of patient as needed, considering:

    a. Play therapist;

    b. Occupational therapist;

    c. Physical therapist;

    d. Clinical nurse specialist, orthopedic;

    e. Subspecialist, pediatric orthopedic surgeon;

    f. Social worker;

    g. Psychiatric nurse specialist;

    h. Dietitian.

3. Consider patient and family preferences in planning to meet desired mobility goals.

4. Encourage family members, especially parents, to participate in care of patient according to needs and situations (feeding, comfort measures).

5. Provide diversional activities appropriate for age and developmental level.

6. Maintain appropriate safety guidelines according to age and developmental guidelines.

7. Devote appropriate attention to traction or related equipment in use (e.g., weights hanging free, rope knots tight, etc.).

8. Monitor patient and family needs for education regarding patient's situation and any futuristic implications.

9. Attend to intake and output to ensure adequate fluid balance for each 24-hour period.

10. Address related health issues appropriate for patient and family.

WOMEN'S HEALTH

(Note:The following nursing orders apply to those women placed on restrictive activities because of threatened abortions, premature labor, multiple pregnancy, or pregnancy-induced hypertension.)

1. Encourage family and significant others to participate in plan of care for client.

2. When resting in bed, rest in left lateral position as much as possible:

    a. To prevent supine hypotension;

    b. To allow adequate renal and uterine perfusion.

3. Encourage client to list life-style adjustments that need to be made.

4. Teach client relaxation skills and coping mechanisms.

5. Maintain proper body alignment with use of positioning and pillows.

6. Encourage adequate protein intake.

7. Provide diversional activities.

    a. Hobbies such as:

        (1) Needlework

        (2) Reading

        (3) Painting

        (4) Television

    b. Job-related activities as tolerated (that can be done in bed)

        (1) Reading

        (2) Writing

        (3) Telephone conferences

    c. Activities with children

        (1) Reading to child

        (2) Painting or coloring with child

        (3) Allowing child to ''help'' mother

           (a) Bringing water to mother

(b) Assisting in fixing meals for mother, etc.
d. Encourage help and visits from friends and relatives
   (1) Visit in person
   (2) Telephone visit
   (3) Help with child care
   (4) Help with housework

MENTAL HEALTH

1. Attempt all other interventions before considering immobilizing client as an intervention. (See Violence, Potential for, Chapter 9, for appropriate interventions.)
2. Carefully monitor client for appropriate level of restraint necessary. Immobilize the client as little as possible while still protecting the client and others.
3. Obtain necessary medical orders to initiate methods that limit the client's physical mobility.
4. Carefully explain to client in brief, concise language reasons for initiating this intervention and what behavior must be present for the intervention to be terminated.
5. Attempt to gain client's voluntary compliance with the intervention by explaining to client what is needed and with a ''show of force'' (having the necessary number of staff available to force compliance if the client does not respond to the request).
6. Initiate forced compliance only if there is an adequate number of staff to complete the action safely. (See Violence, Potential for, Chapter 9, for a detailed description of intervention with forced compliance.)
7. Secure the environment the client will be in by removing harmful objects such as accessible light bulbs, sharp objects, glass objects, tight clothing, and metal objects such as clothes hangers or shower curtain rods, etc.
8. If client is placed in four-point restraints, maintain one-to-one supervision.
9. If client is in seclusion or in bilateral restraints, observe client at least every 15 minutes, more frequently if agitated (list observation schedule).
10. Leave urinal in room with client or offer toileting every hour.
11. Offer client fluids every 15 minutes.
12. Discuss with client his or her feelings about the initiation of immobility and review with him or her again, at least twice a day, the behavior necessary to have immobility discontinued.
13. When checking client let him or her know you are checking by calling him or her by name and orienting him or her to day and time. Inquire about client's feelings and implement necessary reality orientation.
14. Provide meals at regular intervals on paper containers providing necessary assistance (amount and type of assistance required should be listed here).
15. If client is in restraints, remove restraints at least every 2 hours, one limb at a time. Have client move limb through a full range of motion and inspect for signs of injury. Apply lubricants such as lotion to area under restraint to protect from injury.
16. Pad the area of the restraint that is next to the skin with sheepskin or other nonirritating material.
17. Check circulation in restrained limbs in the area below the restraint by observing skin color, warmth, and swelling. Restraint should not interfere with circulation.
18. Change client's position in the bed every 2 hours (list schedule for change here).
19. Place body in proper alignment to prevent complications and injury; use pillows for support if client's condition allows.
20. If client is in four-point restraints place on stomach or side to prevent aspiration or choking.
21. Place client on intake and output monitoring to ensure adequate fluid balance is maintained.
22. Have client in seclusion move around the room at least every 2 hours and during this time initiate active range of motion (note schedule for this activity here).
23. Administer medications as ordered for agitation.

24. Monitor blood pressure before administering antipsychotic medications.
25. Assist client with daily personal hygiene. (Record time for this here).
26. Have environment cleaned on a daily basis.
27. Review with client the purpose for restraint or seclusion as required and discuss alternative kinds of behavior that will express feelings without threatening self or others.
28. Remove client from seclusion as soon as the contracted behavior is observed for the required amount of time (both of these should be very specific and listed here). (See Violence, Potential for, Chapter 9, for detailed information on behavior change and contracting specifics.)
29. Schedule time to discuss this intervention with client and his or her support system. Inform support system of the need for the intervention and about special considerations related to visiting with the client. This information must be provided with consideration of client confidentiality. Plan to spend at least 5 minutes with the members of the support system before and after each visit.
30. Arrange consultations with appropriate resources after client is released from mobility limitations to assist client with developing alternative coping behavior. This could include a physical therapist, an occupational therapist, or a social worker.

HOME HEALTH

1. Teach patient and family measures to promote physical mobility.
   a. Use of assistive devices (wheelchairs, crutches, canes, walkers, prostheses, adaptive eating utensils, devices to assist with activities of daily living, etc.).
   b. Providing safe environment (reduce barriers to activity such as throw rugs, furniture in pathway, electric cords on floor, doors, steps, etc.).
   c. Maintaining skin integrity.
   d. Use of safety devices (ramps, lift bars, tub rails, tub or shower seat).
   e. Proper transfer techniques.
2. Assist patient and family in identifying risk factors pertinent to the situation.
   a. Immobility
   b. Malnourishment.
   c. Confusion or lethargy
   d. Physical barriers
   e. Neuromuscular deficit
   f. Musculoskeletal deficit
   g. Trauma
   h. Pain
   i. Medications which affect coordination and level of arousal
   j. Debilitating disease (cancer, stroke, diabetes, muscular dystrophy, multiple sclerosis, arthritis, etc.)
   k. Depression
   l. Lack of or improper use of assistive devices
   m. Casts, slings, traction, IVs, etc.
   n. Weather hazards
3. Assist patient and family in identifying life-style changes that may be required.
   a. Alterations in living space (ramps, assistive devices, etc.)
   b. Changes in role functions
   c. Range of motion exercises
   d. Positioning and transferring techniques
   e. Pain control
   f. Progressive activity
   g. Use of assistive devices
   h. Prevention of injury

   i. Maintenance of skin integrity
   j. Assistance with activities of daily living
   k. Special transportation needs
   l. Financial concerns
4. Consult with or refer to appropriate assistive resources as indicated.
   a. Arthritis Foundation
   b. Diabetes Association
   c. Muscular Dystrophy Association
   d. Multiple Sclerosis Society
   e. Head Injury Association
   f. Parkinson's Disease Association
   g. Rehabilitation
   h. Social service
   i. Occupational therapist
   j. Physical therapist
   k. Nutritionist
   l. Family support groups
   m. Medical equipment supplier
   n. Visiting nurse
   o. Psychiatric nurse clinician
   p. Homemaker
   q. Physician
   r. Occupational counselor
   s. Financial counselor

EVALUATION
OBJECTIVE 1

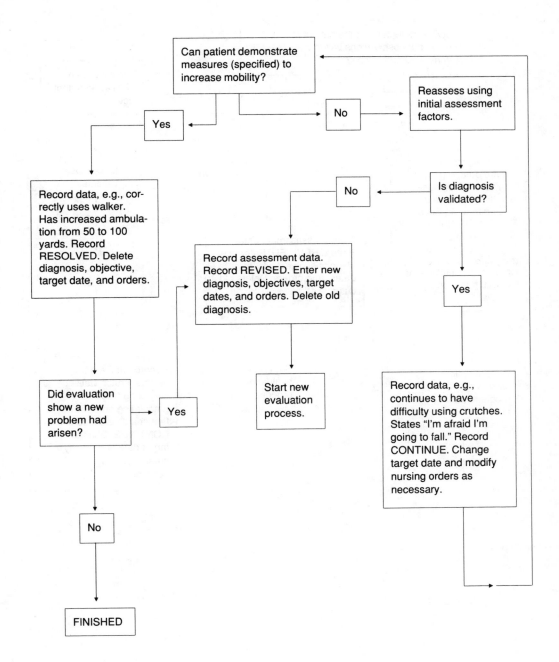

OBJECTIVE 2

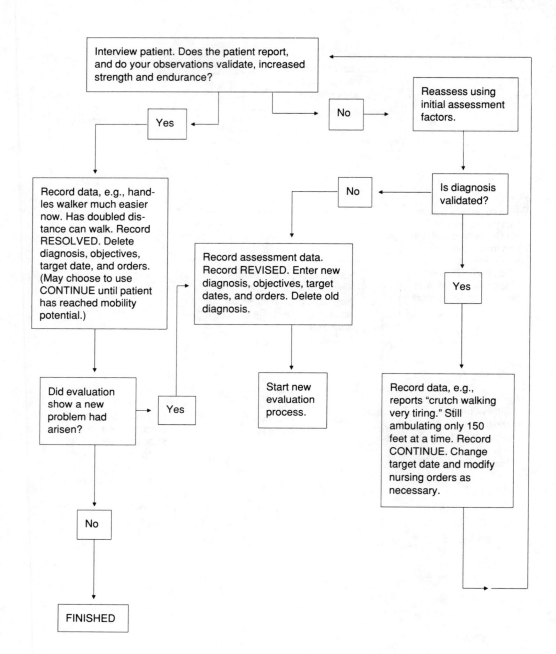

Self-Care Deficit (Bathing-Hygiene, Dressing-Grooming, Feeding, Toileting)

DEFINITION

A state in which the individual experiences an impaired ability to perform or complete feeding activities or bathing hygiene-activities or dressing-grooming activities or toileting activities for oneself (NANDA, 1987, pp. 87,89–91.)

(Note: This diagnosis refers to a decreased ability; it is not intended to be used for describing the normal developmental requirements of infants and children. However, alterations in the normal pattern of growth and development can be related to self-care deficits.)

DEFINING CHARACTERISTICS (NANDA, 1987, pp. 87, 89–91)

The nurse will review the initial pattern assessment for the following defining characteristics to determine the diagnosis of Self-Care Deficit.

1. Self-Care Deficit: Feeding
   a. Major defining characteristics
      (1) Self-feeding deficit (Level 0–4—same code as Physical Mobility, Impaired).
      (2) Inability to bring food from a receptacle to the mouth
   b. Minor defining characteristics
      None given.
2. Self-Care Deficit: Bathing-Hygiene
   a. Major defining characteristics
      (1) Self-Bathing or Self-Hygiene Deficit (Level 0–4—same code as Physical Mobility, Impaired)
      (2) Inability to wash body or body parts
      (3) Inability to obtain or get to water source
      (4) Inability to regulate temperature or flow
   b. Minor defining characteristics
      None given
3. Self-Care Deficit: Dressing-Grooming
   a. Major Defining characteristics
      (1) Self-Dressing or Self-Grooming Deficit (Level 0–4—same code as Physical Mobility, Impaired)
      (2) Impaired ability to put on or take off necessary items of clothing
      (3) Impaired ability to obtain or replace articles of clothing
      (4) Impaired ability to fasten clothing
      (5) Inability to maintain appearance at a satisfactory level
   b. Minor defining characteristics
      None given.
4. Self-Care Deficit: Toileting
   a. Major defining characteristics
      (1). Self-Toileting Deficit (Level 0–4—same code as Physical Mobility, Impaired)
      (2) Inability to get to toilet or commode
      (3) Inability to sit on or rise from toilet or commode
      (4) Inability to manipulate clothing for toileting
      (5) Inability to carry out proper toilet hygiene
      (6) Inability to flush toilet or commode
   b. Minor defining characteristics
      None given.

RELATED FACTORS (NANDA, 1987, pp. 87,89–91)

1. Intolerance to activity
2. Decreased strength and endurance

3. Pain or discomfort
4. Perceptual or cognitive impairment
5. Neuromuscular impairment
6. Musculoskeletal impairment
7. Depression or severe anxiety
8. Impaired transfer ability
9. Impaired mobility status

DIFFERENTIATION

Several other nursing diagnoses may need to be considered in the differential.

Activity Intolerance should be considered if the nurse observes or validates reports of the patient's inability to complete required tasks because of insufficient energy. Physical Mobility, Impaired is appropriate if the patient has difficulty with coordination, range of motion, muscle strength and control, or activity restrictions related to treatment.

Uncompensated Sensory Deficit is of concern when a loss of acuity in vision, touch, smell, hearing, or balance is assessed.

Knowledge Deficit may exist if the family or client verbalizes less-than-adequate understanding of self-care.

The nursing diagnosis of Health Maintenance, Altered should be considered when a client or family fails to adhere to a therapeutic plan.

Oral Mucous Membrane, Altered should be considered if pain in the oral cavity contributes to self-feeding deficit.

If the client exhibits impaired attention span, impaired ability to recall information; impaired perception, judgment, and decision making; or impaired conceptual and reasoning abilities, the nursing diagnosis of Thought Process, Altered should be made.

Individual Coping, Ineffective or Family Coping, Ineffective is suspected if there are major differences between reports by the patient and the family of health status, health perceptions, and health care behavior. Verbalizations by the client or family regarding the inability to cope also indicate this differential nursing diagnosis. Through observing family interactions and communication, the nurse may assess that Family Process, Altered is a consideration. Orally communicated messages, rigidity of family functions and roles, and failure to accomplish expected family developmental tasks are a few observations to alert the nurse to this possible diagnosis.

Urinary Elimination Patterns, Altered or Bowel Elimination, Altered should be investigated if the patient is having difficulty in self-hygiene, self-grooming, or self-toileting.

NURSING ORDERS

ADULT HEALTH

(Note: Self-care deficits range from a total self-care deficit to very specific areas of self-care deficits such as bathing-hygiene, feeding, toileting, etc. The nursing orders presented below are very general in nature and would need to be adapted to fit the exact self-care deficit of the individual. Collaboration with a rehabilitation nurse clinician or review of rehabilitation literature would be excellent sources for current and specific nursing orders related to the specific self-care deficit. Review of other care plans in this book will also be helpful, e.g., Urinary Elimination Patterns, Altered; Activity Intolerance; Physical Mobility, Impaired; Skin Integrity, Impaired, Nutrition, Altered.)

1. Provide extra time for giving care and include:
   a. Emotional support
   b. Teaching
   c. Return demonstration of self-care activities
2. Assist patient and significant others in planning measures to overcome or adapt to self-care deficits:

    a. Gradual increments in self-care responsibility, e.g., getting up in chair independently before ambulating to bathroom by self.
3. Place visual aid in room to help document progress:
    a. Chart which allows placement of stars for each day client accomplishes goal in self-care.
    b. Calendar to document progress on.
4. Provide positive reinforcement for each self-care accomplishment.
5. Perform range of motion exercises, or assist patient with, at least once per shift.
6. Assist significant others to provide assistive devices (e.g., raised toilet seat: buttonhook: knife, fork, or spoon with built-up handles: angled extension on comb and brush).
7. Remind patient to wear corrective appliances (e.g., braces, dentures, glasses, hearing aid).
8. Monitor:
    a. Vital signs every 4 hours while awake;
    b. Ambulation—increase on daily basis to extent possible.
9. Collaborate with physician regarding pain management.
10. Measure intake and output. Total every 8 hours.
11. Monitor bowel elimination at least daily.
12. Establish bowel and bladder retraining programs as necessary. See Bowel and Urinary Elimination, Altered (Chapter 4).
13. Collaborate with dietitian regarding diet (e.g., foods to facilitate self-feeding).
14. Provide privacy and safety for patient to practice self-care.
15. Refer to:
    a. Visiting nurse service
    b. Physical therapist
    c. Occupational therapist
    d. Appropriate self-help group
    e. Rehabilitation nurse clinician
16. Have visiting nurse service assist significant others to adapt home environment to promote self-care and safety:
    a. Nonslip rugs
    b. Ramps
    c. Handrails
    d. Safety strips in tub and shower

CHILD HEALTH

1. Monitor patient's and parent's potential for self-care measures appropriate to age and developmental and situational factors.
2. Allow patient and parents to participate in planning for care when possible to help ensure best compliance.
3. Teach the appropriate skills necessary for self-care in the child's terms with sensitivity to developmental needs for practice, repetition, or reluctance.
4. Collaborate with related health team members as needed to include:
    a. Occupational therapist
    b. Physical therapist
    c. Social worker
    d. Clinical nurse specialist
    e. Pediatrician subspecialists
    f. Community support groups
5. Provide opportunities which will enhance the child's confidence in performing self-care.
6. Monitor teaching needs related to special equipment or aids to enhance self-care activities.
7. Provide reinforcement of successes by stickers or charts to monitor progress.

WOMEN'S HEALTH

1. Encourage client to list life-style adjustments that need to be made.
2. Encourage progressive activity and increased self-care as tolerated:
   a. Ambulation
   b. Bathing
   c. Body image and early exercises
   d. Bowel care
   e. Breast care
   f. Perineal care
3. Encourage client to get adequate rest.
   a. Take care of self and baby only.
   b. Let significant others take care of the housework and other children.
   c. Learn to sleep when the baby sleeps.
   d. Have specific, set times for visiting of friends or relatives.
   e. If breastfeeding, significant other can bring infant to mother at night (mother does not always have to get up every time for infant).

Infant

4. Provide quiet, supportive atmosphere for interaction with infant.
   a. Bonding
   b. Caretaking activities
   c. Feeding
      (1) Breast
      (2) Bottle
5. Instruct client in infant care and encourage return demonstration of:
   a. Bathing
      (1) NEVER leave infant or small child alone in bath.
      (2) Bathe in small area (kitchen sink is good) for first weeks.
         (a) Warm area in house
         (b) Convenient for mother
         (c) Not drafty
         (d) Never run water directly from faucet onto infant, always test with forearm before placing infant in water (warm, but not hot)
   b. Cord care
      (1) Clean with alcohol and cotton swabs when changing diapers.
         (a) Clean around base of cord
         (b) Leave alone until it drops off
         (c) Alert mother that there will be a small amount of spotting (bleeding) at cord site when it drops off
   c. Clothing
      (1) How to determine if infant is warm enough.
         (a) Feel infant's chest or back with hand, never judge infant's body temperature by feeling hands or feet.
      (2) Laundering of infant's clothing
   d. Diapering
      (1) Cloth diapers
      (2) Disposable diapers
      (3) Cleaning of infant when changing diapers
         (a) Female infants
         (b) Male infants

    e. Circumcision care
      (1) Yellen clamp (metal clamp)
        (a) Gently wash penis with water to remove urine and feces
        (b) Reapply fresh, sterile Vaseline gauze around glans
        (c) Best to use cloth diapers until completely healed (approximately 7–10 days).
      (2) Plastic bell
        (a) Gently wash penis with water to remove urine and feces
        (b) Do not apply Vaseline gauze
        (c) Leave plastic circle on penis alone until tissue heals and circle falls off
    f. Taking baby's temperature and reading a thermometer
      (1) Axillary
      (2) Rectal
5. Explain infant alert and rest states and how caretaker can best use these states to interact with infant.

MENTAL HEALTH

1. Determine client's optimum level of functioning and note here.
2. Develop behavioral short-term goals by:
    a. Listing those activities client can assume;
    b. Breaking these activities into their component parts;
    c. Determining how much of each activity client could successfully complete and listing achievable activities here with goal achievement dates;
    d. Discussing expectations with client.
3. Keep instructions simple.
4. Provide support to client during tasks by:
    a. Spending time with client while he or she is completing the task;
    b. Having all items necessary to achieve task readily available;
    c. Assisting client in focusing on the task at hand;
    d. Providing positive verbal feedback as each step of the task is achieved.
5. Keep environment uncluttered, presenting only those items necessary to complete the task in the order needed.
6. Develop a reward schedule for achievement of goals. Discuss with client possible rewards and list those things client finds rewarding here with the goal to be achieved to gain the reward.
7. Schedule adequate time for client to accomplish task. (Depressed client may need 2 hours to bathe and dress).
8. Decrease environmental stimuli to the degree necessary to assist client in focusing on task.
9. Present activities of daily living on a regular schedule and note that schedule here. This schedule should be developed in consultation with the client.
10. Spend (number) minutes with client twice a day discussing feelings and reactions to current progress and expectations. Times for this and person responsible for this activity should be listed here.
11. Allow client to perform activities even though it might be easier at times for staff to complete the task for the client.
12. Communicate expectations and goals to all staff members.
13. Discuss with family and other support systems and the client the plan and goals. Spend at least 5 minutes with family after each visit to answer questions and explain treatment plan.
14. Teach family or support systems how to assist client in achieving established goals.
15. Spend time with client discussing alternative ways of coping with the frustration that may occur while attempting to reach established goals.

16. Collaborate with occupational therapist or physical therapist regarding special adaptations needed to assist client with task accomplishment (i.e., exercises to increase muscle strength when they have not been used for a period of time).
17. Monitor effects medication side effects may have on goal achievement and collaborate with physician regarding problematic areas.
18. Develop goals and schedules with client, communicating that he or she does have responsibility and control in issues related to care.
19. Discuss with client and significant others those things that will facilitate continuance of self-care at home and develop a plan that will assist client in obtaining necessary items.
20. Refer to community resources as necessary for continued support. These could include:
    a. Vocational rehabilitation services
    b. Social services
    c. Financial aid
    d. Physical therapist
    e. Occupational therapist
    f. Psychiatric nurse clinician
    g. Physician
    h. Illness-related support groups

HOME HEALTH

1. Monitor factors contributing to self-care deficits (specify). (This includes items in the etiologies section.)
2. Involve patient and family in planning, implementing, and promoting reduction in the self-care deficit (specify):
    a. Family conference
    b. Mutual goal setting
    c. Communication
3. Assist patient and family to obtain assistive equipment as required:
    a. Raised toilet seat
    b. Adaptive equipment for eating utensils, combs, brushes, etc.
    c. Rocker knife
    d. Suction device under plate or bowl
    e. Wrist or hand splints
    f. Blender, crockpot, microwave
    g. Long-handled reacher
    h. Box on seat of chair
    i. Raised ledge on utility board
    j. Straw and straw holder
    k. Washcloth with soap
    l. Wheelchair, walker, motorized cart, cane
    m. Bedside commode, incontinence undergarments
    n. Bars and attachments and benches for shower or tub
    o. Hand-held shower device
    p. Long-handled sponge
    q. Shaver holder
    r. Medication organizers, magnifying glass
    s. Diet supplements
    t. Hearing aid
    u. Corrective lenses
    v. Dressing aids: dressing stick, zipper pull, buttonhook, long-handled shoehorn, shoe fasteners, Velcro closures

4. Teach patient and family signs and symptoms of overexertion.
   a. Pain
   b. Fatigue
   c. Confusion
   d. Decrease or excessive increase in vital signs
   e. Injury
5. Assist patient and family in life-style adjustments that may be required.
   a. Teach proper use of assistive equipment
   b. Adapting to need for assistance or assistive equipment
   c. Determining criteria for monitoring patient's ability to function unassisted
   d. Time management
   e. Stress management
   f. Development of support systems
   g. Learning new skills
   h. Work, family, social, and personal goals and priorities
   i. Coping with disability or dependency
   j. Provide environment conducive to self-care: privacy, pain relief, social contact, familiar and favorite surroundings and foods
   k. Prevention of injury (falls, aspiration, burns, etc.)
   l. Monitoring of skin integrity
   m. Development of consistent routine
   n. Mechanism for alerting need for assistance
6. Refer to appropriate assistive resources as indicated
   a. Occupational therapist
   b. Physical therapist
   c. Nutritionist
   d. Physician
   e. Meals on Wheels
   f. Support groups
   g. Home aide
   h. Pharmacist
   i. Rehabilitation therapist
   j. Medical appliance manufacturer
   k. Social service
   l. Visiting nurse
   m. Respiratory therapist
   n. Speech therapist
   o. Community transportation
   p. Psychiatric nurse clinician
   q. CPR/first aid training
   r. Job or educational counselor
   s. Foundations such as Diabetes Association, Lung Association, Cancer Society, Muscular Dystrophy Association, Multiple Sclerosis Association, etc.

EVALUATION
OBJECTIVE 1

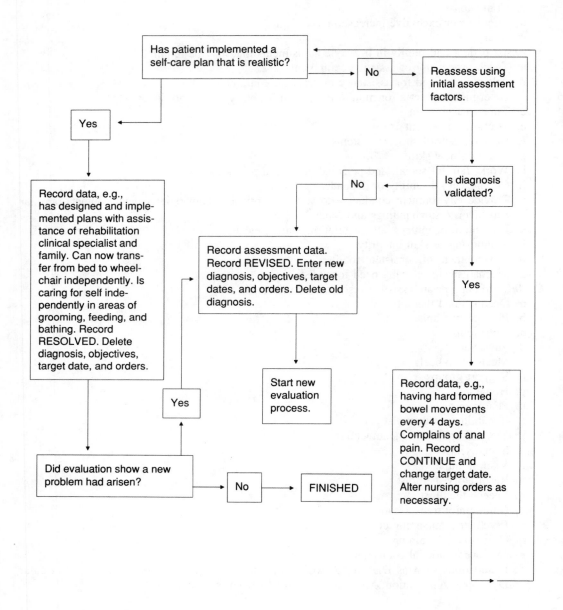

OBJECTIVE 2

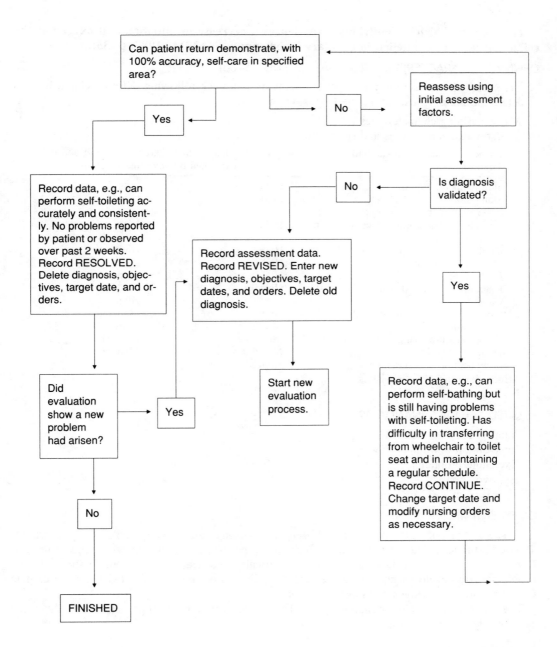

Tissue Perfusion, Altered

DEFINITION

The state in which an individual experiences a decrease in nutrition and oxygen at the cellular level due to a deficit in capillary blood supply (NANDA, 1987, p. 35).

DEFINING CHARACTERISTICS (NANDA, 1987, pp. 35–36)

The nurse will review the initial pattern assessment for the following defining characteristics to determine the diagnosis of Tissue Perfusion, Altered.

1. Major defining characteristics
   a. Estimated sensitivities and specificities:

	Chances that characteristic will be present in given diagnosis	Chances that characteristic will not be explained by any other diagnosis
Skin temperature, cold extremities	High	Low
Skin color	Moderate	Low
Dependent, blue or purple		
Pale on elevation, color does not return on lowering of leg	High	High
Diminished arterial pulsations	High	High
Skin quality: shining	High	Low
Lack of lanugo	High	Moderate
Round scars covered with atrophied skin	High	Moderate
Gangrene	Low	High
Slow-growing, dry, brittle nails	High	Moderate
Claudication	Moderate	High
Blood pressure changes in extremities	Moderate	Moderate
Bruits	Moderate	Moderate
Slow healing of lesions	High	Low

2. Minor defining characteristics
   None given.

RELATED FACTORS (NANDA, 1987, p. 36)

1. Interruption of arterial flow.
2. Interruption of venous flow.
3. Exchange problems.
4. Hypovolemia.
5. Hypervolemia.

DIFFERENTIATION

Tissue Perfusion, Altered has to be differentiated from Cardiac Output, Altered: Decreased. Tissue Perfusion, Altered relates to deficits in the peripheral circulation with cellular impact. Cardiac Output, Altered: Decreased relates specifically to a heart malfunction. Tissue perfusion problems may develop secondary to decreased cardiac output but can also exist without cardiac output problems (Doenges & Moorhouse, 1985).

In either diagnosis, close collaboration will be needed with a medical practitioner to ensure the best possible interventions.

OBJECTIVES

1. Will have no signs or symptoms of altered tissue perfusion by (date).

AND/OR

2. Will implement a plan to decrease the likelihood of future alterations in tissue perfusion by (date).

TARGET DATE

A maximum target date would be 2 days from the date of service admission because of the dangers involved. A patient who develops this diagnosis should be referred to a medical practitioner immediately.

NURSING ORDERS

ADULT HEALTH

1. Monitor, at least every 4 hours:
    a. Peripheral pulses;
    b. Capillary refill;
    c. Skin temperature;
    d. Edema—measure circumference with tape measure;
    e. Motor and sensory status;
    f. Vital signs;
    g. For signs and symptoms of pulmonary edema.
2. Weigh daily at 7:30 AM.
3. Measure intake and output. Total each 8 hours.
4. Provide skin and foot care at least once per shift:
    a. Cleanse and dry well
    b. Apply lotion
    c. Do not massage if possibility of emboli exists
    d. Collaborate with enterstomal therapist regarding care of open lesions:
       (1) Cleansing
       (2) Medicated ointments, etc.
       (3) Dressings
5. Exercise extremities at least every 4 hours:
    a. Range of motion
    b. Buerger-Allen exercises
    c. Collaborate with physical therapist regarding gradually increasing total exercise program.
6. Apply supportive or antiembolic hose. Remove for at least 30 minutes each shift and cleanse skin underneath.
7. Collaborate with physician regarding frequency of each of the following laboratory examinations and monitor results:
    a. Electrolytes
    b. Arterial blood gases
    c. Blood urea nitrogen
    d. Cardiac enzymes
    e. Coagulation time
8. Administer, as ordered, and monitor results of medications:
    a. Analgesics
    b. Anticoagulants
    c. Vasodilators
    d. Antilipemics
9. Position patient carefully and change position at least every hour while awake:
    a. Arterial interference—head and chest elevated, extremities in dependent position.
    b. Venous interference—extremities elevated.
    c. Combined arterial-venous interference—supine.
    d. Apply sheepskin, alternating air mattress, or egg crate mattress to bed.
    e. Provide heel and elbow protectors.
    f. Provide bed cradle to avoid linen pressure on extremities.

    g. Do not use knee gatch or pillows under knees.

10. Apply, and monitor closely, warm packs for phlebitis.
11. Collaborate with dietitian regarding dietary adaptations:
    a. Calorie restriction
    b. Low cholesterol
    c. Decreased saturated fats
    d. Decreased caffeine and alcohol intake
12. Teach patient, and assist in implementation at least once per shift:
    a. Stress management techniques;
    b. Relaxation techniques.
13. Teach patient and significant others:
    a. Exercise program;
    b. Dietary adaptation;
    c. Stopping smoking;
    d. Avoiding extremes in temperature;
    e. Avoiding prolonged standing, sitting, or crossing of legs;
    f. Avoiding use of over-the-counter medications;
    g. Continued use of stress management and relaxation techniques;
    h. Skin and foot care;
    i. Prescribed medication regimen—effects, toxicity.
14. Monitor bowel elimination at least daily.
15. Refer to visiting nurse service.

Additional Information (Cunningham, 1981; Kavanagh and Riegger, 1983)

Perfusion is the movement of blood to and from a body part. Adequate perfusion determines cell survival and depends on an adequate pump and vascular volume as well as adequate functioning of the precapillary sphincters. Factors affecting the adequacy of these structures include vasomotor, metabolic, and neural factors.

The basic function of the cardiovascular system is to transport water, oxygen, nutrients, and hormones to the cells and to remove carbon dioxide, waste products, and heat from the cells. The size of the blood vessels decreases along the length of the arterial system, which increases resistance to fluid flow. To perfuse the cells adequately, the mean arterial blood pressure is maintained within a relatively narrow range by such regulatory systems as the baroreceptors, sympathetic nerves, and the cardiac branch of the vagus nerve.

CHILD HEALTH

1. Perform appropriate monitoring and documentation for contributory factors to include:
    a. Circulatory monitoring of anatomic site or general signs and symptoms related to peripheral pulses.
    b. Apical pulse, blood pressure, temperature, and respiration (monitor at least every hour or as ordered, and check cardiac monitor if applicable).
    c. Related intake and output every hour.
    d. Nausea, vomiting.
    e. Constipation, diarrhea.
    f. Tolerance of feeding.
    g. Pain or discomfort.
    h. Skin color—temperature, breakdown.
    i. Circulatory pattern. Notify physician for change in circulatory pattern to suggest lack of oxygenation, especially cyanosis, arterial blood gas results, or related symptoms.
    j. Appropriate functioning of equipment such as ventilator, arterial line, or intravenous pump.
    k. Maintenance of intravenous line for administration of fluids.

l. Positional demands.

m. Pain or discomfort.

n. Sensory input appropriate for age and developmental status.

o. Offer small, frequent feedings as appropriate.

p. Monitor fluid and electrolytes.

2. Plan for nursing care through collaboration of health team members to include:

    a. Pediatrician or sub specialist such as neonatologist or pediatric cardiologist

    b. Pediatric clinical nurse specialist

    c. Respiratory therapist

    d. Physical therapist

    e. Occupational therapist

    f. Family counselor

    g. Support group

    h. Community nurse specialist

    i. Psychiatrist or nurse specialist

    j. Genetic counselor

    k. Social service worker

    l. Crippled Children Service Agent for congenital anomaly, such as cardiac defect

3. Provide for appropriate availability of resuscitative equipment as needed, including:

    a. Ambu bag

    b. Crash cart for pediatrics with drugs and defibrillator

    c. Appropriate respiratory intubation equipment

4. Allow for parental and child health teaching needs by allowing 10–15 minutes per 8-hour shift for verbalization of concerns.

5. Allow for parental participation in care of child at appropriate level, such as by comfort measures, assisting with feeding, or related activity.

6. Encourage rest by scheduling procedures together with devotion to ample time between activities.

7. Allow patient and parental preferences in plan of care.

8. Deal with appropriate related factors associated with altered tissue perfusion, such as minimizing crying by anticipating needs.

9. Administer medications as ordered.

10. Provide appropriate safety for age.

11. Maintain proper use of equipment, such as Clinitron bed or special K-pads to offer aids to circulation.

12. Provide for appropriate follow-up via scheduled appointments after hospitalization.

13. Provide patient with teaching appropriate to needs of illness and family.

14. Ensure that parents have attended CPR classes previous to hospital dismissal.

WOMEN'S HEALTH

1. Assist patient in identifying life-style adjustments that may be needed due to changes in physiological function or needs during experiental phases of life (e.g., pregnancy, birth, postpartum and related to gynecology).

2. Avoid prolonged sitting, sitting with crossed legs, or standing.

3. Develop exercise plan for cardiovascular fitness during pregnancy.

4. Avoid wearing constrictive clothing.

5. Maintain a balanced diet with adequate hydration.

6. Avoid constipation and bearing down to prevent hemorrhoids.

7. Monitor client for signs of pregnancy-induced hypertension (PIH).

    a. Prenatal

        (1) Weight

      (2) Blood pressure
      (3) Presence of edema
      (4) Proteinuria
   b. Preeclampsia
      (1) Headaches
      (2) Visual changes such as blurred vision
      (3) Increased edema of face and pitting edema of extremities
      (4) Oliguria
      (5) Hyperreflexia
      (6) Nausea or vomiting
      (7) Epigastric pain
   c. Eclampsia
      (1) Convulsions
      (2) Coma
  8. Monitor for edema.
   a. Swelling of hands, face, legs, or feet.
      (1) Caution—may have to remove rings.
      (2) May need to wear loose shoes or a bigger shoe size.
      (3) Schedule rest breaks during day where she can put her feet up.
      (4) When lying down, lie on left side to promote placental perfusion and prevent compression of vena cava.
  9. In collaboration with physician (as appropriate), monitor:
   a. Intake and output (urinary output not less than 30 ml/hr or 120 ml/4 hr)
   b. Magnesium sulfate ($MgSO_4$) and hydralazine hydrochloride (Apresoline) therapy (Have antidote for $MgSO_4$ [calcium gluconate] available at all times during $MgSO_4$ therapy.)
   c. Deep tendon reflexes (DTR)
   d. Respiratory rate, pulse and BP as often as needed
   e. Seizure precautions
   f. Bed rest and reduction in noise level in patient's environment
   g. Fetal heart rate and well-being
 10. Provide quiet, nonstimulating environment for client.
 11. Monitor fetal heart tones as often as necessary.
 12. Provide client and family factual information and support as needed.
 13. Teach client to report any symptoms of PIH immediately (Jensen & Boback, 1985, p. 962).
   a. Rapid rise in BP
   b. Rapid weight gain
   c. Marked hyperreflexia, especially transient or sustained ankle clonus
   d. Severe headache
   e. Visual disturbances
   f. Epigastric pain
   g. Increase in proteinuria
   h. Oliguria, with urine output of less than 30 ml/hr
   i. Drowsiness
 14. In collaboration with dietititan:
   a. Obtain nutritional history;
   b. Provide high-protein diet (80–100 gm protein);
   c. Provide low-sodium diet (not above 6 gm daily or below 2.5 gm daily).

Oral Contraceptive Therapy

 15. Monitor for factors that contraindicate use of oral birth control pills:
   a. Family history of stroke, diabetes, or reproductive cancer.

b. History of thromboembolic disease or vascular problems, hypertension, hepatic disease, and smoking.

c. Presence of any breast disease, nodules, or fibrocystic disease.

Premenstrual Syndrome

16. Assist client to identify symptoms that occur premenstrually which interfere with normal activities of daily living.
    a. Constipation
    b. Bloating (abdominal)
    c. Edema in hands and feet
    d. Headaches or vertigo
    e. Oliguria
    f. Irritability
    g. Depression
17. Provide client with literature on premenstrual syndrome
18. Refer to self-help, support group in community
19. In collaboration with dietitian:
    a. Obtain nutritional history;
    b. Provide diet high in complex carbohydrates and protein;
    c. Provide low-sodium diet (not above 6 gm daily or below 2.5 gm daily).
20. Teach and encourage client to:
    a. Utilize an exercise program;
    b. Utilize biofeedback for severe symptoms;
    c. Stop smoking;
    d. Utilize relaxation techniques to reduce stress.

MENTAL HEALTH

(Note: The nursing orders in this section reflect alteration in tissue perfusion related to the cerebral and peripheral vascular systems, since these are the ones most commonly affected in the mental health setting. Information related to altered tissue perfusion for the cardiopulmonary, gastrointestinal, and renal system is presented in the section on adult health.

1. Check on orthostatic hypotension by taking blood pressure while client is lying down, then taking blood pressure just after client stands or sits up (provide support for client to prevent injury from a fall).
2. Monitor client's mental status. If compromised, provide information in a clear, conscise manner.
3. Discuss with client causes of decreased cerebral blood flow.
4. Have client get out of bed slowly by:
    a. Sitting up;
    b. Swinging legs over edge of bed;
    c. Resting in this position for at least 2 minutes;
    d. Standing up slowly;
    e. Walking slowly.
5. Tell client to avoid situations in which he or she changes position quickly (i.e., bending over to pick something up off the floor, standing quickly from a sitting position).
6. Have client supported while changing positions that cause vertigo until problem is resolved.
7. Assist client in getting in and out of the bathtub.
8. Collaborate with physician regarding alterations in medications.
9. If situation persists have client:
    a. Sleep sitting up or with head elevated;
    b. Use elastic stockings that are waist high

(1) Apply them while client is still in bed

(2) Have client raise legs for several minutes

(3) Apply stockings slowly and evenly

(4) Remove stockings after client is lying down at least every 8 hours

10. Develop with client a plan for daily exercise that is very modest (i.e., walking the length of one hall for 15 minutes twice a day for 3 days, then increasing distance and time gradually until client is walking for 30 minutes twice a day). Note client's exercise regime here.

11. Develop with the client a reward schedule for implementing exercise plan. List rewards and the reward schedule here.

12. Provide the client with positive verbal support for goal accomplishment.

13. Do not allow client to participate in unit activities that could produce injury until the condition is resolved (i.e., cooking, using sharp objects while standing, etc.).

14. Discuss with client the effects of alcohol and smoking on blood flow and assist client to develop alternative coping behavior if necessary.

15. Provide decaffeinated beverages for the client. Consult with dietary department about this adaptation.

16. Increase client's fluid intake during times of increased loss such as exercise or periods of anxiety. Instruct client in the need for this.

17. Observe client carefully after injecting medications that have a high potential for producing hypotension. This is especially true for those clients who are very agitated and physically active.

18. Inform client of need to change position slowly after injecting medication.

19. Teach client and support system about over-the-counter medications that alter blood flow (i.e., cold medications, antihistamines, diet pills, etc.).

Peripheral

20. Monitor peripheral pulses on affected limbs every 8 hours.

21. Avoid and teach client to avoid pressure in points on affected limbs to include:
    a. Changing position frequently when sitting or lying down and avoiding pressure in the area behind the knees.
    b. Not crossing legs while sitting.
    c. Making sure shoes fit properly and do not rub feet.
    d. Elevating feet when sitting to reduce pressure on backs of legs.

22. Keep feet clean and dry and teach client to do same by assessing foot condition once a day. This assessment should include:
    a. Washing feet;
    b. Checking for sores, reddened areas, and blisters;
    c. Keeping toenails trimmed and caring for ingrown nails;
    d. Applying lotion to feet;
    e. Rubbing reddened areas if client does not have a history of emboli;
    f. Applying clean, dry socks;
    g. Teaching significant others to assist with foot care of elderly client;
    h. Keeping limbs warm (but do not use external heating sources such as heating pads or hot water bottles).

23. Develop with the client an exercise program and note that program here. Begin slowly and gradually increase time and distance (i.e., walk for 15 minutes 2 times per day for 1 week. This should be increased until client is walking 1 mile in 30–45 minutes 3 times a week). Note client's specific exercise plan here to include times and amounts.

24. Instruct client to discontinue exercise if:
    a. Pulse does not return to resting rate within 3 minutes after exercise;
    b. Shortness of breath continues for more than 10 minutes after stopping exercise;

    c. Fatigue is excessive;

    d. Muscles are painful;

    e. Client experiences dizziness, pain in the chest, lightheadedness, loss of muscle control, or nausea.

25. Encourage client's exercise by:

    a. Walking with him or her;

    b. Determining things that the client would find rewarding and supplying these as goals are achieved;

    c. Providing positive verbal support as goals are achieved;

    d. Note client's specific reward system here.

26. Monitor client's nutritional status and refer to nutritionist for teaching if necessary.

27. Discuss with client the effects of smoking on peripheral blood flow and assist him or her in decreasing or eliminating this by:

    a. Referring to a stop-smoking group;

    b. Encouraging him or her not to smoke before meals or exercise;

    c. Decreasing amount smoked per day.

28. Discuss special needs with client and support system before discharge.

29. Refer to community agencies to provide ongoing care as needed. These could include:

    a. Visiting nurse

    b. Social services

    c. Nutritionist

    d. Walking clubs

    e. Financial counseling

HOME HEALTH

(Note: If this diagnosis is suspected when caring for a client in the home, it is imperative that a physician referral be obtained immediately. If the client has been referred to home health care by a physician, the nurse will collaborate with the physician in the treatment of the client).

1. Teach patient and family appropriate monitoring of signs and symptoms of alteration in tissue perfusion.

    a. Pulse (lying, sitting, standing)

    b. Skin temperature, turgor

    c. Edema

    d. Motor status

    e. Sensory status

    f. Blood pressure (lying, sitting, standing, pulse pressure)

    g. Respiratory status (dyspnea, cyanosis, rate)

    h. Weight fluctuations

    i. Urinary output

    j. Leg pain with walking

2. Assist patient and family in identifying life-style changes that may be required.

    a. Eliminating smoking

    b. Decreasing caffeine

    c. Decreasing alcohol

    d. Avoiding over-the-counter medications

    e. Protecting skin and extremites from injury due to decreased sensation (burns, frostbite, etc.)

    f. Protecting skin from pressure injury (frequent position changes, sheepskin for pressure areas, foot cradle)

    g. Improving arterial blood flow (keep extremities warm, elevate head and chest, avoid crossing legs or sitting for long periods of time, wiggle fingers and toes every hour, range of motion exercises)

    h. Performing exercise program as tolerated

    i. Improving venous blood flow (elevate extremity, use antiembolus stockings, avoid pressure behind knees: pillows, gatch bed, etc.)

    j. Performing skin and foot care

    k. Decreasing cholesterol and saturated fat

    l. Performing diversional activities as needed

    m. Practicing stress management

3. Teach family basic CPR.
4. Teach patient and family purposes, side effects, and proper administration technique of medications.
5. Assist patient and family to set criteria to help them to determine when a physician or other intervention is required.
6. Consult with or refer to appropriate assistive resources as indicated.

    a. American Red Cross

    b. Visiting nurse

    c. Homemaker

    d. Stop-smoking group

    e. Physical therapist

    f. Occupational therapist

    g. Nutritionist

    h. Physician

    i. Social service

    j. Occupational counselor

EVALUATION
OBJECTIVE 1

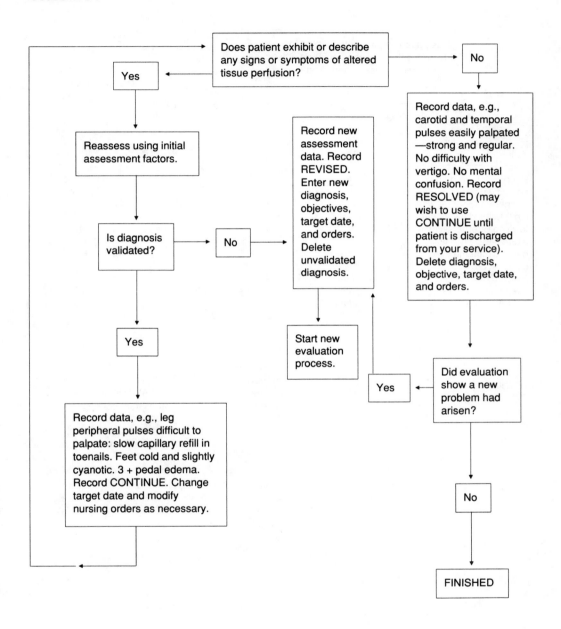

Does patient exhibit or describe any signs or symptoms of altered tissue perfusion?

No

Yes

Reassess using initial assessment factors.

Is diagnosis validated?

No

Yes

Record data, e.g., leg peripheral pulses difficult to palpate: slow capillary refill in toenails. Feet cold and slightly cyanotic. 3 + pedal edema. Record CONTINUE. Change target date and modify nursing orders as necessary.

Record new assessment data. Record REVISED. Enter new diagnosis, objectives, target date, and orders. Delete unvalidated diagnosis.

Start new evaluation process.

Record data, e.g., carotid and temporal pulses easily palpated —strong and regular. No difficulty with vertigo. No mental confusion. Record RESOLVED (may wish to use CONTINUE until patient is discharged from your service). Delete diagnosis, objective, target date, and orders.

Yes

Did evaluation show a new problem had arisen?

No

FINISHED

OBJECTIVE 2

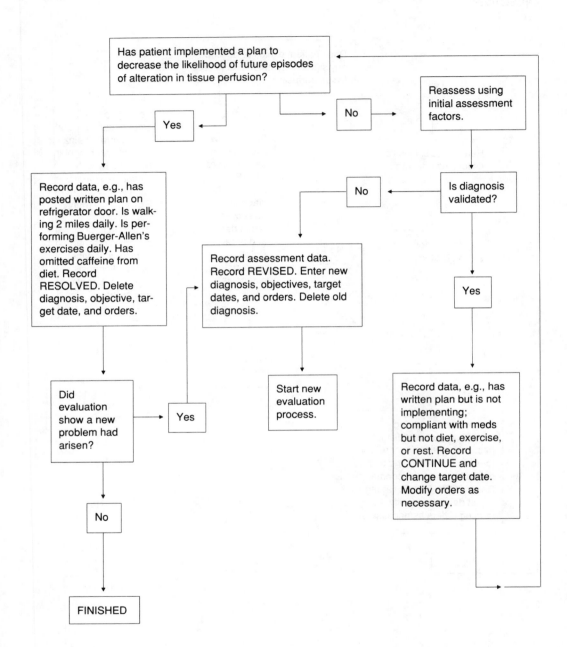

REFERENCES

Cunningham, S. (1981). Circulatory and fluid-electrolyte status. In P. Mitchell & A. Loustau (Eds.), *Concepts basic to nursing*. New York: McGraw-Hill.

Doenges, M., & Moorhouse, M. (1985). *Nurse's pocket guide: Nursing diagnoses with interventions*. Philadelphia: F. A. Davis.

Gordon, M. (1985). *Manual of nursing diagnosis*. New York: McGraw-Hill.

Jensen, M. D., & Bobak, I. M. (1985). *Maternity and gynecologic care: The nurse and the family*. St. Louis: C. V. Mosby.

Kavanagh, J., & Riegger, M. (1983). Assessment of the cardiovascular system. In W. Phipps, B. Long, & N. Woods (Eds.), *Medical-surgical nursing: Concepts and clinical practice*. St. Louis: C. V. Mosby.

Kelly, M. A. (1985). *Nursing diagnosis source book*. East Norwalk, CT: Appleton-Century-Crofts.

Kitzinger, S. (1984). *The experience of childbirth* (5th ed.). London: Cox & Wyman (Pelican Books).

Lentz, M. (1981). Selected aspects of deconditioning secondary to immobilization. *Nursing Clinics of North America, 16*, 729–737.

Lindan, R., Joiner, E., Freehafer, A., & Hazel, C. (1980). Incidence and clinical features of autonomic dysreflexia in patients with spinal cord injury. *Paraplegia, 18*, 285–292.

Mitchell, P. (1981). Motor status. In P. Mitchell & A. Loustau (Eds.), *Concepts basic to nursing*. New York: McGraw-Hill.

Murray, R., & Zentner, J. (1985). *Nursing assessment and promotion through the life span*. Englewood Cliffs, NJ: Prentice-Hall.

Noble, E. (1982). *Essential exercises for the childbearing year* (2nd ed.). Boston: Houghton Mifflin.

North American Nursing Diagnosis Association. (1987). *Taxonomy I with complete diagnoses*. St. Louis: Author.

North American Nursing Diagnosis Association. (1988). *Proposed nursing diagnoses*. St. Louis: Author.

Pardue, N. (1984). Immobility. In J. Flynn & P. Heffron (Eds.), *Nursing: From concept to practice*. Bowie, MD: Brady Communication.

Potter, P., & Perry, A. (1985). *Instructor's manual for use with fundamentals of nursing: Concepts, process, and practice*. St. Louis: C. V. Mosby.

Schuster, C., & Ashburn, S. (1986). *The process of human development: A holistic approach*. Boston: Little, Brown.

SUGGESTED READINGS

Allman, R., Laprade, C., Noel, L., Walker, J., Moorer, C., Dear, M., & Smith, C. (1986). Pressure sores among hospitalized patients. *Annals of Internal Medicine, 105* (3), 337–342.

American Nurses' Association. (1986). *Standards of home health nursing practice*. Kansas City, MO: Author.

Bassuk, E., & Schoonover, S. (1977). *The practitioner's guide to psychoactive drugs*. New York: Plenum.

Bohachick, P. (1987). Pulmonary embolism in neurological and neurosurgical patients. *Journal of Neuroscience Nursing, 19*, 191–197.

Buergin, P. (1983). Interventions for the person with motor problems. In W. Phipps, B. Long, & N. Woods (Eds.), *Medical-surgical nursing: Concepts and clinical practice*. St. Louis: C. V. Mosby.

Carpenito, L. (1983). *Nursing diagnosis: Application to clinical practice*. New York: J. B. Lippincott.

Crittenden, R. (1983). *Discharge planning*. Bowie, MD: Robert J. Brady.

Crittendon, F. (1983). *Discharge planning for health care facilities*. Los Angeles: University of California Extension Allied Health Publications.

Drayton-Hargrove, S., & Reddy, M. (1986). Rehabilitation and longterm management of the spinal cord injured adult. *Nursing Clinics of North America, 21*. 599–610.

Earnhardt, J., & Frye, B. (1984). Understanding dysreflexia. *Rehabilitation Nursing, 9* (2), 28–30.

Feuer, L. (1987). Discharge planning. Home caregivers need your support, too. *Nursing Management, 18*, 58–89.

Fogel, C. I., & Woods, N. F. (1981). *Health care of women: A nursing perspective*. St. Louis: C. V. Mosby.

Gettrust, K., Ryan, S. & Engelman, D. (1985). *Applied nursing diagnosis. Guides for comprehensive care planning*. New York: John Wiley & Sons.

Gordon, M. (1982). *Nursing diagnosis: Process and application*. New York: McGraw-Hill.

Griffith-Kenney, J. (1986). *Contemporary women's health: A nursing advocacy approach*. Menlo Park, CA: Addison-Wesley.

Hadeka, M. (1987). *Clinical judgment in community health nursing*. Boston: Little, Brown.

Hinz, M. D., & Masten, Y. (1986). Unpublished manuscript.

Humphrey, C. (1986). *Home care nursing handbook*. East Norwalk, CT: Appleton-Century-Crofts.

Iyer, P., Taptich, B., & Bernocchi-Losey, D. (1986). *Nursing process and nursing diagnosis*. Philadelphia: W. B. Saunders.

Jaffe, M., & Skidmore-Roth, L. (1988). *Home health nursing care plans*. St. Louis: C. V. Mosby.

Jones, D., Lepley, M., & Baker, B. (1984). *Health assessment across the lifespan*. New York: McGraw-Hill.

Kneisl, C., & Wilson, H. (1984). *Handbook of psychosocial nursing care*. Menlo Park, CA: Addison-Wesley.

Lederer, J., et al. (1985). *Care planning pocket guide: A nursing diagnosis approach*. Menlo Park, CA: Addison-Wesley.

Luckmann, J., & Sorensen, K. (1980). *Medical-surgical nursing* (2nd ed.). Philadelphia: W. B. Saunders.

McClelland, E., Kelly, K., & Buckwalter, K. (1985). *Continuity of care: Advancing the concept of discharge planning*. Orlando, FL: Grune & Stratton.

McFarland, G., & Wasli, E. (1986). *Nursing diagnoses and process in psychiatric mental health nursing*. Philadelphia: J. B. Lippincott.

McKay, S. R. (1980). Maternal position during labor and birth: A reassessment. *Journal of Obstetric, Gynecologic and Neonatal Nursing, 9* ,288–291.

National League for Nursing. (1986). *Policies and procedures*. New York: Accreditation Division for Home Care, National League for Nursing.

National League for Nursing. (1988). *Accreditation program for home care and community health: Criteria and standards*. New York: Author.

Neeson, J. D., & May, K. A. (1986). *Comprehensive maternity nursing: Nursing process and the childbearing family*. Philadelphia: J. B. Lippincott.

O'Keefe, D. F. (1985). When the accident victim is pregnant. *Contemporary OB/GYN, 26*, 148–163.

Orem, D. (1985). *Nursing: Concepts of practice* (3rd ed.). Boston: Little, Brown.

Rinke, L. (1988). *Outcome standards in home health*. New York: National League for Nursing.

Sande, D., & Billingsley, C. (1985). Language development in infants and toddlers. *Nurse Practitioner, 10*, 39–47.

Schuster, C. (1977). Normal physiological parameters through the life cycle. *Nurse Practitioner, 2*, 25–28.

Shrock, P. (1986). Feeling fit. *Lamaze Parent's Magazine*, 25–27, 68.

Smitherman, C. (1981). *Nursing actions for health promotion*. Philadelphia: F. A. Davis.

Steffi, B., & Eide, I. (1978). *Discharge planning handbook*. New York: Charles B. Slack.

Stuart, G., & Sundeen, S. (1988). *Pocket nurse guide to psychiatric nursing*. St. Louis: C. V. Mosby.

Tompkins, E. (1980). Effect of restricted mobility and dominance on perceived duration. *Nursing Research, 29*, 333–338.

Watson, J. (1985). *Nursing: The philosophy and science of caring*. Boulder, CO: Colorado Associated University Press.

Whaley, L. and Wong, D. (1987). *Nursing care of infants and children*. St. Louis: C.V. Mosby.

CHAPTER SIX

Sleep-Rest Pattern

Pattern Description

The nurse may care for patients who have preexisting sleep disturbances as well as for patients who develop sleep problems as a result of specific health alterations. A sleep disturbance may be the reason a client seeks health care or it may be a problem partially resolved by the client. In either instance the nurse must individualize care to meet the specific alteration in sleep or rest according to the patient's needs.

The sleep-rest pattern includes relaxation in addition to sleep and rest. The pattern is based on a 24-hour day and looks specifically at how the individual rates or judges the adequacy of his or her sleep, rest and relaxation in terms of both quantity and quality. The pattern also looks at the patient's energy level in relation to the amount of sleep, rest, and relaxation described by the patient.

Pattern Assessment

1. Any problems with sleep?
   a. Difficulty going to sleep
   b. Frequent awakening during night
   c. Early awakening
2. Does client feel rested after sleep?
3. Does client use any sleep aids?
   a. Over-the-counter medications
   b. Prescription drugs
   c. Relaxation techniques
   d. Audio tapes
   e. Other
4. Does client have scheduled rest and relaxation periods?
   a. When
   b. Activities during period
5. Does client have frequent sensation of fatigue?
   a. Relationship to activities
   b. Time of day

Conceptual Information

A person at rest feels mentally relaxed, free from anxiety, and physically calm. Rest need not imply inactivity, and inactivity does not necessarily afford rest. Rest is a reduction in bodily work which results in the person feeling refreshed and with a sense of readiness to perform activities of daily living.

Sleep is a state of rest that occurs for sustained periods. The reduced consciousness during sleep provides time for essential repair and recovery of body systems. A person who sleeps has temporarily reduced interaction with the environment. Sleep restores a person's energy and sense of well-being.

Recent studies confirm that sleep is a cyclical phenomenon. The most common sleep cycle is the 24-hour, day-night cycle. This 24-hour cycle is also referred to as the circadian rhythm. In general, the 24-hour circadian rhythm is governed by light and darkness. Additional factors that influence the sleep-wake cycle of the individual are biological cycle such as hormonal and thermoregulation cycles. Most individuals attempts to synchronize activity with the demands of modern society. The two specialized areas of the brainstem which control the cyclical nature of sleep are the reticular activating system in the brainstem, spinal cord, and cerebral cortex, and the bulbar synchronizing portion in the medulla. These two systems function intermittently by activating and suppressing the higher centers of the brain.

After falling asleep, a person passes through a series of stages which afford rest and recuperation physically, mentally, and emotionally. A person's age, general health status, culture, and emotional well-being will dictate the amount of sleep required. On the whole, older persons require less sleep while young infants require the most sleep. As the nurse assesses the patient's needs for sleep and rest, every effort is made to individualize the care plan. A major emphasis is to provide client education regarding the influence of disease process on sleep-rest patterns when applicable.

Various factors influence a person's capability to gain adequate rest and sleep. For the home setting it is appropriate for the nurse to assist the client in developing behavior conducive to rest and relaxation. In a health care setting such as the hospital, the nurse must be able to provide ways of promoting rest and relaxation in a stressful environment. Loss of privacy, unfamiliar noises, frequent examinations, tiring procedures, and a general upset in daily routines culminate in a threat to the client's achievement of essential rest and sleep.

Developmental Considerations

In general, as age increases the amount of sleep per night decreases. The length of each sleep cycle—active (rapid eye movement, REM) and quiet (non-rapid eye movement, NREM)—changes with age. For adults, there is no particular change in the actual number of hours slept, but there is a change in the amount of deep sleep and light sleep. As age increases, the amount of deep sleep decreases and the amount of light sleep increases. This helps explain why the older patient awakens more easily and spends time in sleep throughout the day and night. REM sleep decreases in amount from the time of infancy (50%) to late adulthood (15%). The changes in sleep pattern with development are (Lee, 1981):

Infant: Awake 7 hours; NREM sleep, 8.5 hours; REM sleep, 8.5 hours.
Age 1: Awake 13 hours; NREM sleep, 7 hours; REM sleep, 4 hours.
Age 10: Awake 15 hours; NREM sleep, 6 hours; REM sleep, 3 hours.
Age 20: Awake 17 hours; NREM sleep, 5 hours; REM sleep, 2 hours.
Age 75: Awake 17 hours; NREM sleep, 6 hours; REM sleep, 1 hour.

Infant

The newborn begins life with a regular schedule of sleep and activity that is evident during periods of reactivity. For the first hour infants born of unmedicated mothers spend 60% of the time in the quiet, alert state and only 10% of the time in the irritable, crying state. Five distinct sleep-activity states for the infant are listed by Whaley and Wong (1987, p. 316). These states are:

1. Regular sleep;
2. Irregular sleep;
3. Drowsiness;
4. Alert inactivity;
5. Waking and crying.

The newborn and young infant spend more time in REM sleep than adults.

As the infant's nervous system develops the infant will have longer periods of sleep and wakefulness that become more regular. At approximately 8 months of age the infant goes through the stage of separation anxiety with potentially altered sleep patterns. Teething, ear infections, or other alteration affect sleep patterns. Respirations are quiet with minimal activity noted during deep sleep. The infant sleeps an average of 12–16 hours/day.

Toddler

The toddler needs approximately 10–12 hours of sleep at night with an approximate 2-hour nap in the afternoon. The percentage of REM sleep is 25%. Rituals for preparation for sleep are important, with bedtime associated as separation from family and fun. Quiet time to gradually unwind, a favorite object for security, and a relatively consistent bedtime are suggested. Nightmares may begin to occur due to magical thinking.

The preschooler sleeps approximately 10–12 hours/day. Dreams and nightmares may occur at this time and resistance to bedtime rituals is also common. Unwinding or slowing down from the many activities of the day is recommended to lessen sleep disturbances. Actual attempts to foster relaxation by mental imaging at this age have proved successful. The percentage of REM sleep is 20%.

Special needs may be prompted for the toddler during hospitalization. When at all possible the mother's presence should be encouraged throughout nighttime to lessen fears. Limit setting with safety in mind is also necessary for the toddler due to the surplus of energy and the desire for constant activity. The pre-schooler may be at risk for fatigue. Sleep may not be necessary at nap time, but rest without disturbance is recommended to supplement night sleep and to prevent fatigue.

School-Age Child

The school-aged child seems to do well without a nap and requires approximately 10 hours of sleep per day, with REM sleep being approximately 18.5%. Individualized rest needs are developed by this age with a reliable source being the child who can express feelings about rest or sleep. Health status would also determine to a great extent how much sleep the child at this age requires. Permission to stay up late must be weighed in view of potential upset to routine and demands of the next day. When bedtime is assigned a status, peer pressure and power issues may ensue.

When the school-ager alters the usual routines of sleep and rest, fatigue may be a result. Attempts should be made to maintain usual routines even when school is not in session to best maintain the usual sleep-rest pattern.

Adolescent

Irregular sleep patterns seem to be the norm for the adolescent due to high activity levels and usual peer-related activities. There may be a tendency to overexertion which is made more pronounced by the numerous physiologic changes which create increased demands on the body. Fatigue may be most likely during this time. On the average, the adolescent sleeps approximately 8–10 hours/day with REM sleep being 20%.

Rest may be necessary to supplement sleep to best prevent illness or the risk of illness. Extracurricular activities may also need to be limited.

Young and Middle-Aged Adult

The young adult sleeps approximately 8 hours/day with REM sleep being 22%. Sleep patterns may be subject to young infants or children in the household or after-hours professional and social demands.

The young adult may be at high risk for fatigue due to increasing role expectations, especially in the instance of a new baby being cared for. It is wise that sleep deprivation not be allowed as a means of trying to cope with the many expectations the young adult may feel, whether related to daily living as a professional or not.

Older Adult

The older adult requires less sleep on the average approximately 5–7 hours/day. The percentage of REM sleep is 20–23%. The actual decrease in sleep needs may serve as an upsetting factor for the older adult. Specific concerns for insomnia are associated with institutionalized older adults who may not all sleep from 9 PM to 6 AM or whatever expectations the schedule seems to dictate. Safety needs during sleep time or rest must be kept in mind.

The actual decreased need for sleep may be upsetting to the older adult and result in fatigue. Division of sleep time between day and night may prove beneficial. Individualized attention to sleep and potential fatigue is critical to best prevent further loss of activity and self-worth for this client.

Applicable Nursing Diagnosis

Sleep Pattern Disturbance

DEFINITION

Disruption of sleep time causes discomfort or interferes with desired life-style (North American Nursing Diagnosis Association [NANDA] 1987, p. 83).

DEFINING CHARACTERISTICS (NANDA, 1987, p. 83)

The nurse will review the initial pattern assessment for the following defining characteristics to determine the diagnosis of Sleep Pattern Disturbance.

1. Major defining characteristics
    a. Verbal complaints of difficulty falling asleep.
    b. Awakening earlier or later than desired.
    c. Interrupted sleep.
    d. Verbal complaints of not feeling well rested.
    e. Changes in behavior and performance (increasing irritability, restlessness, disorientation, lethargy, listlessness).
    f. Physical signs (mild fleeting nystagmus, slight hand tremor, ptosis of eyelid, expressionless face, dark circles under eyes, frequent yawning, changes in posture).
    g. Thick speech with mispronunciation and incorrect words.
2. Minor defining characteristics
    None given.

RELATED FACTORS (NANDA, 1987, p. 83)

1. Sensory alterations
    a. Internal—illness, psychological stress
    b. External—environmental changes, social cues

DIFFERENTIATION

Sleep pattern disturbance rarely requires differentiation from other diagnoses. One possible differentiation, however, is Individual Coping, Ineffective. In many instances, patients will use sleep as an avoidance mechanism and might report a sleep pattern disturbance when in reality there is no disturbance. The patient has a normal sleep pattern but desires to increase the amount of sleep to avoid having to deal with the stress, anxiety, fear, etc.

Differentiation is based on assessment of the comparison between the usual sleep-rest pattern and the current sleep-rest pattern as described by both the patient and at least one other significant other. An increase in the amount of time spent in sleeping would more likely indicate a coping problem rather than a true sleep pattern disturbance. The presence of recent or current situational or maturational crises resulting in more rather than less sleep would assist in validating Individual Coping, Ineffective versus Sleep Pattern Disturbance.

OBJECTIVES

1. Will demonstrate at least 6–8 hours of uninterrupted sleep each night by (date).

AND/OR

2. Will verbalize decreased number of complaints regarding loss of sleep by (date).

TARGET DATE

The suggested target date is no less than 2 days after the date of diagnosis and no more than 5 days. This length of time will allow for modification of circadian rhythm.

NURSING ORDERS

ADULT HEALTH

1. Maintain room temperature at 68°–72° F.
2. Close door to room; limit traffic into room beginning at least 1 hour prior to scheduled sleep time.
3. Teach relaxation exercises.
4. Suggest sleep preparatory activities such as quiet music, warm fluids, decreased active exercise at least 1 hour prior to scheduled sleep time.
5. Notify operator to hold telephone calls after 9 PM.
6. Provide warm, noncaffeinated fluids after 6 PM; limit fluids after 9 PM.
7. Assist to bathroom or bedside commode, or offer bedpan at 9 PM.
8. Ensure adherence, as closely as possible, to patient's usual bedtime routine.
9. Place in preferred sleeping position; support position with pillows.
10. Schedule all patient therapeutics prior to 9 PM.
11. Administer required medication (e.g., analgesics, sedative, if appropriate) after all daily activities and therapeutics are completed.
12. Give massage immediately after administering medication.
13. Assess effectiveness of medication 30 minutes after time of administration.
14. Provide night light.
15. Once client is sleeping, place "do not disturb" sign on door. Increase exercise and activity during day as appropriate for patient's condition.
16. As appropriate, discuss reasons for sleep pattern disturbance; teach appropriate coping mechanisms.

CHILD HEALTH

1. Give warm bath 30 minutes to 1 hour before scheduled sleep time.
2. Feed 15–30 minutes before scheduled sleep time—formula, snack of protein and simple carbohydrate, no fats.
3. Implement usual bedtime routine—rocking, patting, favorite stuffed animal or blanket.
4. Read soporific story to child.
5. Provide environment conducive to sleep—room temperature of 74°–78° F; soft, relaxing music; night light.
6. Restrict loud physical activity at least 2–3 hours before scheduled sleep time.
7. Schedule therapeutics around sleep needs.
8. Assist parents with defining and standardizing general waking and sleeping schedule.
9. Teach parents and child appropriate age-related relaxation techniques.
10. Discuss with parents difference between inability to sleep and fears related to developmental crises.
    a. Infant and toddler—separation anxiety
    b. Preschooler—fantasy versus reality
    c. School age—ability to perform at expected levels
    d. Adolescent—role identity versus role diffusion
11. Ensure child's safety according to developmental and psychomotor abilities (e.g., infant placed on abdomen; no plastic, loose-fitting sheets; bed rails to prevent falling out of bed).

WOMEN'S HEALTH

1. Assist patient to schedule rest breaks throughout day.
2. Teach relaxation exercises.
3. Maintain proper body alignment with use of positioning and pillows. Have patient return demonstrate proper positioning when appropriate.

4. Review daily schedule with patient and assist patient to adjust sleep schedule to coincide with infant's sleep pattern.
5. Identify a support system which can assist patient in alleviating fatigue.
6. Assist patient in identifying life-style adjustments that may be needed due to changes in physiologic function or needs during experiential phases of life (e.g., pregnancy, postpartum, menopause).
   a. Possible lowering of room temperature.
   b. Layering of blankets or covers that can be discarded or added as necessary.
   c. Practicing relaxation immediately before scheduled sleep time.
   d. Establishing a bedtime routine (bath, food, fluids, activity).
7. Involve significant others in discussion and problem-solving activities regarding life-cycle changes that are affecting work habits and interpersonal relationships (e.g., hot flashes, pregnancy, postpartum fatigue).
8. Teach client to experiment with restful activities when she cannot sleep at night rather than lying in bed and thinking about not sleeping.

MENTAL HEALTH

1. Provide only decaffeinated drinks during all 24 hours.
2. Spend (amount of time) with patient in activity of patient's choice at least twice a day.
3. Provide appropriate positive reinforcement for achievement of steps toward reaching objective.
4. Assist client with bedtime routine. Suggested activities include:
   a. Taking a warm bath;
   b. Having a backrub;
   c. Doing relaxation exercises;
   d. Reading;
   e. Ensuring quiet environment;
   f. Drinking warm milk.
5. Talk patient through deep muscle relaxation exercise for 30 minutes at 9 PM.
6. Sit with patient for (amount of time) three times a day in a quiet environment and provide positive reinforcement for patient's accomplishments. (*Note: This for patients with increased activity.*)
7. Go to patient's room and walk with him or her to the group area three times a day.
8. Spend time out of the room with the patient until he or she demonstrates ability to tolerate 30 minutes of interacting with others. (*Note: For patients with depressed mood.*)
9. Spend 30 minutes with client discussing concerns 2 hours at bedtime.
10. Dim lights, decrease environmental noise, and decrease activity in area by 9 PM.
11. If patient does not fall asleep within 45 minutes after retiring, have him or her get up and move around unit, sit at nurses' station and read, or engage in some other activity that does not focus on working or going to sleep, but that is not exciting for the patient.
12. Administer sleep medication if needed.

HOME HEALTH

1. Teach patient and family to provide restful environment and to promote sleep routine.
2. Involve patient and family in planning, implementing, and promoting restful environment and sleep routine.
3. Close door to room.
4. Turn room lights off and provide small night light.
5. Pull blinds to shield from street lights (at night) or sunlight (daytime).
6. Limit activity in room beginning at least 30 minutes before scheduled sleep time.
7. Unplug telephone in room or adjust volume control on bell.
8. Coordinate family activities and patient's sleep needs to maximize both schedules.

9. Request that visits and calls be at specified times so that sleep time is not interrupted.
10. Maintain pain control via appriopriate medications, body positioning, and relaxation.
11. Provide favorite music, pillows, bedclothes, teddy bears, etc.
12. Provide optimal room temperature and ventilation.
13. Support usual bedtime routine as much as possible in relation to medical diagnosis and patient's condition.
14. Schedule nursing therapuetics to minimize disruption of sleep (i.e., hygiene measure, vital signs, dressing changes, etc.).
15. Assist patient with bedtime routine as necessary.
16. Encourage self-care, exercise, and activity as appropriate and based on medical diagnosis and patient condition.

EVALUATION
OBJECTIVE 1

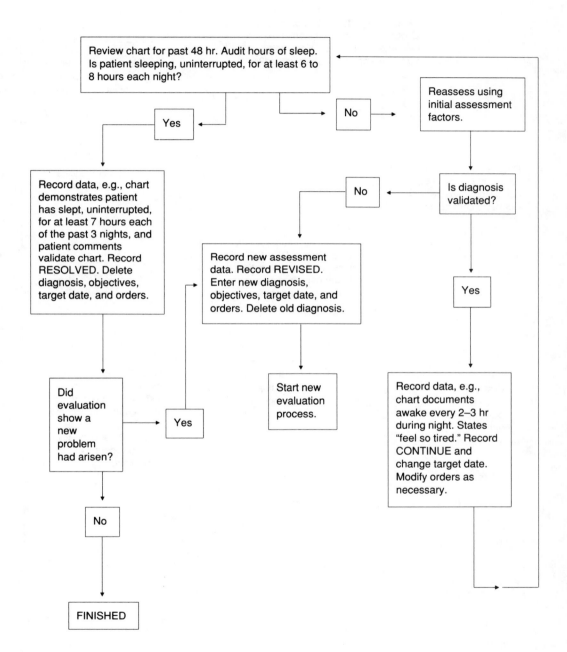

OBJECTIVE 2

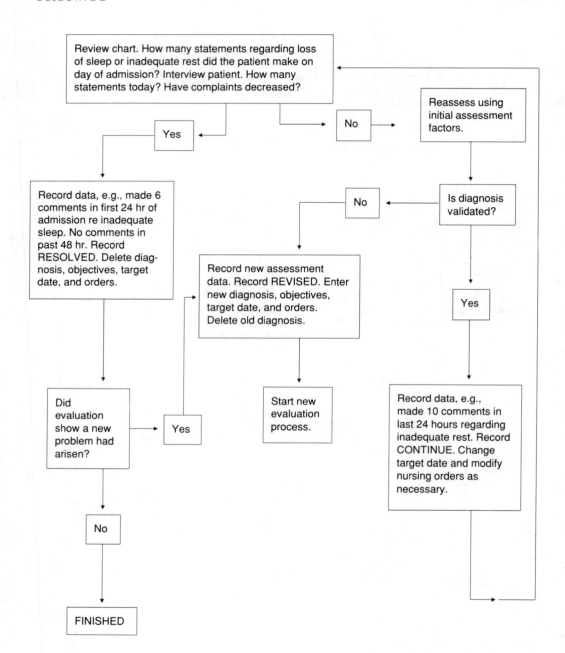

REFERENCES

Lee, K. (1981). Rest status. In P. H. Mitchell and A. Loustau (Eds.), *Concepts basic to nursing* (3rd ed.) (pp. 603–621). New York: McGraw-Hill.

North American Nursing Diagnosis Association. (1987). *Taxonomy I with complete diagnoses*. St. Louis: Author.

Whaley, L., & Wong, D. (1987). *Nursing care of infants and children*. St. Louis: C. V. Mosby.

SUGGESTED READINGS

Brill, E., & Kitts, D. (1986). *Foundations for nursing*. East Norwalk, CT: Appleton-Century-Crofts.

Crittendon, R. (1983). *Discharge planning*. Bowie, MD: Robert J. Brady.

Hadeka, M. (1987). *Clinical judgment in community health nursing*. Boston: Little, Brown.

Humphrey, C. (1986). *Home care nursing handbook*. East Norwalk, CT: Appleton-Century-Crofts.

Jaffe, M., & Skidmore-Roth, L. (1988). *Home health nursing care plans*. St. Louis: C. V. Mosby.

McClelland, E., Kelly, K., & Buckwalter, K. (1984). *Continuity of care: Advancing the concept of discharge planning*. Orlando, FL: Grune & Stratton.

McFarland, G., & Wasli, E. (1986). *Nursing diagnoses and process in psychiatric mental health nursing*. Philadelphia: J. B. Lippincott.

Murray, R., & Zentner, J. (1988). *Nursing assessment and health promotion through the lifespan*. Philadelphia: Prentice-Hall.

National League for Nursing. (1986). *Policies and procedures*. New York: Accreditation Division for Home Care, National League for Nursing.

National League for Nursing. (1988). *Accreditation program for home care and community health: Criteria and standards*. New York: Author.

North American Nursing Diagnosis Association. (1988). *Proposed nursing diagnoses*. St. Louis: Author.

Rinke, L. (1988). *Outcome standards in home health*. New York: National League for Nursing.

Steffi, B., & Eide, I. (1978). *Discharge planning handbook*. New York: Charles B. Slack.

Walsh, J., Persons, C., & Wieck, L. (1987). *Manual of home health care nursing*. Philadelphia: J. B. Lippincott.

CHAPTER SEVEN

Cognitive-Perceptual Pattern

Pattern Description

Rationality, the ability to think, has often been described as the defining attribute of human beings. Thus, the Cognitive-Perceptual Pattern becomes the essential premise for all other patterns used in the practice of nursing. Since this pattern deals with the adequacy of the sensory modes and adaptations necessary to negate inadequacies in the cognitive functional abilities, any failure in recognizing alterations in this pattern will hamper assessment and intervention in all of the other patterns. The nurse must be cognizant of the Cognitive-Perceptual Pattern as an integral and important part of holistic nursing.

The Cognitive-Perceptual Pattern deals with thought, thought processes, and knowledge as well as the way the patient acquires and applies knowledge. A major component of the process is perceiving. Perceiving incorporates the interpretation of sensory stimuli. Understanding how a patient thinks, perceives, and incorporates these processes to best adapt and function is paramount in assisting the patient to return to or maintain the best health state possible. The nurse will do well to assess for alterations in the process of cognition and perception as an initial step in any assessment.

Additionally, the nurse-patient relationship posits the human response as a major premise for the nursing process. Ultimately, then, it is this very notion of thought and learning potential which facilitates the ultimate self-actualization of human beings.

Pattern Assessment

1. Patient's description of adequacy of special senses:
   a. Vision—Glasses? Contact lenses? Regular checkups? Results of test with Snellen chart.
   b. Hearing—Any changes? Difficulty? Hearing aid? Results of testing.
   c. Taste—Any changes? Any persistent taste sensation, e.g., "everything tastes sour"? Results of testing.
   d. Touch—Any decreased (numbness) or increased (tingling) sensations? Results of testing.
   e. Smell—Any changes? Any persistent odor, e.g., "all smells the same"? Results of testing.
2. Patient's description of pain. Ranking (0–10) of pain acuity. What has been used to relieve pain? Adequacy of this measure?
3. Any problems with learning? Memory? Decision making? Are these problems of recent origin? Highest formal educational level (e.g., 3rd grade, high school graduate)? College graduate?
4. Person states he or she feels distressed related to uncertainty about choices.
5. Person verbalizes undesired consequences of alternative actions being considered.
6. Person exhibits vacillation between choices, with extreme being paralysis of analysis.
7. Delayed decision-making.
8. Verbal questioning or actual discussion of specific values being questioned.

9. Physical manifestations of resultant tension due to inability to make a decision, such as increased heart rate, restlessness, tenseness, failure to relax and carry out usual role.
10. Inability to feel at ease regarding the threat of the need to make the decision to resolve a conflict.

Conceptual Information

A person who is able to carry out usual cognitive-perceptual pattern experiences conscious thought, is oriented to reality, solves problems, is able to perceive via sensory input, and responds appropriately in carrying out the usual activities of daily living in the fullest level of functioning. All of these functions rely on a healthy nervous system containing receptors to detect input accurately, a brain which can interpret the information correctly, and transmitters which can transport decoded information. Bodily response is also a basic requisite to respond to the sensory and perceptual demands of the individual.

Cognition is the process of obtaining and using knowledge about one's world through the use of perceptual abilities, symbols, and reasoning. For this reason it includes the use of human sensory capabilities to receive input about the environment. This process usually leads to perception, which is the process of extracting information in such a way that the individual transforms sensory input into meaning. Cognition incorporates knowledge and the process used in its acquisition; therefore, ideas (concepts of mind symbols) and language (verbal symbols) are two of its tools. Learning may be considered the dynamic process in which perceptual processing of sensory input leads to concept formation and change in behavior. Cognitive development is highly dependent on adequate, predictable sensory input.

There are two general approaches to contemporary cognitive theory. The information-processing approach attempts to understand human thought and reasoning processes by comparing the mind to a sophisticated computer system that is designed to acquire, process, store, and use information according to various programs or designs.

The second approach is based on the work of the Swiss psychologist Jean Piaget, who considered cognitive adaptation in terms of two basic processes: assimilation and accommodation. Assimilation is the process by which the person integrates new perceptual data or stimulus events into existing schemata or existing patterns of behavior. In other words, in assimilation, a person interprets reality in terms of his or her own model of the world based on previous experience. Accommodation is the process of changing that model the individual has of the world by developing the mechanisms to adjust to reality. Piaget believed that representational thought does not originate in a social language but in unique symbols that provide a foundation later for language acquisition (Murray & Zentner, 1979, p. 21).

The American psychologist Jerome Bruner broadened Piaget's concept by suggesting that the cognitive process is effected by three modes: the enactive mode involves representation through action, the iconic mode uses visual and mental images, and the symbolic mode uses language.

Cognitive dissonance is the mental conflict which takes place when beliefs or assumptions are challenged or contradicted by new information. The unease or tension the individual may experience as a result of cognitive dissonance usually results in the person resorting to defense mechanisms in an attempt to maintain stability in his or her conception of the world and self.

In a broad sense, thinking activities may be considered internally adaptive responses to intrinsic and extrinsic stimuli. The thought processes serve to express inner impulses; but they also serve to generate appropriate goal-seeking behavior by the individual. This behavior is enhanced by perceptual processes as well.

Perception is the process of extracting information in such a way that the individual transforms sensory input into meaning. The senses which serve as the origin of perceptual stimuli are as follows:

1. Exteroceptors (distance sensors)
   a. Visual

   b. Auditory
2. Proprioceptors (near sensors)
   a. Cutaneous (skin senses which detect and communicate or transduce changes in touch, e.g., pressure, temperature, and pain.)
   b. Chemical sense of taste.
   c. Chemical sense of smell.
3. Interoceptors (deep senses)
   a. Kinesthetic sense which tranduces changes in position of the body and motions of the muscles, tendons, and joints.
   b. Static or vestibular sense which transduces changes related to maintaining position in space and the regulation of organic functions such as metabolism, fluid balance, and sensual stimulation.

It is important to note that since perceptual skill processing is an internal event, its presence and development are inferred by changes in overt behavior.
(Note: The need for further data regarding the normal physiology of the nervous system is acknowledged as the prerequisite for full appreciation of this cognitive-perceptual pattern.)

Developmental Considerations

Infant

The neonate is born able to use the senses, generally speaking. The neonate should have a pupillary reflex in response to light and a corneal reflex in response to touch. The sensory myelinization is best developed at birth for hearing, taste, and smell.

Vision. With regard to vision, the eye is not structurally completely differentiated from the macula. The newborn has the capacity to momentarily fixate on a bright or moving object held within 8 inches and in the midline of the visual field. By approximately 4 months of age, the infant is capable of 20/200 visual acuity. Binocular fixation and convergence to near objects is possible by approximately 4 months of age. In a supine position, the infant follows a dangling toy from the side to past midline.

Hearing. The neonate is capable of detecting a loud sound of approximately 90 decibels and reacts with a startle. At birth all of the structural components of the ear are fully developed. However, the lack of cortical integration and full myelination of the neural pathways prevents specific response to sound. The infant will usually search to locate sounds. By approximately 15 months of age the infant is beginning eye-hand coordination and is capable of accommodation to near objects. Of concern at this age would be any abnormalities noted in any of these tasks plus rubbing of eyes, self-rocking, or other self-stimulating behavior. By approximately 2 months the infant will turn to the appropriate side when a sound is made at ear level. By approximately 20 months the infant will localize sounds made below the ear. A cause for concern might be failure to be awakened by loud noises or any of the above findings being abnormal. Speech or the uttering of sounds by age of 6–8 months would also be a component.

Smell. Smell seems to be a factor in breast-fed infants' response to the mother's engorgement and leaking. Newborns will turn away from strong odors such as vinegar and alcohol. By approximately 6–9 months, the infants associate smell with different foods and familiar people of their circle of activity. Avoidance of strong, unpleasant odors occurs also.

Taste. The newborn responds to various solutions with the following gustofacial reflexes:

1. A tasteless solution elicits no facial expression.
2. A sweet solution elicits an eager suck and a look of satisfaction.
3. A bitter liquid produces an angry, upset expression.

By 1 year of age the infant shows marked preference with similar responses to different flavors as did the young neonate.

Touch. At birth the neonate is capable of perception of touch with mouth, hands, and soles of feet being most sensitive. There is increasing support for the notion that touch and motion are essential to normal growth and development.

By a year of age the infant has a preference for soft textures over rough, grainy textures. The infant relies on the sense of touch for comforting. Overresponse or underresponse to stimuli (e.g., pain) is cause for concern.

Proprioception. The infant at birth is limited in perceiving itself in space, as this requires deep myelination and total integration of cortical activity. There is momentary headcontrol. In general, referral to more exacting neurologic reflexes of the neonate will provide in-depth supplementary data. In essence, primitive reflexes, which are protective in nature, serve to assist the neonate in adjustment to extrauterine life and identification of congenital anomalies. A critical appreciation of organic and operational synergy for the CNS is necessary as sensory deficits are considered.

By approximately 3 months of age the infant will, when suspended in a horizontal prone position with the head flexed against the trunk, reflexly draw up the legs—this is known as the Landau reflex. It remains present until approximately 12–24 months of age. Another related reflex is the parachute reflex in which the infant, on being suspended in a horizontal prone position and suddenly thrust downward, will place hands and fingers forward as an attempt to protect himself or herself from falling. This reflex appears at approximately 7 months and persists indefinitely.

The neonate responds with total body reaction to a painful stimulus. The primitive reflexes demonstrate this, especially the Moro or startle response to sudden loss of support or loud noises. The neonate is dependent on others for protection from pain. The mother of a newborn is most often the person who assumes this task, along with father and other primary caregivers. For this reason, management of pain must also include the parents. Distraction is useful in dealing with painful stimuli, as with a pacifier.

The infant gradually offers localized reaction in response to pain at approximately 6–9 months of age. Still, the cognitive abilities of the infant remain limited with respect to pain. Often a physical tugging of the painful body part proves to be the clue of pain for the infant, as with an earache. The infant is incapable of offering cooperation in procedures and must be physically restrained, as resistance to painful stimuli is mainifested. Crying and irritability may also be manifestations of pain, particularly when the nurse is sure other basic needs have been attended to.

If chronic pain comes to be a way of life for the infant soon after birth or before much development has occurred, there may be potential alterations in any of the subsequent development. In some instances, infants adapt and develop high tolerances for pain.

The neonate will be dependent on others for appropriate care and health maintenance. Values for health care are being formed through this provision of care by others.

The infant will gradually continue to learn values of health care. Safety becomes an ongoing need as has been previously acknowledged. Parents or primary caregivers assume this responsibility. The infant is capable of object permanence but cannot be expected to remember abstract notions.

The neonate subjected to hypoxia in the perinatal period is at risk for possible future developmental delays. Apgar scores are typically used as a criterion, in addition to neurologic reflexes. Seizures during the neonatal period must also be followed. In a general sense, the premature infant of less than 38 weeks gestation should also be considered at risk for developmental delays. It is paramount that close examination be performed for basic primitive reflexes and general neonatal status as well as identification of any genetic syndromes or congenital anomalies.

The infant gradually incorporates symbols and interacts with the world through primary caregivers. Any major delays in development should be cause for further close follow-up. Sensory-perceptual deficiencies may indeed bring about impaired thought processes.

Toddler

Vision. Binocular vision is well established by now. The toddler can distinguish geometric shapes and can demonstrate beginning depth perception. Marked strabismus should be treated at this time to prevent ambylopia. The toddler is able to begin to name colors.

Hearing. Smell, taste, and touch all become more related as the toddler initially sees an object and handles it while enjoying via all the senses what it is to "know." Regression to previous tactile behavior for comfort is common in this group, as exemplified by a preference for being patted and rocked to sleep during times of stress such as illness. Concerns by this time would be for secondary deficits in development to show themselves. There is also a great concern for the toddler who shows greater response to movement than sound or who avoids social interaction with other children. By this time speech should be sufficiently developed to validate a basic sense of the toddler's ability to use symbols. Proprioception is not perfected, but "toddling" represents a major milestone. Falls at this age are common.

There is an even greater incorporation of sensory activity in sequencing for the preschooler, in whom major myelination for the most part is fully developed. There is refinement of eye-hand coordination with reading readiness apparent. Visual acuity begins to approach 20/20 and the preschooler will know colors. After age 5 there is minimal potential for development of ambylopia. Language becomes more sophisticated and serves to provide social interaction. By this age the child will remember and exercise caution regarding potential dangers, such as hot objects.

The toddler may regress to previous behavior levels with physical resistance in response to painful stimuli. This will be especially true with invasive procedures. On occasion a toddler may demonstrate tolerance for painful procedures on the basis of understanding benefits offered, for example, young children with a medical diagnosis of leukemia. This is not the usual case, however. Temper tantrums, outbursts, and avoidance of painful stimuli describe the usual behavior of the toddler. Once the toddler must deal with chronic pain there may be regression to previous behavior as a means of coping.

The preschooler views any invasive procedure as mutilation and attempts to withdraw in response to pain. The preschooler cries out in pain and will express feelings in his or her own terms as descriptors of pain. The interpretation of pain is influenced greatly by the parental and familial value systems. In severe pain the potential for regression to previous behavior is high. The nurse should be aware that fears of abandonment, death, or the unknown will be brought out by pain for this age group. Also, the effect the pain has on others may serve to further frighten the child.

Play is an ideal noninvasive means of assessment. Difficulties in gait, balance, or the use of upper limbs in symmetry with lower limbs should be noted, as well as related holistic developmental components including speech, motor, cognitive, perceptual, and social components. Allowance should be made for regression to prior patterns as needed in times of stress such as illness and hospitalization. If a deficit exists, parents should be encouraged to continue appropriate follow-up and intervention.

The preschooler may be aware of how he or she is different from peers, although egocentrism continues. Of importance is the mastery of separation from parents for increasing periods of time. The likelihood of sibling integration should be considered also. At this time a known neglect of one side of the body may be problematic, as the child may rebel and fail to comply with desired therapy.

The toddler gradually learns to care for himself or herself and is strongly influenced by the family's value system. There is capacity for expression of beginning thoughts.

The preschooler has capacity for magical thinking and enjoys role-play of the parent of the same sex. At this age, beginning resistance to parental authority is common and the child is still egocentric in thought. This makes it difficult to apply universal understanding of use of language and symbols for children of this age (e.g., death may be perceived as "sleep").

By this age there should be a general notion of the cognitive capacity for the child. The child explores the world in a meaningful fashion and still relies closely on primary care-givers. If there are marked delays, these should be monitored with a focus on maintaining optimum functioning with developmental sequencing.

The preschooler will enjoy activity and is beginning to enjoy learning colors, using words in sentences, and gradually forming relationships with persons outside the immediate family. If there are delays, they should continue to be monitored. By now major deficits in cognition become more obvious.

School-Age Child

The school-ager has a significant ability to perform logical operations. More complete myelination and maturation enhance the basic physiologic functioning of the central nervous system. Generally, the school-age child can establish and follow simple rules. There is self-motivation with a gradual grasp of time in a more abstract nature. The concept of death is recognized as permanent.

The school-age child begins to interpret the experience of pain with a cognitive component—the cause or source of pain, as well as implications for possible recurrence. The child of this developmental category will attempt to hold still as needed, with an appearance of bravery. Expression of the experience of pain is to be expected by a school-ager. If the school-ager is particularly shy, special attempts should be made to establish a trusting relationship to best manage pain. A major fear is loss of control. The nurse must consider the need to completely evaluate chronic pain. In some instances, it may signal other altered patterns, especially a distressed family or inability to cope as well. Lower performance in school can be an indicator for chronic pain. Also, the nurse should be aware of the increased complexity required for daily activities of living. The child of this age may feel negative about himself or herself if he or she is unable to perform as peers do. The importance of group activities cannot be overstressed.

The school-age child will blossom with a sense of accomplishment. When school does not bring success, frustration follows. It is mandatory that caution be exercised in assessing for deficits versus behavioral manifestations of not liking school.

Adolescent

Vision. Acuity of 20/20 is reached by now. Squinting should be investigated, as should any symptoms of prolonged eye-strain.

Hearing. Further investigation should be done on any adolescent who speaks loudly or who fails to respond to loud noises.

Touch. Overreaction or underreaction to painful stimuli is cause for further investigation.

Taste. The adolescent may prefer food fads for length of time, but concern would be appropriate if the adolescent overuses spices, especially salt or sugar, or complaints of foods not "tasting as they used to."

Smell. The adolescent should distinguish a full range of odors. The nurse should be concerned if the adolescent is unresponsive to noxious stimuli.

Proprioception. There may be temporary clumsiness associated with marked growth spurts. Concern would be held for patterns of deteriorating gross and fine motor coordination and ataxia.

By now the adolescent is capable of formal operational thought and is able to move beyond the world of concrete reality to abstract possibilities and ideas. Problem solving is evident with inductive and deductive capacity. There is an interest in values with a tendency toward idealism. Attention must be given to the adolescent's sensitivity to others and potential for rejection if body image is altered. Of particular importance at this time are sports and peer-related activities. As feelings are explored more cautiously there is a tendency to draw into oneself at this stage. There may be major conflicts over independence exaggerated when self-care is not possible.

The adolescent fears mutilation and attempts to deal with pain as an adult might. Self-control is strived for with allowance for capitalization on gains from pain. Sexuality factors of role performance enter into this group as pain occurs. As with the adult, an attempt to discover the cause and implication of the pain is made. The adolescent experiencing chronic pain will be at risk for normal peer interaction and may potentially endure altered self-perception.

The adolescent will most often remain steady in cognitive functioning if there are no major emotional or sensory problems. Of concern at this age would be substance abuse which could impair thought processes.

Adult and Older Adult

Vision. The adult is capable of 20/20 vision with a gradual decline in acuity and accommodation after approximately 40 years of age. There is a tendency toward farsightedness. Color discrimination decreases in later ages with blues being the major hues affected. Depending on the cause, there is a great potential for the use of corrective aids. In examples of degenerative processes, though, such is not the case, as with macula degeneration. Eventually depth perception is also affected. There may also be a sensitivity to light as with cataract formation. The nurse should be alert for all etiologic components, but especially the retinopathy associated with diabetic alterations.

Hearing. The adult has a sensitivity to accurately discriminate 1600 different frequencies. There should be equal sensation of sounds for the left and right ear. The Rinne test may be done to validate air and bone conduction via a tuning fork. The Weber test may be used to assess lateralization. Equilibrium assessment will provide data regarding the vestibular branch.

With time, the acuity of what is heard gradually diminishes, with detection of high pitch frequencies especially affected. The nurse should be concerned with a lack of response to loud noises, increased volume of speech, and universal nodding of head when someone speaks.

Smell. There may be a gradual deterioration in sensitivity for smell after approximately age 60, although for the most part the sense of smell remains functional in the absense of organic disease. There may be altered gastrointestinal enzyme production, which ultimately interferes with usual perception of smells.

Taste. The ability to taste is well differentiated in adulthood. Sweet and sour can be detected bilaterally. Concern may be raised if the client states the sense of taste has diminished or changed. There is a gradual loss of acuity in taste as aging occurs in later life. This is due in part to decreased enzymatic production and utilization in digestive processes. Oversalting or spicing of foods may serve as a clue to this loss of taste sensation.

Touch. The adult is able to discriminate on a wide range of tactile stimuli, including pressure, temperature, texture, and pain or noxious components. With aging there is a decrease in subcutaneous fat, loss of skin turgor, increase in capillary fragility, and a decrease in conduction of impulses. All of these changes influence the sense of touch with a loss of acuity in aging.

Proprioception. The adult is well coordinated and has a keen sense of perception of his or her body in space. There are multiple protective mechanisms which aid in maintaining balance. Typically, even with eyes closed, the individual is able to stand and maintain balance.

By now the tolerance and threshold one has for pain is well established. Nonetheless, because an increased potential for awareness of ways to cope with the pain exists, the adult may potentially be equipped with a more stable base from which to respond. Paradoxically the adult may also experience unresolved conflicts of previous development levels as well. For this reason the required change may be subject to associated changes as the multiple demands of daily living are affected by pain and its response by the adult.

The adult is equipped to solve problems and apply principles to everyday living. There is emphasis on seeking a mate for life who is able to satisfy basic companionship needs. There may be difficulties in accepting life's challenges as parents or as adults juggling the many roles necessary. There is, in later life, a gradual decline in problem-solving capacity which may be exaggerated by illness.

Allowance for potential decreases in bodily perception and functioning with age must be considered. As assessment is carried out, focus should be on risk factors such as chronic illness, financial deficits, resolution of ego integrity versus despair, and obvious etiologic components. The nurse should assist the patient to maintain self-care as the patient desires.

With aging there is a gradual loss of balance, perhaps most related to the concurrent vascular changes. For this reason proprioceptive data may provide an immediate basis for safety needs of the geriatric client.

In the absence of adversity, the adult enjoys the daily challenges of living. If coping is altered for whatever reason, a risk for impaired thought process exists. With aging, there may be potential risks for impaired thought process. In addition, there may be potential risks for some regarding degenerative brain and CNS disorders which include impaired thought processes also.

Applicable Nursing Diagnoses

Comfort, Altered: Pain

DEFINITION

A state in which an individual experiences and reports the presence of severe discomfort or an uncomfortable sensation. (North American Nursing Diagnosis Association [NANDA], 1987, p. 105).

DEFINING CHARACTERISTICS (NANDA, 1987, pp. 105–106)

The nurse will review the initial pattern assessment for the following defining characteristics to determine the diagnosis of Comfort, Altered: Pain.

1. Pain
   a. Major defining characteristics
      (1) Subjective
         (a) Communication (verbal or coded) of pain descriptions
      (2) Objective
         (a) Guarding behavior, protective
         (b) Self-focusing
         (c) Narrowed focus (altered time perception, withdrawal from social contact, impaired thought processes)
         (d) Distraction behavior (moaning, crying, pacing, seeking out other people or activities, restlessness)
         (e) Facial mask of pain (eyes lack luster, "beaten look," fixed or scattered movement, grimace)
         (f) Alteration in muscle tone (may span from listless to rigid)
         (g) Autonomic responses not seen in chronic stable pain (diaphoresis, blood pressure and pulse change, pupillary dilation, increased or decreased respiratory rate).
2. Chronic pain
   a. Definition: A state in which the individual experiences pain that continues for more than 6 months in duration.
   b. Major defining characteristics
      (1) Verbal report or observed evidence of pain experienced for more than 6 months
   c. Minor defining characteristics
      (1) Fear of reinjury
      (2) Physical and social withdrawal
      (3) Altered ability to continue previous activities
      (4) Anorexia
      (5) Weight changes
      (6) Changes in sleep patterns
      (7) Facial mask
      (8) Guarded movement

RELATED FACTORS (NANDA, 1987, pp. 105–106)

1. Pain
   a. Injuring agents (biological, chemical, physical, psychological)
2. Chronic pain
   a. Chronic physical or psychosocial disability

DIFFERENTIATION

In most instances the subjective component of expression of pain serves as the single most universal differential for pain versus other diagnoses. It is highly likely that other contributory or related components of potentially all other patterns will need to be explored. A unique challenge is offered when the patient is unable to speak or express the painful experience while still being pain-ridden. A time factor will aid in separating Sleep Pattern Disturbance or Role-Relationship Alterations from Comfort, Altered. There may be those unique instances in which an emotional or psychological component must be dealt with as a major factor of the pain experience. Examples of this are the stoic individual who negates pain and the individual who capitalizes on the pain experience as a means of gaining desired goals.

OBJECTIVES

1. Will verbalize a decreased number of complaints of pain by (date).

AND/OR

2. Will require no more than one medication for pain per 24 hours by (date).

TARGET DATE

For the majority of health disruptions, pain will begin to resolve within 72 hours after the client has sought health care assistance. Thus, the suggested target date is 3 days after the date of diagnosis.

NURSING ORDERS

ADULT HEALTH

1. Monitor for pain at least every 2 hours on (even/odd) hour. Have patient rank pain on a scale of 0–10 at each incidence of pain. Review and have patient review activity engaged in prior to each pain episode and document. Request patient to share thoughts and feelings prior to onset of painful episode.
2. Teach patient to report pain as soon as it starts. Allow patient to talk about pain experience in as much detail as desired.
3. Administer pain medication as ordered. Monitor and record amount of pain relief within 30 minutes after administration. Have patient rerank pain (0–10). If not relieving pain, collaborate with physician regarding change in medication.
4. Give massage immediately following administration of each pain medication and after each turning.
5. Turn at least every 2 hours on (even/odd) hour. Maintain anatomical alignment with pillows or other padded support.
6. Provide calm, quiet environment. Limit activity for at least 2 hours following pain medication administration.
7. Monitor vital signs at least every 4 hours while awake.
8. Monitor sleep-rest pattern. Promote rest periods during day and at least 8 hours sleep each night (see care plan for Sleep Pattern Disturbance).
   a. Warm bath before retiring.
   b. Warm fluids before retiring.
9. Offer 2–3 ounces of wine before each meal and at bedtime.
10. Promote activity and exercise to extent possible (i.e., so long as it does not result in pain). Provide range of motion at least every 4 hours while awake.
11. Apply heat or cold (on 2 hours; off 2 hours). Select heat, cold, dry, moist, according to what patient states provides the best pain relief.
12. Check bowel elimination at least once per shift.
13. Encourage fluid intake every 2 hours while awake, up to 3000 ml per day.
14. Provide oral hygiene every 4 hours while awake.
15. Allow time for patient to discuss fears and anxieties related to pain by scheduling at least 15 minutes once per shift to visit with patient on one-to-one basis. Provide accurate information to patient regarding:
    a. Pain threshold

b. Pain tolerance

c. Addiction

d. Medication effectiveness and ineffectiveness

e. Expressing pain

16. Apply mentholated or aspirin ointment to affected area every 4 hours and when needed, as appropriate.

17. Use noninvasive pain relief techniques as appropriate:

a. Biofeedback

b. Progressive relaxation

c. Guided imagery

d. Rhythmic breathing

e. Distraction

f. Contralateral stimulation

18. Collaborate with physician regarding use of transcutaneous electrical nerve stimulation (TENS).

19. Teach patient and significant others:

a. Cause of pain

b. Self-administration of pain medication

c. Avoiding and minimizing pain

    (1) Splinting

    (2) Gradual increase in activities

d. Use of alternate noninvasive techniques

    (1) Progressive relaxation

    (2) Stress management techniques

    (3) Biofeedback

    (4) Self-hypnosis

    (5) Guided imagery

    (6) Distraction

e. Combining techniques (e.g., medication with relaxation technique).

f. To try various pain relief measures and to alternate pain relief measures.

g. To express anger, frustration, and grief with pain management and change in life-style.

h. To be more active in his or her own pain arrangement program. Note successes, minimize failure.

i. Value of adequate rest and maintaining weight within normal range.

20. Refer to or collaborate with other health professionals:

a. Occupational therapist

b. Physical therapist

c. Pain clinic

d. Home health nurse

e. Psychiatric nurse clinician

Additional Information

Keep current on comparative doses of analgesics, true effect of so-called potentiators, and noninvasive means of pain relief. Do not worry about a patient becoming addicted. With the average length of stay being 5–7 days, it is doubtful addiction could occur. Current research in this area shows an extremely low rate of addiction due to medication administration in a health care setting. The same research indicates we undermedicate for pain rather than overmedicate. Undermedication is particularly true in the case of infants and children. See Margo McCaffery's publication (1979) for a discussion on this research as well as further information on pain control.

CHILD HEALTH

1. Monitor for contributory factors to pain at least every 8 hours or as required:

a. Physical injury or surgical incision

  b. Stressors
  c. Fears
  d. Knowledge deficit
  e. Anxieties
  f. Fatigue
  g. Description of exact nature of pain whether per McGill or Elkind tools.
  h. Temperature, pulse, respirations, and blood pressure.
  i. Response to medication as ordered.
  j. Meaning of pain to child and family.
2. Provide appropriate support in management of pain for the patient and significant others by:
  a. Validation of the pain;
  b. Maintaining self-control to extent feasible;
  c. Providing education to deal with specifics applicable. Assist patient and family to ventilate about the pain experience by allowing at least 30 minutes per shift for such ventilation.
  d. Allowing parents to be present and participate in comforting of patient. Assist child and parents to develop a plan of care which addresses individual needs and is likely to result in a better coping pattern (particularly for chronic pain).
  e. Appropriate diversional activities for age and developmental level.
  f. Attention to controlling external stimuli such as noise, light, etc.
  g. Use of relaxation techniques appropriate for child's capacity.
  h. Appropriate follow-up of pain tolerance and response to medication as ordered:
    (1) Encourage pain medication route to be oral if there is no IV.
    (2) If IV route is utilized, monitor for respiratory and blood pressure depression.
    (3) Monitor intake and output for decrease due to hypomotility or spasm.
    (4) Monitor for possible drug allergies.
  i. Appropriate emotional support during painful procedure or experience.
    (1) Explanations in child's level of openness and honesty.
    (2) Use of puppets to demonstrate procedure.
    (3) Explanation to parents that even if child cries excessively, their presence is encouraged.
    (4) Comforting before, during, and after procedure.
    (5) Reward the child for positive behavior according to developmental need, for example, stars on a chart.
    (6) Discuss and encourage parents and child to share feelings about the painful experience.
  j. Collaborate with or refer to appropriate health team members such as:
    (1) Pediatrician, surgeon, subspecialist
    (2) Clinical nurse specialist
    (3) Psychologist
    (4) Social worker
    (5) Play therapist
    (6) Family therapist
    (7) Community support group
    (8) National Arthritis Foundation
    (9) School nurse
  k. Teach patient and family ways to follow up at home or school with needed pain regimen, including:
    (1) Appropriate timing of medication;
    (2) Appropriate administration of medication;
    (3) Need not to substitute acetaminofen for aspirin in arthritics.
    (4) Monitor for stomach alterations or other complications, especially respiratory depression, secondary to administration of pain medication.
  l. Develop daily plans for pain management to determine those which might be suited for patient to use on a regular basis.

m. Identify need to have several alternate plans to deal with pain.

n. Be astute for possible increased tolerances or sensitivities to pain medication.

(Note: Chronic pain holds a likelihood of recurrence; therefore, a need for long-term follow-up is especially critical. This places the patient at risk for developmental delays as a resultant pattern.)

WOMEN'S HEALTH

(Note: The majority of pain experienced by women is associated with the pelvic area and the reproductive organs. Determining the origin of the pain is one of the most difficult tasks facing nurses dealing with the gynecological client. An organic explanation for the pain is never found in approximately 25% of women. Because of the close association with the reproductive organs, gynecologic pain can be extremely frightening, can connote social stigma, affect the perception of the feminine role, cause anger and guilt, and totally dominate the woman's existence. "Pain is culturally more acceptable in certain parts of the body and may elicit more sympathy than pain in other sites" [Fogel & Woods, 1981, p. 230].)

1. Identify factors in client's life-style that could be contributing to pain.
2. Record accurate menstrual cycle and obstetric, gynecologic, and sexual history, being certain to note problems, previous pregnancies, descriptions of previous labors, previous infections or gynecologic problems and any infections as a result of sexual activities.
3. Assist the client to describe her perception of pain as it relates to her.
4. Describe dysmenorrhea pain pattern, being certain to determine if the pain occurs before, during, or after menstruation.
5. Monitor disturbance of client's daily routine as a result of pain.
6. Describe the location of the pain (i.e., lower abdomen, legs, breasts, or back).
7. Describe any edema, especially "bloating" at specific times during the month.
8. Describe the location, onset, and character of the pain (i.e., mild cramping or severe).
9. Ascertain if pain is associated with nausea, vomiting, or diarrhea.
10. Identify any precipitating factors associated with pain (i.e., emotional upsets, exercise, or medication).
11. Explore the client's perception of pain associated with menstruation.
12. Assist client in identifying various methods of pain relief, including exercise (pelvic rock), biofeedback, relaxation, and medication (analgesics, antiprostaglandins).
13. Encourage client to describe her perception of labor pain as it related to her previous laboring experiences.
14. Provide factual information about the laboring process.
15. Refer client to childbirth preparation group.
16. Describe methods of coping with labor pain (i.e., relaxation, imaging, breathing, and medication).
17. Provide support during labor.
18. Encourage involvement of significant others as support during labor process.
19. Encourage client to describe her perception of pain associated with postpartum.
20. Provide information for pain relief (i.e., Kegel exercises, sitz baths, medications).
21. Explain etiology of "afterbirth pains" to involution of uterus.
22. Explain relationship of breastfeeding to involution and uterine contractions.
23. Assist patient in putting on supportive bra.
24. Encourage early, frequent breast feedings to enhance letdown reflex.
25. Support patient and provide information on correct breastfeeding techniques.
    a. Nurse at both breasts each feeding.
    b. Change positions from one feeding to next to distribute sucking pressure and prevent sore nipples.
26. Check baby's position on breast; be certain areola is in mouth and not just the nipple.
27. Provide warm, moist heat for relief of engorged breasts.

28. Provide analgesics for discomfort of engorged breasts.
29. Pump after infant nurses until breast is relieved. (Do not empty breasts, as this will cause more engorgement if infant is not able to empty breasts at each feeding).
30. Encourage client to nurse on least sore side first to encourage let-down reflex.
31. Apply ice to nipple just before nursing to decrease pain.

MENTAL HEALTH

1. Monitor nurse's response to the client's perception of pain. If the nurse has difficulty understanding or coping with the client's expression of pain this should be discussed with a colleague in an attempt to resolve the nurse's concerns. (This is important because the nurse's response to the client can be communicated and have an effect on the client's level of anxiety which can then affect the pain response.)
2. Note any recurring patterns in the pain experience such as time of day, recent social interactions, physical activity, etc. If a pattern is present begin a discussion of this observation with the client to initiate client awareness and assess client's perceptions of the observation.
3. Determine effects pain has had on client's life, including role responsibilities, financial impact, cognitive and emotional functioning, and family interactions.
4. Review client's beliefs and attitudes about the pain and the role pain is assuming in client's life. If pain is assuming an important role then it might be difficult for the client to "give up" all of the pain and this should be considered in all further interventions. If pain is very important to client's definition of self the following interventions are used:
   a. Assure client that you are not requiring him or her to give up the pain by indicating that you are only interested in that pain that causes undue discomfort or by indicating that you recognize that this client's pain is special and that it would be difficult if not impossible for the health care team to get rid of it.
   b. Spend brief, goal-directed time with the client when he or she is focusing conversation on pain or pain-related activities.
   c. Schedule time with the client when he or she is not complaining about pain. List this schedule here. These interactions should be pleasant and provide positive feedback to the client about an aspect of himself or herself that is not pain-related. This could include special activities in which the client is involved, follow-up on a non-pain-related conversation the client seemed to enjoy, etc.
   d. Find at least one non-pain-related activity the client enjoys that can be the source of positive interaction between client and others and encourage client participation in this activity with positive reinforcement (list client-specific positive reinforcers here along with the activity).
   e. Discuss with client alternatives for meeting personal need currently being met by pain. (May need to refer client to another, more specialized care provider if this is a problem of long standing or if client demonstrates difficulty in discussing these concerns. Refer to Self-Concept, Disturbance in for specific interventions related to perceptions of self.)
   f. Develop with the client a plan to alter those factors that intensify the pain experience (i.e., if the pain increases at 4 PM. each day and the client associates this with his boss's daily visit at 5 PM, then the plan might include limiting the visits from the boss or having another person present when the boss visits). List specific interventions here.
5. Provide a calm, quiet environment.
6. Discuss with client his or her concerns about hospitalization and the plan of care to decrease fear and anxiety.
7. Use touch interventions that decrease the experience of pain. This could include:
   a. Backrubs;
   b. Massage of those areas affected if potential for clots is not present (this can be a light touch or deep massage, whichever the client finds most useful);

    c. Therapeutic touch;

    d. Acupressure holding points for specific areas of pain;

    e. Application of cold (first 24–48 hours after trauma);

    f. Application of heat (48 hours after trauma);

    g. Application of transcutaneous electrical nerve stimulation (TENS).

8. Develop with client plan for learning relaxation techniques and have client practice technique 30 minutes two times a day at (note practice times here). Remain with client during practice session to provide verbal cues and encouragement as necessary. These techniques can include:

    a. Meditation;

    b. Progressive deep muscle relaxation;

    c. Visualization techniques that require the client to visualize scenes that enhance the relaxation response (such as being on the beach or having the sun warm the body, etc.);

    d. Biofeedback;

    e. Prayer;

    f. Autogenic training.

9. Have client begin using the relaxation technique 30 minutes before a situation that has been identified as intensifying pain experiences.

10. Teach client diaphragmatic breathing and have client practice this technique 30 minutes tᵥ .ce a day at (note times here). Remain with client during practice sessions to provide verbal support and direction. Have client use this technique each time an analgesic is requested or administered.

11. Monitor interaction of analgesic with other medications the client is receiving, especially antianxiety, antipsychotic, and hypnotic drugs.

12. Review client's history for indication of illicit drug use and the effects this may have on client's tolerance to analgesics.

13. If client is to be withdrawn from the analgesic, discuss the alternative coping methods and how they will assist client with this process. Assure client that support will be provided during this process; help client identify those items that will be most difficult; and schedule one-to-one time with client during these times.

14. If client demonstrated altered mood refer to Individual Coping, Ineffective for interventions.

15. Consult with occupational therapy to assist client in developing diversional activities. Note time for these activities here as well a list of special equipment that may be necessary for the activity.

16. Involve client in group activities by sitting with him or her during a group activity such as a game, or assign client a responsibility for preparing one part of a unit meal. Begin with activities that require little concentration and then gradually increase the task complexity.

17. Consult with physician for possible referral for use of hypnosis in pain management.

18. Sit with the client and the family during at least two visits to assess family interactions with the client and the role pain plays in family interactions.

19. Discuss with the client the role of distraction in pain management and develop a list of those activities the client finds distracting and enjoyable. These could include listening to music, watching TV or special movies, or physical activity. Develop with the client a plan for including these activities in the pain management program and list that plan here.

20. Discuss with the client the role that exercise can play in pain management (encourages release of natural endorphins) and develop an exercise program with the client. This should begin at or below the client's capabilities and could include a 15-minute walk twice a day or 10 minutes on a stationary bicycle. Note the plan here with the type of activity, length of time, and time of day it is to be implemented.

21. Provide positive reinforcement to the client for implementing the exercise program by spending time with the client during the exercise, providing verbal feedback and allowing client the rewards that have been developed. These rewards are developed with the client.

22. Monitor family and support system understanding of the pain and perceptions of the client. If they demonstrate the attitude that the client is closely perceived with the pain then develop a plan to include them in the experiences described above. List that plan here. Consider referral to a clinical specialist in mental health nursing or a family therapist to assist family in developing non-pain-related interaction patterns.
23. Provide ongoing feedback to client or support system on progress.
24. Refer to outpatient support systems and assist with making arrangements for the client to contact these before discharge. These systems could include:
    a. Occupational therapist
    b. Physical therapist
    c. Clinical nurse specialist in mental health nursing
    d. Visiting nurse services
    e. Hypnotherapist
    f. Financial counseling
    g. Disease-related support groups
    h. Family therapist
    i. Social services

HOME HEALTH

1. Teach patient and family measures to promote comfort:
    a. Proper positioning
    b. Appropriate use of medications (e.g., narcotics as ordered if pain is severe, non-narcotic analgesics, anti-inflamatories)
    c. Knowledge regarding source of pain or of disease process
    d. Self-management of pain and of care as much as is appropriate
    e. Relaxation techniques
    f. Therapeutic touch
    g. Massage (if not contraindicated)
    h. Meaningful activities
    i. Distraction
    j. Breathing techniques
    k. Heat (if not contraindicated)
    l. Regular activity and exercise
    m. Planning and goal setting
    n. Biofeedback
    o. Yoga, tai chi
    p. Imagery, hypnosis
    q. Group or family therapy
2. Teach patient and family factors which decrease tolerance to pain and methods for decreasing these factors.
    a. Lack of knowledge regarding disease process or pain control methods
    b. Lack of support from significant others regarding the severity of the pain
    c. Fear of addiction or fear of loss of control.
    d. Fatigue
    e. Boredom
    f. Improper positioning
3. Involve patient and family in planning, implementing, and promoting reduction in Comfort, Altered: Pain.
    a. Family conference
    b. Mutual goal setting
    c. Communication

    d. Support for caregiver

4. Assist patient and family in life-style adjustments that may be required.
    a. Occupational changes
    b. Family role alterations
    c. Comfort measures for chronic pain
    d. Financial situation
    e. Responses to pain (mood, concentration, ability to complete activities of daily living)
    f. Coping with disability or dependency
    g. Mechanism for altering need for assistance
    h. Providing appropriate balance of dependence and independence
    i. Stress management
    j. Time management
    k. Obtaining and using assistive equipment (e.g., for arthritis)
    l. Regular rather than as needed schedule of medications for pain

5. Teach patient and family purposes, side effects, and proper administration techniques of medications.

6. Consult with or refer to appropriate assistive resources as indicated.
    a. Physical therapist
    b. Occupational therapist
    c. Social service
    d. Family counselor
    e. Psychiatric nurse clinician
    f. YMCA/YWCA for relaxation classes (yoga, massage. etc.)
    g. Visiting nurse
    h. Physician, neurologist, anesthesiologist.
    i. Acupuncturist or acupressurist, biofeedback therapist
    j. Imagery or hypnotherapist
    k. Support groups, respite or day care
    l. Pain specialist
    m. Financial counselor
    n. Spiritual counselor
    o. Pharmacist
    p. Hospice
    q. Rehabilitation counselor
    r. Community transportation

EVALUATION
OBJECTIVE 1

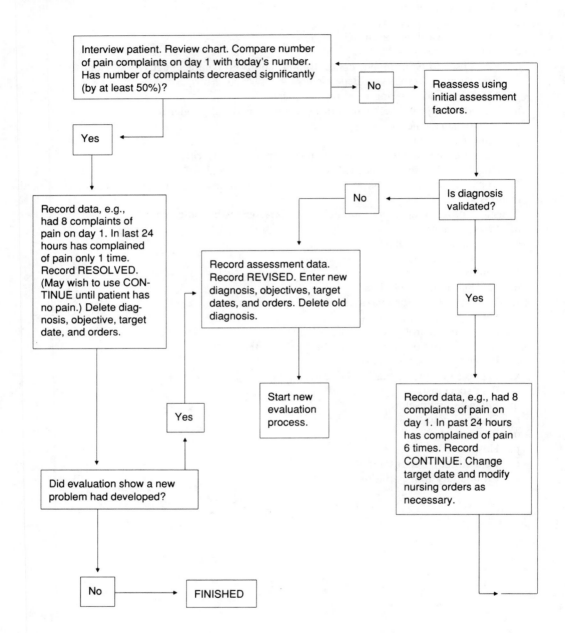

OBJECTIVE 2

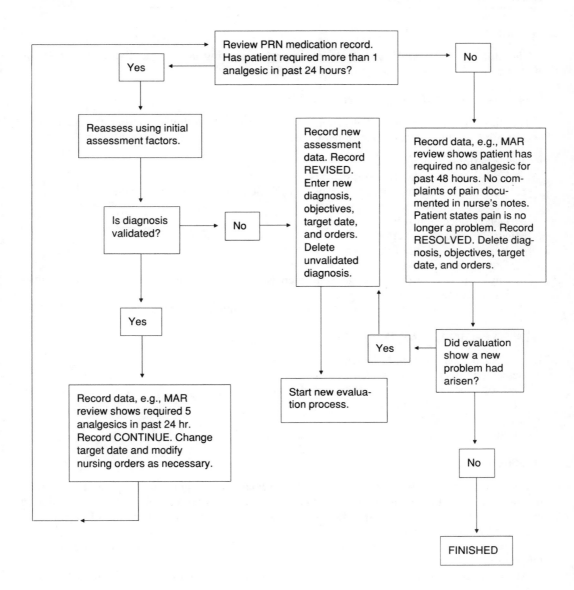

Decisional Conflict

DEFINITION

The state of uncertainty about choice among competing actions involving risk, loss, or challenge to personal life values (NANDA, 1988).

DEFINING CHARACTERISTICS (NANDA, 1988)

The nurse will review the initial pattern assessment for the following defining characteristics to determine the diagnosis of Decisional Conflict.

1. Major defining characteristcs
   a. Verbalized uncertainty about choices
   b. Verbalization of undesired consequences of alternative actions being considered
   c. Vacillation between alternative choices
   d. Delayed decision making
2. Minor defining characteristics
   a. Verbalized feeling of distress
   b. Self-focusing
   c. Physical signs of distress or tension (increased heart rate, increased muscle tension, restlessness, etc.)
   d. Questioning personal values and beliefs while attempting to make a decision

RELATED FACTORS (NANDA, 1988)

1. Unclear personal values or beliefs.
2. Perceived threat to value system.
3. Lack of experience or interference with decision making.
4. Lack of relevant information.
5. Support system deficit.
6. Multiple or divergent sources of information.

DIFFERENTIATION

Decisional Conflict is differentiated from the various other cognitive-perceptual diagnoses by nature of the client's verbalization of feeling that, given appropriate information, a decision or choice of a plan to deal with a specific issue cannot be made, or that risk of loss of personal life values exists in the decision.

Altered Self-Perception or Self-Concept is related to an increased level of arousal with a perceived threat to the self or significant relationships.

Anxiety may be considered as a feeling of threat which may not be known by the person as a specific causative factor.

Individual Coping, Ineffective is closely related in that adaptive behavior and problem-solving abilities are not able to meet the demands of the client's needs.

Role-Relationship patterns would be differentiated by the person being able to function in usual role-relationship activities of daily living despite decisional conflict.

Each of these other patterns may be contributory and must be explored for potential concurrent existence.

OBJECTIVES

1. Will verbalize at least one concrete personal decision by (date).

AND/OR

2. Will return demonstrate at least (number) conflict resolution techniques by (date).

TARGET DATE

Value clarification, belief examination, and learning decision making processes will require a considerable length of time and will require much support. Therefore, target dates in increments of weeks would be appropriate.

NURSING ORDERS

ADULT HEALTH

1. Instruct patient in stress-reduction techniques. Have patient return demonstrate specific techniques at least daily.
2. Assist patient to focus on problem-solving processes. Help patient to verbalize alternatives and advantages and disadvantages of solutions. Help patient to realistically appraise situations and set realistic short-term objectives.
3. Support patient's values. Do not be judgmental. Help patient to clarify values and beliefs.
4. Assist patient to seek, find, and interpret relevant information about problem; refer to community resources for support.
5. Refer to psychiatric nurse clinician.

CHILD HEALTH

(Note: the care plan for a child under this diagnosis is the same as for an adult within the developmental parameters for the child, or when this is not feasible, as the parents might intervene on behalf of the infant or child.)

1. Determine who will intervene on behalf of the infant or child or mother, father, or appointed legal guardian as applicable.
2. In instances of conflicting decision makers, ensure that the child's rights are protected according to legal statutes.
3. Ensure that appropriate documentation is carried out according to situational needs.
4. Although the child may be ill-equipped or unable to participate fully in decision making, encourage developmentally appropriate components for care to assist in learning.
5. Be certain that choices or options indeed exist when the child is allowed to exercise decision making.
6. Provide behavioral reinforcement which best fosters learning with appropriate follow-up when the child is involved in decisional conflict.
7. Consider potential long-term residual or subsequent effects related to specific decisional conflict for the child or family.

WOMEN'S HEALTH

1. Provide an atmosphere that encourages client to view her options in the event of an unwanted pregnancy.
2. Allow client to discuss beliefs and practices in a non-threatening atmosphere.
3. Give clear, concise, complete information to the client, describing the choices available to her.
   a. Carrying the pregnancy
   b. Adoption of infant
   c. Abortion
4. Include significant others in conversation and decision as the client desires.
5. Assure the client of confidentiality.
6. Discuss with the client the advantages and disadvantages of each option.
7. Refer client to proper agency for guidance and treatment.

8. Discuss and view with client the different methods of birth control.
9. Provide factual information, listing the advantages and disadvantages of each method.
10. Explore with client her and her partner's likes and dislikes during sexual act.
11. Assess the client's ability to use correctly the different methods of birth control.
12. Provide client information on obtaining her method of choice.
13. Explore with client and significant other their views on children and family.

MENTAL HEALTH

(Note: The client who is experiencing a decisional conflict is faced with confusion about alternative solutions. When assisting these clients the nurse should be careful not to connote the client's confusion negatively. Various authors have supported the positive role confusion plays in the change process [Erickson, 1983; Keeney, 1983; Watzlawick, Weakland, & Fisch, 1974]. Milton Erickson frequently encouraged confusion as a way to distract the conscious mind and allow the unconscious to develop solutions. It is from this theoretical base that the following interventions are developed.)

1. Assure the client that the difficulty he or she is experiencing in decision making is positive in that it has placed him or her in a position to look for new creative solutions. If he or she were not experiencing this difficulty, he or she might be tempted to remain in the same old problem solution set.
2. Assist client in reducing the pressure of time on making a decision. Have client expand the time he or she has given himself or herself to make a decision. Asking the client the following question may assist in this process: "What is the worst that will happen if a decision is not made right now?"
3. Assist client in verbalizing all information that he or she currently has on the choices.
4. Have client explore feelings related to the choices and the information related to the choices. This process may extend over several days. The client may be reluctant to verbalize negative feelings related to certain choices if a trusting relationship has not yet been developed with the nurse.
5. Have the client discuss how significant others think and feel about the various choices. Have client evaluate the impact of the feelings of significant others on his or her decision making process.
6. Have client fantasize an ideal choice.
7. Have client construct a list of solutions (at least 20) that would produce the ideal choice. (These solutions are not to be evaluated at this time. Encourage client to develop some unrealistic solutions. This may be promoted by asking the client what he or she might tell a friend to do in this situation or by having client generate three magic-wish solutions, i.e., "If you had a magic wand, what would you do to resolve this situation?")
8. Sort through developed list with client generating solutions from the ones listed. At this time the client can begin to combine and eliminate ideas after evaluation. Carefully evaluate each solution before it is eliminated. What appears to be a bizarre solution can become useful when combined or altered with another idea.
9. As each idea is evaluated, provide all information necessary to evaluate the idea.
10. Explore client's thoughts and feelings about each idea.
11. Remind client that there are no perfect answers and each of us makes the best choice that can be made at the time.
12. Remind client that if a choice that is made does not resolve the problem alternative solutions can then be tried.
13. Remind client that solution that does not work provides more information about the problem that can be used in developing future solutions.
14. Meet with client and support system to allow the support system to be a part of the decision making process if this is appropriate.

15. Discuss with client and support system any secondary gains from not making a decision.
16. Once a decision is made, have client develop a behavioral plan for implementation.

HOME HEALTH

1. Teach patient and family measures to decrease decisional conflict.
   a. Providing appropriate health information
   b. Joining a support group
   c. Clarifying values
   d. Performing stress reduction activities
   e. Seeking spiritual or legal assistance as needed.
   f. Identifying useful sources of information.
2. Assist patient and family in identifying risk factors pertinent to the situation.
   a. Lack of knowledge
   b. Developmental or situational crisis
   c. Role confusion
   d. Excess stress
   e. Excess stimuli
3. Consult with or refer to appropriate assistive resources as indicated.
   a. Support group
   b. Psychiatric nurse clinician
   c. Stress reduction
   d. Health education
   e. Family counselor
   f. Spiritual adviser
   g. Attorney

EVALUATION
OBJECTIVE 1

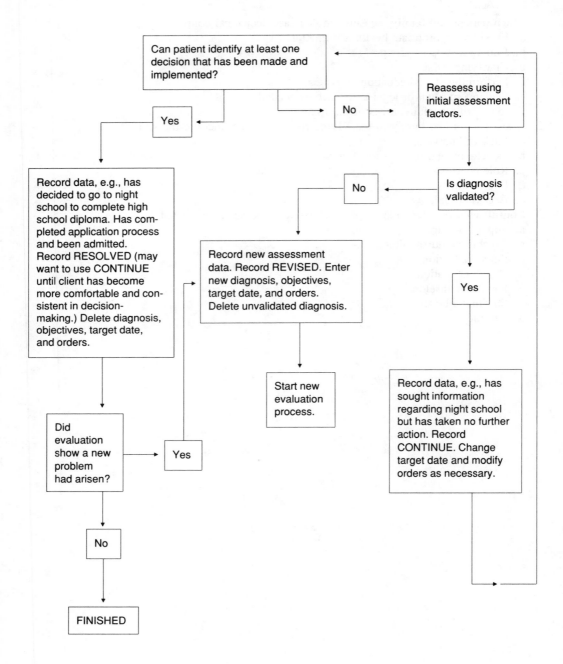

OBJECTIVE 2

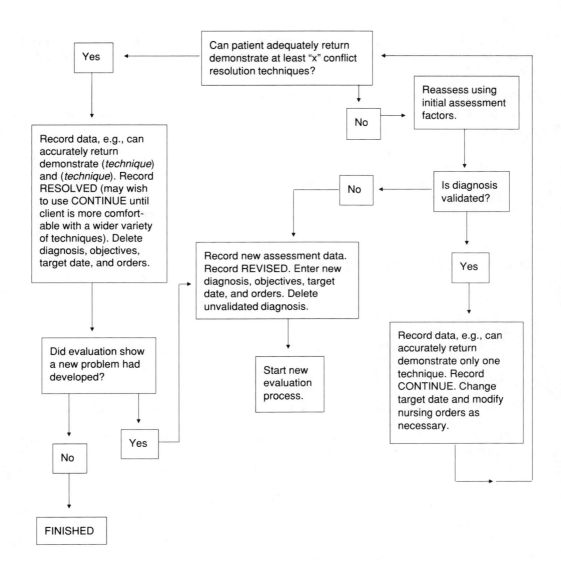

Can patient adequately return demonstrate at least "x" conflict resolution techniques?

Yes

No

Reassess using initial assessment factors.

Record data, e.g., can accurately return demonstrate (*technique*) and (*technique*). Record RESOLVED (may wish to use CONTINUE until client is more comfortable with a wider variety of techniques). Delete diagnosis, objectives, target date, and orders.

No

Is diagnosis validated?

Yes

Record new assessment data. Record REVISED. Enter new diagnosis, objectives, target date, and orders. Delete unvalidated diagnosis.

Did evaluation show a new problem had developed?

Start new evaluation process.

Record data, e.g., can accurately return demonstrate only one technique. Record CONTINUE. Change target date and modify nursing orders as necessary.

No

Yes

FINISHED

Knowledge Deficit

DEFINITION

The situation in which the individual experiences a lack of information or has difficulty in applying information, thus increasing the risk of actual compromise in health care. (NANDA, 1987, p. 103)

DEFINING CHARACTERISTICS (NANDA, 1987, p. 103)

The nurse will review the initial pattern assessment for the following defining characteristics to determine the diagnosis of Knowledge Deficit.

1. Major defining characteristics
   a. Verbalization of the problem
   b. Inaccurate follow-through of instruction
   c. Inaccurate performance of test
   d. Inappropriate or exaggerated behavior (e.g., hysterical, hostile, agitated, apathetic).
2. Minor defining characteristics
   None given.

RELATED FACTORS (NANDA, 1987, p. 103)

1. Lack of exposure.
2. Lack of recall.
3. Information misinterpretation.
4. Cognitive limitation.
5. Lack of interest in learning.
6. Unfamiliarity with information resources.

DIFFERENTIATION

The major differential diagnoses are Noncompliance; Thought Process, Altered; Powerlessness; and Health Maintenance, Altered.

In Noncompliance the patient can return demonstrate skills accurately or verbalize the regimen needed, but does not follow through on self care.

Thought Process, Altered would be evident by lack of immediate recall on return demonstration rather than inaccurate or limited demonstration and recall.

Powerlessness would be indicated by statements reflecting "how will this help?"; "control"; "have to rely on others" rather than statements related to "don't really understand"; "not really sure now"; "is this right?"

Health Maintenance, Altered may include Knowledge Deficit but is broader in scope and includes such aspects as limited resources and mobility factors.

OBJECTIVES

1. Will return demonstrate (knowledge deficit activity) by (date).

AND/OR

2. Will restate (knowledge deficit material) by (date).

TARGET DATE

Individual learning curves vary significantly. A target date ranging from 3 to 7 days could be appropriate based on the individual's previous experience with this material, education level, potential for learning, and energy level.

NURSING ORDERS

ADULT HEALTH

1. Contract with patient regarding what the patient wants and needs to learn. Be sure to include a time frame in the contract. Have patient sign contract to ensure patient consent for teaching.
2. Design teaching plan specific to patient's deficit area (e.g., self-administration of medication) and specific to patient's level of education (e.g., 8th grade reading level). Include significant others in teaching sessions. Be sure plan includes content, objectives, methods, and evaluation.
3. Explain each procedure, rationale for procedure, and patient's role.
4. Teach only absolutely relevant information first.
5. Provide positive reinforcement as often as possible for patient's progress.
6. Design teaching to stimulate as many of the patient's senses as possible (e.g., visuals, audio, touch, smell). Have patient return demonstrate any psychomotor activities; have patient restate, in own words, cognitive materials.
7. Provide quiet, well-lighted, temperature-controlled teaching environment.
8. Ensure that basic needs are taken care of before and immediately after teaching sessions.
   a. Food and fluids
   b. Toileting
   c. Pain relief
9. Pace teaching according to patient's rate of learning and preference.
10. Encourage patient's verbalization of anxiety, concern, etc. about self care. Listen carefully. Redesign plan to incorporate patient's concerns.
11. Incorporate into teaching plans, in addition to specifics:
    a. Normal body functioning
    b. Signs and symptoms of altered functioning
    c. Diet (food and fluid)
    d. Exercise and activity
    e. Growth and development
    f. Self-examination
    g. Impact on environment, stress, and change in life-style on health.
12. After first teaching session, start each teaching session with revalidation of the previous session. End each session with a summary.
13. Collaborate with and refer to appropriate assistive resources:
    a. Home health
    b. Physical therapist
    c. Occupational therapist

CHILD HEALTH

1. Review what the patient's and family's level of knowledge is regarding illness, hospitalization, situation, and cultural and value beliefs.
2. Plan to meet educational needs based on nursing order 1.
3. Determine if there are ambiguities in the minds of parents or child.
4. Encourage patient and family to express concerns or fears regarding health care.
5. Determine the readiness of patient and family for education.
6. Identify the learning capacity for the patient and family.
7. Determine the scope and appropriate presentation for patient and family based on all of the above, plus developmental crises for each and all—do not overwhelm the patient.
8. Evaluate appropriately the effectiveness of the teaching-learning experience by:
   a. Brief verbal discourse to provide concrete data;
   b. Written examination in brief to show progress;

    c. Observation of skills critical for care (e.g., change of dressing according to sterile technique);

    d. Allowing child to perform skills in general fashion with use of dolls.

  9. Provide collaboration with health team members as needed.

10. Allow for continuity in care with same nurses to enhance learning.

11. Allow patient and family sufficient time and application opportunities while still in hospital.

12. Offer appropriate community resources for follow-up support (e.g., Diabetic Association, Easter Seals, etc.).

13. Monitor on an ongoing basis for changes which may necessitate further education.

14. Provide continued educational components of care.

15. Provide care as needed with gradual assumption of care by patient and family as tolerated.

16. Offer clarification in a nonjudgmental, nonthreatening manner.

17. Offer reinforcement and sincere support in successes of learning and application.

WOMEN'S HEALTH

1. Teach normal physiologic changes new mother can expect.
   - a. Lochia flow
     - (1) Normal
       - (a) Rubra 1–3 days
       - (b) Serosa 3–10 days
       - (c) Alba 10–14 days
     - (2) Abnormal
       - (a) Bright red blood and clots with firm uterus
       - (b) Foul odor
       - (c) Pain, fever
       - (d) Persistent lochia serosa or pink to red discharge after 2 weeks
   - b. Breast changes
     - (1) Breastfeeding
       - (a) Engorgement
       - (b) Comfort measures
       - (c) Clothing
       - (d) Positions for mother and infant comfort
       - (e) Hygiene
     - (2) Non-breastfeeding
       - (a) Suppression of lactation
         - (1) Medications
         - (2) Clothing—tight fitting bra
         - (3) Comfort measures
       - (b) Importance of holding baby while bottle feeding
         - (1) Do not prop bottle
         - (2) Burp baby often
       - (c) Formulas
         - (1) Different kinds
         - (2) Preparation
   - c. Perineum and rectum
     - (1) Episiotomy
     - (2) Hemorrhoids
     - (3) Hygiene
     - (4) Medications
     - (5) Comfort measures
2. Demonstrate infant care to new parents.

    a. Bathing

    b. Feeding

    c. Cord care

    d. Holding, carrying, etc.

    e. Safety

3. Discuss infant care, taking into consideration age and cultural differences of parents.
   a. Teenagers
      (1) Involve significant others
      (2) Have mother return demonstrate infant care
   b. First-time older mothers
      (1) Allow verbalization of fears
      (2) Involve significant others
      (3) Provide encouragement
   c. Adjust teaching to take into consideration different cultural caretaking activities such as:
      (1) Preventing the evil eye in the hispanic culture
      (2) Mother not holding the baby for (number) days immediately

4. Demonstrate newborn skills to parents
   a. Utilize different assessment skills to teach parents about their newborn's capabilities.
      (1) Gestational Age Assessment
      (2) Physical examination of newborn
      (3) Brazelton Neonatal Assessment Scale
   b. Encourage parents to hold and talk to newborn.

5. Discuss different methods of birth control and the advantages and disadvantages of each method.
   a. Chemical
      (1) Spermicides
      (2) Pills
   b. Mechanical
      (1) Condom
      (2) Diaphragm
      (3) Intrauterine device (IUD)
   c. Behavioral
      (1) Abstinence
      (2) Temperature, ovulation, cervical mucus (Billing's method)
      (3) Coitus interruptus
   d. Sterilization
      (1) Vasectomy
      (2) Tubal ligation
      (3) Hysterectomy

MENTAL HEALTH

1. Discuss with client his or her perceptions of the problem and possible solutions.
2. Discuss with client his or her values and beliefs related to the area of concern.
3. Ask client about previous learning experiences in general and about those related to the current area of concern (i.e., has client learned that he or she is a poor learner, that he or she does not have the intellectual ability to learn the type of information that is currently required, or that the smallest mistake in the activity to be learned could be fatal).
4. Monitor client's current level of anxiety. If level of anxiety will inhibit learning, assist client with anxiety reduction. Refer to Anxiety for detailed interventions.
5. Determine what client thinks is most important in the current situation.
6. Assist client in meeting those needs that present lower-level needs on Maslow's hierarchy so attention can be focused on the area of learning to be addressed (i.e., if client is concerned

that children are not being cared for while he or she is hospitalized he or she may not be able to focus on learning). List the needs to be met here.

7. Provide client with both written and verbal information. Make sure this information is in the language client communicates in most effectively.
8. Provide information in a manner client can understand (remove medical terms and use words for body parts and functions client understands).
9. Divide learning task into portions the client can easily master and develop a schedule for presenting this information to the client. Note this schedule here along with the person responsible for presenting the information to the client.
10. Keep health care team informed of client's progress on the learning task in daily verbal reports at the change of shift. Any alterations or changes in the learning plan should be noted here.
11. Spend (number) minutes each shift at (note times here) reviewing learning with client. During this time client may ask questions or practice new behavior.
12. Provide rewards to client each time a portion of the task is mastered. These rewards should be client-specific and listed here. Positive verbal reinforcement should also be provided.
13. Begin by presenting information that causes client the least amount of anxiety and progress from there.
14. Establish an environment that ensures enhancement of learning experience (i.e., if teaching involves diet alterations consult with dietitian so meals served in the hospital are congruent with the teaching plan, or if medications are to be given at home have schedule and manner of administration fit with the plan that is to be implemented at home).
15. As client learns information, challenge learning by presenting potential problems to client to be solved. Have these challenges be at the client's level of understanding and abilities (e.g., "O.K., now you know how you should take your pills at home. What would you do if you dropped one on the floor?").
16. Spend (number) minutes three times a day with client while he or she practices those psychomotor skills necessary to accomplish learning. These practice periods should be in at least 30-minute blocks.
17. Select, with client's assistance, those significant others that can participate in the learning process with the client.
18. Include support system in at least one practice session each day.
19. As teaching progresses, continually monitor client's emotional response to information and alter plan accordingly.
20. Encourage client to suggest adaptations in procedures that would facilitate implementation at home by asking client how it will be to perform each of the learning tasks in the home environment. Clients with outdoor plumbing will have difficulty with procedures that require access to running water in the house.
21. Include client in group learning experiences (i.e., medication groups).
22. Have client assume increasing responsibility for performing task to be learned while in hospital. Note client's level of responsibility here.
23. Refer client to appropriate community support groups (i.e., Alcoholics Anonymous, I Can Cope, etc.).
24. Refer client to community resources as necessary for continued support. These could include:
    a. Visiting nurse
    b. Psychiatric nurse clinician
    c. Physical therapist
    d. Occupational therapist
    e. Vocational rehabilitation
    f. Nutritionist
    g. Social services

h. Financial counselor

HOME HEALTH

(Note: Much of the interactions between patients, families, and the nurse during the course of home health care is related to health education. Proper assessment by the nurse of the potential for or actual knowledge deficit is imperative. The nurse should use techniques based on learning theory to design teaching interventions which will be appropriate to the situation at hand. These techniques include, but are not limited to, readiness of participant, repetition of the material using several senses, reinforcement of learner's progress, positive and enthusiastic approach, decreasing barriers to learning, e.g., language, pain, physical illness, etc.)

1. Teach patient and family measures to reduce knowledge deficit by seeking the following information and learning conditions:
   a. Information regarding disease process
   b. Rationale for treatment interventions
   c. Techniques for improving learning situation (motivation, teaching materials that match cognitive level of participants, reduction of discomfort, e.g., control of pain, familiar surroundings, etc.)
   d. Enhancement of self-care capabilities
   e. Written materials to supplement oral teaching (written materials are appropriate to cognitive level and to self-care management)
   f. Addressing patient and family questions
2. Design teaching program that is appropriate for situation and for learners involved.
3. Coordinate the teaching activities of other health care professionals which may be involved. Reinforce the teaching of range of motion by the physical therapist, for example.
4. Provide an environment which enhances learning.
   a. Decrease anxiety.
   b. Reduce external stimulation (noise, interruption, etc.).
   c. Provide appropriate supporting materials and supplies (e.g., anatomical pictures, required needles, vials, syringes, etc.).
   d. Encourage a positive attitude.
   e. Direct learning to specific and unique needs of learners.
5. Involve patient and family in planning, implementing, and promoting reduction in knowledge deficit.
   a. Family conference
   b. Mutual goal setting
   c. Communication
   d. Family members responsible for specific tasks or information
6. Consult with or refer to assistive resources as indicated:
   a. Community resources such as library, community college, university, extension service, YMCA/YWCA
   b. Professional organizations such local nurses association, local medical association
   c. Community groups such as American Cancer Society, American Diabetes Association, American Heart Association, American Lung Association, etc.
   d. Physical therapist
   e. Occupational therapist
   f. Nutritionist
   g. Physician

EVALUATION
OBJECTIVE 1

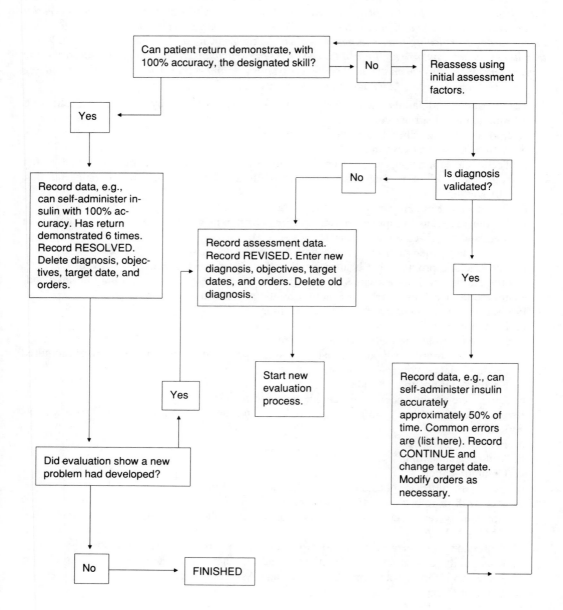

OBJECTIVE 2

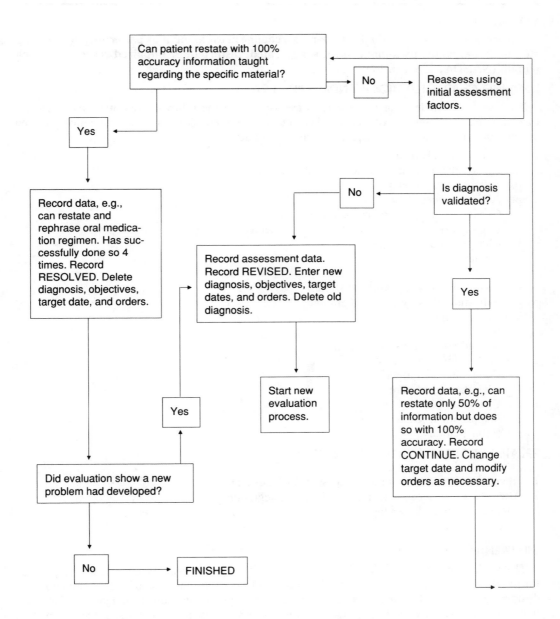

Sensory-Perceptual Alterations

DEFINITION

A state in which an individual experiences a change in the amount or patterning of incoming stimuli accompanied by a diminished, exaggerated, distorted, or impaired response to such stimuli (NANDA, 1987, p. 97).

DEFINING CHARACTERISTICS (NANDA, 1987, p. 97)

The nurse will review the initial pattern assessment for the following defining characteristics to determine the diagnosis of Sensory-Perceptual Alteration. Note that this alteration may be visual, auditory, kinesthetic, gustatory, tactile, or olfactory.

1. Major defining characteristics
   a. Disoriented in time, in place, or with persons
   b. Altered abstraction
   c. Altered conceptualization
   d. Change in problem-solving abilities
   e. Reported or measured change in sensory acuity
   f. Changes in behavior pattern
   g. Anxiety
   h. Apathy
   i. Change in usual response to stimuli
   j. Indication of body-image alteration
   k. Restlessness
   l. Irritability
   m. Altered communication patterns
2. Minor defining characteristics
   a. Complaints of fatigue
   b. Alteration in posture
   c. Change in posture
   d. Inappropriate responses
   e. Hallucinations

RELATED FACTORS (NANDA, 1987, p. 97)

1. Altered environmental stimuli, excessive or insufficient.
2. Altered sensory reception, transmission, or integration.
3. Chemical alterations, endogenous (electrolyte) or exogenous (drugs, etc.)
4. Psychologic stress.

DIFFERENTIATION

The subjective component will be a major factor to separate primary and secondary patterns for the Sensory-Perceptual Alteration. In addition, a heavy substantiation of organic function and dysfunction should assist the nurse in developing the appropriate nursing diagnosis. There are potential contributory components from all other patterns. It therefore is critical that this pattern be assessed with caution and steadfastness. Of particular importance is the close relationship of the emotional component in sensory functioning. For this reason, caution against judging prematurely is called for. Unlike some of the other patterns, the sensory alterations may need to be considered on an ongoing basis to best be facilitated.

OBJECTIVES

1. Will identify and initiate at least two adaptive ways to compensate for (specific sensory deficit) by (date).

AND/OR

2. Will verbalize fewer problems with (specific sensory deficit) by (date).

TARGET DATE

Assisting the patient in dealing with an uncompensated sensory deficit is a long-term process. Also, the patient may never accept the deficit but can be helped to adapt to the deficit. Therefore, an appropriate target date would be no sooner than 5–7 days from the date of diagnosis.

NURSING ORDERS

ADULT HEALTH

(Note: The following orders are general in nature. The orders should be individualized toward the specific sensory deficit, i.e., vision, hearing, touch, smell, kinesthesia.)

1. Provide calm, nonthreatening environment:
   a. Orient to room.
   b. Check safety factors frequently:
      (1) Siderails
      (2) Uncluttered room
      (3) Lighting—dim at night; increased during day
      (4) Arrange environment to assist in compensating for specific deficit
      (5) Avoid extremes in noise volume
   c. Place bedside table, overbed table in same position each time and within easy reach. Ascertain which items patient wants on these tables and where the items are to be placed. Place items in same place each time.
   d. Have significant others bring familiar items from home to enhance physical and psychologic comfort.
   e. Promote consistency in care (e.g., same nurse, as near same routine as possible) to decrease unessential stimuli.
   f. Follow patient's own routine as much as possible (e.g., bath, bedtime, meals, grooming). Pace activities to patient's preference.
   g. Promote comfort (e.g., turning, massage, etc).
2. Monitor, at least once per shift:
   a. Intake and output
   b. Vital signs
   c. Circulatory status
   d. Neurologic status
   e. Sleep-rest amounts
   f. For signs and symptoms of sensory overload or sensory deficit
3. Encourage activity and exercise to extent possible and interspace with rest periods. Do range of motion at least every 4 hours while awake.
4. Collaborate with occupational therapist regarding appropriate diversionary activity.
5. Explain all procedures and rationales for procedures.
   a. Face patient and speak slowly
   b. Use simple, clear, concise instructions
6. Assist patient to eat to extent necessary (e.g., feed totally or cut up food and open packages).
7. Provide reality orientation as necessary:
   a. Keep clock and calendar in room.
   b. Touch patient frequently.
   c. Check orientation to person, time, and place at least once per shift.
   d. Listen carefully.
8. Promote adaptation to deficit:

    a. Encourage patient to use prosthetic or assistive devices such as glasses.

    b. Make health teaching specific to deficit

    c. Stimulate senses to appropriate level (e.g., different visuals in room, variety of sounds [music, radio, TV], variety of odors, encourage visitors)

  9. Avoid extremes in temperature:

    a. Room

    b. Food

    c. Bath

10. Refer to appropriate assistive resources:

    a. Home health

    b. Support groups according to specific alteration

CHILD HEALTH

1. Determine how the parent and child perceive the deficit addressed by setting aside adequate time (30 minutes) each shift for discussion and listening.
2. Provide educational materials and reinforcement of use of prosthetics or aids as applicable, in patient's and parents terms.
3. Stress the importance of follow-up evaluation for any suspected sensory deficits of infants and young children.
4. Allow for extra anticipatory safety needs according to sensory deficit and child's developmental capacity.
5. Administer medications as needed and ordered.
6. Provide adaptive environmental and daily care milieu according to sensory deficit.
7. Make appropriate referrals to health care professionals to best deal with sensory deficits.

    a. Pediatrician, neurologist, ear and nose specialist

    b. Subspecialists such as pediatric surgeon

    c. Pediatric clinical nurse specialist

    d. Play therapist

    e. Specific community resource—Lighthouse for the Blind

    f. Community or public health nurse

    g. Teachers, school system

    h. Social worker

    i. Psychologist

    j. Developmental specialist

    k. Occupational therapist

    l. Physical therapist

    m. Early childhood programs

    n. Ophthalmologist or audiologist

    o. Genetic screening

8. Initiate plans for home dismissal at least 4 days before discharge to allow time for confidence in performance of necessary tasks according to deficit.
9. Provide attention to family coping as it may relate to the deficit:

    a. Assessment of usual dynamics

    b. Identification of impact on parent and siblings

    c. Presence of mental deficits

    d. Values regarding the deficit

    e. Support systems

10. Provide for appropriate follow-up appointments before dismissal.
11. Review for appropriate immunization, especially rubella, mumps, and measles.
12. In presence of ear infections, exercise caution regarding use of ototoxic medications such as gentamycin.

13. Correlate medical history for potential risk factors such as chronic middle ear infections, upper respiratory infections, or allergies.
14. Provide appropriate sensory stimulation for age, beginning slowly so as not to overload child.
15. Deal with other contributory factors such as nutrition, illness, etc.
16. Include parents in plans for rehabilitation whenever possible by:
    a. Using basic plan for care;
    b. Adapting intervention as required for child;
    c. Supporting them in their role;
    d. Pointing out opportune times for interaction;
    e. Informing them of appropriate safety precautions for age and situation;
    f. Encouraging gentle handling and comforting of infant.
17. Provide continuity in staffing for nursing care of child and family.
18. In instances of handicapped child, provide appropriate attention to developing sequencing to best actualize potential offered.
19. Especially note on follow-up the home environment for nurturing aspects and support systems.

WOMEN'S HEALTH

Vision

1. Monitor client for signs of pregnancy-induced hypertension.
2. Monitor for signs and symptoms of preeclampsia (i.e., headaches, visual changes such as blurred vision, increased edema of face, oliguria, hyperreflexia, nausea or vomiting, and epigastric pain).
3. Teach client the importance of reporting the above signs and symptoms, as they can be precursors to eclampsia.

Smell

Morning Sickness (Nausea and Vomiting of Early Pregnancy)
4. In collaboration with dietitian:
    a. Obtain dietary history
    b. Assist patient in planning diet which will provide adequate nutrition for her and her fetus' needs
5. Teach methods for coping with gastric upset, nausea, and vomiting.
    a. Eating bland, lowfat foods
    b. Increasing carbohydrate intake
    c. Eating small frequent meals
    d. Having dry crackers or toast before getting out of bed
    e. Taking vitamins and iron with snack before going to bed
    f. Supplementing diet with high-protein liquids (e.g., soups, eggnog)

Touch

Pregnancy
6. Be aware of expectant mother's sensitivity to extraneous touching.
    a. Shyness
    b. Protectiveness of unborn child
    c. Uterine sensitivity during pregnancy and particularly during labor
7. Maternal touch.
    a. Encourage visual and tactile contact between mother and infant to enhance attachment.
    b. Provide conducive atmosphere for continual mother-infant contact.

c. Delay newborn eye treatment for 1 hour, so that baby can see mother's face.

Kinesthesia

8. Be aware of expectant mother's increased vulnerability related to physical size of body in 3rd trimester.
   a. Protectiveness of unborn child.
   b. Heavy movement
   c. Possible slowed reflexes
   d. Tires easily
9. Assist in and out of difficult furniture that is too low.
10. Encourage correct body mechanics when lying down or sitting up.
11. Encourage to wear seat belt when traveling in auto (shoulder belt best).

New Mother

12. Identify factors in client's daily activities which could be contributing to sense of isolation.
13. Monitor client's pattern of activities of daily living.
    a. Care of self.
       (1) Rest when infant rests.
       (2) Contact friends who have children of same age such as other members of childbirth class.
       (3) Have a day out, away from infant.
           (a) Relatives
           (b) Friends
           (c) Mother's Day Out programs (usually run by different church groups)
    b. Care of infant.
       (1) Allow expression of anger and frustration.
       (2) Contact nurse, physician's office, hospital, or childbirth educator for answers to questions about infant care.
    c. Identify client's support systems.
       (1) Encourage use of formal support systems.
           (a) Hospital (many postpartum or nursery units have special callback lines for their new mothers)
           (b) Physician offices
               (i)   Obstetrician
               (ii) Pediatrician
               (iii) Family practitioner
           (c) Nurses
               (i) Childbirth educators
               (ii) Nursing centers (some specialize in maternal and newborn care)
       (2) Encourage use of informal support systems.
           (a) Friends from childbirth class
           (b) Friends with infants same age as client's
           (c) Family (especially grandparents)
    d. Allow mother and father to verbalize their perception of birth and postpartum experience.
    e. Encourage communication between mother and father.
    f. Encourage professional women to keep in contact with their professional friends (if staying home for an extended period before returning to work).

Rural Women

14. Encourage at least yearly contacts for health maintenance.
    a. Physician
    b. Clinic

c. Health care facility
15. Help establish network for:
    a. Social contact
    b. Emergencies
    c. Support
16. Allow client to verbalize her perception of her life-style.
17. Provide as pleasant an atmosphere as possible.
    a. Indirect lighting (when direct lighting is not necessary)
    b. Windows with curtains that allow outside light (if windows are present)
    c. Music (if couple prefers)
    d. Adequate seating for significant others (father or family)

MENTAL HEALTH

1. Provide client with appropriate prosthesis if the deficit has been previously diagnosed and a prosthesis provided.
2. Maintain prothesis to ensure optimal functioning.

Auditory Deficits

3. Clean ear with wet washcloth over finger.
4. If eardrops are ordered, warm to body temperature before instilling into the ear.
5. Speak in low tones to allow for alterations in hearing high-frequency sounds.
6. Allow client extended time to respond to verbal messages.
7. Decrease background noise as much as possible to avoid confusion.
8. Do not shout when talking with client; this only accentuates vowel sounds while decreasing consonant sounds.
9. Use nonverbal cues as much as possible to enhance verbal messages.
10. Provide message board to use with client.
11. Replace batteries in hearing aids as necessary.
12. Clean ear wax from ear mold of hearing aid as necessary.
13. Stand where the client can watch your lips when you are speaking to him or her.
14. Make lips visible to the client by clipping moustaches away from lips (males) or wearing a lipstick that highlights lips (females).
15. Teach client and family proper maintenance of hearing aid.
16. Teach client and family proper care of ears (i.e., use of ear plugs when in an environment with loud noises, protecting the ear from water while swimming, blowing the nose with mouth and both nostrils open, etc.).
17. Teach client to turn better ear toward speaker. Note here client's better ear so staff can stand on that side when speaking to client.
18. Assist client with activities of daily living as necessary. Note the activity as well as the type of assistance needed here.

Visual Deficit

19. Provide client with his or her eyeglasses or contact lenses during waking hours. Note here where they are to be kept when client is not using them and place them in that place when client removes them.
20. Provide written information in large print or audio recorded format.
21. Provide telephone dials and other equipment necessary for the client with large numbers on nonglare surfaces. Last special equipment that is necessary for this client here and when the client may need it so it can be provided at appropriate times.
22. Provide an environment with adequate, nonglare lighting.
23. Place client in social or group situations so they are not looking directly into an open window.
24. Provide nonglare work surfaces.

25. Identify stairs with contrasting tape or paint.
26. Identify client's room with large numbers or client's name in large print.
27. Identify door frames from doors with contrasting tape or paint.
28. Provide large-screen TV and pictures with large, colorful images.
29. Orient client to the environment locating bathrooms, furniture, steps, exits, etc.
30. Verbally address client when entering client's proximity.
31. Approach client from the front.
32. Do not alter the client's physical environment without telling him or her of the changes.
33. Address client by name to clearly identify who you are talking to. Remove loose rugs and furniture from walkways.
34. Ask client about special environmental adaptations he or she prefers or uses (list those here).
35. Provide client with talking books and large-print periodicals.
36. Enter client's environment every hour to make contact with the client and provide assurance that he or she is a matter of concern to the nursing staff. Note times here.
37. Teach client and family proper maintaince of eyeglasses and other prosthesis.
38. Teach client and family methods to improve environmental safety.
39. Assist client with activities of daily living as necessary. List the activites that require assistance here along with the type of assistance that is needed.

Touch and Kinesthesia Deficit

40. Remove sharp objects from the client's environment.
41. Protect client from exposure to excessive heat and cold by:
    a. Checking temperature of heat and cold packs carefully before application.
    b. Teaching client to check the temperature of bath and other water to be placed on the skin with a thermometer.
    c. Checking temperature of bath water for client while he or she is on the nursing unit.
    d. Teaching client to wear protective clothing whenever he or she goes out doors in the winter time.
    e. Teaching client not to use heating pads or hot water bottles.
    f. Have client and family lower the setting on the hot water heater in the home to 124° F.
42. Instruct client not to smoke unless someone is with him or her.
43. Have client change position every 2 hours (note times for change here).
44. Monitor condition of skin every 4 hours, and note any alterations in integrity. (Note times for assessment here.)
45. Have client wear well-fitting shoes when walking.
46. Teach client to visually inspect skin on a daily basis, observing for alterations in integrity.
47. Trim toenails and fingernails for client. Maintain these at a safe length.
48. Assist client in determining if clothing is fitting properly without abrading the skin.
49. Perform foot care on a daily basis to include:
    a. Bathing feet in warm water;
    b. Applying moisturizing lotion;
    c. Trimming nails as needed;
    d. Checking skin for abrasions or reddened areas.
    (Note time for foot care here.) This process should be taught to the client and the client should be assuming primary responsibility for this care before discharge. This should be done with nursing supervision.
50. Provide client with assistance with movement in the environment until he or she is able to make the necessary adaptations to alterations in sensations.
51. Consult with physical therapist regarding teaching client appropriate adaptations for safe and effective movement.
52. Assist client with care of affected body parts.

53. Assist client with activities of daily living to include:
    a. Eating
    b. Bathing
    c. Dressing and grooming
54. Note type and amount of assistance needed here.
55. Refer to occupational therapy for assisting with learning new self-care behavior.

Smell Deficit

56. Assess for extent of neurologic dysfunction.
57. Determine effect this has on client's appetite and work with dietitian to make meals visually appealing to compensate for loss of smell.

General Interventions for All Deficits

58. Monitor client's neurologic status as indicated by current condition and history of deficit (i.e., if deficit is recent assessment would be conducted on a schedule that could range from every 15 minutes to every 8 hours). Note frequency and times of checks here. If checks are to be very frequent then it might be useful to keep a record of these checks on a flow sheet.
59. If deficit is determined to result from a psychologic rather than a physiologic dysfunction, refer to Individual Coping, Ineffective; Body Image Disturbance; Anxiety; and Self-Esteem Disturbance for detailed care plans. *(Note: A comprehensive physical examination and other diagnostic evaluations should be completed before this determination is made. Each of these deficits can be symptoms of severe physiologic or neurologic dysfunction and should be approached with this understanding, especially in a mental health environment where the clients may be assigned without careful assessment. This is a great risk for the client who has a history of mental health problems.)*
60. If deficit is related to a psychologic dysfunction, attend to needs resulting from the identified sensory deficit in a matter-of-fact manner, providing basic care and having client do the majority of the care.
61. If deficit is related to a psychologic dysfunction, spend 15 minutes every hour with the client in an activity that is not related to the sensory deficit. If the client begins to focus on the deficit terminate the interaction.
62. Spend 1 hour twice a day discussing with the client the effects the deficit will have on his or her life and developing alternative coping behavior. Note times for conversations here. If family is involved in the client's care they should be included on a planned number of these interactions.
63. Refer to appropriate mental health professional if client is going to require long-term assistance in adapting to the deficit or if current emotional adaptation becomes complicated.
64. Discuss with client and support system the necessary alterations that may be necessary in the home environment to facilitate daily living activities.

HOME HEALTH

1. Teach patient and family measures to prevent sensory deficit.
    a. Use of protective gear (goggles, sunglasses, earplugs, special clothing in hazardous conditions to prevent radiation, sun, or chemical burns)
    b. Avoidance of sharp or projectile toys
    c. Prevention of injuries to eyes, ears, skin, nose, and tongue
    d. Prevention of nutritional deficiencies
    e. Close monitoring of medications that may be toxic to the 8th cranial nerve
    f. Correct usage of contact lenses
    g. Prevention of fluid and electrolyte imbalances
2. Involve patient and family in planning, implementing, and promoting correction or compensation for sensory deficit (specify) by (date).

    a. Family conference

    b. Mutual goal setting

    c. Communication

3. Assist patient and family in life-style adjustments that may be required.

    a. Assistance with activities of daily living

    b. Adjustment to and usage of assistive devices: hearing aid, corrective lenses, magnifying glasses

    c. Providing safe environment (protect kinesthetically impaired from burns, for example)

    d. Stopping substance abuse

    e. Changes in family and work role relationships

    f. Techniques of communicating with individual with auditory or visual impairment

    g. Providing meaningful stimulation

    h. Special transportation needs

    i. Special education needs

4. Consult with or refer to appropriate assistive resources as indicated.

    a. Visiting nurse

    b. Audiologist

    c. Speech therapist

    d. Physical therapist

    e. Occupational therapist

    f. Social service

    g. Community resources for the handicapped

    h. Physician

    i. Financial counselor

    j. Family counselor

    k. Psychiatric nurse clinician

    l. Rehabilitation

EVALUATION
OBJECTIVE 1

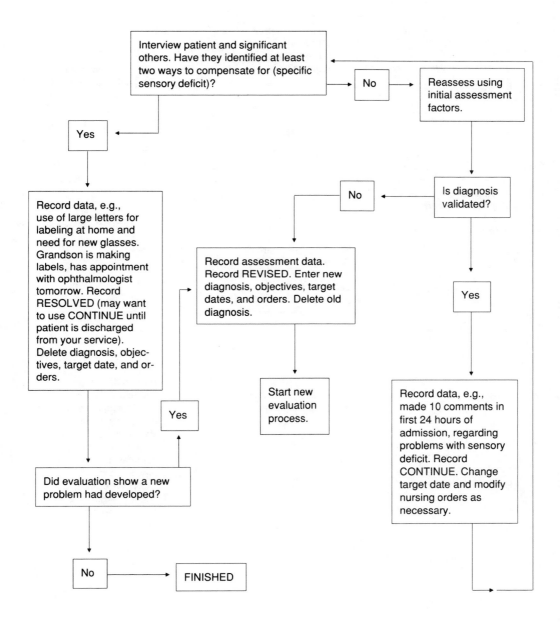

Interview patient and significant others. Have they identified at least two ways to compensate for (specific sensory deficit)?

No → Reassess using initial assessment factors.

Yes

Record data, e.g., use of large letters for labeling at home and need for new glasses. Grandson is making labels, has appointment with ophthalmologist tomorrow. Record RESOLVED (may want to use CONTINUE until patient is discharged from your service). Delete diagnosis, objectives, target date, and orders.

Is diagnosis validated?

No → Record assessment data. Record REVISED. Enter new diagnosis, objectives, target dates, and orders. Delete old diagnosis.

Yes

Start new evaluation process.

Yes

Did evaluation show a new problem had developed?

Record data, e.g., made 10 comments in first 24 hours of admission, regarding problems with sensory deficit. Record CONTINUE. Change target date and modify nursing orders as necessary.

No → FINISHED

OBJECTIVE 2

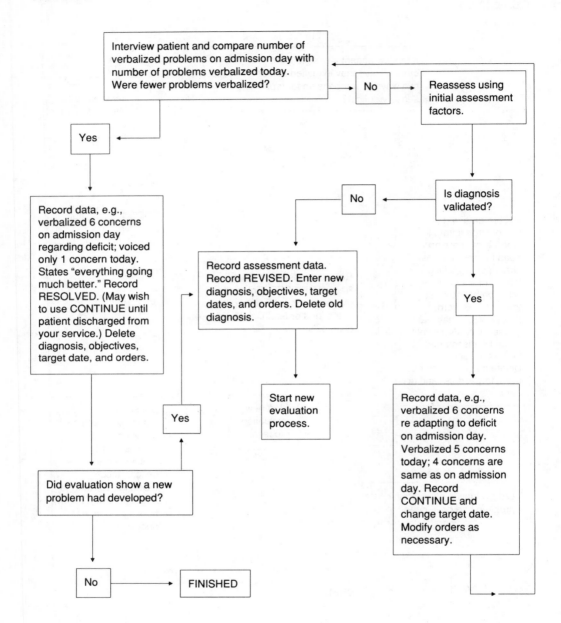

Thought Process, Altered

DEFINITION

A state in which the individual experiences a disruption in cognitive operations and activities. (NANDA, 1987, p. 104)

DEFINING CHARACTERISTICS (NANDA, 1987, p. 104)

The nurse will review the initial pattern assessment for the following defining characteristics to determine the diagnosis of Thought Process, Altered.

1. Major defining characteristics
   a. Inaccurate interpretation of environment
   b. Cognitive dissonance
   c. Distractibility
   d. Memory deficits or problems
   e. Egocentricity
   f. Hyper or hypovigilance
2. Minor defining characteristics
   a. Inappropriate nonreality-based thinking

RELATED FACTORS (NANDA, 1987, p. 104)

None given.

DIFFERENTIAL

This diagnosis may have contributory aspects from any of the other diagnoses or patterns. Uniquely though in this pattern, amelioration of other problems may not significantly change the impairment in thought process. In combination with altered coping this pattern requires much more time than is typically the case for hospitalization.

OBJECTIVES

1. Will have at least a (number) % decrease in signs and symptoms of impaired thought process.

AND/OR

2. Will be oriented to time, person, and place by (date).

TARGET DATE

A target date of 5 days would be acceptable since this can be a very long-range problem.

NURSING ORDERS

ADULT HEALTH

1. Monitor, at least every 4 hours while awake:
   a. Vital signs
   b. Neurologic status, particularly for signs and symptoms of IICP.
   c. Laboratory values for metabolic alkalosis, hypokalemia, increased ammonia levels, infection.
2. Collaborate with psychiatric nurse clinician and rehabilitation nurse specialist.
3. Provide safe, calm environment:
   a. Provide side rails on bed.
   b. Keep room uncluttered.
   c. Reorient client at each contact.
   d. Reduce extraneous stimuli e.g., limit noise, visitors, reduce bright lighting.
   e. Use touch judiciously.
   f. Prepare for all procedures by explaining simply and concisely.

    g. Provide good but not intensely bright lighting.

    h. Have family bring clock, calendar, and familiar objects from home.

4. Design communications according to patient's best means of communication (e.g., writing, visuals, sound):

    a. Give simple, concise directions.

    b. Listen carefully.

    c. Present reality consistently.

    d. Do not challenge illogical thinking.

5. Encourage patient to use prosthetic or assistive devices (e.g., glasses, dentures, hearing aid, walker, etc.).

6. Provide frequent rest periods.

7. Provide consistent approach in care:

    a. Nurse

    b. Routine

8. Encourage self-care to the extent possible.

9. Involve significant others in care and include in teaching sessions.

10. Refer to and collaborate with appropriate assistive resources:

    a. Home health

    b. Support groups

    c. Occupational therapist

    d. Physical therapist

CHILD HEALTH

1. Monitor cognitive capacity according to age and developmental capacity.

2. Note discrepancies in chronologic age and mastery of developmental milestones.

3. Determine, according to situation, what etiologic factors may contribute to altered thought process; especially those related to behavioral and mental processes, and potential for substance abuse.

4. Collaborate with health professionals in formulating a plan of care, to include:

    a. Clinical nurse specialist

    b. Pediatrician, subspecialists

    c. Psychiatrist

    d. Sociologist

    e. Play therapist

    f. Family therapist

    g. Community health nurse

5. Provide ongoing reality orientation by encouraging family to visit, time emphasis, personal awareness, and gradual resumption of daily routine to degree possible.

6. Provide anticipatory safety to reflect greater range of potentials according to psychomotor capacity.

7. Encourage family members to express concerns of child's condition by allowing 30 minutes each shift for ventilation purposes.

8. Provide for primary health needs, including administration of medications, comfort measures, and control of environment to aid in child's adaptation.

9. Structure the room in a manner which befits the child's needs.

10. Allow for ample rest periods.

11. Monitor for existence of other patterns, especially altered coping and role performance.

12. Assist family in dismissal plans by utilization of appropriate state and community resources.

13. If institutionalization is required, assist family in learning about related issues.

14. Maintain ethical and legal confidentiality on patient's behalf.

15. Allow for culturally unique aspects in management of care.

16. Provide for appropriate follow-up by making appointments for next clinic visits.
17. Allow family members opportunities for learning necessary care and mastery of content for long-term needs.
18. Make appropriate referrals for family as needed for follow-up.

WOMEN'S HEALTH

This nursing diagnosis will pertain to the woman the same as to any other adult. The reader is referred to the other sections (Adult Health, Home Health, and Mental Health) for specific nursing orders pertaining to women and altered thought process.

MENTAL HEALTH

1. Monitor client's level of anxiety and refer to Anxiety care plan for detailed interventions related to this diagnosis.
2. Speak to client in brief, clear sentences.
3. Keep initial interactions short but frequent. Interact with client for (number) minutes every 30 minutes. Begin with 5-minute interactions and gradually increase the times of interactions.
4. Assign the client a primary care nurse on each shift to assume responsibility for gaining a relationship of trust with the client.
5. Be consistent in all interactions with the client.
6. Set limits on inappropriate behavior that increase the risk of the client or others being harmed. Note the limits here as well as revisions to the limits.
7. Initially place client in an area with little stimulation.
8. Orient client to the environment and assign someone to provide one-on-one interaction while client orients to unit.
9. Do not make promises that cannot be kept.
10. Inform client of your availability to talk with him or her; do not pry or ask many questions.
11. Do not argue with the client about delusions or hallucinations; inform client in a matter-of-fact way that this is not your experience of the situation (e.g., "I do not hear voices talking about killing you," or "I do not think I am angry with you").
12. Recognize and support client's feelings (e.g., "You sound frightened").
13. Respond to the feelings being expressed in delusions or hallucinations.
14. Initially have client involved in one-to-one activities; as condition improves gradually increase the size of the interaction group. Note current level of functioning here.
15. Have client clarify those thoughts you do not understand. Do not pretend to understand that which you do not.
16. Do not attempt to change delusional thinking with rational explanations. This may encourage client to cling to these thoughts.
17. After listening to delusion or information about hallucination once do not engage in conversations related to this material.
18. Focus conversations on here and now content related to real things in the environment or to activities on the unit.
19. Do not belittle or be judgmental about the client's delusional beliefs or hallucinations.
20. Avoid nonverbal behavior that indicates agreement with delusional beliefs or hallucinations.
21. When client's behavior and anxiety level indicate readiness, place client in small group situations so feedback can be given on delusional beliefs by peers. Client will spend (number) minutes in group activities (number) times a day (time and frequency will increase as client's ability to cope with these situations improves).
22. Develop a daily schedule for the client that encourages focus on "here and now" and is adapted to client's level of functioning so success can be experienced. Note daily schedule here.

23. Assign client meaningful roles in unit activities. Provide roles that can be easily accomplished by client to provide successful experiences. Note client responsibilities here.
24. Primary nurse will spend (amount) minutes with client twice a day to discuss client's feelings and the effects of the delusions on the client's life. (Number of minutes and the degree of exploration of client's feelings will increase as client develops relationship with nurse.)
25. Provide rewards to client for accomplishing task progression on the daily schedule. These rewards should be ones the client finds rewarding.
26. Spend (number) minutes twice a day walking with client. This should start at 10 minute intervals and gradually increase. This can be replaced by any physical activity the client finds enjoyable. A staff member should be with client during this activity to provide social reinforcement to the client for accomplishing the activity.
27. Arrange a consultation with occupational therapist to assist client in developing or continuing special interests.
28. Observe client for cue of hallucinating (intent listening for no apparent reason, talking to someone when no one is present, muttering to self, etc.).
29. Monitor delusional beliefs and hallucinations for potential of harming self or others.
30. Note any change in behavior that would indicate a change in the delusional beliefs or hallucinations that could indicate a potential for violence.
31. If hallucinations place client at risk for self-harm or harm to others, place client on one-on-one observation or seclusion.
32. If client is placed in seclusion interact with client at least every 15 minutes to provide reality orientation and assist client in controlling hallucinations and delusions.
33. If client appears to be hallucinating, engage client in here and now reality-oriented conversation or involve client in a concrete activity.
34. Have client tell staff when hallucinations are present or when they are interfering with client's ability to interact with others.
35. Provide medication as ordered.
36. Maintain environment in a manner that does not enhance hallucinations (e.g., television programs that validate client's hallucinations, abstract art on the walls, wallpaper with abstract designs or designs that enhance imagination).
37. Maintain environment that does not stimulate client's delusions (i.e., if client has delusions related to religion limit discussions of religion and religious activity on unit to very concrete terms); limit interaction with persons who stimulate delusional thinking.
38. Teach client to control hallucinations by:
    a. Checking ideas out with trusted others;
    b. Practicing thought-stopping by singing to self, telling the voices to go away (this done quietly to self).
39. Primary nurse will assist client in identifying signs and symptoms of increasing thought disorganization and in developing a plan to cope with these situations before they get out of control. This will be done in the regular scheduled interaction times between the primary nurse and client (see nursing order 24 above).
40. As client's condition improves primary nurse will assist client to identify onset of hallucinations and delusions with periods of increasing anxiety.
41. As connection is made between thought disorder and anxiety client will be assisted to identify specific anxiety-producing situations and learn alternative coping behaviors. See Anxiety for specific interventions.
42. Refer client to outpatient support groups.
43. Refer client and support system to appropriate support systems such as family therapy, social services, financial counseling, occupational therapy, or vocational rehabilitation.
44. Refer to outpatient support systems and assist with making arrangements for the client to contact these before discharge. These systems could include:

a. Visiting nurse
b. Adult day care
c. Disease-related support groups
d. Outpatient mental health services
e. Crisis intervention hot lines
f. Family therapy
g. Mental health nurse clinical specialist
h. Occupational therapy
i. Social services

HOME HEALTH

1. Teach patient and family to monitor for signs and symptoms of impaired thought processes:
   a. Poor hygiene
   b. Poor decision-making or judgment
   c. Regression in behavior
   d. Delusions
   e. Hallucinations
   f. Changes in interpersonal relationships
   g. Distractibility
2. Involve patient and family in planning, implementing, and promoting appropriate thought processing.
   a. Family conference
   b. Mutual goal setting
   c. Communication
3. Assist patient and family in life-style adjustments that may be necessary:
   a. Providing safety and prevention of injury
   b. Frequent orientation to person, place, and time
   c. Reality testing and verification
   d. Alterations in role functions in family or at work
   e. Alterations in communication
   f. Stopping substance abuse
   g. Setting limits
   h. Learning new skills
   i. Avoiding potential for violence
   j. Suicide prevention
   k. Possible chronicity of disorder
   l. Finances
   m. Reducing sensory overload
   n. Stress management
   o. Relaxation techniques
   p. Support groups
4. Assist patient and family to set criteria to help them to determine when professional intervention is required.
5. Teach patient and family purposes, side effects, and proper administration techniques of medications.
6. Consult with or refer to appropriate assistive resources as required.
   a. Psychiatric nurse clinician
   b. Family counseling
   c. Mental health and mental retardation centers
   d. Sheltered workshops
   e. Occupational or recreational therapist

f. Job counselor
g. Social service
h. Physician
i. Visiting nurse
j. Substance abuse assistance (e.g., Alcoholics Anonymous, drug rehabilitation)
k. Crisis center
l. Financial counseling

EVALUATION
OBJECTIVE 1

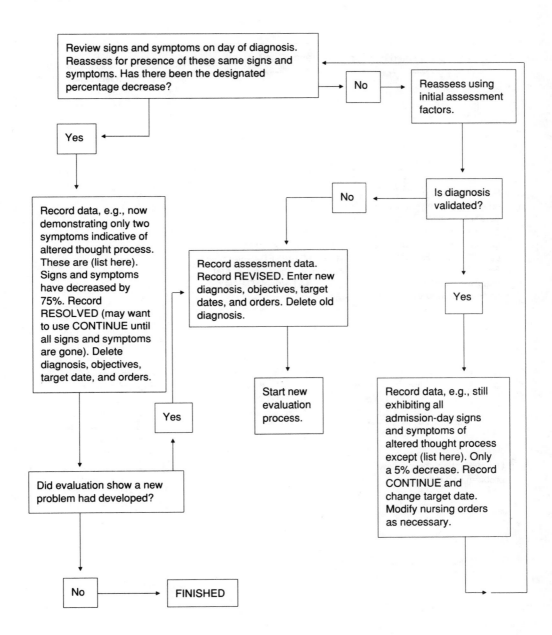

Review signs and symptoms on day of diagnosis. Reassess for presence of these same signs and symptoms. Has there been the designated percentage decrease?

No

Reassess using initial assessment factors.

Yes

Record data, e.g., now demonstrating only two symptoms indicative of altered thought process. These are (list here). Signs and symptoms have decreased by 75%. Record RESOLVED (may want to use CONTINUE until all signs and symptoms are gone). Delete diagnosis, objectives, target date, and orders.

No

Is diagnosis validated?

Record assessment data. Record REVISED. Enter new diagnosis, objectives, target dates, and orders. Delete old diagnosis.

Yes

Yes

Start new evaluation process.

Record data, e.g., still exhibiting all admission-day signs and symptoms of altered thought process except (list here). Only a 5% decrease. Record CONTINUE and change target date. Modify nursing orders as necessary.

Did evaluation show a new problem had developed?

No   FINISHED

OBJECTIVE 2

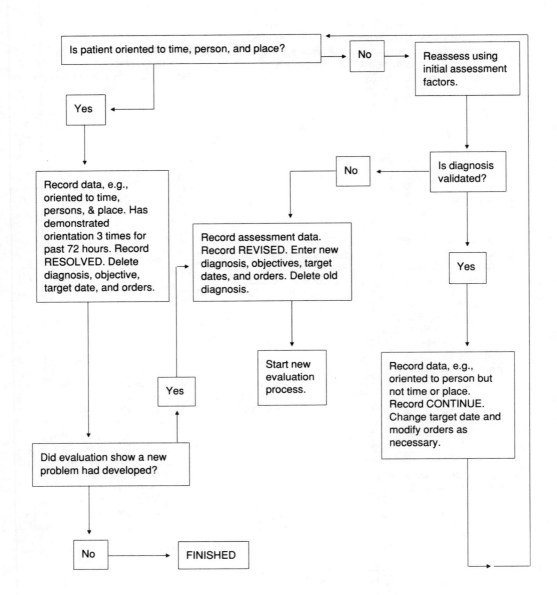

Unilateral Neglect

DEFINITION

The state in which an individual is perceptually unaware of and inattentive to one side of the body (NANDA, 1987, p. 98).

DEFINING CHARACTERISTICS (NANDA, 1987, p. 98)

The nurse will review the initial pattern assessment for the following defining characteristics to determine the diagnosis of Unilateral Neglect.

1. Major defining characteristics
   a. Consistent inattention to stimuli on an affected side
2. Minor defining characteristics
   a. Inadequate self-care
   b. Positioning or safety precautions in regard to the affected side
   c. Does not look toward the affected side
   d. Leaves food on plate on the affected side

RELATED FACTORS (NANDA, 1987, p. 98)

1. Effects of disturbed perceptual abilities (e.g., hemianopsia, one-sided blindness, neurologic illness, or trauma).

DIFFERENTIATION

A major premise for the diagnosis to exist is that of denial of existence of the affected side or limb of the body or failure to utilize or attend to same. Spatial involvement may also occur. There may be situations in which psychological or emotional hysteria must be differentiated on the basis of onset and relational symptomatology.

In altered sensory or perceptual patterns there will be a difference in actual manifestation according to the nerves involved. Caution should be exercised in assessing for the appropriate pattern.

OBJECTIVES

1. Will return demonstrate at least (number) measures to reduce the effect of unilateral neglect by (date).

AND/OR

2. Will have decreased signs and symptoms of unilateral neglect by (date).

TARGET DATE

A target date between 5 and 7 days would be appropriate to evaluate initial progress.

NURSING ORDERS

ADULT HEALTH

1. Frequently remind patient to attend to both sides of his or her body.
2. Assist patient to touch and feel neglected side of body. Help patient become more aware of and articulate sensations on neglected side.
3. Assist patient with range of motion exercises to neglected side of body. Teach extent of movement of each joint on neglected side of body.
4. Help patient to position neglected side of body in a similar way as attended side of body.
5. Remind patient to turn plate to notice all of food.
6. Turn every 2 hours on the (odd/even) hour. Monitor skin condition on each turning.
7. Refer to rehabilitation nurse clinician.

CHILD HEALTH

(See nursing orders applicable under Sensory-Perceptual Alterations in addition to those listed below.)

1. Allow 30 minutes every shift for patient and family to express how they perceive the unilateral neglect.
2. Determine how the unilateral neglect affects the usual expected behavior or development for the child.
3. Monitor for presence of secondary or tertiary deficits.
4. Establish with family input appropriate anticipatory safety guidelines which are based on the unilateral neglect and the developmental capacity of the child.
5. Stress appropriate follow-up prior to dismissal from hospital with appropriate time frame for family.

WOMEN'S HEALTH

This nursing diagnosis will pertain to women the same as to any other adult. The reader is referred to the other sections (Adult Health, Home Health, and Mental Health) for specific nursing orders and objectives pertaining to women and Unilateral Neglect.

MENTAL HEALTH

Nursing interventions for this diagnosis are those described in Adult Health.

HOME HEALTH

1. Monitor for factors contributing to unilateral neglect (e.g., disturbed perceptual abilities, neurologic disease, or trauma).
2. Involve patient and family in planning, implementing, and promoting reduction in effects of unilateral neglect:
   a. Family conference
   b. Mutual goal setting
   c. Communication
   d. Support for caregiver
3. Teach patient and family measures to decrease effects of unilateral neglect:
   a. Active and passive range of motion exercises
   b. Ambulation with assistive devices (canes, walkers, crutches)
   c. Placing objects within field of vision and reach
   d. Assistive eating utensils
   e. Assistive dressing utensils
   f. Provide safe environment (e.g., remove objects from area outside field of vision)
4. Assist family and patient to identify life-style changes that may be required.
   a. Change in role functions
   b. Coping with disability or dependency
   c. Obtaining and using assistive equipment
   d. Coping with assistive equipment
   e. Maintaining safe environment
5. Consult with appropriate assistive resources as indicated:
   a. Occupational therapist
   b. Physical therapist
   c. Rehabilitation therapist
   d. Community transportation
   e. Psychiatric nurse clinician
   f. Respite or day care
   g. Social services

h. Job or education counselor
i. Neurologist
j. Visiting nurse
k. Support groups
l. Psychologist

EVALUATION
OBJECTIVE 1

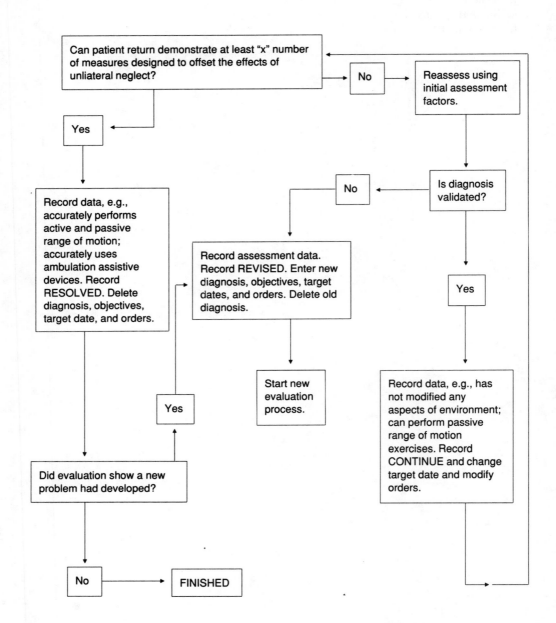

OBJECTIVE 2

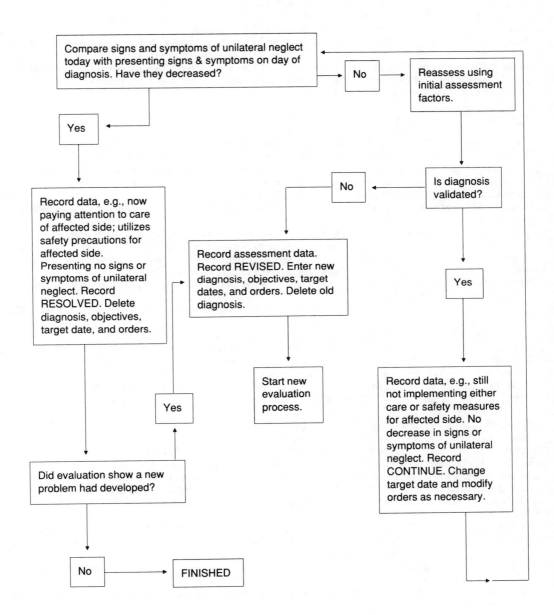

REFERENCES

Erickson, M. (1983). *Healing in hypnosis*. New York: Irvington.

Fogel, E. I., & Woods, N. F. (1981). *Health care of women: A nursing perspective*. St. Louis: C. V. Mosby.

Keeney, B. (1983). *Aesthetics of change*. New York: The Guilford Press.

Murray, R., & Zentner, J. (1979). *Nursing assessment and health promotion through the lifespan*. Englewood Cliffs, NJ: Prentice-Hall.

North American Nursing Diagnosis Association. (1987). *Taxonomy I with complete diagnoses*. St. Louis: Author.

North American Nursing Diagnosis Association. (1988). *Proposed nursing diagnoses*. St. Louis: Author.

Watzlawick, P., Weakland, J., & Fisch, R. (1974). *Change*. New York: W. W. Norton.

SUGGESTED READINGS

Ahmann, E. (1984). The child at home with chronic pain. *Maternal Child Nursing, 9,* 164–266.

American Nurses' Association (1986). *Standards of home health nursing practice.* Kansas City, Mo: Author.

Brown. C. C. (Ed.). (1986). *The many facets of touch*. Skillman, NJ: Johnson & Johnson Baby Products.

Carpenito, L. J. (1983). *Nursing diagnosis: Application to clinical practice*. New York: J. B. Lippincott.

Crittendon, R. (1983). *Discharge planning*. Bowie, MD: Robert J. Brady.

Doenges, M., & Moorhouse, M. (1985). *Nurse's pocket guide: Nursing diagnosis with interventions*. Philadelphia: F. A. Davis.

Endometriosis Association. (1983). *Brochure: Education support research*. Milwaukee, WI: Author.

Escobar, P. (1985). Management of chronic pain. *Nurse Practitioner, 8,* 24–32.

Feuer, L. (1987). Discharge planning: Home caregivers need your support, too. *Nursing Management, 18,* 58–59.

Flavell, J. H. (1974). *Cognitive development*. Englewood Cliffs, N.J.: Prentice-Hall.

Gettrust, K., Ryan, S., & Engleman, D. (1985). *Applied nursing diagnosis: Guides for comprehensive care planning*. New York: John Wiley & Sons.

Griffith-Kenney, J. (1986). *Contemporary women's health: A nursing advocacy approach*. Menlo Park, CA: Addison-Wesley.

Hadeka, M. (1987). *Clinical judgment in community health nursing*. Boston: Little, Brown.

Heidrich, G., & Perry, S. (1982). Helping the patient in pain. *American Journal of Nursing, 82,* 1828–1833.

Humphrey, C. (1986). *Home care nursing handbook*. East Norwalk, CT: Appleton-Century-Crofts.

Jacox, A. K. (1977). *Pain. A source book for nurses and other health professionals*. Boston: Little, Brown.

Jaffe, M., & Skidmore-Roth, L. (1988). *Home health nursing care plans*. St. Louis: C. V. Mosby.

Jensen, M. D., & Bobak, I. M. (1985). *Maternity and gynecologic care: The nurse and the family*. St. Louis: C. V. Mosby.

Kelly, M. A. (1985). *Nursing diagnosis source book*. East Norwalk, CT: Appleton-Century-Crofts.

Kneisl, C., & Wilson, H. (1984). *Handbook of psychosocial nursing care*. Reading, MA: Addison-Wesley.

Kodadek, S. (1985). Working with the chronically ill. *Nurse Practitioner, 8,* 45–47.

Lara, M. (1985). Intractable pain: Is medication the only answer? *Nursing Life, 5,* 44–47.

Lerner, R. M. (1976). *Concepts and theories of human development*. Menlo Park, CA: Addison-Wesley.

Luckmann, J., & Sorensen, K. (1980). *Medical-surgical nursing*. Philadelphia: W. B. Saunders.

Malinski, V. (1986). *Explorations on Martha Roger's science of unitary human beings*. East Norwalk, CT: Appleton-Century-Crofts.

McCaffery, M. (1979). *Nursing management of the patient with pain* (2nd ed.). Philadelphia: J. B. Lippincott.

McClelland, E., Kely, K., & Buckwalter, K. (1984). *Continuity of care: Advancing the concept of discharge planning*. Orlando, FL: Grune & Stratton.

McFarland, G., & Wasli, E. (1986). *Nursing diagnoses and process in psychiatric mental health nursing*. Philadelphia: J. B. Lippincott.

Meinhart, N., & McCaffery, M. (1983). *Pain: A nursing approach to assessment and analysis*. East Norwalk, CT: Appleton-Century-Crofts.

Meissnek, J. E. (1980). McGill-Mezack pain questionnaire. *Nursing '80, 10* (1), 50–51.

Miller, T., & Jay, L. (1985). Cognitive-behavioral and pharmaceutical approaches to sensory pain management. *Topics in Clinical Nursing, 4,* 34–43.

National League for Nursing. (1986). *Policies and procedures*. New York: Accreditation Division for Home Care, National League for Nursing.

National League for Nursing. (1988). *Accreditation program for home care and community health: Criteria and standards*. New York: Author.

Neeson, J. D., & May, K. A. (1986). *Comprehensive maternity nursing: Nursing process and the childbearing family*. New York: J. B. Lippincott.

Peduzzi, T. (Ed.). (1985). Alterations in sensory perception: Nursing implications. *Topics in Clinical Nursing,* *6*(4), VII.

Reich, N., & Otten, P. (1987). *Manual of psychiatric nursing care plans.* Boston: Little, Brown.

Rinke, L. (1988). *Outcome standards in home health.* New York: National League for Nursing.

Schultz, J., & Dark, S. (1982). *Manual of psychiatric nursing care plans.* Boston: Little, Brown.

Scott, J., & Radford, K. (1984). Factors affecting the management of pain. *Maternal Child Nursing, 9,* 253–255.

Sheredy, C. (1984). Factors to consider when assessing responses to pain. *Maternal Child Nursing, 9,* 250–252.

Steffi, B., & Eide, I. (1978). *Discharge planning handbook.* New York: Charles B. Slack.

Van Arsdale, K. (1987). Fantasy: It's more than just a nice thought. *Archives of Psychiatric Nursing, 1*(4), 264–268.

Walk, R. D. (1975). *Perceptual development.* Monterrey, CA.: Brooks Cole Publishing.

Walsh, J., Persons, C., & Wieck, L. (1987). *Manual of home health care nursing.* Philadelphia: J. B. Lippincott.

Watson, J. (1985). *Nursing: The philosophy and science of caring.* Boulder, CO: Colorado Associated University Press.

Weaver, M. (1985). Acupressure: An overview of theory and application. *Nurse Practitioner, 8,* 38–42.

Whaley, L. & Wong, D. (1987). *Nursing care of infants and children.* St. Louis: C. V. Mosby.

CHAPTER EIGHT

Self-Perception and Self-Concept Pattern

Pattern Description

As the nurse interacts with the client the most important knowledge the client brings is self-knowledge. It is this knowledge that determines the individual's manner of interaction with others. This knowledge base is most often labeled self-concept. One's self-concept is composed of beliefs and attitudes about the self, body image, self-esteem, and information about abilities. The individual's behavior is not only affected by those experiences prior to interactions with the health care system but also by interactions with the health care system.

Pattern Assessment

1. Describe the client's general behavior and appearance.
   a. Personal hygiene and manner of dress.
   b. Response to nurse and others.
   c. Posture, gait, facial expression, and speech pattern.
2. Describe the client's attention and concentration. This could include the ability to remember a series of words or to perform some type of complex activity such as repeating the months of the year backwards. This assessment can also be done by evaluating the client's ability to follow a conversation.
3. Describe the client's capacity for abstraction. This is usually assessed by asking the client to state the meaning of proverbs, but this capacity can also be assessed in the course of a conversation by determining the client's ability to develop meaningful, complex concepts in the conversation.
4. Assess the client's fund of knowledge. What the client knows about the world, information about current events, awareness of local or national politics, and familiarity with the geographic location in which the client lives all contribute to this information assessment.
5. Describe the client's insight into the present illness. This includes client's perception of what brought him or her into contact with the health care system and what he or she can contribute to improve the situation.
6. Assess the level of consciousness for the client who appears to have a deficit in this area.
7. Assess the client's orientation. Is the client oriented to person, place, and time? A realistic assessment of this area considers the information available to the client that would allow him or her to keep current in this area.
8. Assess short-term memory. This includes memory of information received in the last 5 minutes and can be assessed by determining the client's ability to follow a conversation or to remember the interviewer's name.

9. Assess social judgment. This is usually done with a series of specific questions but can also be done in the course of the interview by observing the client's ability to differentiate the socially acceptable response to situations.
10. Describe the client's feelings and mood (also referred to as mood and affect).
11. Describe the content of the client's thought. This would include any particular themes, illusions, delusions, or hallucinations that are contained in the client's conversations.

Conceptual Information

Definition of the self and of a self-concept has been an issue of debate in philosophy, sociology, and psychology for many years, and many publications are available on this topic. The complexity of the problem of defining self is enhanced by the knowledge that external observation provides only a superficial glimpse of the self and introspection requires that the "knower" knows himself or herself so that information actually gained is self-referential. In spite of these problems the concept continues to be pervasive in the literature and in the universal experience of "self" or "not self." Intuitively one would say, of course, "There is a self because I have experiences separate from those around me, I know where I end and they begin." The importance of self is also emphasized by the language and the multitude of self-referential terms such as self-actualization, self-affirmation, ego-involvement, and self-concept. Turner (1968) addresses society's need for the individual to conceptualize the self-as-object. Recognizing the self-as-object allows society to place responsibility, which becomes a very valuable asset in maintaining social control and social order. This returns us to the initial problem of what the self is and how we can understand ourselves and others' selves (Gordon & Gergen, 1968)

In this section the assumption is made that self-concept refers to the individual's subjective cognitions and evaluations of self; thus, it is a highly personal experience. This indicates that the self is a personal construct and not a fact or hard reality. It is further assumed that the individual will act, as stated earlier, in congruence with the self-concept. This conceptualization is consistent with the authors that will be discussed and with the assumptions utilized in psychological research (Gordon & Gergen, 1968). It is also important to recognize that language assists in developing a conceptualization. This becomes crucial when thinking about the concept of self in English because the English language comes from a tradition of Cartesian dualism which does not express integrated concepts well. Often it will appear that the information presented is separating the individual into various parts when, in fact, an integrated whole is being addressed. For example, James (1968) talks about an I and Me. If these terms were taken at face value it would appear that the individual is being divided into multiple parts when, in fact, an integrated whole is being discussed and the words describe patterns of the whole. Unless otherwise stated it can be assumed that the concepts presented in this book reflect on the individual as an integrated whole.

Symbolic interaction theory provides a basis for understanding the self. The foundation for the self in this theoretical model is developed by James (1968) and Mead (1968). James outlines the internal working of the self with his concepts of "I" and "me." "I" is the thinker or the state of consciousness. "Me" is what the "I" is conscious of and includes all of what people consider theirs. This "me" contains three aspects: the "material me," the "social me," and the "spiritual me." The self-construction outlined by Mead indicates that there is the "knower" part of the self and that which the "knower" knows. Mead conceptualizes the thoughts themselves as the "knower" to resolve the metaphysical problem of who the "I" is. In Mead's conceptualization the consciousness of self is a stream of thought in which the "I" can remember what came before and continue to know what was known. The development of these memories and how they affect one's behavior is expressly addressed by Mead.

Mead (1968) describes the self-concept as evolving out of interactions with others in social contexts. This process begins at the moment of birth and continues throughout a lifetime. The definition of self can only occur in a social context, for one's self only exists in relation to other selves (p. 56). The individual is continually processing the reactions of others to his or her actions and reactions. This processing is taking place in a highly personalized manner, for the information is experienced through the individual's selective attention, which is guided by the current needs that are struggling to be expressed. This results in an environment that is constructed by one's perceptions. Mead's conceptualization leads to an interesting recursion in that we can only perceive self as we perceive others perceive us. This continues to reinforce the idea that the self-concept is highly personalized.

Many authors have addressed the process of developing a concept of self (Mead, 1968; Turner, 1968; James, 1968). The model developed by Harry Stack Sullivan will be presented here because it is consistent with the information presented in the symbolic interaction literature and is used as the theoretical base in much of the nursing literature.

Sullivan (1968) describes the self-concept as developing in interactions with significant others. Development of the self-concept is seen by Sullivan as a dynamic process resulting from inter-personal interactions that are directed toward meeting physiologic needs. This process has its most obvious beginnings with the infant and becomes more complex as the individual develops. This increasing complexity results from the layering of experiences that occurs in the developing individual. The biological processes become less and less important in governing the individual the further away from birth one is, and the importance of interpersonal interactions increases. The initial interpersonal interaction is between the infant and the primary caregivers. An infant expresses discomfort with a cry and the "parenting one" responds. This response, whether it be tender or harsh, begins to influence the infant's beliefs about itself and the world in general. If the interaction does not provide the infant with a feeling of security, anxiety results and interferes with the progress toward other life goals. Sullivan makes a distinction between the inner experience and the outer event and describes three modes of integration of experience. The first developmental experience is the prototaxic mode. In this mode the small child experiences self and the universe as an undifferentiated whole. At 3–4 months the child moves into the parataxic mode. The parataxic mode presents experiences as separated but without recognition of a connectedness or logical sequence. Finally, the individual enters the syntaxic mode, in which consensual validation is possible. This allows for events and experiences to be compared with others' experiences and for establishing mutually understandable communication instead of the autistic thinking that characterizes the previous stages (Bruch, 1968; Perry & Gawel, 1953).

As one experiences the environment through these three modes of thought the self system or self-concept is developed. Sullivan conceptualized three parts of the self. The part of the self that is associated with security and approval becomes the "good me." That which is within one's awareness but is disapproved of becomes the "bad me." The "bad me" could include those feelings, needs, or desires that stimulate anxiety. Those feelings and understandings that are out of awareness are experienced as "not me." These "not me" experiences are not nonexistent, but are expressed in indirect ways that can interfere with the conduct of the individual's life (Bruch, 1968; Sullivan, 1968).

As the social sciences adopted a cybernetic world view this theoretical perspective has been applied to developing a concept of self. Glasersfeld (1985) spoke of the self as a relational entity that is given life through the continuity of relating that provides the intuitive knowledge that our experience is truly ours. This reflects the perspective of knowing presented at the beginning of this section.

Alan Watts (1966) describes what many authors feel is the self as it can be understood through a cybernetic world view. Self is the whole, for it is part of the energy that is the universe and cannot be separated. "At this level of existence 'I' am immeasurably old; my forms are infinite and their comings and goings are simply the pulses or vibrations of a single and eternal flow of energy" (p. 12). Within this paradigm an individual is connected to every other living being in the universe. This places the self in an unique position of responsibility. The self then becomes responsible to everything because it is everything. This conceptual model resolves the issue of responsibility to society without delineating an individual self to which responsibility is assigned.

Although the conceptual model represented here by Watts fits with current theoretical models being utilized in nursing and the social sciences, it is not congruent with the experience of most persons in Western society. This limits its usefulness when working with clients in a clinical setting. It is presented here to provide the practitioner with an alternative model for themselves.

Sidney Jourard (1968) provides direction for interventions related to an individual's self-concept. The healthy self-concept allows individuals to play roles they have satisfactorily played while gaining personal satisfaction from this role enactment. This person also continues to develop and to maintain a high level of physical wellness (p. 423). This high level of wellness is achieved by gaining knowledge of oneself through a process of self-disclosure. Jourard states that

> If self-disclosure is one of the means by which healthy personality is both achieved and maintained, we can also note that such activities as loving, psychotherapy, counseling, teaching and nursing, all are impossible—without the disclosure of the client (p. 427).

Elaboration of this thought reveals that for the nurse to effectively meet the needs of the client, an understanding of the client's self must be achieved. This understanding must go beyond the interpretation of overt behavior, which is an indirect method of understanding, and access the client's understanding of self through the process of self-disclosure.

Dufault and Martocchio (1985) present a conceptual model for hope that provides a useful perspective for nursing intervention. Hope is defined as multidimensional and process-oriented. Hopelessness is not the absence of hope but is the product of a context that does not activate the process of hoping. Vaillot (1970) supports the contextual view presented by Dufault and Martocchio with the existential philosophical perspective that hope arises from relationships and the beliefs about these relationships. One believes that help can come from the outside of oneself when all internal resources are exhausted. Hopelessness arises in an environment where hope is not communicated. This model supports nursing interventions from a systems theory perspective, because it validates the ever-interacting system, the whole. In this perspective the nurse as well as the client contributes to the "hopelessness" and thus the responsibility of nurturing hope is shared (Dufault and Martocchio, 1985; McGee, 1984; Miller, 1985; Vaillot, 1970; Watson, 1985).

Developmental Considerations

Infant

In general the sources of anxiety begin in a very narrow scope with the infant and broaden out as one matures. Initially the relationship with the primary caregiver is the source of gratification for the infant, and disruptions in this relationship result in anxiety. As one matures, need gratification occurs from multiple sources and therefore the sources of anxiety expand. Specific developmental considerations are as follows:

The primary source of anxiety for the infant appears to be a sense of "being left." This response begins at about 3 months. Sullivan, as indicated earlier, would contend that the infant could experience anxiety even earlier with any disruption in having needs met by the primary caregiver. At age 8–10 months, separation anxiety peaks for the first time. At 5–6 months the infant begins to demonstrate stranger anxiety. Primary symptoms include disruptions in physiologic functioning and could include colic, sleep disorders, failure to thrive syndrome, and constipation with early toilet training. Stranger anxiety and separation anxiety may be demonstrated with screaming, attempting to withdraw, and refusing to cooperate. Both stranger anxiety and separation anxiety are normal developmental responses and should not be considered pathologic as long as they are not severe or prolonged and if the parental response is appropriately supportive of the infant's need.

Fear is a normal protective response to external threats and will be present at all ages. It becomes dysfunctional at the point that it is attached to situations that do not present a threat or when it prevents the individual from responding appropriately to a situation. Thus, it is important that children have certain fears to protect them from harm. The hot stove, for example, should produce a fear response to the degree that it prevents the child from touching the stove and being injured. Fear is a learned response to situations and children learn this response from their caregivers. Thus, it becomes the caregivers' responsibility to model and teach appropriate fear. If a mother cannot tolerate being left alone in the house at night with her children, these children will learn to fear being in this situation. When this home is located in a low-crime area with supportive neighbors and appropriate locks this becomes an inappropriate fear response and the children may be affected by it for a lifetime.

Various developmental stages have characteristic fears associated with them. In the mind of the child these characteristic fears present threats so the fears can be seen both as a source of "fear" and as a source of anxiety. The characteristic fears result from strong or noxious environmental stimuli such as loud noises, bright lights, or sharp objects against the skin. The response to fears produces physiologic symptoms. The most immediate and obvious response is crying and pulling away from the stressful object or situation.

Erickson (Evans, 1976, p. 293; Watson, 1985) indicated that he thought hope evolved out of the successful resolution of this first developmental stage, basic trust versus mistrust. Hope was perceived by Erickson to be a basic human virtue (Evans, 1976, p. 293). The type of environment that has been identified as promoting the development of this basic trust is warm and loving where there is respect and acceptance for personal interests, ideas, needs, and talents (McGee, 1984). Several environmental conditions have been associated with early childhood and are seen as increasing the perceptions consistent with hopelessness. These conditions are economic deprivation; poor physical health; being raised in a broken home or a home where parents have a high degree of conflict; having a negative perception of parents; or having parents who are not mentally healthy (McGee, 1984). From an existential perspective, Lynch (McGee, 1984) identified five areas of human existence that can produce hopelessness. If these areas are not acknowledged in the developmental process, the individual is at greater risk of frustration and hopelessness because hope is being intermingled with a known area of hopelessness. The five areas that Lynch identified are death, personal imperfections, imperfect emotional control, inability to trust all people, and personal areas of incompetence. This supports Erickson's contention that hope evolves out of the first developmental stage, because these basic areas of hopelessness are issues primarily related to the resolution of trust and mistrust. It should be remembered that previously resolved or unresolved developmental issues must be renegotiated throughout life.

Each developmental stage has a set of specific etiologies and symptom clusters related to hopelessness. Since the relationship between self-concept strength and degree of hopefulness is seen as a positive link, many of the etiologies and symptoms of hopelessness at the various developmental stages are similar to those of Self-Esteem Disturbance (McGee, 1984).

As conceptualized by Erickson (Evans, 1976) infancy is the primary age for developing a hopeful attitude about life. If the infant does not experience a situation in which trust in another can be developed, then the base of hopelessness has begun. Thus, if the infant experiences frequent changes in caregivers or has a caregiver that does not meet the basic needs in a consistent and warm manner the infant will become hopeless. Research (Lynch, 1974) has indicated that children who have been raised in an environment of despair are at greater risk for experiencing hopelessness. The situations that appear to promote a hopeless perception of life are economic deprivation, children who have had poor physical health, children from broken homes or homes where the parents quarreled extensively, children who perceived their parents' behavior negatively or whose parents were not mentally healthy. Symptoms of hopelessness in infants resemble infant depression or failure to thrive. Since symptoms in infants are a general response, the diagnosis of Hopelessness must be considered equally with other diagnoses that produce similar symptom clusters such as Powerlessness and Ineffective Coping.

One's perceptions of place in the larger system and of influence in this system begins at birth. These perceptions are developed through interactions with those in the immediate environment and continue throughout life with each new interaction in each new experience. Thus, the child learns from primary caregivers that his or her expressions may or may not have an effect on those around him or her, and also learns what must be done to have an effect. If the caregiver responds to the earliest cries of the infant a sense of personal influence has begun. The two areas that consistently influence one's perceptions of influence are discipline and communication styles.

Implementation of discipline in a manner that provides the child with a sense of control over the environment while teaching appropriate behavior can produce a perception of mutual system influence. Harsh, overcontrolling methods can produce the perception that the child does not have any influence in the system if acting in a direct manner. This produces an indirect influencing style. An example of indirect influence is the child that always becomes ill just before his parents leave for an evening on the town. The parents, out of concern for the child, decide to remain at home and thus never have time together as a couple. Authoritarian styles of interaction can also produce perceptions of powerlessness in adults in unfamiliar environments. If the hospital staff acts in an authoritarian manner, the client may develop perceptions of powerlessness.

Double-bind communication can place the individual in a position of feeling that "no matter what action I take, it appears to be wrong," and also can produce a perception of powerlessness. They are "damned if they do and damned if they don't." If the individual cannot influence this system in a direct manner again, indirect behavior patterns are chosen. Bateson (1972) proposes that this is the process behind the symptom cluster identified as schizophrenia (pp. 271–278). This suggests that if the child is continually placed in the position of being wrong no matter what he or she has done, the child could develop the perception that his or her position is one of powerlessness and carry this attitude with him or her throughout life.

Infants have a need for consistent response to having physiologic needs met, and the most important relationship becomes that with the "parenting one." If this relationship is disrupted and needs are not met, symptoms related to infant depression or failure to thrive could communicate a perception related to powerlessness.

It is important to remember that self-concept, including body image, is developed throughout life.

For the infant, the primary source of developing self-concept and body image is physical interaction with the environment. This includes both the environment's response to physical needs and the body's response to environmental stimuli.

Toddler and Preschooler

The basic sources of anxiety remain the same as with the infant. Separation anxiety appears to peak again at 18–24 months and stranger anxiety peaks again at 12–18 months. Loss of significant others is the primary source of anxiety at this age. In addition to the physiologic responses mentioned above, the child may demonstrate anxiety by motor restlessness and regressive behavior. The preschooler can begin to tolerate longer periods away from the parenting one and enjoys having the opportunity to test his or her new abilities. Lack of opportunity to practice independent skills can increase the discomfort of this age group. Increased anxiety can be seen in regressive behavior, motor restlessness, and physiologic response.

Sources of anxiety can include concerns about the body and body mutilation, concerns about death and concerns about loss of self-control. These concerns can be expressed in the ways discussed above as well as with language and dramatic play as language abilities increase. This could include playing out anxiety-producing situations with dolls or other toys. This play can assume a very aggressive nature. The anxieties of the day can also be expressed in dreams and result in nightmares or other sleep disturbance.

Fears of this age group evolve from real environmental stimuli and from imagined situations. Typical fears of specific age groups are fear of sudden loud noise (2 years), fear of animals (3–4 years), fear of the dark (4–5 years), and fear of the dark and of being lost (6 years). Symptoms of fears include regressive behavior, physical and verbal cruelty, restlessness, irritability, sleep disturbance, dramatic play around issues related to the fear, and increased physical closeness to the caregiver.

Alterations to the body or its functioning place a child at this age at the greatest risk of experiencing hopelessness. If the child experiences a difference between self and other or is ashamed about body functioning, in a nonsupportive environment hopelessness can develop. A specific issue encountered at this stage is toilet training. If the child is placed in a position of being required to gain control over bowel and bladder functions before the ability to physically master these functions has developed, the child can experience hopelessness in that he or she truly cannot make his or her body function in the required manner. Peer interactions are also important at this time because they foster the beginnings of trust in someone other than the ''mothering'' one, thus understanding that hope can be gained elsewhere.

Struggle between self-control and control by others becomes the primary psychosocial issue. If appropriate expansion of self-control is encouraged, the child will develop perceptions related to mutual systemic influence. This appropriate support is crucial if the child is to develop a perception of a personal role in the system. If this struggle for self-control is thwarted the child can express themes of overcontrol in play or become overly dependent on the primary caregiver and withdraw completely from new situations and learning.

For the preschooler there is a continuation and refinement of a sense of personal influence. Varying approaches are explored and a greater sense of what can be achieved is developed. One of the primary sources of anxiety during this stage is loss of self-control. Symptoms of difficulties in this area include playing out situations with personal influence as a theme and aggressive play.

Sources of the self-concept perceptions are the responses of significant others to exploration of new physical abilities and to the toddler's place in these relationships. The primary concept of self is related to physical qualities, motor skills, sex-type, and age. A concept of physical differences and of physical integrity is developed. Thus, situations that threaten the toddler's perception of physical wholeness can pose a threat. This would include physical injury. Toilet training poses a potential threat to the successful development of a positive self-concept or body image. Failure at training could produce feelings of personal incompetence or of the body being shameful.

In the preschooler, physical qualities, motor skills, sex-type, and age continue to be the primary components of self-concept. Peers begin to assume greater importance in self-perceptions. Physical integrity continues to be important and physical difference can have a profound effect on the preschool child.

School-Age Child

Typical fears are strange noises, ghosts and imagined phantoms, natural elements such as fire, drowning, or thunder (6 years); not being liked or being late for school (7 years); and personal failure or inadequacy (8–10 years). Symptoms of these fears include physical symptoms of autonomic stimulation, increased verbalization, withdrawal, aggression, sleep disturbance, or needing to repeat a specific task many times.

Concerns about imagined future events produce the anxieties of the school-age child. The specific concern varies with the developmental age. Early school-age children demonstrate concerns related to the unknowns in their environment such as dark rooms and natural elements such as fire or tornadoes. Middle school-age children have anxieties related to personal inadequacies. Late school-age brings increasing concerns about the evaluation of peers and concerns about the acceptance of peers. Expression of anxiety can occur in the ways discussed in the previous levels, with the addition of increased verbalization and compulsive behavior such as repeating a specific task many times.

Peers' perceptions of the individual assume a role in the development of attitudes related to personal hopefulness and influence within the larger social system. This is built on the perceptions achieved during earlier stages of development. The sense of a strong peer group can produce perceptions of help coming from the outside as long as the child thinks and believes along with the group but can produce perceptions of exaggerated personal influence. Problems at this developmental stage can be demonstrated by withdrawal, daydreaming, increased verbalizations of helplessness and hopelessness, angry outbursts, aggressive behavior, irritability, and frustration.

Self-perception expands to include ethnic awareness, ambition, ideal self, ordinal position, and conscience. There is increasing awareness of self as different from peers. Peers become increasingly important in developing a concept of self, and there is increased comparison of real to ideal self.

Adolescent

The developmental theme that elicits anxiety in this age group revolves around the development of a personal identity. This is facilitated by peer relationships, which can also be the source of anxiety. Expression of this anxiety can occur in any of the ways previously discussed and with aggressive behavior. This aggression can take both verbal and physical forms. A certain amount of "normal" anxiety is experienced as the adolescent moves from the family into the adult world. Anxiety would only be considered abnormal if it violates societal norms and is severe or prolonged. Parental education and support during this developmental crisis can be crucial.

Peer relationships, independence, authority figures, and changing roles and relationships can contribute to fears for adolescents. Expression of these fears produce the symptoms discussed under Pattern Assessment.

The cognitive development of adolescents would suggest that their perceptions of situations are guided by hypothetico-deductive thought and as a result they could develop reasonable models of hopefulness. This cognitive process occurs in conjunction with a lack of a variety of life experience and self-discipline and with a heightened state of emotionality. This can result in a situation in which the immediate goal can overshadow future consequences or possibilities. An adolescent who appears very hopeful when cognitive functioning is not overwhelmed by emotions can be filled with despair when involved in a very emotional situation. Consideration of this ability is important when caring for this age group. It is important to distinguish problem behavior from normal behavior and mood swings. Kinds of behavior that could indicate problems in this area include withdrawal and increased or amplified testing of limits. Situations that affect the peer group hope can place the adolescent at great risk.

Again, issues of dependence-independence assume a primary role. The focus of this struggle is dependence on peers and independence from family.

Body image becomes a crucial area of self-evaluation due to changing physical appearance and heightened sexual awareness. This evaluation is based on the cultural ideal as well as that of the peer group. Perceived personal failures are often attributed to physical differences.

Adult and Elderly

Changes in role and relationship patterns generate the fears specific to these age groups. These could include parenthood, marriage, divorce, retirement, or death of a spouse. Fear expression in these age groups produces the symptoms discussed under Pattern Assessment.

A specific developmental crisis can produce a perception of hopelessness and powerlessness. The situations that place the adult at risk are marriage, pregnancy, parenthood, and divorce.

In the older age group the potential of experiencing multiple losses in the areas of biologic, social, and psychologic well-being places this age group at risk for hopelessness. Hopelessness can result if several losses occur in a short period of time. The symptoms are similar to those discussed under the general description of this diagnosis.

In this age group, change in physical health can increase the perceptions of powerlessness. Such things as sensory deficits, motor deficits, and financial loss contribute to increased dependency and perceptions of powerlessness.

Concerns about role performance assume an important role in self-perceptions. Perceived failures in meeting role expectations can produce negative self-evaluation. The number of roles a person has assumed and the personal, cultural, and support system value placed on the identified roles determines the threat that negative evaluation of performance can be to self-perception. Cultural value and personal identity formation determine the degree to which body image remains important in providing a positive evaluation of self. The adult endows unique significance to various body parts. This valuing process is personal and is often not in personal awareness until there is a threat to the part.

Elderly

Loss of body function contributes to many of the self-perception issues in this age group. These losses also can affect role performance and perception of role performance.

Applicable Nursing Diagnoses

Anxiety

DEFINITION

A vague, uneasy feeling whose source is often nonspecific or unknown to the individual (North American Nursing Diagnosis Association [NANDA], 1987, p. 107).

DEFININING CHARACTERISTICS (NANDA, 1987, p. 107)

The nurse will review the initial pattern assessment for the following defining characteristics to determine the diagnosis of Anxiety.

1. Major defining characteristics
   a. Subjective
      (1) Increased tension
      (2) Apprehension
      (3) Painful and persistent increased helplessness
      (4) Uncertainty
      (5) Fearfulness
      (6) Feeling scared
      (7) Regretfulness
      (8) Overexcitedness
      (9) Being rattled
      (10) Distress
      (11) Jitteriness
      (12) Feelings of inadequacy
      (13) Shakiness
      (14) Fear of unspecified consequences
      (15) Expressed concerns about changes in life events
      (16) Worry
      (17) Anxiety
   b. Objective
      (1) Sympathetic stimulation
          (a) Cardiovascular excitation
          (b) Superficial vascoconstriction
          (c) Pupil dilation
      (2) Restlessness
      (3) Insomnia
      (4) Glancing about
      (5) Poor eye contact
      (6) Trembling, hand tremors
      (7) Extraneous movement (foot shuffling, hand or arm movements)
      (8) Facial tension
      (9) Voice quivering
      (10) Self-focus
      (11) Increased wariness
      (12) Increased perspiration

RELATED FACTORS (NANDA, 1987, p. 107)

1. Unconscious conflict about essential values or goals of life.

2. Threat to self-concept.
3. Threat of death.
4. Threat to or change in health status.
5. Threat to or change in role functioning.
6. Threat to or change in interaction patterns.
7. Situational or maturational crisis.
8. Interpersonal transmission or contagion.
9. Unmet needs.
10. Threat to or change in environment.

DIFFERENTIATION

Anxiety should be differentiated from Fear; Spiritual Distress, Grieving; Dysfunctional, Individual Coping, Ineffective; and Self-Concept, Disturbance in.

Fear is the response to an identified threat, while Anxiety is the response to one that cannot be easily identified. Fear is probably the diagnosis that is most often confused with Anxiety. An example of a situation in which Fear would be an appropriate diagnosis would be: After being released from jail the prisoner threatened to kill the judge who placed him or her in jail. The judge, if experiencing psychologic stress, could receive the diagnosis of Fear.

Self-Concept, Disturbance in, is the appropriate alternative diagnosis if the individual's symptoms are related to a general disturbance in the perception of self. Anxiety would be used when the discomfort is related to a specific area and is a perceived threat to the self.

Grieving, Dysfunctional would be considered an appropriate diagnosis if the loss was real, whereas the diagnosis of Anxiety is used when the loss is a threat that is not necessarily real. If the potential loss is real then Grieving, Anticipatory would be the appropriate diagnosis.

Individual Coping, Ineffective would be the appropriate diagnosis if the individual is not making the necessary adaptations to daily life. This may or may not occur with Anxiety.

Spiritual Distress occurs if the individual experiences a threat to his or her value or belief system. This threat may or may not produce Anxiety. If the primary concerns expressed are related to the individual's value or belief system then the appropriate diagnosis would be Spiritual Distress.

OBJECTIVES

1. Will design and implement a plan to reduce anxiety by (date).

AND/OR

2. Will verbalize at least a (number) % decrease in anxiety by (date).

TARGET DATE

A target date of 3 days would be realistic to start evaluating progress. The sooner anxiety is reduced, the sooner other problems can be dealt with.

NURSING ORDERS

ADULT HEALTH

1. Monitor anxiety behavior and relationship to activity, events, people, etc.
2. Reassure patient anxiety is normal. Help patient learn to recognize and identify anxiety.
3. Assist patient to develop coping skills:
   a. Review past coping behavior and success
   b. Help identify and practice new coping strategies:
      (1) Progressive relaxation
      (2) Guided imagery
      (3) Rhythmic breathing
      (4) Balancing exercise and rest

(5) Appropriate food and fluid intake (e.g., reduced caffeine intake)

(6) Distraction

   c. Challenge unrealistic assumptions or goals

   d. Place limits on maladaptive behavior

   e. Focus on one topic at a time

4. Provide at least 20–30 minutes every 4 hours for focus on anxiety reduction:

   a. Encourage client to express feelings verbally and through activity.

   b. Answer questions truthfully.

   c. Offer realistic reassurance and positive feedback.

5. Provide calm, nonthreatening environment:

   a. Explain all procedures and rationale for procedure in clear, concise, simple terms.

   b. Decrease sensory input and distraction (e.g., lighting, noise).

   c. Encourage significant other(s) to stay with patient but not force conversation, etc.

6. Administer antianxiety medication as ordered. Monitor and document effects of medication within 30 minutes of administration.

7. Monitor vital signs at least every 4 hours while awake.

8. Collaborate with psychiatric nurse clinician regarding care. (See Mental Health Care Plan.)

9. Refer to and collaborate with appropriate community resources:

   a. Home health

   b. Outpatient clinics

   c. Support groups.

CHILD HEALTH

1. Obtain a through history for indentification of all possible contributing factors to anxiety.

2. Ascertain how the child and parents cope with usual daily changes and crises.

3. Provide appropriate collaboration with health team members to develop an individualized plan of care to include:

   a. Pediatrician

   b. Clinical nurse specialist

   c. Play therapist

   d. Social worker

   e. Family therapist

   f. Community health nurse

4. Indentify ways to assist parents to assist child in coping with anxiety.

5. Adapt routine to best help child regain control.

6. Modify procedures as possible to best reduce anxiety (e.g., do not use intramuscular injection when alternative routes are possible).

7. Use child's developmental needs as a basis for plan of care, especially for ventilation of anxiety.

8. Allow child and parents adequate time and opportunities to handle required care issues and thus reduce anxiety.

9. Reassess for level of anxiety at least every 8 hours.

10. Encourage family to assist with care as appropriate, including feeding, comfort measures, stories, etc.

11. Offer sufficient opportunities for rest according to age and sleep requirements.

12. Attend to primary physical needs promptly.

13. Indentify knowledge needs and address these.

14. Provide ongoing follow-up for future health needs by scheduling appointments and planning and dismissal.

15. Point out and reinforce successes in conquering anxiety.

16. Assist patient and family to apply coping in future potential anxiety-producing situations.

WOMEN'S HEALTH

Acute Anxiety Attack

1. Do not leave the client alone.
2. Sustain a realistic, tranquil atmosphere.
3. Speak softly using short, simple commands.
4. Be firm but kind.
5. Be prepared to make decisions for the client.
6. Decrease external stimuli and provide a "safe" atmosphere.
7. In collaboration with physician, administer antianxiety medication.

Mild or Moderate Anxiety

8. Guide the client in verbalizing and describing what she felt was going to happen.
9. Tell the client what actually happened and compare with her version of the incident.
10. Assist the client in problem solving.
11. Assist the client in describing ways she can more clearly express her needs.
12. Assist the client in changing unrealistic expectations.
13. Encourage the client to participate in assertiveness training.

Pregnancy and Childbirth

14. Provide the client with factual information about the physical and emotional changes experienced during pregnancy.
15. Review daily schedule with the client and assist the client in identifying life-style adjustments that may be needed for coping with pregnancy.
    a. Practicing relaxation techniques when stress begins to build.
    b. Establishing a routine for relaxing after work.
16. Involve significant others in discussion and problem solving activities regarding life-style changes (pregnancy) that are affecting work habits and interpersonal relationships.
17. Refer to a support group (e.g., childbirth education classes, MCH nurses in the community).
18. Provide the client with factual information about sexual changes during pregnancy.
    a. Answer questions promptly and factually.
    b. Meet people who have had similar experiences.
    c. Discuss fears about sexual changes.
    d. Discuss aspects of sexuality and intercourse during pregnancy.
       (1) Positions for intercourse during different stages of pregnancy
       (2) Frequency of intercourse
       (3) Effect of intercourse on pregnancy or fetus
    e. Describe healing process postpartum and timing of resumption of intercourse.
19. Provide client support during birthing process (e.g., Montrice, support person, coach, etc.).
20. Provide support for significant others during this process.
    a. Allow verbalization of fears.
    b. Answer questions factually.
    c. Demonstrate equipment.
    d. Explain procedures.

MENTAL HEALTH

1. Provide a quiet, nonstimulating environment (for the client experiencing severe or panic anxiety this may be a seclusion setting).
2. Provide frequent, brief interactions that assist the client with orientation. Verbal information should be provided in simple, brief sentences.
3. If the client is experiencing severe or panic anxiety, provide support in a nondemanding atmosphere.

4. If the client is experiencing severe or panic anxiety, provide a here-and-now focus.
5. Provide the client with a simple repetitive activity until anxiety decreases to the level at which learning can begin.
6. If the client is hyperventilating, guide him or her in taking slow, deep breaths. If necessary, breathe along with him or her and provide ongoing, positive reinforcement.
7. Approach the client in a calm, reassuring manner, assessing the caregiver's level of anxiety and keeping this to a minimum.
8. Provide a constant, one-on-one interaction for the client experiencing severe or panic anxiety. This should preclude use of physical restraints, which tend to increase the client's anxiety.
9. Provide the client with alternative outlets for physical tension (this should be stated specifically and could include walking, running, talking with a staff member, using a punching bag, listening to music, doing a deep muscle relaxation sequence) (number) times per day at (state specific times). The outlets should be selected with the client's input.
10. Sit with the client (number) times per day at (include specific times) for (number) minutes to discuss feelings and complaints. As the client expresses these openly the nurse can then explore the onset of the anxiety with the purpose of identifying the sources of the anxiety.
11. After the source of the anxiety has been identified, the time set aside above can be utilized to assist the client in developing alternative coping styles.
12. Provide (number) times per day to discuss with the client interests in the external environment (especially with those clients who tend to focus strongly on nonspecific physical complaints).
13. Talk with the client about the advantages and disadvantages of the current condition. (Help the client to identify secondary gain from the symptoms.) This would be done in the individual discussion sessions or in group therapy when a trusting relationship has been developed.
14. Provide the client with feedback on how his or her behavior affects others (this could be done in an individual or group situation).
15. Provide positive feedback as appropriate on changed behavior. (The target behavior and goals should be listed here.)
16. Provide appropriate behavioral limits to control the expression of aggression or anger. (These limits should be specific to the client and listed here on the care plan, e.g., client will be asked to go to seclusion room for 15 minutes when he raises his voice to another client. The client should be informed of these limits and the limits should not exceed the client's capability. The client should be informed of the limits of the limit, e.g., the limit of the limit for raising his voice is 15 minutes. No limit should be set for an indefinite time. All staff should be aware of the limits so they can be enforced consistently with consistent consequences.)
17. Provide the client with an opportunity to discuss the situation after the consequences have been met.
18. Interact with the client in social activities (number) times per day for (number) minutes. (This will provide the client with staff time other than that which is used to set limits. The activities selected should be done with the client's input and stated here in the care plan.)
19. Provide medication as ordered and observe for appropriate side effects (these should be listed here).
20. Inform the client of community resources that provide assistance with crisis situations and provide a phone number before the client leaves the unit.
21. Develop a list of alternative coping strategies that the client can use at home and have the client practice them before leaving the unit.
22. Provide the client with a written list of appointments that have been scheduled for outpatient follow-up.

HOME HEALTH

1. Teach the patient and family appropriate monitoring of signs and symptoms of anxiety.
   a. Increased pulse

    b. Sleep disturbance

    c. Fatigue

    d. Restlessness

    e. Increased respiratory rate

    f. Inability to concentrate

    g. Short attention span

    h. Feeling of dread

    i. Faintness

    j. Forgetfulness

2. Involve the patient and family in planning and implementing strategies to reduce and cope with anxiety.

    a. Family conference

    b. Mutual goal setting

    c. Communication

3. Assist the patient and family in life-style adjustments that may be required.

    a. Relaxation techniques: yoga, biofeedback, hypnosis, breathing techniques, imagery

    b. Problem-solving techniques

    c. Crisis intervention

    d. Maintaining the treatment plan of health care professionals guiding the therapy

    e. Redirecting energy to meaningful or productive activities: active games and hobbies, walking, sports

    f. Decreasing sensory stimulation

4. Assist the patient and family to set criteria to help them determine when the intervention of a health care professional is required.

5. Teach the patient and family purposes, side effects, and proper administration techniques of medications.

6. Consult with or refer to assistive resources as indicated.

    a. Psychiatric nurse clinician

    b. Physician

    c. Occupational therapist

    d. Social service

    e. Visiting nurse

    f. Relaxation trainer

    g. Family counselor

    h. Mental health center

    i. Crisis intervention

EVALUATION
OBJECTIVE 1

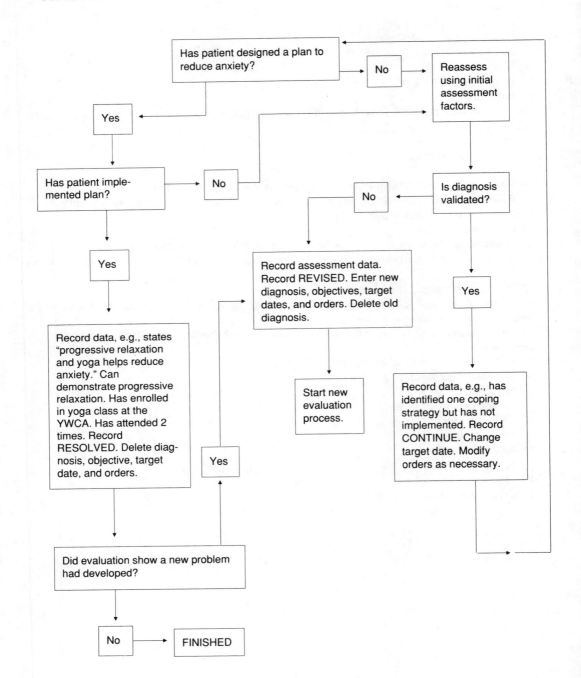

OBJECTIVE 2

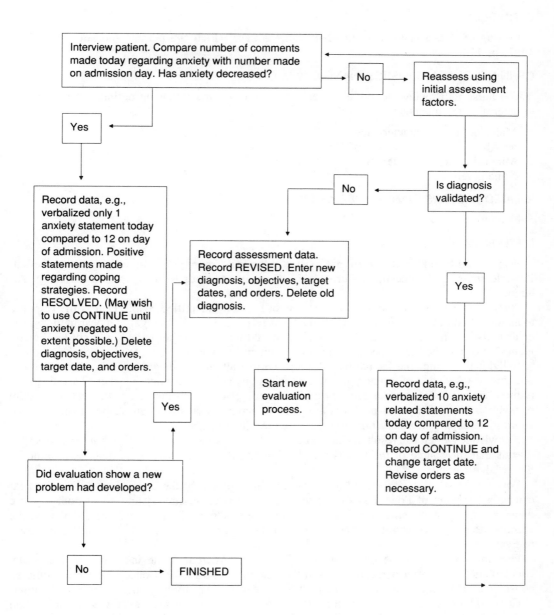

Fear

DEFINITION

Feeling of dread related to an identifiable source which the person validat
1987, p. 112).

DEFINING CHARACTERISTICS (NANDA, 1987, p. 112)

The nurse will review the initial pattern assessment for the following defining (
to determine the diagnosis of Fear.

1. Major defining characteristics
   a. Ability to identify object of Fear.
2. Minor defining characteristics
   None given.

RELATED FACTORS (NANDA, 1987, p. 112)

None given.

DIFFERENTIATION

Fear should be differentiated from Anxiety; Individual Coping,Ineffective; Knowledge Deficit;
Powerlessness; Self-Concept, Disturbance in; Comfort, Altered: Acute Pain; and Parenting, Altered.

Anxiety is the response to a threat that cannot be easily identified, while Fear is the response
to an identified threat. Thus, if the individual was responding to the thought of a bear in the woods
or actually confronting the bear the diagnosis would be Fear. If the threat could not be directly
identified or attached to a specific situation the diagnosis would be Anxiety.

Individual Coping, Ineffective would be the correct alternative diagnosis if the individual was
not able to respond appropriately to life's expectations in an appropriate manner. This diagnosis
is more appropriate for an ongoing problem in coping for which the automatic nervous system
response is less acute. Fear produces an acute autonomic nervous system response and inhibits
appropriate coping in a very time-limited, circumscribed manner.

Knowledge Deficit can result in Fear. If the initial diagnosis appears to be Fear but the assessment
reveals that the source of the fear is a lack of information, the appropriate diagnosis would be
Knowledge Deficit.

Powerlessness can be expressed in a manner that is similar to the expression of Fear, or Fear
can be a symptom of Powerlessness. If the individual is expressing symptoms of both of these
diagnoses along with indications that he or she feels helpless in a specific situation, then the
appropriate diagnosis would be Powerlessness or Powerlessness along with the parallel diagnosis
of Fear.

Fear may be part of the response to Self-Concept, Altered. If the individual indicates any
concern about his or her perception of self then the diagnosis of Self-Concept, Altered should be
considered. This assessment can be difficult because of the sensitivity of the area of investigation.

Comfort, Altered: Pain should be considered if the symptoms of fear are expressed in conjunction
with any expression of pain (see Chapter 7 for defining characteristics).

Parenting, Altered should be considered as the appropriate diagnosis when the child's fears
result from the parent's modeling or reinforcing a child's fear or when the parent is not providing
the appropriate support for the developmental fears. An example might be the child who becomes
uncontrollable in the clinic each time an injection is indicated. During the assessment the nurse
discovers that the parent tells their children that if they do not behave the doctor will give them
a shot as a reinforcer to discipline at home. In this situation the parent's inappropriate use of the
threat of the injection produced a fear in the child.

OBJECTIVES

1. Will design and implement a plan to reduce fears by (date).

AND/OR

2. Will be able to identify source of fear by (date).

TARGET DATE

A target date of 2–3 days would be acceptable, since the sooner the fear can be reduced the sooner other problems can be resolved.

NURSING ORDERS

ADULT HEALTH

1. Assist patient to correct any sensory deficits.
2. Provide information to patient in both written and verbal form.
3. Collaborate with psychiatric nurse clinician regarding care. (see Mental Health Care Plan).
4. Monitor, at least every 4 hours while awake:
   a. Vital signs;
   b. Degree of confusion;
   c. Degree of reality orientation.
5. Maintain calm, safe environment:
   a. Use frequent reassurance
   b. Touch patient frequently
   c. Have someone remain with patient
6. Provide at least 15–20 minutes every 4 hours for patient to ask questions and verbalize fears:
   a. Listen carefully
   b. Support positive coping
   c. Give clear, concise, straightforward information
7. Assist patient to increase development of decision-making skills:
   a. Review decision-making process with patient
   b. Provide opportunity for decision making regarding care
   c. Give positive feedback regarding decision making
   d. Involve significant others in promoting patient's decision making
8. Teach patient and significant others:
   a. Use of progressive relaxation and guided imagery
   b. Use of exercise balanced with rest
   c. Proper food and fluid intake
9. Administer antianxiety medications as ordered. Observe and record response to medication within 30 minutes after administration.
10. Refer to appropriate community resources for assistance.

CHILD HEALTH

1. Offer brief interactions that assist the patient and family with orientation.
2. In instances of severe fear:
   a. Provide support in a non demanding atmosphere;
   b. Provide a here and now focus;
   c. Provide one-on-one care;
   d. Offer simple, direct, repetitive tasks according to potential.
3. Provide patient and family with alternative outlets for physical tension (this should be stated specifically and could include walking, talking, etc.) (number) times per day at (specify times). These outlets should be designed with input from patient.

4. Sit with the patient and parents (number) times per day at (specify time) for (number) minutes to discuss feelings and complaints. (As the client expresses these openly, the nurse can explore the possible onset of fear with the purpose of individualizing the plan according to patient's needs.)
5. Provide feedback to patient and parents to clarify and reexplore changes regarding feelings about fear.
6. Provide appropriate behavioral limits to control the expression of aggression or anger. (These limits should be specific in time, expected behavior, and consequences.)
7. Provide the patient and parents with opportunities to discuss the situation after consequences have been met.
8. Provide opportunities for socialization appropriate for patient and family.
9. Teach patient and family about community resources to aid in handling crises and ensure that patient has phone number of same before dismissal.
10. Develop a list of alternative coping strategies to be practiced by patient and family before dismissal.
11. Ensure follow-up appointments.
12. Assist patient and family to view situation represented as something which can be managed; encourage positive reinforcement of desired behavior patterns.

WOMEN'S HEALTH

(Note: Phobias affect approximately 2–5% of the adult population, and 80% of the affected group are female. The most common phobias among women are agoraphobia, fear of animals, and fear of social situations [Fogel & Woods, 1981; Griffith-Kenney, 1986].)

1. Provide the client a comfortable, unjudging atmosphere in which to discuss her fears.
2. Obtain a detailed history of client's fear.
    a. Encourage client to discuss signs and symptoms or precipitating event.
    b. Ascertain how often problem occurs.
    c. Have client describe her reaction.
    d. Identify coping mechanisms which have previously helped.
    e. Identify those factors or coping mechanisms which *do not* help.
    Birthing Process
3. Allow the client to discuss her plans and fears for the birth of her child.
4. Provide a comfortable atmosphere to encourage the client to relate her fears of:
    a. The unknown;
    b. Safety for herself and her baby;
    c. Pain during the birthing process;
    d. Mutilation during the birthing process;
    e. Of "losing control" during the birthing process.
5. Refer client to appropriate support groups for information:
    a. Childbirth education classes in the community
    b. Schools of nursing (students in obstetrics that have follow-through [case study] of families of pregnant women)
    c. Special national organizations
        (1) International Childbirth Education Association, (ICEA) P.O. Box 20048, Minneapolis, MN 55420
        (2) American Society for Psychoprophylaxis in Obstetrics, (ASPO) 1411 K Street NW, Washington, DC 20005
        (3) American Academy for Husband Coached Childbirth, (AAHCC) Box 5224, Sherman Oaks, CA 91413

(4) National Association of Parents and Professionals for Safe Alternatives in Childbirth, (NAPSAC) P.O. Box 267, Marble Hill, MO 63764

(5) La Leche League International (LLL),9616 Minneapolis Ave., Franklin Park, IL 60131

(6) *National Organization of Mothers of Twins*, 5402 Amberwood Lane, Rockville, MD 20853

(7) Vaginal Birth after Cesarean (VBAC) Information, Nancy Cohen, Great Plain Terrace, Needham, MA 02192

(8) Nurses Association of the American College of Obstetricians and Gynecologists (NAACOG), 600 Maryland Ave. SW, Suite 200 East, Washington, DC

(9) Cesareans/Support Education and Concern, (C/Sec) 22 Forest Road, Framingham, MA 01701

6. Encourage use of relaxation and prepared chidbirth techniques during labor.

7. Monitor client's level of confidence using prepared childbirth techniques during labor.

8. Provide ongoing information during the labor and birth process.

9. Provide accurate information to the significant others during the labor and birth process.

10. Allow significant others to verbalize fears.

11. Assist client in using "imagery" to overcome fears during the birthing process.

12. Provide continuity of care by remaining with the laboring woman throughout the birthing process.

13. Provide physical comforts to the laboring woman.

14. Provide clear answers to client's questions.

15. Keep client informed of her progress in the birthing process.

16. Provide client and significant others with as many opportunities as possible to make decisions about her care during the birthing process.

MENTAL HEALTH

1. Provide a quiet, nonstimulating environment for the client. (This would include removing persons and objects that the person perceives as threatening. If the person is experiencing a thought disorder with delusions and hallucinations, attention should be paid to the details of the environment that could be misinterepreted. At times a same-sex caregiver can increase fear in the client.)

2. Obtain the client's understanding of the threat.

3. Provide a one-on-one relationship for the client with a member of the nursing staff. This should be maintained until the symptoms return to normal levels.

4. Provide clear answers to client's questions.

5. Carry on conversations in the client's presence or vision in a voice that the client can hear.

6. Inform the client of plans related to care before the plans are implemented. If possible discuss these with the client (e.g., if it is necessary to move the client to another room or institution the client should be informed of this change before it takes place).

7. Orient the client to the environment.

8. Maintain a consistent environment and routine (record client's daily routine here along with notes about client's special reactions to visitors and staff members).

9. Provide a primary care nurse for the client on each shift.

10. Sit with the client (number) minutes (number) times per shift (initially the times should reflect short, frequent contacts. This can change with the client's need).

11. Provide the client with objects in the environment that promote security. (These may be symbolic items from home or religious objects. List significant ones here.)

12. Note the client's desired personal space and respect these limits (the general guidelines should be stated here).

13. Assist the client with sorting out the fearful situation by:

a. Recognizing that the experience is real for the client even though that is not your experience of the situation (''I can see that you are very upset; I can understand how those thoughts could make you fearful'');

b. Providing feedback about distorted thoughts (''No, I am not going to punish you, I am here to talk with you about your concerns'');

c. Encouraging client to develop an understanding of the threat by talking about it in specific terms and not vague generalizations (''When you say your family is out to get you who and what do you mean?'');

d. Focusing conversations in the here and now (this would include information about the effects of the client's behavior on those around him, your experience of the client, your perceptions of the environment);

e. Not arguing about client's perceptions; instead, provide feedback in the here and now with your perceptions of the situation. (Client tells you that you must be angry with him or her because of the look you had on your face while reviewing the client's chart. Your response is, ''I am not angry with you, when I was looking at your chart, I was thinking about the conversation we had this morning about your job'').

14. Provide the client with as many opportunities as possible to make decisions about his or her care and current situation.

15. Assist the client in developing a list of potential solutions to the threatening situation.

16. Review developed list of solutions with the client and assist in evaluating the benefits and costs of each solution.

17. Rehearse with the client, if necessary, the solution selected or have client practice a new response to the threatening situation.

18. Provide positive feedback to the client about efforts to resolve the threatening situation.

19. Assist the client in developing alternative outlets for the feelings generated by the threatening situation and provide the opportunity for the use of these outlets (these would be noted in the chart so other staff members would be aware of them and could encourage their use when they notice the client's discomfort increasing).

20. Assist the client in identifying early behavioral cues that indicate fear or that they are entering a fearful situation.

21. Encourage the client in alternative coping strategies developed by:
    a. Providing the necessary environment;
    b. Providing the appropriate equipment;
    c. Spending time with the client doing the activity;
    d. Providing positive reinforcement for the use of the strategy (this could be verbal as well as with special privileges).

22. If fear is related to a specific object or situation, teach the client to use deep muscle relaxation and then teach this along with progressively real mental images of the threatening situation (this is for those situations that will not cause the client harm if they are approached, such as riding in elevators). This could also include other methods of relaxation such as:
    a. Music
    b. Deep breathing
    c. Thought stopping
    d. Fantasy
    e. Assertiveness training
    f. Audio tapes with relaxation images or sequences
    g. Yoga
    h. Hypnosis
    i. Meditation

23. Explore ways to increase client's feeling of control in threatening situation (e.g. a fear of elevators could be altered by the client only riding in elevators with emergency phones and

only riding when he or she could stand near the phone). The fear may also indicate the client is feeling out of control in an unrelated area of his or her life. If this is suspected this should be explored and ways of increasing control should be explored (e.g., a woman's fear of driving could indicate that she feels out of control in her marriage and increased assertive behavior with her husband removes the fear).

24. If the method to increase control involves interactions with the health care team, these should be noted in specific terms on the care plan.
25. Assist the client in developing strategies to be used in the community after discharge, and role play various situations with the client for at least 1 hour for at least 2 days.

HOME HEALTH

1. Teach the patient and family appropriate monitoring of signs and symptoms of fear.
    a. Increased pulse
    b. Flushed face
    c. Sweaty palms
    d. Shortness of breath
    e. Muscle tightness
    f. Nausea, vomiting, diarrhea
    g. Sleep disturbance
    h. Fainting
    i. Sweating
    j. Urinary frequency, urgency
    k. Crying
2. Involve the patient and family in planning and implementing strategies to reduce and cope with fear.
3. Assist the patient and family in life-style adjustments that may be required.
    a. Relaxation techniques: yoga, biofeedback, hypnosis, breathing techniques, imagery
    b. Providing a secure environment: familiar objects and familiar people, predictable events without surprises
    c. Communication techniques: responses that reflect reality; orient to person, time and place; explain activities; provide predictable and consistent situations; and maintain visual, auditory, and tactile contact
    d. Problem-solving strategies
    e. Providing a sense of mastery (i.e. accomplishable goals in secure environment)
    f. Maintain the treatment plan of the health care professional guiding the therapy
4. Assist the patient and family to set criteria to help them to determine when the intervention of a health care professional is required.
5. Consult with or refer to assistive resources as indicated:
    a. Psychiatric nurse clinician
    b. Physician
    c. Occupational therapist
    d. Social service
    e. Visiting nurse
    f. Relaxation trainer
    g. Support groups
    h. Desensitization therapist
    i. Family counselor
    j. Mental health center

EVALUATION
OBJECTIVE 1

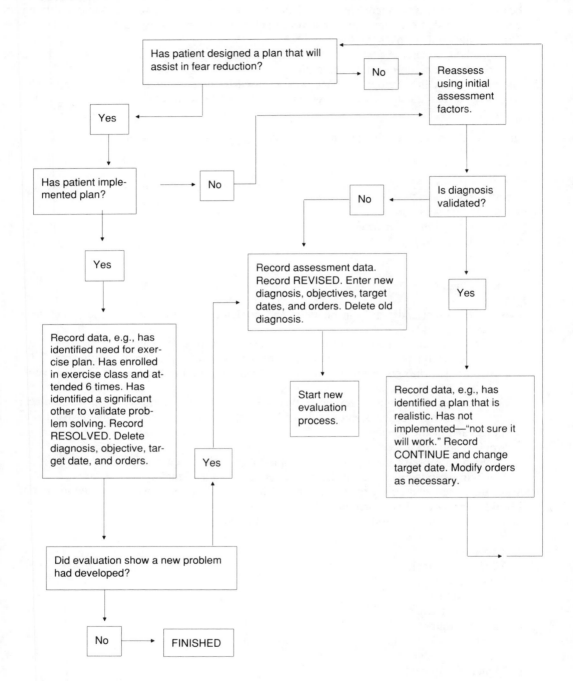

OBJECTIVE 2

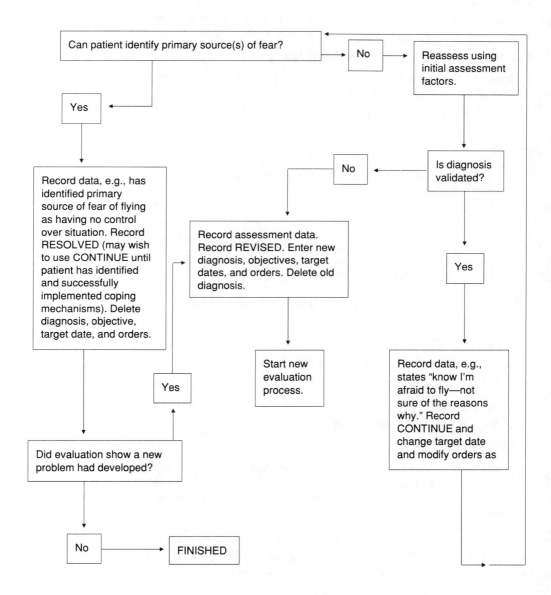

Hopelessness

DEFINITION

A state in which an individual sees limited or no alternatives or p(
is unable to mobilize energy on his or her own behalf (NANDA, 19(

DEFINING CHARACTERISTICS (NANDA, 1987, p. 99).

A nurse will review the initial pattern assessment for the following
determine the diagnosis of Hopelessness.

1. Major defining characteristics
   a. Passivity
   b. Decreased verbalization
   c. Decreased affect
   d. Verbal cues (despondent content, ''I can't,'' sighing)
2. Minor defining characteristics
   a. Lack of initiative
   b. Decreased response to stimuli
   c. Turning away from speaker
   d. Closing eyes
   e. Shrugging in response to speaker
   f. Decreased appetite
   g. Increased sleep
   h. Lack of involvement in care, or passively allowing care
   i. Decreased affect

RELATED FACTORS (NANDA, 1987, p. 99)

1. Prolonged activity restriction creating isolation.
2. Failing or deteriorating physiologic condition.
3. Long-term stress.
4. Abandonment.
5. Lost belief in transcendent values or God.

DIFFERENTIATION

Hopelessness should be differentiated from Anxiety; Individual C(
Processes, Altered; Fear; Knowledge Deficit; Self-Concept, Disturbar

Powerlessness is present when the individual perceives that his or
a situation regardless of the options that the person may see in a situ
when the individual perceives that there are few or limited choices in
may evolve out of Hopelessness. Powerlessness is the perception that
a difference, while Hopelessness is the perception that there are no
decision about which is the most appropriate diagnosis is based on t
nurse about which symptoms predominate.

Anxiety may have as a component a perception of Hopelessness. T
narrowed perception of the anxious client. Hopelessness may have as
situation could develop when the client is feeling overwhelmed with t
no alternatives in a difficult situation. The primary diagnosis evolves f
If Anxiety is the predominant symptom cluster it should be the prima
strong influence it has on the client's perceptions.

Ineffective Individual Coping can result from Hopelessness. A per
limited options in a situation can result in the belief that personal actio

:havior may not be initiated. If Ineffective Individual Coping is determined
:d lack of options then Hopelessness would be the primary diagnosis.
Altered can produce a sense of Hopelessness because of the individual's
.ssess the situation. Thus, the most appropriate diagnosis would be Thought

.i sense of Hopelessness. If the client is fearful in a situation perception can
.ternative options may be overlooked. When Fear and Hopelessness occur
.d be the primary diagnosis.
.n evolve in a situation when the client has insufficient knowledge about options.
.rmined to be the situation, Knowledge Deficit would be the primary diagnosis.
can evolve in situations where Self-Concept, Disturbance in is profound. In these
.ndividual perceives self in a manner that limits perceptions of options. When
Hopelessness and Self-Concept, Disturbance in occur together, Self-Concept, Disturbance in would
be the primary diagnosis.

OBJECTIVES

1. Will initiate a realistic plan to reduce perception of hopelessness by (date).

AND/OR

2. Will verbalize a decrease in complaints regarding hopelessness by (date).

TARGET DATE

A target date ranging between 3 and 5 days would be appropriate for initial evaluation. A target date over 5 days might lead to increased complications such as potential for self-injury. A target date sooner than 3 days would not provide a sufficient length of time for realizing the effects of intervention.

NURSING ORDERS

ADULT HEALTH

1. Establish a therapeutic and trusting relationship with patient and family.
2. Support patient's efforts at objectively describing feelings of hopelessness.
3. Assist the patient to find alternatives.
4. Assist the patient to engage in social interaction.
5. Identify religious, cultural, or community support groups.
6. As health status permits, increase activity level.
7. Encourage food and fluid intake.
8. Moderate sleep-wake cycles.
9. Encourage active participation in activities of daily living.
10. Refer to psychiatric nurse clinician.

CHILD HEALTH

1. Monitor for etiologic components contributing to hopelessness pattern.
2. Identify other primary nursing needs and deal with these as needed.
3. Encourage patient and family to verbalize feelings about current status with 30 minutes set aside each shift for this purpose.
4. Assist patient and family to explore growth potential afforded by this specific experience.
5. Identify resources in the community which may be of assistance such as national and local organizations (e.g., Red Cross).
6. Collaborate with related health team members to include:
   a. Pediatrician
   b. Subspecialist
   c. Psychiatrist

   d. Clinical nurse specialist
   e. Social Service
   f. Family therapist
   g. Community health nurse
   h. Play therapist
   i. Legal counsel
   j. Child protective services
 7. Provide appropriate follow-up with appointments for post hospital checkups.
 8. Allow for gradual assumption of daily routine with planning input from patient and family.
 9. Allow for preferences in day-by-day decisions when appropriate to help restore sense of being in control.
10. Provide explanations and educational offering for procedures and treatments.
11. Allow for opportunities for child to "play out" feelings under appropriate supervision if possible.
   a. Play with dolls for toddler
   b. Art and puppets for preschooler
   c. Peer discussions for adolescents

WOMEN'S HEALTH

(Note: All nursing orders in Adult Health, Mental Health, and Home Health can apply to women with the following additions.)

Infertility

(See Chapter 10 for detailed information on infertility. The following nursing orders are for the couple, man, or woman who has been proven, for whatever reason, to have no hope to be able to conceive a child.)

1. Provide a nonjudgmental atmosphere to allow the infertile couple to express their feelings:
   a. Anger
   b. Denial
   c. Inadequacy
   d. Guilt
   e. Depression
   f. Grief
2. Provide the infertile couple with accurate information on:
   a. Adoption;
   b. Living without children.
3. Refer to support groups in the community.
4. Support and allow couple to work through grieving process
   a. Grief for loss of fertility
   b. Grief for loss of children
   c. Grief for loss of idealized life-style
   d. Grief for loss of feminine life experiences such as:
      (1) Pregnancy
      (2) Birth
      (3) Breastfeeding
5. Encourage couple to talk honestly with one another about feelings.
6. Encourage couple to seek professional help if necessary to deal with feelings:
   a. Sexual relationship
   b. Conflicts
   c. Anxieties
   d. Parenting
   e. Coping mechanisms used for dealing with loss of fertility

7. Assist couple to explore:
   a. Their expectations;
   b. Relatives expectations;
   c. Society's expectations.
8. Be alert for signs of:
   a. Depression;
   b. Anger;
   c. Frustration;
   d. Impending crisis.

MENTAL HEALTH

1. Monitor health care team's interactions with client for behavior (verbal and nonverbal) that would encourage the client not to be hopeful. If situations are identified they should be noted here and the team should discuss alternative ways of behaving in the situation. The actions that are determined to be needed to support the client's hope should be noted on the care plan.
2. Sit with client (number) times per day at (specify times) for 30 minutes to discuss feelings and perceptions the client has about the identified situation. These times should also include discussions about the client's significant others, times the client has enjoyed with these persons, projects or activities the client was planning with or for these persons that have not been accomplished, client's values and beliefs about health and illness, and the attitudes about the current situation.
3. Identify with client's significant others times that they can talk with the staff about the current situation. Themes that should be explored during this interaction should be their thoughts and feelings about the current situation, ways in which they can support the client, the importance of their support for the client, questions they may have about the client's situation, and possible outcomes. (Note the time for this interaction here as well as the name of the person who will be talking with the significant others.)
4. Note times when significant others will be visiting and schedule this time so there will be a private time for them to interact with the client. (Note these times here and designate those times that are scheduled as private visitation times.) Inform client and significant others of those places on the unit where they can have privacy to visit.
5. Identify with client preferences for daily routine and place this information on the care plan to be implemented by the staff. (It is vital to this client to have the information shared with all staff so that it will not appear that the time spent in providing information was wasted.)
6. Provide information to questions in an open, direct manner.
7. Provide information on all procedures at a time when the client can ask questions and think about the situation.
8. Allow client to participate in decision making at the level to which he or she is capable (the client who has never made an independent decision would be overwhelmed by the complexity of the decisions made daily by the corporation executive). If necessary, offer decision situations in portions that the client can master successfully (the amount of information that the client can handle should be noted here as well as a list of decisions the client has been presented with).
9. Provide positive reinforcement for behavior changed and decisions made (those things that are reinforcing for this client should be listed here along with the reward system that has been established with the client; e.g., play one game of cards with the client when a decision about ways to cope with a specific problem has been made).
10. Provide verbal social reinforcements along with behavioral reinforcements.
11. Keep promises (specific promises should be listed in the care plan so that all staff will be aware of this information).

12. Accept client's decision if the decision was given to the client to make. These decisions should be noted on the care plan.
13. Provide ongoing feedback to client on progress.
14. Spend 30 minutes a day talking with client about current coping strategies and exploring alternative coping methods. Note time for this discussion here as well as the person responsible for this interaction. When alternative coping styles have been identified this time should be used to assist client with necessary practice. The alternative styles that the client has selected should be noted on the care plan and the staff should assist the client in implementing the strategy when appropriate. These could include deep muscle relaxation, visual imagery, prayer, or talking about alternative ways of coping with stressful events.
15. Allow client to express anger and assist with discovering constructive ways of expressing this feeling (e.g., talking about this feeling, using a punching bag, playing ping pong, throwing or hitting a pillow). Talk with client about signs of progress and assist him or her in recognizing these as they occur with verbal reminders or by keeping a record of steps taken toward progress.
16. Assist client in establishing realistic goals and realistic expectations for situations. The goals should be short-term and be stated in measurable behavioral terms. (Usually dividing the goal set by the client in half provides an achievable goal; this could involve dividing one goal into several smaller goals.) Note goals and evaluation dates here.
17. Determine times with the client to evaluate progress toward these goals and to discuss their observations about this progress. These specific times should be listed here with the name of the person responsible for this activity. Initially this may need to be done on a daily basis until the client develops competency in making realistic assessments.
18. Assist client in developing a list of contingencies for possible blocks to the goals. These would be "what if" and "if then" discussions to provide direction for the client with an opportunity to mentally rehearse situations that could require alteration of goals. This protects the client from all-or-none situations. This would be done in the goal-setting session and a record of the alternatives discussed would be made in the chart for future reference.
19. Discuss with client values and beliefs about life and assess importance of formal religion in the client's life. If client requires contact with a person of his or her belief system, arrange this and note necessary information for contacting this person here. Provide client with the time necessary to perform those religious rituals that are important to him or her. Note the rituals here with the times scheduled and any assistance that is required from the nursing staff.
20. Provide the client with opportunities to enjoy aesthetic experiences that have been identified as important such as listening to favorite music, having favorite pictures placed in the room, enjoying favorite foods, having special flowers in the room. Spend 5 minutes three times a day discussing these experiences and assisting the client in becoming involved in the enjoyment of them. Note here those activities that have been identified by the client as important and times when they will be discussed with the client.
21. Assist client in developing an awareness and an appreciation for the here and now by helping him or her focus attention in the present by pointing out to him or her the beauty in the flowers in the room, the warmth of the sunshine as it comes through the window, the calmness or aliveness of a piece of music, the taste and smell of a special food item, the odor of flowers, etc.
22. Establish a time to talk with client about maximizing potential at his or her current level of functioning. Note date and time for this discussion here. This may need to be done in several stages during more than one time depending on the client's level of denial. Note person responsible for these discussions here.

HOME HEALTH

1. Monitor for factors contributing to the hopelessness (e.g., psychologic, social, economic, spiritual, environmental, etc.).
2. Involve patient and family in planning, implementing, and promoting reduction or elimination of hopelessness.
   a. Family conference
   b. Mutual goal setting
   c. Communication
   d. Support for the caregiver
3. Assist patient and family in life-style adjustments that may be required.
   a. Use relaxation techniques: yoga, biofeedback, hypnosis, breathing techniques, imagery.
   b. Provide assertiveness training.
   c. Provide opportunities for individual to exert control over situation; give choice when possible; support and encourage self-care efforts.
   d. Provide sense of mastery: accomplishable and meaningful goals in secure environment.
   e. Look for meaning in situation.
   f. Provide treatment for physiologic condition.
   g. Provide grief counseling.
   h. Provide spiritual counseling.
   i. Prevent suicide.
4. Consult with or refer to assistive resources as indicated:
   a. Psychiatric nurse clinician
   b. Physician
   c. Occupational therapist
   d. Religious leader or counselor
   e. Hospice
   f. Social service
   g. Support groups
   h. Relaxation trainer
   i. Family counseler
   j. Mental health center
   k. Financial counselor
   l. Crisis center

EVALUATION
OBJECTIVE 1

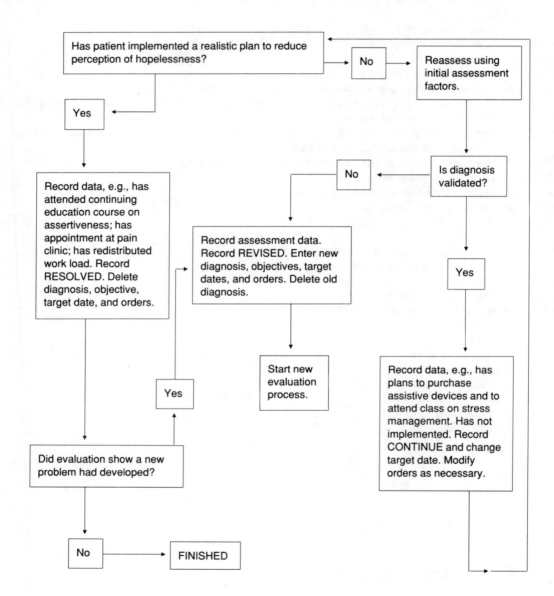

OBJECTIVE 2

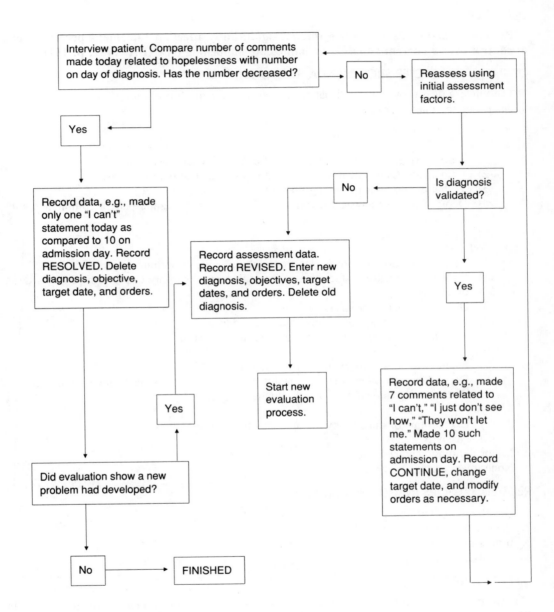

Powerlessness

DEFINITION

Perception that one's own action will not significantly affect an outcome; a of control over a current situation or immediate happening (NANDA, 1987

DEFINING CHARACTERISTICS (NANDA, 1987, p. 101)

The nurse will review the initial pattern assessment for the following defin to determine the diagnosis of Powerlessness.

1. Major defining characteristics
   a. Severe
      (1) Verbal expressions of having no control or influence over situation
      (2) Verbal expressions of having no control or influence over outcome
      (3) Verbal expressions of having no control over self-care
      (4) Depression over physical deterioration which occurs despite patient compliance with regimens
      (5) Apathy
   b. Moderate
      (1) Nonparticipation in care or decision-making when opportunities are provided
      (2) Expressions of dissatisfaction and frustration over inability to perform previous tasks or activities
      (3) Does not monitor progress
      (4) Expression of doubt regarding role performance
      (5) Reluctance to express true feelings, fearing alienation from caregivers
      (6) Passivity
      (7) Inability to seek information regarding care
      (8) Dependence on others that may result in irritability, resentment, anger, and guilt
      (9) Does not defend self-care practices when challenged
   c. Low
      (1) Expressions of uncertainty about fluctuating energy levels
      (2) Passivity
2. Minor defining characteristics
   None given

RELATED FACTORS (NANDA, 1987, p. 102)

1. Health care environment.
2. Interpersonal interaction.
3. Illness related regimen.
4. Life-style of helplessness.

DIFFERENTIATION

Powerlessness should be differentiated from Anxiety; Individual Coping, Ineffective; Thought Processes, Impaired; Fear; Knowledge Deficit; Self Concept, Disturbance in.

Anxiety may have as a component a perception of Powerlessness. This would evolve into a situation where the anxious client would not attempt to resolve the situation. Powerlessness can also have as a component anxiety. Deciding on the primary diagnosis is based on the clinical judgment of the nurse about which symptoms predominate.

Individual Coping, Ineffective can result from Powerlessness. A perception of Powerlessness can produce Ineffective Individual Coping, because if one perceives that one's own actions cannot influence a situation appropriate actions may not be taken. If Individual Coping, Ineffective is determined to result from a perceived lack of influence then Powerlessness would be the primary diagnosis.

Thought Processes, Impaired can produce a sense of Powerlessness because of the individual's inability to accurately assess the situation. Thus, the most appropriate diagnosis would be Thought Processes, Altered.

Fear can produce a sense of Powerlessness just as Powerlessness can produce Fear. Differentiation is based on the predominant symptom sequence.

If the client lacks sufficient knowledge about a situation a perception of Powerlessness may result. Therefore, Knowledge Deficit would be the primary diagnosis.

Self Concept, Disturbance in can produce perceptions of Powerlessness if the self-perception is disturbed in relation to role performance, personal identity, or self-esteem. Powerlessness may be one of a cluster of symptoms related to a disturbance in self-concept. Differentiation is based on the pervasiveness of the perception. Pervasive disruptions would be related to disturbance in self-concept.

OBJECTIVES

1. Will describe areas of control over self by (date).

AND/OR

2. Will initiate a plan to deal with feelings of powerlessness by (date).

TARGET DATE

A target date of 3 days would be realistic to check for progress toward reduced feeling of powerlessness.

ADDITIONAL INFORMATION

The paradox of the metaphor of power has been presented in the literature. Systems theorists and cyberneticians have presented the most useful information when one is planning intervention strategies. Keeney (1983) presents a summary of the debate over the power metaphor. In sum, most cyberneticians find this to be an invalid metaphor when discussing systems of interaction. The process of a system involves mutual interactions and within a system each member exerts influence over the other members. Therefore, the individual who acts as if he or she is powerless is exerting "power" over the other parts of the system to act in a manner that would increase this "lost" personal power. The "powerless" one is then actually exercising power to motivate other parts of the system to act in certain ways (pp. 130–135). Understanding this conceptual model provides the client with an opportunity to know how one's behavior affects the situation and provides nurses with an opportunity to understand their reactions to and feelings toward the client with the diagnosis of powerlessness. If the power metaphor is not accepted, this affects the concept of internal versus external locus of control that is often discussed in conjunction with powerlessness (Carpenito, 1983, p. 334). The concepts of internal and external loci of control become metaphors for how a person perceives personal influence within an interactional system. Persons with an external locus of control do not understand their influence on the system, whereas persons with an internal locus of control have an understanding of personal influence.

NURSING ORDERS

ADULT HEALTH

1. Plan care with patient:
   a. Likes and dislikes
   b. Where he or she wants personal items placed
   c. Routines, to extent possible, according to patient's own pace and schedule.
   d. Diet selected by patient

2. Avoid:
    a. Reinforcing manipulative behavior;
    b. Using negative feedback (e.g., arguing with patient);
    c. Overuse of health care terminology.
3. Provide calm, safe environment:
    a. Answer questions truthfully
    b. Explain all procedures and rationale for procedures
    c. Give positive reinforcement to extent possible
    d. Reduce sensory input
4. Involve significant others in care
5. Encourage patient to provide as much of self-care as possible.
6. Monitor, at least once per shift:
    a. Vital signs;
    b. Exercise;
    c. Sleep-rest periods;
    d. Food and fluid intake;
7. Refer to appropriate community resources:
    a. Psychiatric nurse clinician
    b. Home health
    c. Support groups

CHILD HEALTH

1. Perform a thorough assessment appropriate for patient's developmental needs to identify specific factors which are causing "powerlessness."
    a. Use art if needed and appropriate
    b. Use puppetry
    c. Use group therapy if appropriate
2. Plan care with paraprofessionals to best deal with individual's and family needs as appropriate.
3. Provide options *when* they exist in nursing care.
4. Provide continuity in care with same staff to degree possible.
5. Attend to primary needs promptly.
6. Allow family to participate in care as they are able and choose to.
7. Adopt plan of care to best meet child's and family's needs by including them in voicing preferences whenever appropriate.
8. Identify and address educational needs which might be contributing to powerlessness.
9. Balance high technology with high touch and appropriate attention.
10. Respect cultural and religious preferences, especially in dietary and daily routines.
11. Allow for adequate rest.
12. Provide for appropriate diversional activities as appropriate.
13. Refer to patient by preferred name or nickname. List that name here.
14. Allow for privacy and need to withdraw to family as a unit.
15. Keep patient and family informed as changes occur.
16. Maintain appropriate safety-minded environment.
17. Provide opportunities for parents to demonstrate appropriate care for child to aid in feeling in control on dismissal from hospital.
18. Provide for appropriate follow-up appointments as needed.

WOMEN'S HEALTH

1. Provide the client with factual information about the type of care institutions provide during the birthing process.
    a. Traditional obstetric services

      b. Family-centered maternity care units

      c. Single-room maternity care

      d. Mother-baby care

      e. Birthing centers

  2. Identify the client's preferences (birth plan) for the birth of their child.

  3. Refer the client to support groups for information:

      a. Childbirth classes

      b. Sibling classes

      c. La Leche League

  4. Provide answers to questions in an open, direct manner.

  5. Provide information on all procedures so the client can make informed choices.

  6. Assist the client and significant others in establishing realistic goals (list goals with evaluation dates here).

  7. Allow the client and significant others to participate in decision making at the level to which she is capable.

  8. Identify the client's needs and how they are being met.

  9. Provide the client continuous feedback on her progress in labor.

10. Provide positive reinforcement for mothering tasks.

11. Assist the client in identifying infant behavior patterns and understanding how they allow her infant to communicate with her.

12. Assist the client's decisions (e.g., to breastfeed or not to breastfeed, who she wants as significant others during the birthing process).

13. Allow the client maximum control over the environment. This could include husband staying in postpartum room to assist with infant care, keeping the newborn with the mother at all times, using different positions for birth (i.e., squatting or hand knee position), having grandparents and siblings in the room with mother and newborn, etc.

14. Reassure the new mother that it takes time to become acquainted with her infant.

15. Support and reassure the mother in learning infant care (i.e., breastfeeding, bathing, changing, holding a newborn, cord care, bottle feeding).

16. Allow the client (new mother or new father) to verbalize fears and insecure feelings about her or his new role of being a mother or father.

17. Assist the client in identifying life-style adjustments that may be needed due to the incorporation of a newborn into the family structure.

18. Involve significant others in discussion and problem-solving activities regarding role changes within the family.

19. Assist the client to use relaxation techniques during the birthing process (labor).

MENTAL HEALTH

  1. Sit with the client (number) times per day at (specify times) for 30 minutes to discuss feelings and perceptions the client has about the identified situation.

  2. Identify client preferences for daily routine and place this information on the care plan to be implemented by the staff. (It is vital to this client to have the information shared with all staff so that it will not appear that the time spent in providing information was wasted.)

  3. Provide information to questions in an open, direct manner.

  4. Provide information on all procedures at a time when the client can ask questions and think about the situation.

  5. Allow the client to participate in decision making at the level to which he or she is capable (the client who has never made an independent decision would be overwhelmed by the complexity of the decisions made daily by the corporation executive). If necessary, offer decision situations in portions that the client can master successfully (the amount of information

that the client can handle should be noted here as well as a list of decisions the client has been presented with).

6. Identify the client's needs and how these are currently being met. If these involve indirect methods of influence discuss alternative direct methods of meeting these needs (the client who requests medication for headache every 15 minutes is requesting attention and is encouraged to approach the nurse and ask to talk when the need for attention arises).

7. Provide positive reinforcement for behavior changed and decisions made (those things that are reinforcing for this client should be listed here along with the reward system that has been established with the client; e.g., play one game of cards with the client when a decision about what to eat for dinner is made or walk with client on hospital grounds when a decision is made about grooming).

8. Provide verbal social reinforcements along with behavioral reinforcements.

9. Keep promises (specific promises should be listed in the care plan so that all staff will be aware of this information).

10. Assist the client in identifying current methods of influence and in understanding that influence is always there by providing feedback on how influence is being used in the client's interactions with the nurse.

11. Accept the client's decisions if the decisions were given to the client to be made (i.e., if the decision to take or not take medication was left with the client, the decision not to take medication should be respected).

12. Allow the client maximum control over the environment (this could include where clothes are kept, how room is arranged, times for various activities). Note preferences here.

13. Spend 30 minutes 2 times per day at (note specific times) allowing the client to role play interactions that are identified as problematic (the specific situations as well as new behavior should be noted here).

14. Provide opportunities for significant others to be involved in care as appropriate (careful assessment of the interactions between client and significant others must be made to determine best balance of influencing behavior between client and support system). Specific situation should be listed here.

15. Monitor the health care team's interactions with the client for behavior patterns that would encourage the client to choose indirect methods of influence (this could include interactions that encourage the adult client to assume a childlike role). If situations are identified they should be noted here.

16. Provide on-going feedback to the client on progress.

17. Assist the client in establishing realistic goals. List goals with evaluation dates here (usually dividing the goal set by the client in half provides an achievable goal; this could also involve dividing one goal into several smaller goals).

18. Refer the client to outpatient support systems and assist with making arrangements for the client to contact these before discharge (these could be systems that would assist the client in maintaining a perception of influencing ability and could include assertiveness training groups, battered wives' programs, legal aid, etc.).

HOME HEALTH

1. Involve the patient and family in planning and implementing strategies to reduce powerlessness:
   a. Family conference
   b. Mutual goal setting
   c. Communication

2. Assist the patient and family in life-style adjustments that may be required.
   a. Relaxation techniques: yoga, biofeedback, hypnosis, breathing techniques, imagery
   b. Providing opportunities for individual to exert control over situation: give choices when possible; support and encourage self-care efforts

   c. Problem solving and goal setting
   d. Providing sense of mastery: accomplishable goals in secure environment
   e. Maintaining the treatment plan of the health care professionals guiding therapy
   f. Obtaining and providing accurate information regarding condition
3. Consult with or refer to assistive resources as indicated:
   a. Psychiatric nurse clinician
   b. Physician
   c. Occupational therapist
   d. Social service
   e. Relaxation trainer
   f. Support groups
   g. Family Counselor
4. Assist the patient and family to set criteria to help them determine when the intervention of a health care professional is required.

EVALUATION
OBJECTIVE 1

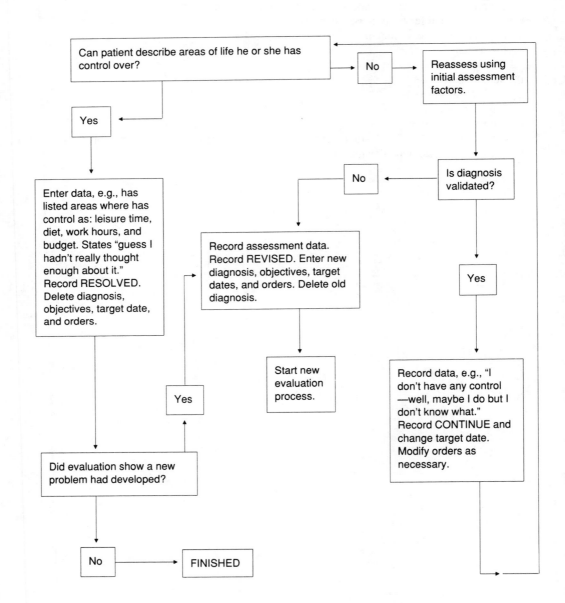

OBJECTIVE 2

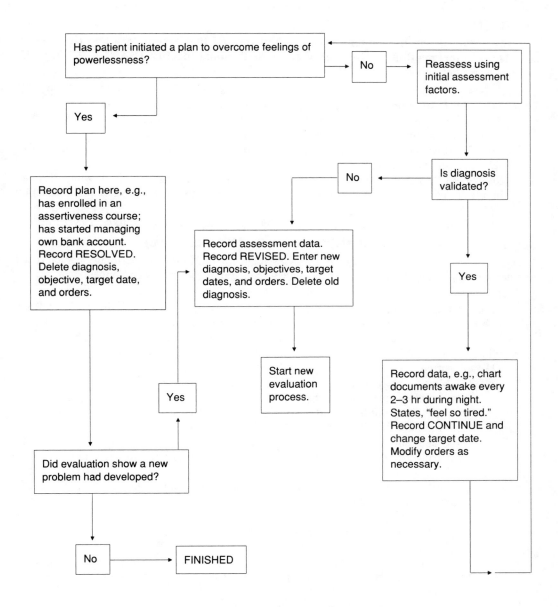

Self-Concept Disturbance in (Body Image, Self-Esteem, Personal Identity)

DEFINITION

A disruption in the individual's perception of the self that results in a negative view of self. This can include Body Image, Self-Esteem, or Personal Identity. (NANDA, 1987, p. 93)
Component definitions:

1. Body Image: Disruption in the way one perceives one's body image (NANDA, 1987, p. 93).
2. Self-Esteem: Disruption in the way one perceives one's self-esteem (NANDA, 1987, p. 95).
   a. Self-Esteem Disturbance: Negative self evaluation or feelings about self or self capabilities, which may be directly or indirectly expressed (NANDA., 1988).
   b. Chronic Low Self-Esteem: Longstanding negative self-evaluational feelings about self or self capabilities (NANDA, 1988).
   c. Situational Low Self-Esteem: Negative self evaluation or feelings about self which develop in response to a loss or change in an individual who previously had a positive self-evaluation (NANDA, 1988).
3. Personal Identity: Inability to distinguish between self and nonself (NANDA, 1987, p. 96).

DEFINING CHARACTERISTICS (NANDA, 1987, p. 95; 1988, pp. 93–96)

The nurse will review the initial pattern assessment for the following defining characteristics to determine the diagnosis of Self Concept, Disturbance in or one of its components.

1. Body Image
   a. Major defining characteristics—A *or* B must be present to justify the diagnosis of Body Image, Altered: A, verbal response to actual or perceived change in structure or function; B, nonverbal response to actual or perceived change in structure or function. The following clinical manifestations may be used to validate the presence of A *or* B.
      (1) Objective
         (a) Missing body part
         (b) Actual change in structure or function
         (c) Not looking at body part (intentional or unintentional)
         (d) Trauma to nonfunctioning part
         (e) Change in social involvement
         (f) Change in ability to estimate spatial relationship of body to environment
         (g) Not touching body part
         (h) Hiding or overexposing body part (intentional or unintentional)
      (2) Subjective verbalization of:
         (a) Change in life-style
         (b) Fear of rejection or of reaction by others
         (c) Focus on past strength, function, or appearance
         (d) Negative feelings about body
         (e) Feelings of helplessness, hopelessness, or powerlessness
         (f) Preoccupation with change or loss
         (g) Emphasis on remaining strengths, heightened achievement
         (h) Extension of body boundary to incorporate environmental objects
         (i) Personalization of part or loss by name
         (j) Depersonalization of part or loss by impersonal pronouns
         (k) Refusal to verify actual change
   b. Minor defining characteristics
      None given.
2. Self-Esteem
   a. Major defining characteristcs

   (1) Inability to accept positive reinforcememnt
   (2) Lack of follow-through
   (3) Nonparticipation in therapy
   (4) Not taking responsibility for self care (self-neglect)
   (5) Lack of eye contact
   (6) Self-destructive behavior
   b. Minor defining characteristics
       None given.
3. Self-Esteem Disturbance
   a. Major defining characteristics
       (1) Makes self-negating statements
       (2) Uses expressions of shame or guilt
       (3) Evaluates self as unable to deal with events
       (4) Rationalizes away or rejects positive feedback and exaggerates negative feedback about self
       (5) Is hesitant to try new things or situations
       (6) Denies problems obvious to others
       (7) Projects blame or responsibility for problems
       (8) Rationalizes personal failures
       (9) Is hypesensitive to slight or criticism
       (10) Is grandiose
   b. Minor defining characteristics
       None given.
4. Chronic Low Self-Esteem
   a. Major defining characteristics
       (1) Makes self-negating statements
       (2) Uses expressions of shame or guilt
       (3) Evaluates self as unable to deal with events
       (4) Rationalizes away or rejects positive feedback and exaggerates negative feedback about self
       (5) Is hesitant to try new things or situations
   b. Minor defining characteristics
       (1) Frequently lacks success in work or other life events
       (2) Is overly conforming, dependent on other's opinions
       (3) Lacks eye contact
       (4) Is nonassertive, passive
       (5) Is indecisive
       (6) Excessively seeks reassurance
5. Situational Low Self-Esteem
   a. Major defining characteristics
       (1) Episodic occurrence of negative self-appraisal in response to life events in a person with a previously positive self-evaluation
       (2) Verbalization of negative feelings about the self (helplessness, uselessness)
   b. Minor defining characteristics
       (1) Makes self-negating statements
       (2) Uses Expressions of shame or guilt
       (3) Evaluates self as unable to handle situations and events
       (4) Has difficulty making decisions
6. Personal Identity
   a. Major defining characteristics
       None given.

   b. Minor defining characteristics
      None given.

RELATED FACTORS (NANDA, 1987, pp. 93–97, 1988)

1. Body Image
   a. Biophysical
   b. Cognitive, perceptual
   c. Psychosocial
   d. Cultural or spiritual
2. Self-Esteem
   None given.
3. Self-Esteem Disturbance
   None given.
4. Chronic Low Self-Esteem
   None given.
5. Situtional Low Self-Esteem
   None given.
6. Personal Identity
   None given.

DIFFERENTIATION

The primary issues related to differentiation occur within the main category in relationship to the subcategories of Self-Esteem Disturbance, Body Image Disturbance, and Personal Identity Confusion.

Self-Esteem Disturbance addresses the lack of confidence in one's self and is characterized by negative self-statements, lack of concern about personal appearance, and withdrawal from others not related to physical problems or attributes.

Body Image Disturbance relates to alterations in perceptions of self related to actual or perceived alterations in body structure or function. If the primary alteration in self-perception is related to body structure or function, this diagnosis is primary.

Personal Identity is a disturbance in the individual's ability to perceive self and non-self. If the client demonstrates an inability to differentiate self from the environment or others, this would be the appropriate diagnosis. An example would be the client who perceives a life support machine as part of the self.

Self-Concept, Disturbance in should be differentiated from Anxiety; Individual Coping, Ineffective; Powerlessness; Sensory-Perceptual Alteration; Social Isolation; and Spiritual Distress.

Anxiety presents with a nonspecific threat. If the threat is specific and is identified with one of the Disturbed Self-Concept categories then the identified threat becomes the diagnosis.

Individual Coping, Ineffective results from the client's inability to cope appropriately with stress. If the client demonstrates a decreased ability to cope appropriately with the disturbance in self-concept the diagnosis may appear as Powerlessness, but rather than the individual acting out of a general belief about personal influence, it is a specific situation.

Sensory-Perceptual Alteration could produce a disturbance in Personal Identity and should be the primary diagnosis if the disturbance is produced by either a deficit or an excess in sensory input.

Social Isolation is aloneness perceived as imposed by others and may result from a Disturbance in Self-Concept, if the individual feels unworthy of interactions with others. If the Social Isolation evolves from Disturbance in Self-Concept, then the self-concept diagnosis would be appropriate.

Spiritual Distress is a questioning of one's life principles or values rather than questioning the self. If the doubt is focused only on the value-belief system, then Spiritual Distress would be the appropriate diagnosis.

OBJECTIVES

1. Will verbalize an increased number of positive self-concept statements by (date).

AND/OR

2. Will list at least (number) positive aspects about self by (date).

TARGET DATE

A target date of 3–5 days would be acceptable to begin monitoring of the program.

NURSING ORDERS

ADULT HEALTH

1. Collaborate with psychiatric nurse clinician regarding care (see Mental Health Care plan).
2. Teach the patient and significant others patient's self-care requirements.
3. Control pain.
4. Use anxiety-reducing techniques to assist patient in adapting self-concept.
5. Use frequent contact with patient to encourage verbalization of feelings:
   a. Be honest with patient
   b. Point out and limit self-negation statements
   c. Do not support denial
   d. Focus on reality and adaptation (not necessarily acceptance)
   e. Set limits on maladaptive behavior
   f. Focus on realistic goals
   g. Be aware of own nonverbal communication and behavior
   h. Avoid moral, value judgments
6. Promote calm, safe environment.
7. Allow patient to progress at own rate. Start with simple, concrete tasks. Reward success.
8. Encourage client to try to note differences in situations and events.
9. Help client to ascertain why he or she can maintain self-esteem in one situation and not in another situation.
10. Build on coping mechanisms or interpretations that maintain or increase self-esteem. Assist to find alternative coping mechanisms.
11. Encourage patient to use available resources:
    a. Prosthetic devices
    b. Assistive devices
    c. Reconstructive and corrective surgery
    d. Occupational therapy
    e. Physical therapy
12. Refer to and collaborate with community resources:
    a. Home health
    b. Support group
    c. Rehabilitation facilities
13. Encourage assertive behavior; assist to review passive and aggressive behavior.

CHILD HEALTH

1. Monitor for contributory factors related to poor self-concept, including:
   a. Family crisis;
   b. Lack of adequate parenting;
   c. Lack of sensory stimulation;
   d. Physical scars, malformation; or disfigurement;
   e. Altered role performance;
   f. Social isolation;

    g. Developmental crisis.
2. Identify ways patient can formulate or reestablish a positive self-concept according to developmental needs to address:
    a. Coping skills;
    b. Communication skills;
    c. Role expectations;
    d. Self-care;
    e. Daily activities of living;
    f. Basic physiologic needs, primary health care;
    g. Expression of self;
    h. Peer and social relationships;
    i. Feelings of self-worth;
    j. Decision-making;
    k. Validation of self.
3. Praise and reinforce positive behavior.
4. Explore value conflicts and their resolution.
5. Collaborate with health team members as needed to include:
    a. Pediatric subspecialist, psychiatrist
    b. Pediatric clinical nurse specialist
    c. Family therapist
    d. Play therapist
    e. School nurse
    f. Community health nurse
    g. School counselor
    h. Religious clergy person
    i. Social worker
    j. Peer support group members
    k. Legal counsel
    l. Child protective services
6. Meet primary health needs in an expedient manner.
7. Provide appropriate attention to other nursing pattern alterations, especially those directly affecting this pattern as Potential for Violence or Ineffective Parenting.
8. Provide for follow-up previous to dismissal from hospital as indicated.
9. Use developmentally appropriate strategies in care of these children:
    a. Infants and toddlers—play therapy, puppets
    b. Preschoolers—art
    c. School-agers—art, role playing
    d. Adolescents—discussion, role-playing
10. Carry out teaching of appropriate health maintenance (this could be the appropriate way of dealing with crisis related to shyness or poor communication skills).

WOMEN'S HEALTH

Body Image: Hysterectomy

1. Assist the client facing gynecologic surgery in identifying life-style adjustments that may be needed.
2. Provide explanation of medical procedure and resultant nursing care.
3. Provide factual information as to physiologic and psychologic changes client will experience.
4. Allow the client to grieve loss of body image (e.g., no longer able to have children).
5. Reassure the client that sexual activities do not need to change (e.g., she will still feel like a woman).

6. Involve significant others in discussion and problem-solving activities regarding life cycle changes that might affect self-concept and interpersonal relationships (e.g., hot flashes, sexual relationships, ability to have children).
7. Dispel "old wives' tales" such as:
    a. You will no longer feel like a woman (reassure client there will be no more pregnancies or menstruation; but hysterectomy *does not* affect sexual performance, enjoyment, or response).
    b. There will be masculinization (no basis for this belief, does not occur).
    c. There will be weight gain (will not occur if client follows former life-style and participates in an exercise routine and follows proper diet).
8. In collaboration with physician provide factual information on estrogen replacement therapy.
9. Monitor woman's response to having a hysterectomy.

Body Image: Mastectomy

10. Assist the the client facing mastectomy in identifying life-style adjustments that may be needed.
11. Provide an explanation of medical procedure and resultant nursing care.
12. Monitor the client's anxiety level and appropiately discuss, preoperatively, the physical and emotional changes she will experience:
    a. Routines related to surgery
        (1) Anesthesia
        (2) Pain
        (3) Time involved for surgery (particularly for significant others)
        (4) Equipment
        (5) Early mobility
        (6) Decreased joint stiffness
        (7) Minimal or no lymphedema
        (8) Faster return to normal functioning
13. Provide an empathetic atmosphere that will allow the client to ventilate fears and concerns and to ask questions:
    a. How will I look?
    b. How will significant others react?
    c. Will I still be able to wear sexy clothes?
14. Provide factual information as to physiologic and psychologic changes client will experience.
15. Allow the client to grieve loss of body parts and loss of body image.
16. Involve significant others in discussion and problem-solving activities regarding changes that might affect self-concept and interpersonal relationships.
17. Refer to appropriate support groups:
    a. Reach to Recovery
    b. Spiritual leader

Body Image: Pregnancy

18. Assist the client in identifying life-style adjustments due to physiologic, physical, and emotional changes that will occur throughout pregnancy and postpartum.
19. List the body changes that occur during pregnancy and the effect on body image (particularly for teenagers).
    a. Weight gain
    b. Breast tenderness and enlargement
    c. Enlargement of abdomen
    d. Change in gait
    e. Chloesma (mask of pregnancy)
    f. Striations (stretch marks) from pregnancy

20. Consider the client's age and preparation for pregnancy, including (particularly for teenagers):
    a. Stress weight loss after delivery usually takes 1 or 2 weeks
    b. Physical development
    c. Attitude toward health care providers
    d. Self-esteem
    e. Emotional support
    f. Life-style interruptions

Postpartum

21. Reassure the client that her prepregnant figure will return.
    a. Emphasize that weight loss usually takes 1 or 2 weeks.
    b. Encourage the client to bring an attractive, loose-fitting dress to wear home.
    c. Caution breastfeeding women against purposeful weight loss while lactating.
    d. Encourage non-breastfeeding mothers to follow low-calorie, high-protein diet for weight loss.
    e. Encourage exercise (begin slowly and work up to desired plan).
    f. Avoid fatigue.

Self-Esteem Disturbance

(Note: Nursing orders for mental health and adult health can apply to women with the following additions.)
22. Allow the client to "relive" birthing experience by listening quietly to her perception of the birthing experience.
23. Encourage the client to express her concerns about her physical appearance.
24. List activities in which the client can engage to gain positive feelings about herself.
    a. Join friends or an exercise group with the same goals as the client.
    b. Encourage in activities outside the home as appropriate (e.g., parenting support groups, women's groups, etc.)
25. Encourage networking with other women with similar interests.
26. Encourage the client to "do something for herself," e.g.,
    a. Buy a new dress
    b. Fix hair differently
    c. Find some time for herself during the day
       (1) Take a walk
       (2) Take a nice bath
       (3) Rest quietly
       (4) Do a favorite thing (e.g., reading, sewing, or some hobby)
       (5) Spend time with spouse, without the children (let grandparents babysit)
27. Encourage the client to engage in positive thinking.
28. Encourage the client to engage in assertiveness training.

MENTAL HEALTH

1. Sit with client (number) minutes (number) times per shift to discuss client's feelings about self.
2. Answer questions honestly.
3. Provide feedback to client about nurses' perceptions of the client's abilities and appearance by:
    a. Using "I" statements;
    b. Using references related to the nurse's relationship to the client;
    c. Describing the client's behavior in situations;
    d. Describing the nurse's feelings in relationship.
4. Provide positive reinforcement (list those things that are reinforcing for the client and when

they are to be used, also list those things that have been identified as nonreinforcers for this client; include social rewards).

5. Provide group interaction with (number) of persons (number) minutes three times a day at (times). (This activity should be gradual within client's ability; i.e., on admission client may tolerate one person for 5 minutes. If the interactions are brief the frequency should be high; i.e., 5-minute interactions should occur at 30-minute intervals).

6. Protect client from harm by:
   a. Removing all sharp objects from environment;
   b. Removing belts and strings from environment;
   c. Providing a one-to-one constant interaction if potential for self-harm is high;
   d. Checking on client's whereabouts every 15 minutes;
   e. Removing glass objects from environment;
   f. Removing locks from room and bathroom doors;
   g. Providing a shower curtain that will not support weight;
   h. Checking to see if client swallows medications.

7. Reflect back to client negative self-statements made by the client. (This should be done with a supportive attitude in a manner that will increase client's awareness of these negative evaluations of self).

8. Set achievable goals for client.

9. Provide activities that the client can accomplish and that the client values (care should be taken not to provide tasks or activities the client finds demeaning or this could reinforce client's negative self-evaluation).

10. Provide verbal reinforcement for achievement of steps toward a goal.

11. Have the client develop a list of strengths and potentials.

12. Define the client's lack of goal achievement or failures as simple mistakes that are bound to occur when one attempts something new (e.g., learning comes with mistakes, if one does not make mistakes one does not learn).

13. Define past failures as the client's best attempts to solve a problem (e.g., if the client had known a better solution he or she would have used it; one does not set out to fail).

14. Make necessary items available for the client to groom self.

15. Spend (number) minutes at (time) assisting the client with grooming, providing necessary assistance and positive reinforcement for accomplishments.

16. Reflect back to the client those statements that discount the positive evaluations of others.

17. Focus the client's attention on the here and now (past happenings are difficult for the nurse to provide feedback on).

18. Present the client with opportunities to make decisions about care and record these decisions on the care plan.

19. Develop with the client alternative coping strategies.

20. Practice new coping behavior with the client (number) minutes at (times).

Body Image

21. Spend (number) minutes with the client at (times) discussing perception of disruption in life-style necessitated by change.

22. Discuss with the client meaning of loss or change from a personal and cultural perspective.

23. Discuss with the client significant other's reaction to loss or change.

24. Set an appointment to discuss with the client and significant others effects of the loss or change on their relationships. (Time and date of appointment and all follow-up appointments should be listed here.)

25. Monitor the nurses's nonverbal reactions to loss or change and provide the client with verbal information when necessary to establish the nurse's acceptance of the change.

26. Spend (number) minutes with the client at (times) to assist with efforts to enhance appearance.

27. Refer to appropriate support groups. (The name of the contact person and times of visits should be listed here and could include ostomy support groups, mastectomy groups, organized sports activities for the physically handicapped, etc.)
28. Approach nursing care of loss or change in a positive, matter-of-fact manner.
29. Provide physical activities two times per day at (times) that provide the client opportunities to define boundaries of body. (These activities should be ones the client identifies as enjoyable and that are easily accomplished by the client. Those activities that are selected should be listed here. If this diagnosis is in conjunction with an eating disorder, adjust exercise to appropriate levels for the client.)
30. Discuss with the client the difference between the cultural ideal of physical appearance and the population norm based on the realities of physiology. (This activity should be done by the primary care nurse who has developed a relationship with the client.)
31. Have the client draw a picture of self before and after body change and discuss this with them. This activity can also be done with clay models constructed by the client. (This activity should be done by the primary care nurse who has developed a relationship with the client.)
32. Have the eating disorder client draw a life-size picture of self on paper hung on the wall, then have the client stand against the picture and trace the real outline and discuss the differences. (This activity should be done by the primary care nurse who has developed a relationship with the client.)
33. When the client has begun to discuss issues related to body change with the primary care nurse, the client can then be asked to discuss reactions to image of self in a mirror. One hour should be allowed for this activity. (This activity should be done by the primary care nurse who has developed a relationship with the client.)
34. Discuss with the client the mental images held of what the altered body is like and what life will be like. (One hour should be allowed for this activity and it should be implemented by the primary care nurse after a relationship has been established).

Self-Esteem

35. Place the client in a therapy group for (number) minutes once a day where the focus is mutual sharing of feelings and support of each other to facilitate the client's awareness of others' thoughts about themselves and him or her.
36. Identify with the client those situations that are perceived as most threatening to self-esteem.
37. Assist the client in identifying alternative methods of coping with the identified situations. (These should be developed by the client and listed here.)
38. Role play with the client once per day for 45 minutes those high-risk situations that were identified and the alternative coping methods.
39. Establish an appointment with the client and significant others to discuss their perceptions of the client's situation (the time of this and follow-up appointments should be listed here).
40. Discuss with the client current behavior and reactions of others to this behavior.
41. Practice with client (number) minutes twice a day making positive "I" statements.

Personal Identity

42. Provide a quiet, nonstimulating environment.
43. Provide frequent interactions that assist the client with orientation. Verbal information should be provided in simple, brief sentences.
44. Sit with the client (number) minutes (number) times per day at (list specific times here) to provide the client with an opportunity to discuss feelings and thoughts.
45. Provide the client with honest, direct feedback in all interactions.
46. Utilize constructive confrontation if necessary to include:
    a. "I" statements
    b. Relationship statements that reflect nurse's reaction to the interaction

    c. Responses that will assist the client in understanding such as paraphrasing and validation of perceptions.
47. Discuss with the client the source of the threat.
48. Develop with the client alternative coping strategies. (Those activities, items, or verbal responses that are rewarding for the client should be listed here).
49. When the client is presented with a threat, assist with progressing through one of the alternative coping methods or practice with the client the alternative coping methods (number) minutes twice a day.
50. Develop achievable goals with the client. (The goals that are appropriate for this client should be listed here.)
51. As the client masters the first set of goals, develop increasingly complex goals and problems.
52. Provide positive reinforcement for accomplishments at any level. (Those activities, items, or verbal responses that are rewarding for the client should be listed here.)
53. Do not argue with the client who is experiencing an alteration in thought process. (Refer to Chapter 7 for related care plan for Thought Process, Altered.)
54. Monitor the client's mental status before attempting learning or confrontation. If the client is disoriented, orient to reality as needed.
55. If disorientation is present related to organic brain dysfunction, distract client from those disorientations that are not corrected with a brief, simple explanation. (Short-term memory loss will assist with changing client's orientation without getting into a strong confrontation.)

HOME HEALTH

1. Involve the patient and family in planning and implementing strategies to reduce and cope with disturbances in self-concept.
   a. Family conference
   b. Mutual goal setting
   c. Communication
2. Assist the patient and family in life-style adjustments that may be required:
   a. Obtaining and providing accurate information
   b. Clarifying misconceptions
   c. Maintaining safe environment
   d. Encouraging appropriate self-care without encouraging dependence or expecting unrealistic independence
   e. Providing opportunity for expressing feelings
   f. Realistic goal-setting
   g. Providing sense of mastery: accomplishable goals in secure environment
   h. Maintaining the treatment plan of the health care professionals guiding therapy
   i. Relaxation techniques: yoga, biofeedback, hypnosis, breathing techniques, imagery
   j. Altering roles
   k. Encouraging touching, viewing, and caring for site which is contributing to body image disturbance
3. Consult with or refer to assistive resources as indicated:
   a. Rehabilitation therapist
   b. Prosthesis manufacturer
   c. Ostomy therapist
   d. Psychiatric nurse clinician
   e. Visiting nurse
   f. Support groups
   g. Physician
   h. Occupational therapist
   i. Physical therapist

j. Relaxation trainer
k. Social service
l. Family counselor
m. Financial counselor

EVALUATION
OBJECTIVE 1

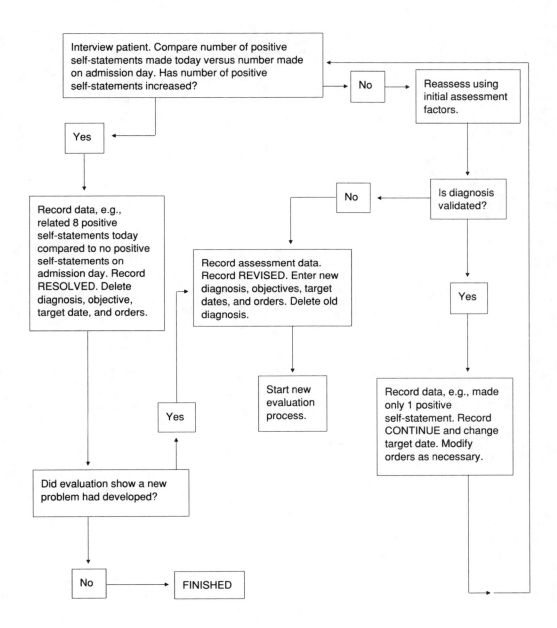

OBJECTIVE 2

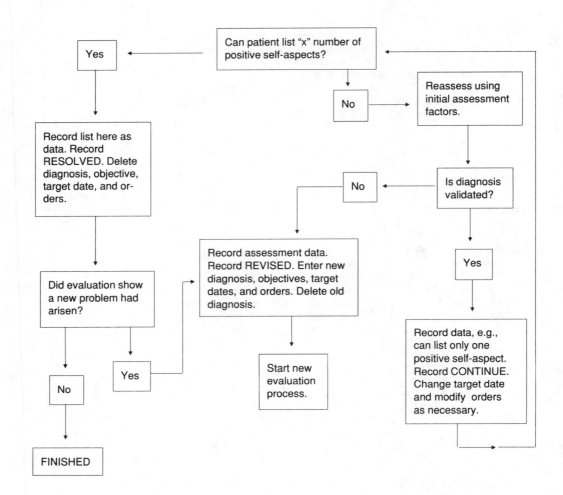

REFERENCES

Bateson, G. (1972). *Steps to an ecology of mind*. New York: Ballantine.

Bruch, H. (1968). Interpersonal theory: Harry Stack Sullivan. In A. Burton (Ed.), *Operational theories of personality*. New York: Brunner-Mazel.

Carpenito, L. J. (1983). *Nursing diagnosis: Application to clinical practice*. New York: J. B. Lippincott.

Dufault, K., & Martocchio, B. (1985). Hope: Its spheres and dimensions. *Nursing Clinics of North America, 20* (2), 379–391.

Evans, R. (1976). *The making of psychology*. New York: Alfred Knopf.

Fogel, E. I., & Woods, N. F. (1981). *Health care of women: A nursing perspective*. St. Louis: C. V. Mosby.

Glasersfeld, E. V. (1985). Cybernetics, experience and the concept of self. In K. J. Gergen & R. E. Davis (Eds.), *The social construction of the person* (pp. 67–113). New York: Springer-Verlag.

Gordon, C., & Gergen, K. J. (Eds.). (1968). *The self in social interaction: Vol. 1. Classic and contemporary perspectives*. New York: John Wiley & Sons.

Griffith-Kenney, J. (1986). *Contemporary women's health: A nursing advocacy approach*. Menlo Park, CA: Addison-Wesley.

James, W. (1968). The self. In C. Gordon & K. J. Gergen (Eds.), *The self in social interaction; Vol. 1. Classic and contemporary perspectives*. (pp.41–49). New York: John Wiley & Sons.

Jourard, S. (1968). Healthy personality and self-disclosure. In C. Gordon & K. T. J. Gergen (Eds.), *The self in social interaction: Vol. 1. Classic and contemporary perspectives*. (pp. 423–434). New York: John Wiley & Sons.

Keeney, B. (1983). *Aesthetics of change*. New York: Guilford.

Lynch, W. F. (1974). *Images of hope: Imagination as healer of the hopeless*. Notre Dame, IN: University of Notre Dame Press.

McGee, R. (1984). Hope: A factor influencing crisis resolution. *Advances in Nursing Science, 7* (4), 34–43.

Mead, G. H. (1968). The genesis of self. In C. Gordon & K. J. Gergen (Eds.), *The self in social interaction: Vol. 1. Classic and contemporary perspectives*, (pp. 51–59). New York: John Wiley & Sons.

Miller, J. (1985). Inspiring hope. *American Journal of Nursing, 85* (1), 22–25.

North American Nursing Diagnosis Association. (1987). *Taxonomy I with complete diagnoses*. St. Louis: Author.

North American Nursing Diagnosis Association. (1988). *Prosposed nursing diagnoses*. St. Louis: Author.

Perry, H. S., & Gawel, M. L. (1953). *The interpersonal theory of psychiatry*. New York: Norton & Co.

Sullivan, H. S. (1968). Beginnings of the self-system. In C. Gordon & K. J. Gergen (Eds.), *The self in social interaction: Vol. 1. Classic and contemporary perspectives* (pp. 171–177). New York: John Wiley & Sons.

Turner, R. (1968). The self-conception in social interaction. In C. Gordon & K. J. Gergen (Eds.), *The self in social interaction: Vol. 1. Classic and contemporary perspectives*, (pp. 93–106). New York: John Wiley & Sons.

Vaillot, M. (1970). Hope the restoration of being. *American Journal of Nursing, 70*(2), 268–273.

Watts, A. (1966). *The book: On the taboo against knowing who you are*. New York: Random House.

Watson, J. (1985). *Nursing: The philosophy and science of caring*. Boulder, CO: Colorado Associated University Press.

SUGGESTED READINGS

Bateson, G. (1979). *Mind and nature*. New York: Bantam.

Crittendon, R. (1983). *Discharge planning*. Bowie, MD: Robert J. Brady.

Doenges, M., & Moorhouse, M. (1985). *Nurse's pocket guide: Nursing diagnosis with interventions*. Philadelphia: F. A. Davis.

Garner, D., & Garfinkel, P. (Eds.).(1985). *Handbook of psychotherapy for anorexia nervosa and bulimia*. New York: The Guilford Press.

Gettrust, K., Ryan, S., & Engleman, D. (1985). *Applied nursing diagnosis: Guides for comprehensive care planning*. New York: John Wiley & Sons.

Haber, J., Leach, A., Schudy, S., & Sideleau, B. (1982). *Comprehensive psychiatric nursing* (2nd ed.). New York: McGraw-Hill.

Hadeka, M. (1987). *Clinical judgment in community health nursing*. Boston: Little, Brown.

Jaffe, M., & Skidmore-Roth, L. (1988). *Home health nursing care plans*. St. Louis: C. V. Mosby.

Jensen, M. D., & Bobak, I. M. (1985). *Maternity and gynecologic care: The nurse and the family*. St. Louis: C. V. Mosby.

Kelly, M. A. (1985). *Nursing diagnosis source book*. East Norwalk, CT: Appleton-Century-Crofts.

McClelland, E., Kelly, K., & Buckwalter, K. (1984). *Continuity of care: Advancing the concept of discharge planning*. Orlando, FL: Grune & Stratton.

National League for Nursing. (1988). *Accreditation program for home care and community health: Criteria and standards.* New York: Author.

Rinke, L. (1988). *Outcome standards in home health.* New York: National League for Nursing.

Schilder, P. (1968). The image and appearance of the human body. In C. Gordon & K. J. Gergen (Eds.), *The self in social interaction* (pp. 107–114). New York: Springer-Verlag.

Schuster, C., & Ashburn, S. (1980). *The process of human development.* Boston: Little, Brown.

Slaby, A., Lieb, J., & Tancredi, L. (1981). *Handbook of psychiatric emergencies* (2nd ed.). New York: Medical Examination Publishing.

Smitherman, C. (1981). *Nursing actions for health promotion.* Philadelphia: F. A. Davis.

Sonstegard, L. J., Kowalski, K. M. & Jennings, B. (1983). *Women's health: Vol. 2 Childbearing.* New York: Grune & Stratton.

Steffi, B., & Eide, I. (1978). *Discharge planning handbook.* New York: Charles B. Slack.

Walsh, J., Persons, C., & Wieck, L. (1987). *Manual of home health care nursing.* Philadelphia: J. B. Lippincott.

Wilson, H., & Kneisl, C. (1983). *Psychiatric nursing* (2nd ed.). Reading, MA: Addison-Wesley.

CHAPTER NINE

Role-Relationship Pattern

Pattern Description

The role-relationship pattern is concerned with how a person feels he or she is performing the expected behavior delineated by the self and others. A disturbance in self-concept or self-image may result in altered self-esteem, questions regarding personal identity, or a change in role performance. For these reasons, the nurse must be cautious in interpreting data for specifying personal values, beliefs, and kinds of behavior the patient may exhibit as to appropriateness in role performance. The reason a patient seeks nursing assistance may be the alteration in role-relationship functioning, or it may be a secondary or resultant consideration of one or more other patterns. It is paramount to identify that actual role-relationship patterns are indeed threatened in times of illness or crisis. The nurse must keenly appreciate the patient's concept of role and self and its impact on the patient as a recipient of nursing care.

Pattern Assessment

1. Patient's description of usual role-relationship functioning:
   a. Daily activities of living
   b. Usual relationships of daily living
   c. Perceived threats, actual changes, or loss in any of the described role-relationship patterns
   d. Factors related to any of the aforementioned, to include self, family, work, finances, social obligations or desires, or situational factors
2. Description of patient's general appearance:
   a. Personal hygiene, attire
   b. Posture, gait, facial expression, or body language
   c. Overt signs of emotional distress:
      (1) Weeping
      (2) Anger, hostility
      (3) Inappropriate affect
   d. Response to nurse and others
3. Description of patient's mental status:
   a. Capacity for ideation, orientation to reality, attention span, and problem-solving capacity
   b. Insight into current situation
   c. Capacity for identification of unresolved conflicts which may be related to current situation
   d. Usual coping strategies

Conceptual Information

The social connotation for role performance and relationships is a major premise for the intended use of this pattern. A role is a comprehensive pattern of behavior which is socially recognized, provides a means of identifying, and places an individual in a society. It also serves as a means of coping with recurrent situations. The term "role" is a borrowed theatrical noun which emphasizes the distinction of the actor and the part. A role remains relatively stable even though there may be a variety of persons occupying the position or role. Uniqueness of style may exist within the boundaries of the role as determined by society.

Because roles are such an integral part of our lives they are seldom analyzed until they become a problem to one's internal or external adaptation to life's demands. Roles which are often associated with stages of development serve as society's guides for meaningful and satisfying relationships in life by facilitating an orderly method for transferring knowledge, responsibility, and authority from one generation to the next.

During the childhood years, an individual will have numerous contacts with different individuals of differing values. The child learns to internalize the values of those significant in his or her life as personal goals are actualized. When the goals are realistic, consistent, and attainable, the individual is assisted in developing a sense of self-esteem as these various roles are mastered. Each new role carries with it the potential for gratification and increased ego-identity if the role is acquired. If the role is not mastered, poor self-esteem and role confusion may ensue. The potential for successful role mastery is diminished with multiple role demands and the absence of suitable role models. Additionally, role acquisition depends on adequate patterns of cognitive-perceptual ability and a healthy sense of self.

Although all roles are learned within the context of one's culture, specific roles are delineated in two ways: acquired and achieved. Acquired roles are those roles with variables over which the individual has no choice such as gender, race, etc. Role achievement allows for some choice by the individual with the result of purposefully earning a role such as choosing to become a professional nurse.

Many roles are not clearly defined as being either acquired or achieved, but rather are a combination of the two. Roles are not mutually exclusive, but are interdependent. The roles an individual assumes usually blend well; however, the roles that a person achieves or acquires may not always make for a harmonious blend. Role conflicts may occur from the most internalized personal level to a generalized societal level.

Roles may be influenced by a multitude of factors, including economics, family dynamics, changing roles of institutions, and gender role expectations. It is hoped that with the increased demands on the individual, society will continue to value human dignity with respect for life itself. Roles should allow for self-actualization.

Symbolic interaction encompasses the roles assumed by humans in their constant interaction with other humans, communicating symbolically in almost all they do. This interaction has meaning to both the giver and the receiver of the action, thus requiring both persons to interact symbolically with themselves as they interact with each other. Symbolic interaction involves interpretation, or ascertaining the meaning of the actions or remarks of the other person, and definition, or conveying indications to another person as to how he or she is to act. Human association consists of a process of such interpretation and definition. Through this process the participants fit their own acts to the on going acts of one another and guide others in doing so (Shibutani, 1970).

To explore further how relationships develop, a brief overview of kinship is offered. A kinship system is a structured system of relationships in which individuals are bound one to another by complex, interlocking relationships. Though functionally differentiated, all these relationships, as compared with extrafamilial relationships, tend to be characterized by a high degree of reciprocal cooperation, loyalty, solidarity, and affection. Despite cultural differences, each of the primary relationships reveals a markedly similar fundamental character in all societies, as a consequence of the universality of the family's basic functions. These relationships with their most typical features are (Murdock, 1949):

Husband and Wife: Economic specialization and cooperation; sexual cohabitation; joint responsibility for support, care, and upbringing of children; well-defined reciprocal rights with respect to property, divorce, spheres of authority.

Father and Son: Economic cooperation in masculine activities under leadership of the father; obligation of material support vested in father during childhood of son and in son during old age of father; responsibility of father for instruction and discipline of son; duty of obedience and respect on part of son, tempered by some measure of comradeship.

Mother and Daughter: Relationship parallel to that between father and son, but with more emphasis on child care and economic cooperation and less on authority and material support.

Father and Daughter: Responsibility of father for protection and material support prior to marriage of daughter; economic cooperation, instruction, and discipline appreciably less prominent than in father-son relationship; playfulness common in infancy of daughter, but normally yields to a measure of reserve with the development of a strong incest taboo.

Elder and Younger Brothers: Relationship of playmates, developing into that of comrades; economic cooperation under leadership of elder; moderate responsibility of elder for instruction and discipline of younger.

Elder and Younger Sisters: Relationship parallel to that between elder and younger brother but with more emphasis on physical care of the younger sister.

Brother and Sister: Early relationship of playmates, varying with relative age; gradual development of an incest taboo, commonly coupled with some measure of reserve; moderate economic cooperation; partial assumption of parental role, especially by the elder sibling.

Adult

As the adult acquires full role responsibility, there may be difficulties related to role diffusion, role confusion, role strain, or related assumption of appropriate roles. Also, the ultimate developmental need for assumption of accountability for self may be unresolved. There may be greater likelihood for the various demands of society on male and female roles to be experienced at this time as women assume the multiple roles of wife, mother, worker, housekeeper, etc., just as men also have assumed more and more roles which were formerly assumed by females. This challenge also brings the potential for growth and fulfillment in self-actualizing individuals.

Older Adult

With aging, there perhaps is the potential for fewer demands being placed on the individual, thus leaving more time and fewer opportunities potentially for role performance. This may also be a time when one is able to fulfill volunteer roles and those of choice versus those of demand. A critical factor may be the freedom one feels as basic needs are provided for. If health is satisfactory and one has children or grandchildren to enjoy, financial stability, and is able to pursue fulfillment via role engagement, this would be a self-actualizing experience. On the other hand, if one's health fails, few meaningful family supports exist, and financial needs arise, self-actualizing role performance is potentially threatened.

A more recent eclectic theory of personality development encompassing role theory is that of symbolic interaction. In this orientation, social interaction has symbolic meaning to the participants in relation to the roles assigned by society. (For further related conceptual information, refer to Chapter 8, Self-Perception and Self-Concept Pattern.) The nurse must exercise great caution in maintaining sensitivity to the individual meaning attached to social roles and the way in which these roles are perceived and assumed.

Developmental Considerations

Neonate and Infant

The newborn period is especially critical for the development of the first attachment which is so vital for all future human relationships. Attachment behavior includes crying, smiling, clinging, following, and cuddling. The infant is dependent on its mother and father for basic needs of survival. This is often demanding and requires parents to place self-needs secondary to the needs of the infant. This makes for a potential role-relationship alteration.

Although dependent on others, the infant is an active participant in role-relationship pattern development from conception on. The infant is capable of influencing the interactions of those caring for him or her. Reciprocal interactions also influence the maternal-paternal-infant relationship. Positive interactions will be greatly influenced by infant-initiated behavior as well as maternal-paternal responses and the reciprocal interaction of all involved. The state of the infant as well as the state of the parent interacting with the infant must be considered as critical.

It is important to note that any alteration in health status of the mother, the neonate, or both has the potential of interfering with the establishment of the maternal-infant relationship. This may not necessarily be the case, but it is often critical that the potential risk be acknowledged early so that residual, secondary problems can be prevented with appropriate nursing intervention. It is also important to keep in mind that the infant is taking in all situational experiences and that as learning occurs through interaction with the environment, a gradual evolution of role-relationship patterns occur.

By approximately 12 months of age, the infant shows fear of being left alone and will search for the parents with his or her eyes. The infant will avoid and reject strangers. There is an obvious increasing interest in pleasing parent. In protest the infant cries, screams, and searches for the parent. In despair the infant is listless, withdrawn, and disinterested with the environment. In detachment or resignation a superficial "adjustment" occurs in which the infant appears interested in surroundings, happy, and friendly for short periods of time. The infant is emotionally changeable from crying to laughing with a beginning awareness of separation from the environment. Still, the infant uses mother as a safe haven from which to explore the world. The infant will have a favorite toy, blanket, or other object which serves to comfort him or her in times of stress. (Sucking behavior may also serve to calm the infant, and eventually the infant will develop self-initiated ways of dealing with the stressors of life, such as thumb-sucking versus the actual taking of formula or milk.)

The infant receives cues from significant others and primary caregivers regarding grief responses such as crying, with a preference for the mother. Depending on age and situational status, the infant may protest by crying for mother. In a weakened state, the infant may make little response of preference for caregivers.

According to family structure, the neonate or infant will adapt to usual socialization routines within reasonable limits. Actual isolation for the infant would occur perhaps if the primary caregiver could not exercise usual role-taking behavior for socialization. If this behavior is arrested for marked periods of time, there is a potential for developmental delays secondary to the lack of appropriate social stimulation.

The newborn period is especially critical for the development of the neonate's first attachment for future human relationship. During this period the infant must depend on others for care and basic needs. This is often a demanding situation for parents who must sacrifice their own needs to best meet the needs of the infant.

The infant is dependent on others for care ranging from required food for physical growth to appropriate sensory and social stimulation. In the absence of the stability usually afforded by the family in its usual functioning pattern, the infant may be at risk for failure to thrive or developmental delay. Ultimately, rather than developing a sense of trust and feeling in the world as a place in which one's needs are met, the infant will doubt and mistrust others. This in turn places the infant at risk for an abnormal pattern of development.

Crying serves as the primitive verbal communication for the neonate and infant. As the infant begins to understand and respond to the spoken word, the world should be symbolized as comforting and safe. With time, basic attempts at verbalization are noted in imitation of what is heard. There is a correlation between parental speech stimulation and the actual development of speech in young children, suggesting a positive effect for early stimulation. Echolalia and attempts at making speech are most critical to note during this time.

The infant may be the recipient of violent behavior and all too often it is because of crying.

The attempt to quiet the infant can take the form of lashing out for those individuals unable to deal with usual role-relationship patterns. The infant is unable to defend itself, and therefore is to be protected by reporting of any suspected abusive or negligent behavior by others. At particular risk would be infants with feeding or digestive disorders, premature or small for gestational age infants who require feedings every 2 hours, or others perceived as "demanding" or "irritable." Also at risk would be infants who are born with congenital anomalies or disfigurement.

Toddler

The toddler has an increasing sense of identity and knows himself or herself as a separate person. The toddler treats other children as if they were objects, and gradually becomes involved in parallel play which then leads to a more interactive play with peers. The sharing of possessions is not yet to be expected for toddlers. The toddler begins to formulate a sense of right and wrong with the ability to conform to some social demands, as exemplified by the capacity for self-toileting. It is reasonable that a toddler would begin to work through problems of family relations with other children in play.

The preschool child talks and plays with an imaginary playmate as a projection. What is offered may be what the child views as bad in himself or herself. The preschooler may have some friends of the same sex, and opportunities for socialization serve critical functions. The preschool child lives in the "here and now" and is capable of internalizing more and more of society's norms. There is a sense of morality and conscience by this age. A strong sense of family exists for the preschooler.

The toddler may be unusually dependent on mother, objects of security, and routines. He or she is capable of magical thinking and may believe in animation of inanimate objects, such as believing an x-ray machine is really a mean monster. Toddlers may be fearful of seeing blood. These fears may be unrelated to actual situations.

The preschooler may be critical of himself or herself and may blame himself or herself for a situation with some attempt at viewing the current situation as punishment for previous behavior or thoughts. He or she will tolerate brief separation from parents in usual functioning. Play or puppet therapy which is appropriate to the situation will help the preschooler in expressing feelings.

The toddler must have room to safely explore with a sense of autonomy evolving in the ideal situation. If social isolation limits these opportunities, the toddler will be limited in role-relationship exposure. This will often result in either social isolation or a form of forced precocious role-taking in which the toddler is perceived as being able to satisfy the companionship needs of adults. The toddler may misinterpret socialization opportunities as abandonment or punishment, so short intervals of parallel play with one peer, to begin with, would be appropriate. Toddlers who are denied opportunities for peer interaction would be at risk for role-relationship problems.

The child of the preschool age group may experience alteration in socialization attempts if overpowered by peers, if there are too many rigid or unrealistic rules, or if the situation places the child in a situation which presents values greatly different from those of the child and his or her family. If the child at this age experiences prolonged social isolation or rejection there could be marked potential for difficulty in forming future relationships. If things do not go well regarding socialization, the child at this age may blame himself or herself.

The toddler will seek out opportunities to explore and interact with the environment, provided there is a safe haven to return to as represented by the family. When this facilitative factor is not present, the toddler may regress and become dependent on primary caregivers or others, or may manifest frustration via extremes in demanding behavior. The child's subsequent development may also be affected by family process alteration.

The preschool child is able to verbalize concerns regarding changes in family process but is unable to comprehend dynamics. It is critical to attempt to view the altered process through the eyes of the preschooler who could blame himself or herself for the change or crisis, or who may think magically and have fears which may be unrelated to the situation. Subsequent development may be altered by family process dysfunction, with regression often occurring.

At this age it is important to stress the need for ritualistic behavior as a means of mastering the environment with adequate anticipatory safety. This period allows for knowing "self" as a separate entity. The toddler is capable of attempting to conform to social demands but lacks ability of self-control.

The importance of setting limits must be stressed with regard to safety and disciplinary management. At this age the child begins to resist parental authority. Methods of dealing with differences of rules from one setting to another must be simple and appropriate to the situation.

For the toddler this time can prove frustrating with a need to be understood despite a limited vocabulary.

For the toddler this time can prove frustrating with a need to be understood despite a limited vocabulary. Jargon and gestures may be misinterpreted with resultant frustration for child and parent. Patience and understanding go far with a child of this age. Pictures and the telling of stories serve as means of enhancing speech as well as instilling an appreciation for reading and speech. Feelings come to be expressed by the spoken word also. The child is able to refer to self as "I," "me," or by name.

By preschool age, the child is able to count to 10, is able to define at least one word, and may name four or five colors. Speech now serves as a part of socialization in play with peers. Wants should be expressed freely as the child broadens his or her contact with persons other than primary family members. This child enjoys stories and television programs and attempts to tell stories of his or her own creation.

If the toddler is unable to fulfil the expectations of parents or caregivers who demand unrealistic behavior, there is risk of abuse. Especially noteworthy would be a desire for the young toddler to be capable of self-toileting behavior when in fact such is not possible. This places the toddler in a target population for abuse also. At this age the toddler may be unable to express hostility or anger in the verbal mode and so a common occurrence may be temper tantrums. At risk for violence would be the toddler who resists parental authority in discipline and cannot meet demands of the parents.

School-age Child

Learning social roles as male or female is a major task for the school-age child with a preference for spending time with friends of the same sex rather than the family. The school-ager is capable of role-taking and values cooperation and fair play. There may be a strict moralism of "black" and "white" with no gray areas noted. The school-ager enjoys simple household chores, likes a reward system, and has the capacity for expressing feelings. Fear of disability and concern for missing school are typical concerns for this age group.

Illness may impose separation from the peer group. Although independent of parents in health, the school-ager may require close parental relationship in illness or crisis. Loss of control and fear of mutilation and death are real concerns. The school-age child may fear disgracing parents if loss of control such as crying occurs. He or she is aware of the severity of his or her prognosis and may even deal with reality better than parents or adults might. The school-age child may use art as a means of expressing his or her feelings.

This child is at risk of social isolation if a situation is different from previous socialization opportunities. He or she may experience value conflict and question the rules. He or she may also be afraid to express desires or concerns regarding socialization needs for fear of punishment. Peer involvement is a most vital component of assisting the school-ager to formulate views of acceptable social behavior.

The school-ager may try to assume the role of a parent if the dysfunction of the family relates to the parent of the same sex. This may be healthy with appropriate acknowledgment of limitations.

At this age, the child is concerned with what other friends may think about the family with some stigma attached in certain cultures to divorce, homosexuality, and altered life-styles. It would be critical for the school-ager to have a close friend who might share the cultural views of his or her own family to best endure the altered family process.

Allowance for increasing interests outside the home should be made with a sensitivity to parental approval or disapproval. The child may rebel against parental authority in an attempt to be like peers.

Confidence in self and a general sense of well-being will promote adequacy in communication development. The child of this age continues to learn vocabulary and takes pride in his or her ability to demonstrate appropriate use of words. At this age jokes and riddles serve as a means of encouraging peer interaction with speech. Reading is a leisure activity for the school-age child.

The child will usually enjoy school and consider peer interaction an enjoyable part of life. In instances in which the child feels inferior there may be a risk for violence or abusive behavior as a coverup for poor self-image or low self-esteem. Often there will be related role-relationship alterations as well. The family serves as a means of valuing the interaction which should foster the appropriate enjoyment of friendships. At risk would be those children with learning disabilities or handicaps, parental conflicts, or related role-relationship alterations.

Adolescent

Vacillation between dependence and independence is a common occurrence for the adolescent who is attempting to establish a sense of identity. The adolescent questions traditional values, especially those of parents. There is a gradual trend to independent functioning which allows the adolescent to assume roles of adulthood, including the development of intensive relationships with members of the opposite sex.

The adolescent will be constantly weighing self-identity versus perceived identity expressed via peers. He or she may be fearful of expressing true feelings or concern for fear of rejection by peers, parents, or significant others. Isolation from peers will place the adolescent at risk for altered self-identity as well as altered role-relationship patterns.

The adolescent is able to assist within the family during times of altered process. It is important to stress that in more and more dual-career or single-parent families, young adolescents spend more and more time alone. Nonetheless, adolescents should still have opportunities for peer interaction and socialization according to the family's needs.

There may be marked vacillation, as the adolescent strives to find self-identity, with dependence and independence issues. Even more marked rebellion against parental wishes may be manifest at this time as peer approval is sought.

Any factors that may interfere with usual speech patterns may prove especially difficult for the adolescent. Bracing of teeth may be common, with the potential for self-image alteration. Also, the eruption of 12-year molars could prove painful as might the possible impaction of wisdom teeth later. Expressed wit is valued in this age group, as might be special colloquial expressions to qualify group or peer identity. Difficulty in expression of self may prove most difficult for this individual. Respect for times of reflection and estrangement should be maintained.

The adolescent may be caught in a crossfire of strife for independence versus dependence. For this group it is paramount that self-control be attained to develop the meaningful relationships so critical for appropriate role-relationship patterns. Often those adolescents who have not acquired appropriate socialization skills resort to drugs or alcohol as a means of feeling better and escaping the reality of life. This may also foster loss of control as reality is distorted. In many instances there may be related juvenile delinquency with resultant records of lawbreaking.

Additionally, any adolescent who is assuming a role which stresses or negates the usual development of self-identity would be at risk for violence as a means of coping. An example of this would be two young teenagers attempting to parent when they themselves still require parenting.

Young Adult

Although biophysical and cognitive skills reach their peak during the adult years, the young adult is still in a period of growth and development. Striving for achievement of an education, job security, meaningful intimate relationships with others, and establishment of a family are the primary focuses of the young adult. While young adults usually have achieved independence, they find themselves learning socially relevant behavior and settling into specific acquired roles within a chosen profession or occupation. They begin to adopt some of the values of the group to which they belong and to assume assured roles such as marriage and parenting.

Cognitively, young adults have reached their peak level of intellectual efficiency, and they are able to think abstractly and to synthesize and integrate their ideas, experiences, and knowledge. Thinking for the adult usually involves reasoning, taking into consideration past experiences, education, and the possible outcomes of a situation more realistically and less egocentrically than the adolescent.

Young adulthood is still a time of great adjustment. The individual is expected to look at self in relation to society, learning how to deal with personal needs and desires as opposed to the needs and desires of others, and managing the economic and physical needs of life. Sexual activity focuses toward the development of a single intimate, meaningful relationship and the establishment of a family. In developing the role of parenting, the young adult often falls back on the parenting patterns and behavior of their own parents.

The young adult begins to assume the responsibility of providing for a family. Most young adults are members of dual-career families and thus face the stresses of multiple roles. Many of these young adults become single parents, and the stresses of multiple responsibilities and roles are greater both at home and at work. Just as during adolescence the negation of development of self-identity can lead to crises, role strain and conflict in the young adult can lead to developmental crises and often failure.

Middle-Age Adult

Middle age or middlescence is often considered the most productive years of an individual. Persons in this age group are usually secure in a profession or career, are in the middle of raising a family, and often must assume responsibility for aging parents.

As biophysical changes occur there is a concurrent adaptation of the cognitive and physical activities of the individual. The body ages in varying stages or degrees, and young middle-age adults usually retain the body structure and activity level they established as young adults. Middle-age adults, with more sedentary life-styles, must establish exercise programs to retain their youthful figures. The greatest changes facing both men and women during this time are those associated with the climacteric and the loss of reproductive capabilities. These biologic and physical changes can affect sexual life-styles either positively or negatively, depending on the perception and orientation of the individual.

Most middle-age adults function well and learn to gradually accept the changes of aging, and with proper nutrition, exercise, and a healthy life-style can experience excellent health and a productive middlescence. Middle-age persons usually begin to face more accidents, illness, and death; they begin to deal with their own aging process and death, as well as that of their parents. There is often a role reversal with the middle-age adult assuming the role of the parent.

This is the time of life when individuals usually review their goals and aspirations, sometimes to find that they did not reach the potential they once dreamed. Most middle-age adults begin to feel that there is not enough time to accomplish all they want to accomplish, and they begin to adjust to the fact that they may not reach all of the goals they set in their youth. This can result in a loss of self-esteem or it can be a motivation to develop previously untapped reservoirs which can lead to self-actualization and personal satisfaction.

Older Adult

The older adult must deal with decreasing function with resultant decreasing socialization potential. This is a time for retrospection and a need to ponder the past with sincere concerns regarding the future and death. In some instances a full functional level is possible, whereas for others life is lived vicariously. Elder role modeling opportunities, with respect for those who have lived life, still exist in many cultures. For these individuals the aging process is welcomed and enjoyed as the fullest potential is actualized for role-relationship patterning, namely the generation of values to the young in society. In those instances where aging is accompanied by loss in whatever form, the potential exists for the individual to become dependent on others. This dependency may range from a minor form to a major form of total dependence on others. For some the onset of dependency may be sudden; for others it may be gradual. In either instance the nurse must recognize the impact of the loss for the patient according to values of the patient and family.

Applicable Nursing Diagnoses

Family Processes, Altered

DEFINITION

The state in which a family that normally functions effectively experiences a dysfunction (North American Nursing Diagnosis Association [NANDA], 1987, p. 67).

DEFINING CHARACTERISTICS (NANDA, 1987, p. 67–68)

The nurse will review the initial pattern assessment for the following defining characteristics to determine the diagnosis of Family Processes, Altered.

1. Major defining characteristics
   a. Family system unable to meet physical needs of its members.
   b. Family system unable to meet emotional needs of its members.
   c. Family system unable to meet spiritual needs of its members.
   d. Parents do not demonstrate respect for each other's views on child-rearing practices.
   e. Family members unable to express or accept wide range of feelings.
   f. Family members unable to express or accept feelings of other members.
   g. Family unable to meet security needs of its members.
   h. Family members unable to relate to each other for mutual growth and maturation.
   i. Family uninvolved in community activities.
   j. Family unable to accept or receive help appropriately.
   k. Family is rigid in function and roles.
   l. Family not demonstrating respect for individuality and autonomy of its members.
   m. Family unable to adapt to change or deal with traumatic experiences constructively.
   n. Family failing to accomplish current or past developmental task.
   o. Family has unhealthy decision-making process.
   p. Family members fail to send and receive clear messages.
   q. Boundary maintenance is inappropriate.
   r. Inappropriate or poorly communicated family rules, rituals, or symbols exist.
   s. Unexamined family myths exist.
   t. Family has inappropriate level and direction of energy.

RELATED FACTORS (NANDA, 1987, p. 68)

1. Situational transition or crises.
2. Developmental transition or crises.

DIFFERENTIATION

This diagnosis would need to be differentiated from Family Coping, Ineffective which has a history of destructive patterns of behavior. For the diagnosis of Family Processes, Altered to be applicable there would be evidence that the usual adequacy in coping is altered in relation to a specific crisis. Related contributory diagnoses might include any of the other role-relationship patterns, self-perception deficits, or related factors from any of the other patterns. Once again it is important to acknowledge that a major stressor for the usual family process is illness.

OBJECTIVES

1. Will verbalize increased satisfaction with family interactional pattern by (date).

AND/OR

2. Will describe specific plan to cope with (specific stressor) by (date).

TARGET DATE

Five to seven days would be the earliest acceptable target date. Even after the objective has initially been met, there may be other precipitating events that will again alter family processes; therefore, a long-term date should also be designated.

NURSING ORDERS

ADULT HEALTH

1. Promote a trusting, therapeutic relationship.
2. Promote open, honest communications among the family members.
3. Assist the family to acknowledge and then accept the problem.
4. Allow the family to grieve.
5. Monitor readiness to learn; then teach family about the precipitating situation, its implications, and the expected response to treatment.
6. Help the family to identify its strengths and weaknesses in dealing with the situation.
7. Help family organize to continue usual family activities.
8. Refer to community assistive resources.
9. See Mental Health nursing orders for more detailed interventions.

CHILD HEALTH

1. Encourage the patient and family to express feelings regarding current family process by spending (specific time) each shift for this purpose.
2. Allow for participation by family members in care of patient as permitted according to patient's status.
3. Assist patient and family in identification of ways of coping with current stressors which interfere with normal family process.
4. Collaborate with health professionals in dealing with patient's altered family process to include:
   a. Family therapist
   b. Child psychologist or psychiatrist
   c. Clinical nurse specialist
   d. Pediatrician
   e. Play therapist
   f. Occupational therapist
   g. Physical therapist
   h. Clergy person
5. Promote for sibling participation in patient's hospitalization and plans for discharge.
6. Provide for cultural preferences when possible, including diet, religious needs, and plans for health care.
7. Assist family to identify support groups which will be of assistance in future.
8. Provide opportunities for family members to role play in care-related issues of patient.
9. Provide reinforcement to appropriately value caretaking behavior.

WOMEN'S HEALTH

(Note: Nursing orders in adult health, home health, and mental health will pertain to women, with the following additions. For nursing orders related to women and their families with restricted activity because of premature labor, multiple pregnancy, or pregnancy-induced hypertension, see Physical Mobility, Impaired in Chapter 5.)

Integration of Newborn into Family

1. Assist client and significant others in establishing realistic goals.
2. Provide positive reinforcement for parenting tasks.

3. Assist client in identifying infant behavior patterns and understanding how they allow her infant to communicate with her.
4. Assist client in verbalizing her perceptions of:
   a. Infant's growth and development;
   b. Individual and family needs;
   c. Stresses of being new parent.
5. Identify support groups:
   a. Formal
      (1) Mother's Day Out (churches)
      (2) Parenting groups
   b. Family
   c. Friends
6. Encourage open communication between mother and father on:
   a. Household tasks;
   b. Discipline;
   c. Fears and anxieties.
7. Help develop a plan for sharing household tasks and child caretaking activities.
   a. Bathing
   b. Feeding
   c. Care of siblings
      (1) Spend quality time with older children.
      (2) Allow older children to assist with newborn care (even the smallest child can do this with parental supervision).
         (a) Bringing a diaper to parent
         (b) Pushing baby in stroller
         (c) Holding baby (while sitting on couch is best)

Less-Than-Perfect Baby (Sick Infant or Infant with Anomaly)

8. Encourage verbalization of fears and questions.
9. Follow-up with home visits after discharge from hospital to:
   a. Monitor infant physically;
   b. Monitor family interactions;
   c. Provide support;
   d. Refer to proper agencies.
10. Teach and reinforce methods of caring for and coping with the emotional and physiologic needs of:
    a. The infant;
    b. Siblings;
    c. Parents;
    d. Other relatives (such as grandparents).

MENTAL HEALTH

1. Provide a role model for effective communication by:
   a. Seeking clarification;
   b. Demonstrating respect for individual family members and the family system;
   c. Listening to expression of thoughts and feelings;
   d. Setting clear limits;
   e. Being consistent;
   f. Communicating with the individual being addressed in a clear manner;
   g. Encouraging sharing of information among appropriate system subgroups.
2. Demonstrate an understanding of the complexity of system problems by:

    a. Not taking sides in family disagreements;

    b. Providing alternative explanations of behavior that recognize the contributions of all persons involved to the problem, including health care providers if appropriate;

    c. Requesting the perspective of multiple family members on a problem or stressor.

3. Include all family members in the first interview.

4. Have each member provide his or her perspective to the current difficulties.

5. Assist the family in defining a problem that can be resolved. (For example, rather than defining the problem as "we don't love each other any more," the problem can be defined as "we do not spend time together in family activities." This definition evolves from the family's description of what they mean by the more general problem description.)

6. Assist family in developing behavioral short-term goals by:

    a. Asking what they would see happening in the family if the situation improved;

    b. Having them break the problem into several parts that combine to form the identified stressor;

    c. Asking them what they could do in a week to improve the situation (this should include a response from each family member).

7. Maintain the nurse's role of facilitator of family communication by:

    a. Having family members discuss possible solutions among themselves;

    b. Having each family member talk about how he or she might contribute to both the problem and the problem's resolution.

8. Provide the family with the information necessary for appropriate problem-solving.

9. Answer all questions in an open, direct manner.

10. Support the expression of affect by:

    a. Having family members share feelings with one another;

    b. Normalizing the expression of emotion (i.e., "most persons experience anger after they have experienced a loss");

    c. Providing a private environment for this expression.

11. Maintain and support functional family roles (i.e., allow parents private time alone, allow children to visit parents, presenting problems to the "family leader"). Schedule a time with the family to discuss how the current situation affects family roles and possible changes that may be necessary.

12. Have family identify those systems in the community that could support them during this time and assist family in contacting these systems. Note systems to be contacted here as well as how they will assist the family.

13. Provide positive verbal reinforcement for the family's accomplishments.

14. Assist family in identifying patterns of interaction that interfere with successful problem resolution (e.g., the husband frequently asks his wife closed ended questions, which discourages her from sharing her ideas; the children interrupt the parents when their level of conflict increases to a certain level; the wife walks out of the room when the husband brings up issues related to finances).

15. Assist family in planning fun activities together. Families in crisis often limit their range of emotional experience. This could include time to play together, exercise together, or engage in a shared project. This also helps the family to have a positive experience together.

16. Teach family methods of anxiety reduction and establish a practice schedule and a schedule for discussing how this method could be used on a daily basis in the family. The selected method along with the schedule for discussion and practice should be listed here.

17. Include family in discussions related to planning care and sharing information about the client's condition.

18. Assist family in developing a specific plan when client is scheduled for a pass or discharge. Note that plan here with the assistance needed from the nursing staff for implementation.

19. Refer family to community resources as necessary for continued support. These could include:

   a. Visiting nurse
   b. Mental health nurse clinician
   c. Physician
   d. Family therapist
   e. Social services
   f. Financial counselor
   g. Specific illness-related support groups

HOME HEALTH

1. Teach patient and family appropriate information regarding the care of family members:
   a. Discipline strategies
   b. Normal growth and development
   c. Expected family life-cycles
   d. Coping strategies for family growth
   e. Care of health deviations
   f. Developing and using support networks
   g. Safe environment for family members
   h. Anticipatory guidance regarding growth and development, discipline, family functioning, responses to illness, role changes, etc.
2. Involve patient and family in planning and implementing strategies to decrease or prevent alterations in family process:
   a. Family conference
   b. Group discussion
   c. Mutual goal setting
   d. Communication
   e. Distribution of family tasks
3. Assist patient and family in life-style adjustments that may be required:
   a. Separation or divorce
   b. Temporary stay in community shelter
   c. Family therapy
   d. Communication of feelings
   e. Stress reduction
   f. Identification of potential for violence
   g. Providing safe environment
   h. Therapeutic use of anger
   i. Seeking and providing support for family members
   j. Coping with catastrophic or chronic illness
   k. Requirements for redistributing family tasks
   l. Changing role functions and relationships
   m. Financial concerns
4. Consult with or refer to assistive resources as required:
   a. Child protection
   b. Social service
   c. Financial counselor
   d. Family counselor
   e. Psychiatric nurse clinician
   f. Physician
   g. Teachers and other school officials
   h. School nurse
   i. Visiting nurse
   j. Community shelters

k. Self-help groups: Alcoholics Anonymous, American Cancer Society, American Heart Association, American Diabetes Association, American Lung Association, Multiple Sclerosis Society, Arthritis Foundation, etc.

EVALUATION
OBJECTIVE 1

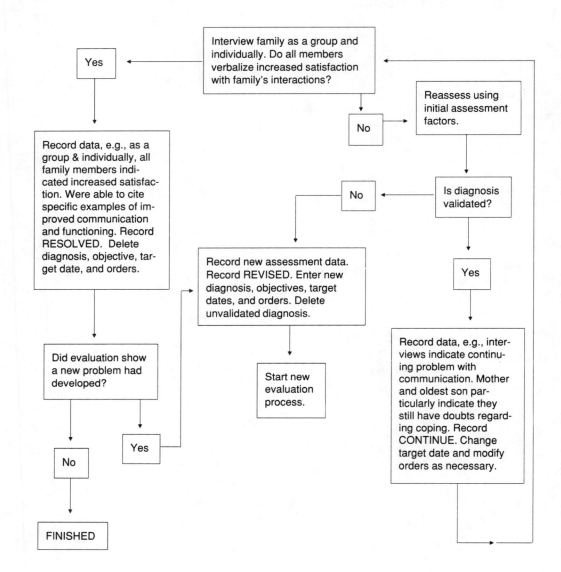

FINISHED

OBJECTIVE 2

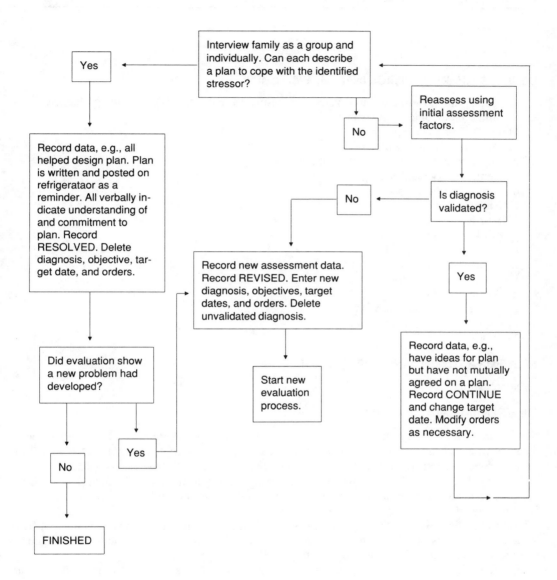

Grieving, Anticipatory

DEFINITION

None given.

DEFINING CHARACTERISTICS (NANDA, 1987, p. 109)

The nurse will review the initial pattern assessment for the following defining characteristics to determine the diagnosis of Grieving, Anticipatory.
1. Major Defining characteristics.
    a. Potential loss of significant object
    b. Expression of distress at potential loss
    c. Denial of potential loss
    d. Guilt
    e. Anger
    f. Sorrow
    g. Choked feelings
    h. Changes in eating habits
    i. Alterations in sleep patterns
    j. Alterations in activity level
    k. Altered libido
    l. Altered communication pattern
2. Minor defining characteristics
    None given.

RELATED FACTORS (NANDA, 1987, p. 109)

None given.

DIFFERENTIATION

Grieving, Anticipatory should be differentiated from Sensory-Perceptual Alteration; Anxiety; Fear; Spiritual Distress; Individual Coping, Ineffective; Self-Concept, Disturbance in; Self-Care Deficit; Sleep Pattern Disturbance; or other patterns substantiated by the assessment data.

Sensory-Perceptual Alteration will be identified according to the patient's change in capacity to exercise judgment or think critically with appropriate sensory-perceptual functioning. This may well be related to Grieving, Anticipatory.

Anxiety is the response the individual has to a threat which is for the most part unidentified. Fear is the response made by an individual to an identified threat. Anxiety and Fear diagnoses may also be related to Grieving, Anticipatory.

Spiritual distress occurs if the individual or family experiences a threat to the existent value system. This may be relevant in the alteration in role-relationship pattern.

Individual Coping, Ineffective would be the appropriate diagnosis if the individual is not making necessary adaptations to daily life. This may also occur in conjunction with the role-relationship pattern.

Self-Concept, Disturbance in and Self-Care Deficit are related by nature of the fact that the role-relationship pattern incorporates the essence of these two. For this reason it would be necessary to exercise caution in selecting the diagnosis according to the actual manifestation of symptoms and the situation represented by the patient or family.

With a Sleep Pattern Disturbance, there is a likely resultant role-relationship alteration, and the reverse is also possible. Physical Mobility, Impaired would also place the individual at risk for alteration in usual role-relationship activities.

In choosing the nursing diagnosis, substantiation of the data to generate the pattern alteration is paramount. It will require collaboration with other members of the health team to correctly intervene and individualize care for this client. There is, as always, the need to continually reassess for changes or modifications to be addressed. As stated previously, any illness or altered state of wellness carries the potential for alteration in role-relationship functions, and therefore all other patterns may potentially result in said alteration.

OBJECTIVES

1. Will verbalize feelings about impending loss by (date).

AND/OR

2. Will identify at least two support systems by (date).

TARGET DATE

A target date ranging from 2 to 4 days would be appropriate in evaluating progress toward achievement of the objective.

NURSING ORDERS

ADULT HEALTH

1. Assist the patient to acknowledge the impending loss by providing one-to-one time at least once per shift.
2. Allow the patient to express grief according to his or her own values, culture, and religion. Avoid making any judgments.
3. Provide a safe, secure environment by establishing the environment according to patient's wishes.
4. Promote a trusting and therapeutic relationship by answering questions fully.
5. Be consistent in approach by frequent updating of the care plan.
6. Offer the patient frequent support and reassurance.
7. Actively listen to the patient. Use touch judiciously.
8. Allow time for the patient to talk or to be silent.
9. Assist the patient to identify and use coping strategies that were successful for him or her in the past.
10. Allow the patient time to work through the grieving process:
    a. Recognize that the work of grieving occurs at different rates for different people and that people may vacillate between and among stages.
    b. Recognize that denial is a necessary response to loss, but do not reinforce denial.
    c. Encourage expression of anger within limits; encourage alternate ways to express anger.
    d. Reduce incoming stimuli; do not expect patient to make major decisions, but help patient to move from simple to more complex decision making.
    e. Reinforce the patient's self-worth.
    f. Acknowledge the person's feelings of guilt but assist the person to explore alternatives to resolve guilt.
    g. Assist patient in expressing life review and to incorporate insights into a new meaning.
11. Include family and significant others in support.
12. Refer to psychiatric nurse clinician as necessary. (Refer to mental health nursing orders for more detailed interventions).

CHILD HEALTH

1. Spend at least 30 minutes every 8 hours (or as situation dictates, but be specific) to address specific anticipated loss by:
   a. Encouraging patient and family to express perception of current situation (may be facilitated by age and developmentally appropriate intervention such as drawing, play or puppet therapy, or the like);

   b. Providing active listening in a quiet, private environment;
   c. Offering clarification of procedures, treatments, or plans for patient and family;
   d. Revising care plan to honor preferences when possible;
   e. Discussing and identifying impact of anticipated loss.
2. Collaborate with appropriate health professional members to meet needs of patient and family in realistically anticipating loss. This may include:
   a. Spiritual leaders;
   b. Family counselors or therapists;
   c. Pediatrician or pediatric subspecialists;
   d. Clinical pediatric nurse specialists;
   e. Psychologists or psychiatrists;
   f. Legal counselors;
   g. Play therapists;
   h. Occupational or physical therapists;
   i. Peers or significant others;
   j. Resource and support groups.
3. Encourage patient and family to realistically develop coping strategies to best prepare for anticipated loss through:
   a. Engaging in diversional activities of choice;
   b. Reminiscing of times spent with loved one or associated with anticipated loss;
   c. Identification of support groups.
4. Encourage optimal function for as long as possible with identification of need for proper attention to rest, diet, and health of all family members at this time of stress.
5. Promote parental and sibling participation in care of infant or child according to situation:
   a. Feedings and selection of menu.
   b. Comfort measures such as holding, backrubs, etc.
   c. Diversional activities, quiet games, stories.
   d. Decisions regarding life support measures and resuscitation.
6. Reassure infant or child that he or she is loved and cared for with ample opportunities to answer questions regarding specific anticipated loss whether related to self or others. According to age and developmental status, provide reassurance that cause for situation is not patient's own doing.
7. Remember that hearing is one of the last of senses to remain functional. Exercise opportunities for loved ones and staff to continue to address patient even though patient may be unable to answer or respond.
8. Provide for appropriate safety and maintenance related to physiologic care of patient.

WOMEN'S HEALTH

Fetal Demise (Pregnancy)

1. Obtain a thorough obstetric history, including previous occurrences of fetal demise.
2. Ascertain if there were any problems conceiving this pregnancy or any attempts to terminate this pregnancy.
3. Assess and record mother's perception of cessation of fetal movements.
4. Monitor and record fetal activity or lack of activity.
5. Inform mother and significant others of antepartal testing and why it is being ordered, and explain results.
   a. Nonstress testing
   b. Oxytocin Challenge Test
   c. Ultrasound
6. Be considerate and honest.
7. Keep client informed. Share information as soon as it becomes available.

8. Allow mother and family to express feelings and begin grieving process.
9. Refer to pastor or spiritual leader if so desired by family.
10. Allow presence of friends and family for support as client desires.
11. With collaboration of physician, facilitate necessary laboratory tests and procedures.
   a. Blood tests such as CBC, type and crossmatch, etc.
   b. DIC screening and coagulation studies
   c. Real time or ultrasound
   d. Amniotomy.
12. Provide emotional support for couple during labor and birth process.
13. Allow expression of fears, guilt, revolt, and inadequacy by the patient.
14. Closely monitor physiologic process of labor.
15. Explain the procedure of induction of labor and the use of:
   a. Pitocin;
   b. IVs;
   c. The uterine contraction pattern.
16. Watch for nausea, vomiting, and diarrhea.
17. Provide comfort measures.
18. Administer analgesics, tranquilizers, and medications for side effects of prostaglandins as ordered.
19. Change patient's position frequently.
20. Observe for full bladder (intake and output recorded).
21. Provide ice chips for dry mouth, lip balm or petroleum jelly for dry lips.
22. Monitor vital signs every 2–4 hours.
23. Utilize breathing and relaxation techniques with patient for comfort.
24. Inform physician of mother's wishes for use of anesthetic for birth.
   a. Awake and aware
   b. Sedated
   c. Asleep

(Note: The following nursing orders can apply to fetal demise, expected poor outcome of delivery [stillbirth], or unexpected stillbirth.)

25. Keep mother and significant others informed at time of delivery.
26. Allow support persons mother desires to be with her at time of delivery.
27. Inform them of sex and weight of infant.
28. Allow them time to see infant if they so desire.
29. Prepare infant for viewing by mother and significant others.
   a. Clean infant as much as possible.
   b. Use clothing to hide gross defects, such as:
      (1) Hat for head defects;
      (2) T-shirt or diapers for trunk defects.
   c. Wrap in soft, clean baby blanket
      (Allow mother to unwrap infant if she desires).
30. Provide time for mother and family to:
   a. See infant;
   b. Hold infant;
   c. Take pictures;
   d. Provide certificate which provides:
      (1) Footprints
      (2) Handprints
      (3) Lock of hair
      (4) Armbands
      (5) Date and time of birth, and weight of infant

(6) Name of infant
31. Provide quiet place where mother and significant others can be with infant.
32. Provide for religious practices such as baptism.
33. Contact religious or cultural leader as requested by mother or significant other.
34. Explain need for autopsy or genetic testing of infant.
35. Refer to appropriate support groups within the community.

Less-Than-Perfect Baby

36. Provide quiet place for mother and family to see infant.
37. Encourage verbalization of fears and questions.
38. Encourage touching and holding of infant by mother and family.
39. Refer to appropriate support groups within community.
40. Refer to appropriate health-care agencies within community.

Infertility

41. Allow time for client to express fears and frustrations.
42. Answer questions honestly.
43. Encourage expressions of:
    a. Anger;
    b. Fear;
    c. Hopelessness;
    d. Guilt;
    e. Inadequacy.
44. Assist in realistic planning for future.
    a. Possible extensive testing
       (1) Fear
       (2) Economics
       (3) Uncertainty
       (4) Embarrassment
       (5) Surgical procedures
       (6) Feelings of inadequacy
    b. Life without children
    c. Adoption

MENTAL HEALTH

(Note: It may take clients anywhere from 6 months to a year to grieve a loss. This should be taken into consideration when developing evaluation dates. In a short-stay hospitalization, a reasonable set of goals would be to assist the client system in beginning a healthy grieving process. It is also important to note the anniversary on which a reaction can be experienced past the 1-year period noted above.)

1. Assign client a primary care nurse and inform client of this decision. (This nurse must have a degree of comfort in discussing issues related to loss and grief.)
2. Primary nurse will spend 30 minutes once a shift with client discussing his or her perceptions of the current situation. These discussions could include:
   a. His or her perceptions of the loss;
   b. His or her values or beliefs about the lost "object";
   c. Client's past experiences with loss and how these were resolved;
   d. Client's perceptions of the support system and possible support system responses to the loss.
3. Primary nurse will schedule 1 hour interactions with client and support system to assist them in discussing issues related to the loss and answering any questions they might have (note time and date of this interaction here).

4. Primary nurse will discuss with client and family role adjustments and other anticipated changes related to the loss.
5. If necessary after the first interaction, primary nurse will schedule follow-up visits with the client and his or her support system (note schedule for these interactions here).
6. Spend (number) minutes (this should begin as 5-minute times and can increase to 10 minutes as client needs and unit staffing permits) with client each hour. If client does not desire to talk during this time, it can be used to give a massage (backrub) or sit with client in silence. Inform client of these times and let him or her know if for some reason this schedule has to be altered and develop a new time for the visit. Inform client that the purpose of this time is for him or her to use as he or she sees fit. The nurse should be seated during this time if he or she is not providing a massage.
7. Provide positive verbal and nonverbal reinforcement to expressions of grief from both the client and the support system. This would include remaining with the client when he or she is expressing strong emotions.
8. Once the client and the support system are discussing the loss, assist them in scheduling time when they can be alone with the client.
9. Answer questions in an open, honest manner.
10. If client support system expresses anger toward the staff and this anger appears to be unrelated to the situation, accept it as part of the grieving process and support the client in its expression by:
    a. Not responding in a defensive manner;
    b. Recognizing the feelings that are being expressed (e.g., ''It sounds like you are very angry right now'', ''It can be very frustrating to be in a situation where you feel you have little control'').
11. Recognize the stages of grief can progress at individual rates and in various patterns. Do not ''force'' a client through stages or express expectations about what the ''normal'' next step should be.
12. If client is in denial related to the loss, allow this to happen and provide client with information about the loss at the client's pace. If client does not remember information given before, simply provide the information again.
13. Allow client and support system to participate in decisions related to nursing care. Those areas in which client decision making is to be encouraged should be noted here along with the client's decision.
14. Normalize client's and support system's experience of grief by telling client that his or her experience is normal and by discussing with him or her potential future responses to loss.
15. Recognize that this is an emotionally painful time for the client and the support system and share this understanding with the client system.
16. Assist client in obtaining the spiritual support needed.
17. Monitor the use of sedatives and tranquilizers. Extensive use of these may delay the grieving process. Consult with physician if overuse is suspected.
18. Monitor the client system's use of alcohol and nonprescription drugs as a coping method. Refer to Individual Coping, Ineffective (Chapter 11) if this is assessed as a problem.
19. Have client and support system develop a list of concerns and problems and assist them in determining those they have the ability to change and those they do not.
20. When they have a list of workable problems have client system list all of the solutions they can think of for a problem, encourage them to include those solutions that they think are impossible or just fantasy solutions. Do this one problem at a time.
21. After solutions have been generated, assist client in evaluating solutions generated. Solutions can be combined, eliminated, or altered. From this list the best solution is selected. It is important that the solution selected is the client's solution.
22. Assist client in developing a plan for implementing this solution. Note any assistance needed from the nursing staff here.

23. Observe client for signs and symptoms of dysfunctional grieving.
24. Monitor client's nutritional pattern and refer to appropriate nursing diagnoses if a problem is identified.
25. Develop an exercise plan for the client. Consult with physical therapist as needed. Develop a reward schedule for the accomplishment of this plan. Note schedule for plan here. This can also include the support system.
26. Provide support for the support system by:
    a. Having them develop a schedule for rest periods;
    b. Providing snacks for them and scheduling periods of high nursing involvement with the client at a time when support persons can obtain meals; this can reassure the support person that client will not be alone while he or she is gone;
    c. Assisting support system in finding cafeteria and transportation;
    d. Suggesting that support persons rest or walk outside or around hospital while client is napping;
    e. Helping support persons discuss with client their feelings.
27. Refer client and support system to community support systems such as:
    a. Hospice groups
    b. The Compassionate Friends, Inc.
    c. The Candlelighters Foundation
    d. The Center for Attitudinal Healing
    e. I Can Cope
28. Refer to outpatient support systems. In addition to those cited above these might include:
    a. Visiting nurse
    b. Social services
    c. Financial counselor
    d. Mental health nurse specialist
    e. Physical therapist

HOME HEALTH

1. Teach patient and family appropriate monitoring of signs and symptoms of anticipatory grief:
    a. Crying, sadness
    b. Alterations in eating and sleeping patterns
    c. Developmental regression
    d. Alterations in concentration
    e. Expressions of distress at loss
    f. Denial of loss
    g. Expressions of guilt
    h. Labile affect
    i. Grieving beyond expected time
    j. Preoccupation with loss
    k. Hallucinations
    l. Violence toward self or others
    m. Delusions
    n. Prolonged isolation
2. Involve patient and family in planning and implementing strategies to reduce or cope with anticipatory grieving:
    a. Family conference
    b. Mutual goal setting
    c. Communication
3. Assist patient and family in life-style adjustments that may be required:
    a. Providing realistic hope

   b. Identifying expected grief pattern in response to loss
   c. Recognizing variety of accepted expressions of grief
   d. Developing and using support networks
   e. Communicating feelings
   f. Providing a safe environment
   g. Therapeutic use of denial
   h. Identifying suicidal potential or potential for violence
   i. Therapeutic use of anger
   j. Exploring meaning of situation
   k. Stress reduction
   l. Promoting expression of grief
   m. Decision making for future
   n. Promoting family cohesiveness

4. Assist patient and family to set criteria to help them to determine when intervention of health care professional is required.
   a. Psychiatric nurse clinician
   b. Support groups
   c. Mental health center
   d. Religious counselor
   e. Family counselor
   f. Visiting nurse
   g. Physician
   h. Social service

EVALUATION
OBJECTIVE 1

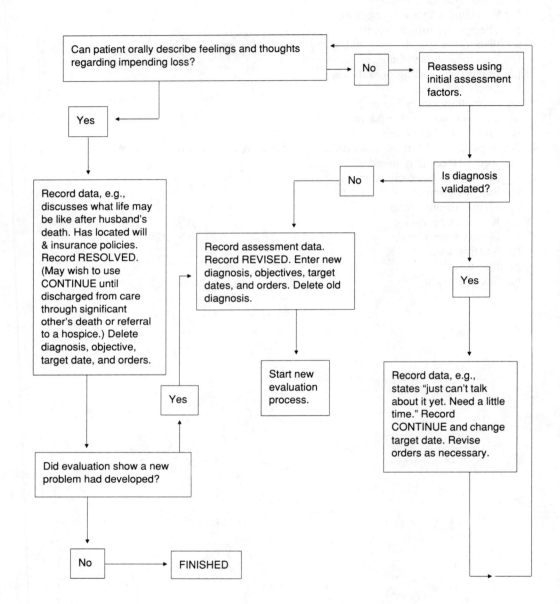

OBJECTIVE 2

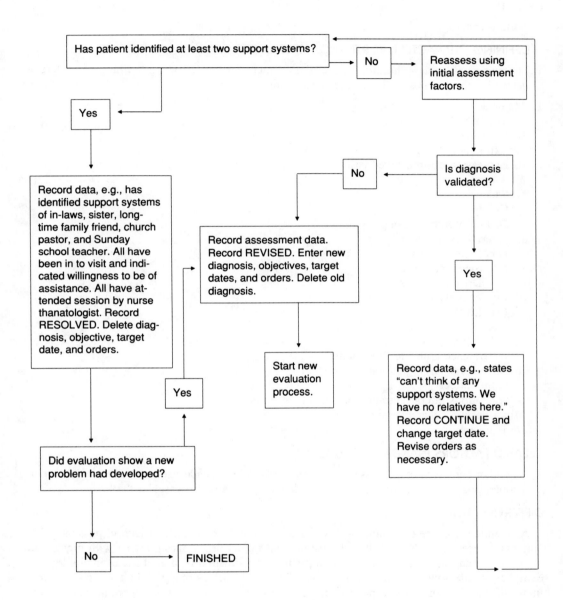

Grieving, Dysfunctional

DEFINITION

None given.

DEFINING CHARACTERISTICS (NANDA, 1987, p. 108)

The nurse will review the initial pattern assessment for the following defining characteristics to determine the diagnosis of Grieving, Dysfunctional.

1. Major defining characteristics
   a. Verbal expression of distress at loss.
   b. Denial of loss.
   c. Expression of guilt.
   d. Expression of unresolved issues.
   e. Anger.
   f. Sadness.
   g. Crying.
   h. Difficulty in expressing loss.
   i. Alterations in:
      (1) Eating habits;
      (2) Sleep patterns;
      (3) Dream patterns;
      (4) Activity level;
      (5) Libido.
   j. Idealization of lost object.
   k. Reliving of past experiences.
   l. Interference with life functioning.
   m. Developmental regression.
   n. Labile effect
   o. Alterations in concentration or pursuits of tasks
2. Minor defining characteristics
   None given.

RELATED FACTORS (NANDA, 1987, p. 108)

1. Actual or perceived object loss (object loss is used in the broadest sense)—objects may include people, possessions, a job, status, home, ideals, parts and processes of the body.

DIFFERENTIATION

As mentioned in the beginning of this chapter for the differential, consider all possible related patterns as needed. Validation that the patient and family are in fact grieving with greater time or severity than might be considered appropriate to the situation is often difficult in children, and extremely challenging with those who do not express themselves freely. All too often this is made more difficult by contributing patterns for a variety of alterations. It is important that the nurse not standardize a 1-year grieving period for all, especially children, as a maximum for normal grief patterns. It is, however, practical to consider this for most instances as a reasonable period of time for grief to be resolved. Actual responses will need to be qualified according to previous coping patterns.

Individual Coping, Ineffective; Anxiety; Fear; Sleep Pattern Disturbance; Nutrition, Altered; Activity-Exercise Alteration; Health Perception-Management Alteration; Cognitive-Perceptual Alteration; and Sexuality Patterns, Altered might also need to be considered as a part of assessment and differentiation for this pattern. The critical validation for existence of dysfunctional grieving is a subjective and objective manifestation of loss being the predominant reason for the patient and family to be unable to assume preloss role-relationship patterns.

OBJECTIVES

1. Will verbalize grief feelings by (date).

AND/OR

2. Will identify ways to appropriately cope with grief by (date).

TARGET DATE

Grief work should begin within 1–2 days after the nurse has intervened; the complete process of grief may take 6 months to a year.

NURSING ORDERS

ADULT HEALTH

1. Promote a trusting relationship.
2. Assist the patient to acknowledge and talk about feelings of the loss.
3. Be consistent, honest, and nonjudgmental in attitude.
4. Encourage the patient in the stages of the grief process.
5. Provide reality orientation.
6. Assist the patient to identify and use support systems.
7. Allow the patient time for life review and to resolve old conflicts.
8. Provide a safe and private environment.
9. Allow the patient to express grief in his or her own way.
10. Refer to psychiatric nurse clinician as necessary (see mental health nursing orders for more detailed interventions).

CHILD HEALTH

(Note: It is difficult to make general assumptions as to how each child views death, but according to previous patterns of behavior, including communication, it would be necessary to allow for developmental patterns previously attained. In young children there may be manifestations of obsessive, ritualistic behavior related to loss or activities surrounding loss. For example, if a loved one died, young children may think that if they fall asleep they may also die. In the event of grieving, regardless of the precipitating event, the child must be allowed to respond in keeping with developmental capacity. At times when the child is in danger of self-injury or injuring others, the potential for violence must also be considered.)

1. Provide opportunities for expression of feelings related to loss or grief according to developmental capacity (e.g., puppets or play therapy for toddlers).
2. Offer support in understanding patient's status for family, with special attention to siblings.
3. Identify impact grief has for family dynamics via assessment of same.
4. Allow for cultural and religious input in care plan, especially related to care of dying patient and care of patient at time of death.
5. Collaborate with professionals and paraprofessionals to aid in resolution of grief according to family preferences:
   a. Clergy
   b. Clinical nurse specialist
   c. Psychologist or psychiatrist
   d. Social worker
   e. Significant others
   f. Pediatrician or subspecialists
6. Identify support groups to assist in resolution of grief, such as Compassionate Friends Organization.

7. Assist family members in identification of coping strategies needed for resultant role-relationship changes.
8. Assist family members to resolve feelings of loss via reminiscing of loved one, positive aspects of situation, or personal growth potential presented.
9. Allow family members time and space to face reality of situation and ponder meaning of loss for self and family.
10. Direct family to appropriate resources regarding positive methods of acknowledging loved one through memorials or related processes.
11. Assist in referral to appropriate resources for funeral planning and arrangements if needed.
12. Provide for follow-up for resolution of grief with appropriate appointments as needed.
13. Have family develop a list of appropriate resources and support groups for long-term resolution of grief before leaving hospital.

WOMEN'S HEALTH

Sudden Infant Death Syndrome (SIDS)

1. Provide opportunity for verbalization of:
   a. How infant's death occurred;
   b. Police investigation;
   c. Sense of guilt;
   d. Feelings of powerlessness;
   e. Questions;
   f. Anger;
   g. Disbelief.
2. Identify impact death or grief has on:
   a. Family members;
   b. Relationship of couple;
   c. Attitude toward other children.
3. Refer to appropriate support groups:
   a. Religious or cultural leaders
   b. Clinical nurse specialists
   c. Pediatrician or obstetrician
   d. Community agencies
   e. Groups concerned with resolution of grief
      (1) Share
      (2) Compassionate Friends

Stillbirth or Fetal Demise

(Note: All nursing orders in Grieving Anticipatory, would apply here with the following additions.)

4. Promote verbalization of fears during subsequent pregnancies.
5. Provide client with information throughout pregnancy.
6. Encourage questions.
7. Be available when client needs to talk:
   a. In person;
   b. By telephone.
8. Refer to appropriate counselor.

Abortion

9. Allow expression of:
   a. Grief;
   b. Anger;

    c. Guilt;
11. Provide factual information.
12. Provide referral to appropriate support group in community.
13. Assist client in realizing:
    a. Grief may not be resolved for over a year;
    b. Situation when decision was made.
14. Assist client in putting event into perspective.

Infertility

(Note: Nursing orders will be the same as in Grieving, Anticipatory with the following additions.)

15. Provide a nonjudgmental atmosphere to allow the infertile couple to express their feelings.
    a. Anger
    b. Denial
    c. Inadequacy
    d. Guilt
    e. Depression
    f. Grief
16. Encourage couple to talk honestly with one another about feelings.
17. Encourage couple to seek professional help if necessary to deal with feelings involving:
    a. Sexual relationship;
    b. Conflicts;
    c. Anxieties;
    d. Parenting;
    e. Coping mechanisms used for dealing with loss of fertility.
18. Assist couple to explore:
    a. Their expectations;
    b. Relatives' expectations;
    c. Society's expectations.
19. Be alert for signs of:
    a. Depression;
    b. Anger;
    c. Frustration;
    d. Impending Crisis.

Rape

(Note: See Chapter 10 for nursing orders related to rape.)

MENTAL HEALTH

1. Monitor source of the interference with the grieving process.
2. Monitor client's use of medications and the effects this may have on the grieving process (sedatives and tranquilizers may delay the grieving process). Consult with physician regarding necessary alterations in this area.
3. Assign a primary care nurse to the client.
4. Provide a calm, reassuring environment.
5. When client is demonstrating an emotional response to the grief, provide privacy and remain with the client during this time.
6. Primary nurse will spend 30 minutes twice a day with the client. These interactions should begin as nonconfrontational interactions with the client. The goal is to develop a trusting relationship so the client can later discuss issues related to the grieving process. A time schedule for these interactions should be listed here.
7. Monitor level of dysfunction and assist client with activities of daily living as necessary. Note type and amount of assistance here.

8. Monitor nutritional status and refer to Nutrition, Altered (chapter 3) for detailed care plan.
9. Monitor significant others' repsonse to the client and have primary nurse set a schedule to meet with them and the client every other day to answer questions and facilitate discussion between the client and the support system. Note schedule for these meetings here.
10. Provide the spiritual support that the client indicates is necessary. Note here the type of assistance needed from the nursing staff.
11. Allow client to express anger and assure him or her that you will not allow harm to come to anyone during this expression.
12. Provide client with punching bags and other physical activity that assists with the expression of anger. Note tools preferred by this client here. Note the specific activities that assist this client with this expression here.
13. Remind staff and support system that client's expressions of anger at this point should not be taken personally even though they may be directed at the person.
14. Answer questions directly and openly.
15. Provide time and opportunity for client to participate in appropriate religious rituals. Note assistance needed from nursing staff here.
16. Sit with client while he or she is talking about the lost object.
17. When client's verbal interactions increase with the primary nurse to the level that group interactions are possible, schedule client to participate in a group that allows expression of feelings and feedback from peers. Note schedule of group here.
18. Assign client appropriate tasks in unit activities. Note type of tasks assigned here. These should be based on the client's level of functioning and should be at a level that the client can accomplish. Note type of tasks to be assigned to client here.
19. If delusions, hallucinations, phobias, or depression are present, refer to Individual Coping, Ineffective (chapter 11) and Thought Process, Altered (chapter 7) for detailed care plans.
20. Primary nurse will engage client and the support system in planning for life-style changes that might result from the loss. Note schedule for these interactions here along with the specific goals.
21. Refer client and support system to appropriate community support services such as:
    a. I Can Cope
    b. Compassionate Friends, Inc.
    c. The Candlelighters Foundation
    d. The Center for Attitudinal Healing
    e. Hospice programs
    f. Social worker
    g. Visiting nurse
    h. Mental health nurse specialist
    i. Financial counselor

HOME HEALTH

1. Teach patient and family appropriate monitoring of signs and symptoms of dysfunctional grief:
    a. Crying, sadness
    b. Alterations in eating and sleeping patterns
    c. Developmental regression
    d. Alterations in concentration
    e. Expressions of distress at loss
    f. Denial of loss
    g. Expressions of guilt
    h. Labile affect
    i. Grieving beyond expected time
    j. Preoccupation with loss

    k. Hallucinations
    l. Violence toward self or others
    m. Delusions
    n. Prolonged isolation

2. Involve patient and family in planning and implementing strategies to reduce or cope with dysfunctional grieving:
    a. Family conference
    b. Mutual goal setting
    c. Communication

3. Assist patient and family in life-style adjustments that may be required:
    a. Providing realistic hope
    b. Identifying expected grief pattern in response to loss
    c. Recognizing a variety of accepted expressions of grief
    d. Developing and using support networks
    e. Communicating feelings
    f. Providing a safe environment
    g. Therapeutic use of denial
    h. Identifying suicidal potential or potential for violence
    i. Therapeutic use of anger
    j. Exploring meaning of situation
    k. Stress reduction
    l. Promoting expression of grief
    m. Decision making for future
    n. Promoting family cohesiveness

4. Assist patient and family to set criteria to help them to determine when intervention of health care professional is required.
    a. Psychiatric nurse clinician
    b. Support groups
    c. Mental health center
    d. Religious counselor
    e. Family counselor
    f. Visiting nurse
    g. Physician
    h. Social service

EVALUATION
OBJECTIVE 1

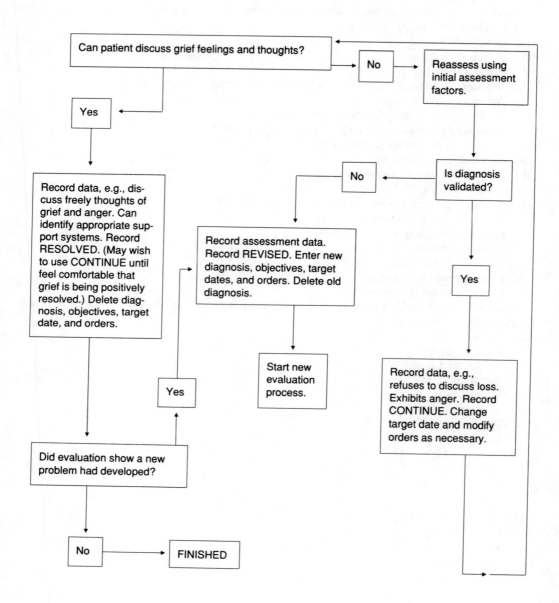

OBJECTIVE 2

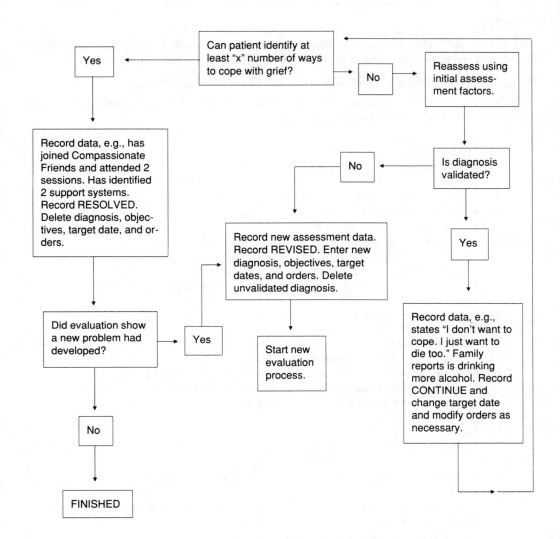

Parenting, Altered: Potential, Actual, Role Conflict

DEFINITION

Ability of nurturing figure(s) to create an environment which promotes the optimum growth and development of another human being (NANDA, 1987, pp. 62, 64).

DEFINING CHARACTERISTICS (NANDA, 1987, pp. 62–65; NANDA, 1988).

The nurse will review the initial pattern assessment for the following defining characteristics to determine the diagnosis of Parenting, Altered.

1. Parenting, Altered: Actual
   a. Major defining characteristics
      (1) Abandonment
      (2) Runaway
      (3) Verbalization of inability to control child
      (4) Incidence of physical and psychologic trauma
      (5) Lack of parental attachment behavior
      (6) Inappropriate visual, tactile, or auditory stimulation
      (7) Negative identification of infant's or child's characteristics
      (8) Negative attachment of meanings to infant's or child's characteristics
      (9) Constant verbalization of disappointment in gender or physical characteristics of the infant or child
      (10) Verbalization of resentment toward the infant or child
      (11) Verbalization of role inadequacy
      (12) Inattentiveness to infant's or child's needs
      (13) Verbal disgust at body functions of infant or child
      (14) Noncompliance with health appointments for self or infant or child
      (15) Inappropriate caretaking behavior (toilet training, sleep and rest, feeding)
      (16) Inappropriate or inconsistent discipline practices
      (17) Frequent accidents
      (18) Frequent illness
      (19) Growth and development lag in the child
      (20) History of child abuse or abandonment by primary caretaker
      (21) Verbalization of desire to have child call parent by first name versus traditional cultural tendencies
      (22) Child receiving care from multiple caretakers without consideration for the needs of infant or child
      (23) Compulsively seeking role approval from others
   b. Minor defining characteristics
      None given.
2. Parenting, Altered: Potential
   a. Major defining characteristics
      Same as items (5) through (23) for Parenting, Altered: Actual.
   b. Minor defining characteristics
      None given.
3. Parental Role Conflict
   a. Definition: The state in which a parent experiences role confusion and conflict in response to crisis.
   b. Major defining characteristics
      (1) Parent expresses concerns or feelings of inadequacy to provide for child's physical and emotional needs during hospitalization or in the home

disruption in caretaking routines

ses concerns about changes in parental role, family functioning, family
n, family health

ng characteristics

Expresses concern about perceived loss of control over decisions relating to child
(2) Reluctant to participate in usual caretaking activities even with encouragement and support
(3) Verbalizes or demonstrates feelings of guilt, anger, fear, anxiety, or frustration about effect of child's illness on family process

RELATED FACTORS (NANDA, 1987, pp. 62–65; NANDA, 1988)

1. Parenting, Altered: Actual
   a. Lack of available role model
   b. Ineffective role model
   c. Physical and psychosocial abuse of nurturing figure
   d. Lack of support between or from significant others
   e. Unmet social or emotional maturation needs of parenting figures
   f. Interruption in bonding process (i.e., maternal, paternal, other)
   g. Unrealistic expectation for self, infant, partner
   h. Perceived threat to own survival, physical and emotional
   i. Mental or physical illness
   j. Presence of stress (financial, legal, recent crisis, cultural move)
   k. Lack of knowledge
   l. Limited cognitive functioning
   m. Lack of role identity
   n. Lack or inappropriate response of child to relationship
   o. Multiple pregnancies
2. Parenting, Altered: Potential
   Same as Parenting, Altered: Actual
3. Parental Role Conflict
   a. Separation from child due to chronic illness
   b. Intimidation with invasive or restrictive modalities (e.g., isolation, intubation), specialized care centers, policies
   c. Home care of a child with special needs (e.g., apnea monitoring, postural drainage, hyperalimentation)
   d. Change in marital status
   e. Interruptions of family life due to home care regimen (treatments, caregivers, lack of respite)

DIFFERENTIATION

Parenting, Altered: Potential or Actual should be differentiated from Family Process, Altered; Family Coping Potential for Growth; Family Coping, Ineffective: Compromised; and Family Coping, Ineffective: Disabling.

Family Processes, Altered would be used if the client could not carry out functions within the family, to include all members of the family or one member of the family, regardless of age or sex. Often there would be a narrow view of roles and dysfunction of those roles within the family. It does not necessarily deal with the role of being a parent, but with the role of being a member of the family group. There is often a breakdown of family growth and development and unhealthy family relationships, and involves the entire family. If the family dysfunction was to cause a mother or father to be unable to nurture their young, then the appropriate diagnosis could be Parenting, Altered: Potential or Actual.

Family Coping, Potential for Growth would be used when a family member effectively adapts and manages the tasks of growth and development within the family and can easily move into self-actualization.

Family Coping, Ineffective: Compromised is used when a key member of the family is unable to facilitate or provide support which allows the family to progress or manage adaptive behavior in the time of crisis.

Family Coping, Ineffective: Disabling is most often used when key family members impede the progress of adaptive behavior of other family members or totally reject or deny the patient's condition, such as a family refusing to accept that a mother is dying.

Any patterns relating to self-concept, coping, and related role-relationship diagnoses may be contributory to alteration in parenting. A key differential note is that one might still be able to parent even though he or she is unable to fulfill the other roles in the associated patterns. Conversely, he or she might be able to fulfill other roles but be unable to adequately fulfill parenting roles.

It is always important to understand what the reasons are for failure to comply with intended regimen, as mentioned in Chapter 2. Often factors such as money, transportation, or knowledge certainly contribute. Additionally, one's own parenting style is primarily determined by previous parenting, thus offering a risk potential for those denied the experience of parental adequacy in their own childhood.

It is always mandatory that a nonjudgmental attitude be maintained by nurses who will be privy to intimate parental-child interactions which are open to interpretation. Objectivity and appreciation of cultural patterns must be maintained. There will be opportunities for validation of potential alteration in parenting. Legal and ethical obligations must also be followed according to local child protective services whenever neglect or abuse is suspected.

OBJECTIVES

1. Will demonstrate appropriate parental role of (specify exactly what, e.g., feeding, administration of medication, etc.) behavior by (date).

AND/OR

2. Will verbalize realistic expectations of self as parent and for child by (date).

TARGET DATE

The diagnosis will require a lengthy amount of time to be totally resolved. However, progress toward resolution could be evaluated within 7 days.

NURSING ORDERS

ADULT HEALTH

1. Provide anticipatory guidance relative to growth and development of self and child.
2. Encourage patient to allow time for own needs.
3. Encourage use of support groups.
4. Provide opportunities for parent to participate in child's care.
5. Assist parent to recognize when stress is becoming distress.
6. Discuss disciplinary methods other than physical.
7. Teach stress management and parenting techniques.
8. Initiate referrals as needed.

CHILD HEALTH

1. Review current level of knowledge regarding parenting of infant or child to include:
   a. Perception of infant or child
   b. Anticipatory development of infant or child

c. Health status of infant or child
d. Current needs of infant or child
e. Infant or child communication
f. Infant or child responsiveness
g. Family dynamics

2. Determine needs for specific health or developmental intervention in collaboration with pediatrician to include:
   a. Clinical nurse specialist
   b. Play therapist
   c. Family therapist
   d. Social worker
   e. Psychiatrist or psychologist
   f. Parenting role models
   g. Support groups such as Parents Anonymous

3. Observe parental readiness and encourage caretaking in a supportive atmosphere in the following ways as applicable:
   a. Feeding
   b. Bathing
   c. Anticipatory safety measures
   d. Clarification of medical or health maintenance regimen
   e. Play and developmental stimulation for age and capacity
   f. Handling and carriage of infant or child
   g. Diapering and dressing of infant or child
   h. Social interaction appropriate for age and capacity
   i. Other specific measures according to patient's status and needs.

4. Encourage parents to verbalize perceived parenting role, both current and desired.

5. Allow parents to gradually assume total care of infant within hospital setting at least 48 hours before dismissal. If more time is required to validate appropriate parenting success, notify pediatrician.

6. Allow parents comfort in expressing true feelings regarding feelings of parenting, especially frustration with seemingly unending demands. Allow for adequate time each 8 hours to provide feedback of daily care the infant requires and see how parent perceives the situation.

7. Assist parents to identify ways of coping with infant and parental demands to include:
   a. Support systems
   b. Respite care, licensed babysitters
   c. Parent education groups
   d. Hotlines for advice or ventilation
   e. Groups which value parenting (church or other groups)

WOMEN'S HEALTH

(Note: Nursing orders that deal with bonding, perception, and caretaking activities of infants are also discussed under Child Health in this section. See also Family Processes, Altered in this chapter; Powerlessness in Chapter 8; and Self-Concept, Disturbance in Chapter 8. The following orders refer to prenatal and postpartum interventions to assist in appropriate parenting.)

Prenatal

1. Assist client in completing the tasks of pregnancy by encouraging verbalization of:
   a. Fears;
   b. Mother's perception of marriage;
   c. Mother's perception of "child within" her;
   d. Mother's perception of changes in her life:

(1) Relationship with partner
(2) Relationship with other children
(3) Effects on career
(4) Effects on family

2. Allow mother to question pregnancy.
   a. "Now" and "Who, me?" (Rubin, 1970).
   b. Assist mother in realizing existence of child by encouraging mother to:
      (1) Note when infant moves;
      (2) Listen to fetal-heart tones during visit to clinic;
      (3) Discuss body changes and their relationship to infant;
      (4) Verbalize any questions she may have.

3. Assist in preparation for birth by:
   a. Encouraging attendance at childbirth education classes;
   b. Providing factual information regarding the birthing experience;
   c. Involving significant others in preparation for birthing process.

4. Assist client in preparing for role transition to parenthood by encouraging:
   a. Economic planning
      (1) Physician fees
          (a) Obstetrician
          (b) Pediatrician
      (2) Hospital
          (a) Normal delivery
          (b) Cesarean section
          (c) Complications
      (3) Prenatal testing fees
          (a) Ultrasound
          (b) Amniocentesis
          (c) Laboratory fees
   b. Social planning
      (1) Changes in life-style
          (a) Consider care of child
          (b) Unable to go out as often
          (c) Fatigue
          (d) Stress of caring for new infant
          (e) Marital relationship

5. Assist client in identifying needs related to family, parent's acceptance of the newborn.
   a. Mother's perceived lack of support by:
      (1) Family (parents, siblings)
      (2) Spouse or partner
      (3) Friends
      (4) Other relatives
   b. Identify stressors present in family.
      (1) Economic
      (2) Housing (living with parents or other family members)
      (3) Drug or substance abuse within family
      (4) Knowledge deficit
          (a) Very young mother
          (b) Older first-time mother
          (c) Mother without her mother to pattern after
      (5) At risk
          (a) Refuses to plan for infant

    (b) No interest in pregnancy or fetal progress
    (c) Overly concerned with own weight and appearance
       (i)   Refuses to gain weight (diets during pregnancy)
       (ii) Negative comments about "What this baby is doing to me!"

Postpartum

6. Assist client and significant others in establishing realistic goals.
7. Provide positive reinforcement for parenting tasks.
   a. Encourage use of birthing rooms; labor, delivery, and recovery (LDR) rooms; and labor, delivery, recovery, and postpartum (LDRP) rooms for birth to allow active participation in birth process by mother and father.
   b. Allow mother and partner time with infant (do not remove to nursery if stable) following delivery.
   c. Provide mother-baby care to allow maximum continuity of mother-infant contact and nursing care.
8. Assist client in identifying different kinds of infant behavior and understanding how they allow her infant to communicate with her.
   a. Perform gestational age assessment with mother and explain significance of findings.
   b. Perform Brazelton neonatal assessment with mother and explain significance of findings.
   c. Demonstrate how to hold infant for maximum communication.
   d. Explain infant reflexes and the importance of understanding them.
      (1) Rooting reflex
      (2) Moro reflex
9. Assist client in identifying support systems.
   a. Friends from childbirth classes
   b. Parents and parents-in-law
   c. Siblings
   d. Nurse specialists
10. Encourage client to reminisce about birthing experience.
11. Assist client in identifying needs related to family functioning.
   a. Identify negative parent behavior
      (1) Maternal
         (a) No interest in new baby
            (i)   Talks *excessively* to friends on phone
            (ii) Is more interested in TV than in feeding infant
            (iii) Refuses to listen to infant teaching
            (iv) Asks no questions
         (b) *Extraordinary* interest in self-appearance
            (i)   *Severe* dieting to gain prepregnancy figure
            (ii) *Overutilization* of exercise to gain prepregnancy figure
         (c) Crying, moodiness
         (d) Lack of interest in family and other children
         (e) Failure to perform physical care for infant
         (f) Noncompliance
            (i)   Breaks appointments with health care providers for self and infant
      (2) Paternal
         (a) Refusal to support wife by:
            (i)   Not assisting in child care;
            (ii) Not sharing household tasks;
            (iii) Keeping "his" social contacts and going out while wife remains at home with child;

      (iv) Not providing financial support;

      (v) Abandonment.

12. Assist client in identifying methods of coping with stress of newborn in family.

    a. Seek professional help.

      (1) Nurse specialist

      (2) Physician (obstetrician or pediatrician)

      (3) Psychiatrist

    b. Identify support system in family or among friends.

    c. Refer to appropriate community or private agencies.

MENTAL HEALTH

1. Monitor the degree to which drugs and alcohol interfere with the parenting process. If this is a factor discuss a treatment program with the client.
2. Ask client who is caring for children while he or she is hospitalized and assess his or her level of comfort with this arrangement. If a satisfactory arrangement is not present refer to social services so arrangements can be made.
3. Discuss with the client expectations and problem perception.
4. Have client identify support systems and gain permission to include these persons in the treatment plan as necessary. This could include spouse, parents, close friends, etc.
5. If client desires to maintain parenting role, arrange to have children visit during hospitalization. Assign a staff member to remain with the client during these visits. The staff person can serve as a role model for the client and facilitate communication between the child and the client. Note schedule for these visits here and the staff person responsible for the supervision of these interactions.
6. Answer client's questions in a clear, direct manner.
7. Spend 30 minutes twice a day with the client discussing his or her perception of the parenting role and his or her expectations for self and children. Note schedule for these interactions here.
8. Arrange 30 minutes a day for interaction between the client and one member of the support system. A staff member is to be present during these interactions to facilitate communication and focus the discussion on parenting issues.
9. Provide client with information on normal growth and development and normal feelings of parents.
10. Assist client in developing a plan for disciplining children. This plan should be based on behavioral interventions and the primary focus should be on positive social rewards. See Patterson (1971) for detailed information on this intervention.
11. Teach client ways of interacting with child that reduce levels of conflict (i.e., providing child with limited choices, spending scheduled time with the child, listening carefully to child).
12. Encourage client to maintain telephone contact with children by providing a telephone and establishing a regular time for the client to call home or have the children call the hospital.
13. Encourage support system to continue to include client in decisions related to the children by having them bring up these issues in daily visits and by assisting client and support system to engage in collaborative decision making regarding these issues.
14. Have client identify parenting models and discuss the effect these persons had on their current parenting style.
15. Observe interaction between parents to assess for problems in the husband-wife relationship that may be expressed in the parenting relationship. If this appears to be happening refer to family therapy.
16. Have client develop a list of problem behavior patterns and then assist him or her in developing a list of alternative behavior patterns. (For example, Current: When I get frustrated with my

child I spank him with a belt. New: When I get frustrated with my child I arrange to send him to the neighbors for 30 minutes while I take a walk around the block to calm down.)

17. Role play with client those situations that are identified as being most difficult and provide opportunities to practice more appropriate behavior. This should be done daily in 30-minute time periods. Note schedule for this activity here and list time periods. Note schedule for this activity here and list those situations that are to be practiced. It would be useful to include spouse.

18. Have client attend group sessions where feelings and thoughts can be expressed to peers and the thoughts and feelings of peers can be heard. Note schedule for the group here.

19. Assist client in identifying personal needs and in developing a plan for meeting these needs at home (e.g., parents will exchange babysitting time with neighbors so they can have an evening out once a month). Note this plan here.

20. Monitor staff attitudes toward client and allow them to express feelings, especially if child abuse is an issue with this client.

21. Assist client with grieving separation from child and refer to Grieving, Anticipatory for a detailed care plan.

22. Provide client with positive verbal support for positive parenting behavior (e.g., ''you demonstrate a great deal of concern for your child's welfare'' ''you have taught your child to be very sensitive''). Make sure these comments are honest and fit the client's awareness of the situation.

23. Assist client in developing stress reduction skills by:
    a. Teaching deep muscle relaxation and practicing this with client 30 minutes a day (note schedule for this practice here).
    b. Discussing with client the role physical exercise plays in stress reduction and developing a plan for exercise (note plan and type of exercise here). Have staff member remain with the client during these exercise periods. Note time for these periods here.
    c. When client's level of tension or anxiety is rising on the unit remind him or her of the exercise or relaxation technique and work through one of these with him or her.
    d. Assist client in identifying the symptoms he or she has of rising tension so he or she can implement the stress reduction activity when client notices this alteration in his or her feelings and behavior.

24. Refer client to community resources such as:
    a. Visiting nurse services
    b. Social services
    c. Mother's Day Out programs
    d. Drop-in crisis centers for young families
    e. Parenting programs
    f. Parents Without Partners
    g. Child development centers
    h. Family therapist
    i. Well-baby clinics

HOME HEALTH

1. Act as role model through use of positive attitude when interacting with the child and parents.
2. Report child abuse and neglect to the appropriate authorities.
3. Teach patient and family appropriate information regarding the care and discipline of children:
    a. Cultural norms
    b. Normal growth and development
    c. Anticipatory guidance regarding psychosocial, cognitive, and physical needs for children and parents
    d. Expected family life cycles

   e. Development and use of support networks
   f. Safe environment for family members
   g. Nurturing environment for family members
   h. Special needs of child requiring invasive or restrictive treatments
4. Involve patient and family in planning and implementing strategies to decrease or prevent alterations (potential or actual) in parenting:
   a. Family conference
   b. Group discussion
   c. Mutual goal setting
   d. Communication
   e. Distribution of family tasks
   f. Promoting parent's self-esteem
5. Assist patient and family in life-style adjustments that may be required:
   a. Development of parenting skills
   b. Use of support network
   c. Establishment of realistic expectations of children and spouse.
6. Refer to appropriate assistive resources such as:
   a. Psychiatric nurse clinician
   b. Visiting nurse
   c. School nurse
   d. Teacher
   e. Religious counselor
   f. Foster placement
   g. Alcoholics Anonymous, substance abuse programs
   h. Home extension unit, church, local college or university for parenting classes
   i. Day care centers
   j. Respite care
   k. Support group for parents of chronically ill children
   l. Parents Without Partners
   m. Home-based care provider
   n. Marriage and family therapist

EVALUATION
OBJECTIVE 1

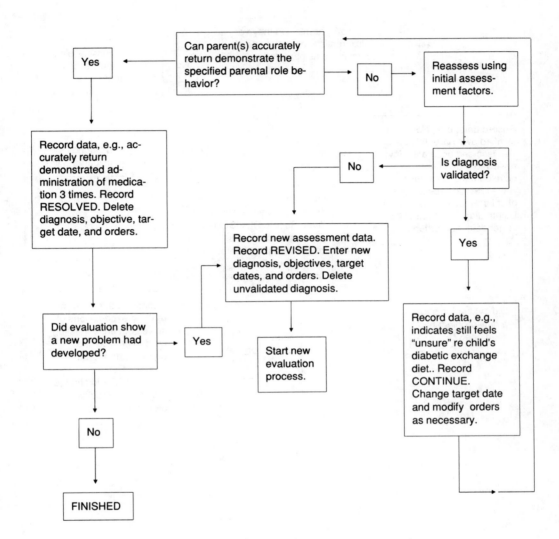

OBJECTIVE 2

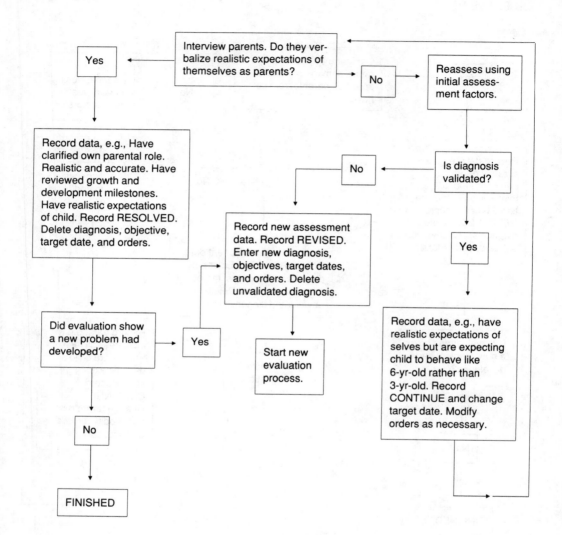

Role Performance, Altered

DEFINITION

Disruption in the way one perceives one's role performance (NANDA, 1987, p 61).

DEFINING CHARACTERISTICS (NANDA, 1987, p 61)

The nurse will review the initial pattern assessment for the following defining characteristics to determine the diagnosis of Role Performance, Altered.

1. Major defining characteristics
   a. Change in self-perception role
   b. Denial of role
   c. Change in other person's perception of role
   d. Conflict in role
   e. Change in physical capacity to resume role
   f. Lack of knowledge of role
   g. Change in usual patterns of responsibility
2. Minor defining characteristics
   None given.

RELATED FACTORS

None given.

DIFFERENTIATION

Role Performance, Altered should be differentiated from Social Isolation and Family Processes, Altered. Alteration usually means change, and although the above diagnoses involve different changes in a patient's life, they are more concerned with system change or change other than in the individual.

Social Isolation involves the patient who, because of physical, communicative, or social problems, chooses to be alone or perceives that he or she is alone and therefore isolated from society. This diagnosis deals mainly with the individual who cannot or will not perform any role.

Family Processes, Altered deals with the family that must in one way or another alter the processes that go on within the family. Many times this will involve altered role performances of the individual family members; however, the overall focus is on the alteration within the family and not with the individual members of the family.

OBJECTIVES

1. Will list at least (number) factors contributing to disturbance in role performance by (date).

AND/OR

2. Will implement plan to offset factors contributing to disturbance in role performance by (date).

TARGET DATE

Target dates for this diagnosis will have to be highly individualized according to each situation. A minimum target date would be 5 days to allow time to identify impinging factors and methods to cope with those factors.

NURSING ORDERS

ADULT HEALTH

1. Encourage patient to express his or her perception of role responsibilities.
2. Help patient and significant others realistically negotiate role responsibilities
3. Help patient identify community resources to assist in role responsibilities (e.g., day care centers, homemakers, etc.).

4. Teach patient regarding role (i.e. parent, caregiver, breadwinner, etc.).
5. Refer to pyschiatric nurse clinician (see mental health nursing orders for more detailed interventions).

CHILD HEALTH

1. Determine how child and parent perceive the role expected for child.
2. Identify confusion or diffusion of role according to child's and parent's expectations versus actual role.
3. Determine value the child has in the family.
4. Determine child's self-perception.
5. Identify ways to alleviate role performance alteration according to actual cause. If child is temporarily unable to participate in certain physical activities, explore other non-physical ways the child can participate.
6. Allow for ventilation of feelings by child via puppetry, art, or other age-appropriate methods at least 30 minutes during each 8 hour shift.
7. Provide patient and parents with options to best facilitate needs for future implications of compromised role performance. (For example, shared experiences with peers who have temporarily had to forsake physical activities due to illness—how they kept up with the team, etc.)
8. Allow for family time by visitation and support for choices to uphold role needs.
9. Provide for safety needs of child and family.
10. Assist in follow-up plans with appropriate appointments for psychiatric or pediatric care.
11. Provide support in identification of risk to normal actualization of potential of child.

WOMEN'S HEALTH

1. Allow client to describe her perception of her role as a mother, wife, and working woman.
2. Identify sources of role stress and strain that contribute to role conflict and fatigue.
3. Assist in developing a schedule that manages time well, both at home and at work.
4. Involve significant others in planning methods of reducing role stress and strain at home by:
   a. Assisting with child care;
   b. Assisting with household duties;
   c. Sharing carpooling and children's activities.
5. Encourage client to use time at work for "work activities" and time at home for "home activities" i.e.,(do not take home work).
6. Look at possibility of job sharing or part-time employment while children are at home.
7. Plan home activities in advance, such as shopping and cooking meals in advance and freezing them for later use.
8. Encourage division of work load by exchanging child care activities with friends or other families in the neighborhood.

MENTAL HEALTH

1. Sit with client (number) minutes (number) times per day to discuss client's feelings about self and role performance.
2. Answer questions honestly.
3. Provide feedback to client about nurse's perceptions of client's abilities and appearance by:
   a. Using "I" statements;
   b. Using references related to the nurse's relationship to the client;
   c. Describing the nurse's feelings in relationship.
4. Provide positive reinforcement (list those things that are reinforcing for the client and when they are to be used; also list those things that have been identified as nonreinforcers for this client; include social rewards).

5. Provide group interaction with (number) persons (number) minutes three times a day at (times). (This activity should be gradual within client's ability, i.e., on admission client may tolerate one person for 5 minutes. If the interactions are brief the frequency should be high, i.e., 5-minute interactions should occur at 30-minute intervals).

6. Protect client from harm by:
   a. Removing sharp objects from environment;
   b. Removing belts and strings from environment;
   c. Providing a one-to-one constant interaction if potential for self-harm is high;
   d. Checking on client's whereabouts every 15 minutes;
   e. Removing glass objects from environment;
   f. Removing locks from room and bathroom doors;
   g. Providing a shower curtain that will not support weight;
   h. Checking to see if client swallows medications.

7. Reflect back to client negative self-statements made by the client. (This should be done with a supportive attitude in a manner that will increase client's awareness of these negative evaluations of self.)

8. Set achievable goals for client.

9. Provide activities that the client can accomplish and that the client values (care should be taken not to provide tasks that the client finds demeaning or this could reinforce client's negative self-evaluation).

10. Provide verbal reinforcement for achievement of steps toward a goal.

11. Have client develop a list of strengths and potentials.

12. Define the client's lack of goal achievement or failures as simple mistakes that are bound to occur when one attempts something new (e.g., learning comes with mistakes; if one does not make mistakes one does not learn).

13. Define past failures as the client's best attempts to solve a problem (e.g., if the client had known a better solution he or she would have used it; one does not set out to fail).

14. Make necessary items available for the client to groom self.

15. Spend (number) minutes at (time) assisting the client with grooming, providing necessary assistance and positive reinforcement for accomplishments.

16. Focus client's attention on the here and now (past happenings are difficult for the nurse to provide feedback on).

17. Present the client with opportunities to make decisions about care and record these decisions on the care plan.

18. Develop with the client alternative coping strategies.

19. Practice new coping behavior with client (number) minutes at (time).

20. Discuss with the client ideal versus current perceptions of role performance.

21. Discuss with the client those factors that are perceived to be interfering with role performance.

22. Have the client develop a list of alternatives for resolving interfering factors. (This list should be noted here.)

23. Establish an appointment with significant others to discuss their perceptions of the client's role performance and their perceptions of the various roles involved in the identified situations. (Date and time of this meeting should be written here.)

24. Discuss with the client and significant others alterations in role that will facilitate successful performance. (Date and time of this meeting should be written here.)

25. Develop a specific list of necessary changes and provide the client system with a written copy.

26. Role play altered role situations with the client system for 1 hour once a day. This would include opportunities for clients to practice those areas of role performance that may be new or unique.

27. If client and client system cannot achieve agreement on the problematic role refer to:

    a. Psychiatric mental health clinical nurse specialist
    b. Family therapist
    c. Social worker
28. If problematic roles involve interactions between client and members of the health care team (nurses, physicians, etc.) request consultation with psychiatric mental health clinical nurse specialist or mental health specialist with experience in the area of resolving system problems (i.e., family therapists, social workers).

HOME HEALTH

1. Monitor for factors contributing to disturbed role performance.
2. Involve patient and family in planning, implementing, and prompting reduction or elimination of disturbance in role function.
    a. Family conference
    b. Mutual goal setting
    c. Clarification of expected role performance of all family members
    d. Communication
3. Assist patient and family in life-style adjustments that may be required.
    a. Treatment of physical or emotional disability
    b. Stress management
    c. Adjustment to changing role functions and relationships
    d. Development and use of support networks
    e. Requirements for redistribution of family tasks
4. Consult with assistive resources as indicated.
    a. Psychiatric nurse clinician
    b. Psychiatrist
    c. Physician
    d. Visiting nurse
    e. Occupational therapist
    f. Financial counselor
    g. Social service
    h. Physical therapist
    i. Support groups
    j. Family counselor

EVALUATION
OBJECTIVE 1

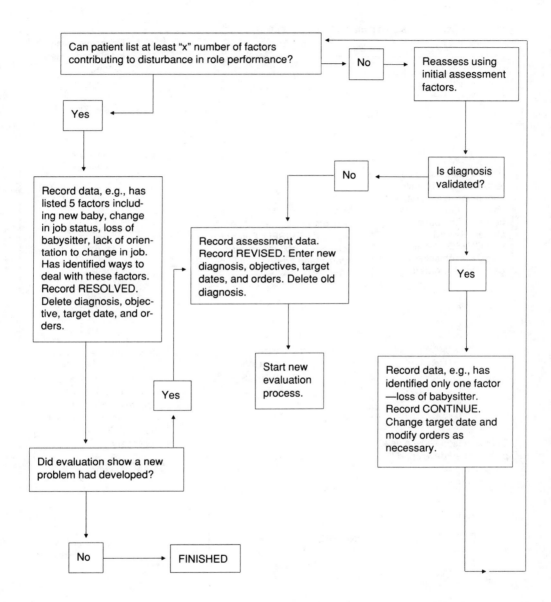

OBJECTIVE 2

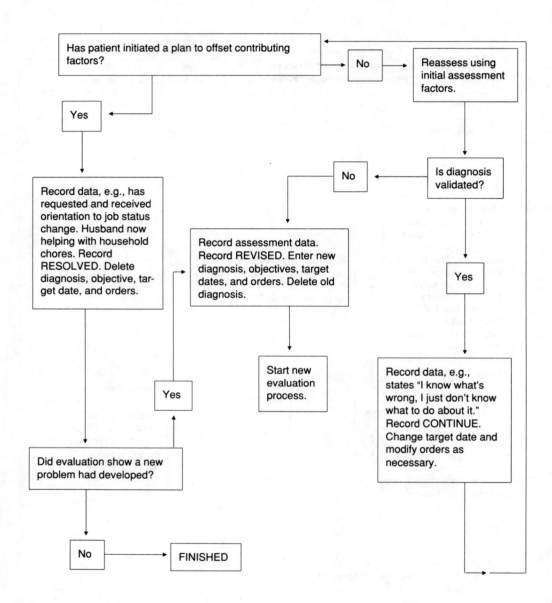

Social Interaction, Impaired

DEFINITION

The state in which an individual participates in an insufficient or excessive quantity or ineffective quality of social exchange (NANDA, 1987, p. 58).

DEFINING CHARACTERISTICS (NANDA, 1987, p 58)

The nurse will review the initial pattern assessment for the following defining characteristics to determine the diagnosis of Social Interaction, Impaired.

1. Major defining characteristics
   a. Verbalized or observed discomfort in social situations
   b. Verbalized or observed inability to receive or communicate a satisfying sense of belonging, caring, interest, or shared history
   c. Observed use of unsuccessful social interaction behavior
   d. Dysfunctional interaction with peers, family, or others
2. Minor defining characteristics
   a. Family report of change of style or pattern of interaction

RELATED FACTORS (NANDA, 1987, p. 58)

1. Knowledge or skill deficit about ways to enhance mutuality
2. Communication barriers
3. Self-concept disturbance
4. Absence of available significant others or peers
5. Limited physical mobility
6. Therapeutic isolation
7. Sociocultural dissonance
8. Environmental barriers
9. Altered thought processes

DIFFERENTIATION

Differentiation for Impaired Social Interaction will be strongly determined by the patient's verbalization of less-than-usual social activities either in quantity or quality. The nurse may also observe a decrease in these activities in terms of visitors, phone calls, or mail.

The diagnosis of Impaired Social Interaction would need to be differentiated from Self-Concept, Disturbance in; Knowledge Deficit; Verbal Communication, Impaired; Physical Mobility, Impaired; Social Isolation; and general problems related to the total patterns of role-relationship and coping–stress tolerance.

Self-Concept, Disturbance in would be determined as the appropriate alternate diagnosis if the individual's symptoms are related to a more general disturbance of the self rather than just social interaction.

Knowledge Deficit, particularly as related to mutuality, would be the appropriate alternate diagnosis if the individual verbalized or demonstrated an inability to attend to significant others' social actions in the context of independent and dependent aspects of their role.

Verbal Communication, Impaired would be the appropriate diagnosis if the individual is unable to receive or send communication, either verbally or nonverbally.

Physical Mobility, Impaired would be the appropriate diagnosis if the physical distance or inability to be near others is the sole determining factor for being unable to carry out one's usual social interactions.

Social Isolation would be the more appropriate diagnosis when the individual is placed in or chooses isolation due to physiologic, sociologic, or emotional concerns. Further assessment is required to completely delineate the exact problem when self-isolation is chosen.

Other role-relationship diagnoses and coping-stress alterations would need to be ruled out or brought in as accompanying diagnoses in many instances. These diagnoses could serve as the reason for the deliberate decision to choose social isolation.

OBJECTIVES

1. Will verbalize satisfaction with quantity and quality of social interactions by (date).

AND/OR

2. Will demonstrate (increased) (decreased) involvement in social interactions by (date).

TARGET DATE

Assisting the patient to modify social interactions will require a significant amount of time. A target date ranging between 7 and 10 days would be appropriate for evaluating progress.

NURSING ORDERS

ADULT HEALTH

1. Role play social interactions with patient.
2. Encourage patient to express how he or she feels or what he or she fears in a social situation.
3. Listen to patient's communication skills and help him or her to find alternative ones.
4. Help patient obtain a realistic perception of self.
5. Help patient participate in group interactions; use crutches, wheelchair, or stretcher to get patient out of his or her room.
6. If patient is in isolation, spend sufficient time with him or her so he or she does not feel so isolated.
7. Involve patient in care; help him or her make decisions about own care.
8. Initiate referrals with support groups.
9. Consult with patient's minister, priest, rabbi.

CHILD HEALTH

1. Monitor for contributory factors to altered social interaction pattern.
2. Determine the effect the altered social interaction has on child, parent, family, and school.
3. Develop a plan of care to best meet child's potential for succeeding with appropriate social interaction—this will be highly qualified by social class and values.
4. Determine if conflict exists between parent's and child's desired social interaction.
5. If conflict exists regarding social interaction, deal with this as needed in values or beliefs pattern.
6. Assist child, parents, and family in ventilation of feelings regarding social interaction impairment, including actual consequences of same.
7. Make referrals as appropriate to professionals best able to assist in dealing with problem (e.g., clinical psychiatric nurse, play therapist, family therapist, etc.).
8. Identify local support groups to appropriately match needs (e.g., parental-child support groups for the handicapped, United Cerebral Palsy Association, Spina Bifida Association).
9. If impaired social interaction also relates to school, include teacher and essential school personnel in plans for resolving the impairment and for best follow-up.
10. Identify follow-up appointment needs and ways to monitor progress for child and family (e.g., stickers as incentives to reinforce desired behavior).
11. Anticipate discrepant or unrealistic expectations by parents of children. Monitor for potential abuse of child according to pattern for this.

WOMEN'S HEALTH

This nursing diagnosis will pertain to women the same as to any other adult. The reader is referred to the other sections (Adult Health, Home Health, and Mental Health) for specific nursing orders.

MENTAL HEALTH

1. If delusions or hallucinations are present, refer to Thought Process, Altered for detailed interventions.
2. Assign primary care nurse to client.
3. Primary nurse will spend (number) minutes twice a day with client. The focus of this interaction will change as a relationship is developed. Initially the nurse should model for the client how to develop a relationship through his or her behavior in developing this relationship with the client. This modeling should include demonstrating respect for the client; consistency in interactions; congruence between thoughts, feelings, and actions; and empathy.
4. Have client identify those persons in the environment that are considered family, friends, and acquaintances. Then have client note how many interactions per week occur with each person. Have client identify his or her thoughts, feelings, and behavior about these interactions.
5. Provide appropriate confrontation with client about his or her behavior patterns that inhibit interaction in relationships with the nurse (See Kneisl & Wilson, 1984 for information about confrontation).
6. Observe client in interactions with others on the unit and identify patterns of behavior that inhibit social interaction.
7. Develop a list of those things the client finds rewarding and provide these rewards as client successfully completes progressive steps in treatment plan.
8. When client is demonstrating socially inappropriate behavior, keep interactions to a minimum and escort client to a place away from activities.
9. When inappropriate behavior stops, discuss the behavior with the client and develop a list of alternative kinds of behavior for the client to use in situations where the inappropriate behavior is elicited. Note those kinds of behavior that are identified as problematic here with the action to be taken if they are demonstrated (e.g., client will spend time out in seclusion or away from group activity).
10. Develop a schedule for gradually increasing time of client in group activities. For example client will spend (number) minutes in the group dining hall during mealtimes or will spend (number) minutes in a group game. Note client's specific activities here.
11. Primary nurse will spend 30 minutes a day with client exploring thoughts and feelings about social interactions and in assisting with reality testing of social interactions (i.e., what others might mean by silence and other nonverbal responses).
12. Identify with client areas of social skill deficit and develop a plan for improving these areas. This could include:
    a. Assertiveness training;
    b. Role playing difficult situations
    c. Teaching client relaxation techniques to reduce anxiety in social situations. (Note plan and schedule for implementation here. This should be a progressive plan with rewards for accomplishment of each step.)
13. Consult with occupational therapist if client needs to learn specific skills to facilitate social interactions (e.g., cooking skills so friends can be invited to dinner, craft skills so client can join others in social interactions around these activities).
14. Include client in group activities on the unit, and assign client activities that can be easily accomplished and that will provide positive social reinforcement from other persons involved in the activities.

15. When client demonstrates tolerance for group interactions, schedule time for the client to participate in a group therapy that provides opportunities for feedback about relationship behavior from peers and for listening to the thoughts and feelings of peers.
16. Discuss with support system ways in which they can facilitate client interaction.
17. Have client identify those activities in the community that are of interest and would provide opportunities for interaction. List those activities here and develop a plan for client to develop necessary skills to ensure opportunities for interactional success during these activities (e.g., practice a card game or tennis while in the hospital).
18. When client reports problems in an interaction, review his or her perceptions of the interaction and an evaluation of when the problems began.
19. Limit amount of time client can spend alone in room. This should be a gradual alteration and done in steps that can easily be accomplished by client. Note specific schedule for client here. Have staff person remain with client during these times until client demonstrates an ability to interact with others.
20. Refer client to appropriate community agencies:
    a. Visiting nurse
    b. Occupational therapist
    c. Social services
    d. Sheltered workshops
    e. Adult day care
    f. Meals on Wheels
    g. Church groups
    h. Social groups that share interests with the client
    i. Mental health nurse clinician
21. Have referral source make contact with client before discharge and schedule a post-discharge meeting.

HOME HEALTH

1. Monitor for factors contributing to the impaired social interaction (e.g., psychologic, physical, economic, spiritual, etc.).
2. Involve patient and family in planning, implementing and promoting reduction or elimination of impaired social interaction.
    a. Family conference
    b. Consistent rules and behavior
    c. Mutual goal setting
    d. Support for care provider
    e. Suicide prevention
3. Assist patient and family in life-style adjustments that may be required.
    a. Providing safe environment
    b. Development and use of support networks
    c. Change in role functions
    d. Prescribed treatments (e.g., medications, behavioral interventions, etc.)
    e. Assistance with self-care activities
    f. Possible hospitalization or placement in half-way house
    g. Treatment of drug or alcohol abuse
    h. Development and practice of social skills
    i. Independent living skills
    j. Finances
    k. Stress management
4. Assist patient and family to develop criteria to determine when crisis exists and professional intervention is necessary.

    a. Violence
    b. Sudden change in ability to care for self
    c. Hallucinations or delusions
5. Consult with or refer to assistive resources as indicated
    a. Respite care
    b. Support groups
    c. Psychiatric nurse clinician
    d. Social worker
    e. Financial counseling
    f. Job counseling
    g. Emergency intervention (e.g., police, emergency room, crisis hotline)

EVALUATION
OBJECTIVE 1

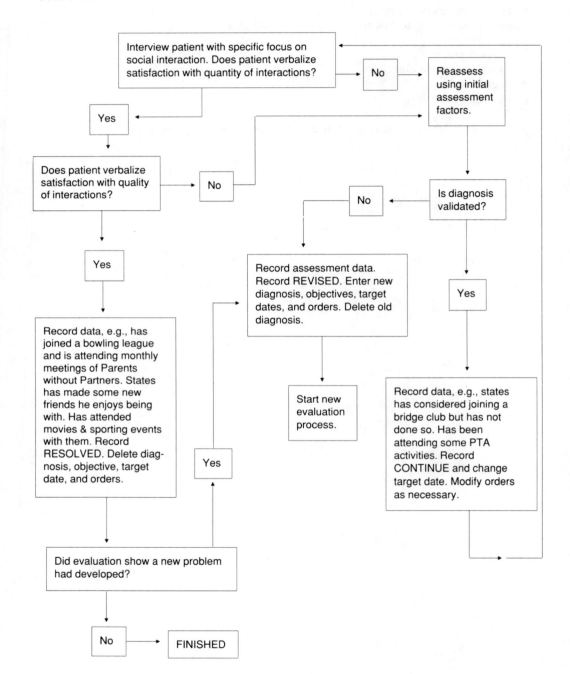

OBJECTIVE 2

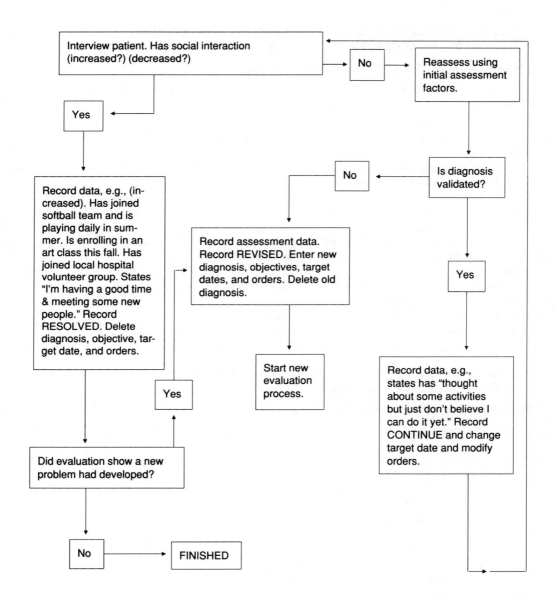

Social Isolation

DEFINITION

Aloneness experienced by the individual and perceived as imposed by others and as a negative or threatened state (NANDA, 1987, p. 59).

DEFINING CHARACTERISTICS (NANDA, 1987, p. 59)

The nurse will review the initial pattern assessment for the following defining characteristics to determine the diagnosis of Social Isolation.

1. Major defining characteristics
   a. Has no supportive significant others (family, friends, group)
   b. Has sad, dull affect
   c. Engages in inappropriate or immature interests and activities for developmental age or stage
   d. Is uncommunicative, withdrawn, no eye contact
   e. Is Preoccupied with own thoughts or with repetitive, meaningless actions
   f. Projects hostility in voice and behavior
   g. Seeks to be alone or exists in a subculture
   h. Has evidence of physical or mental handicap or altered state of wellness
   i. Shows behavior unaccepted by dominant cultural group
2. Subjective
   a. Expresses feelings of aloneness imposed by others
   b. Expresses feelings of rejection
   c. Experiences feelings of difference from others
   d. Feels inadequacy in or absence of significant purpose in life
   e. Express inability to meet expectations of others
   f. Feels insecurity in public
   g. Expresses values acceptable to the subculture but unacceptable to dominant cultural group
   h. Expresses interests inappropriate to the developmental age or stage

RELATED FACTORS (NANDA, 1987, pp.59–60)

Factors contributing to the absence of satisfying personal relationships, such as:

1. Delay in accomplishing developmental tasks
2. Immature interests
3. Alterations in physical appearance
4. Alterations in mental status
5. Unaccepted social behavior
6. Unaccepted social values
7. Altered state of wellness
8. Inadequate personal resources
9. Inability to engage in satisfying personal relationships

DIFFERENTIATION

This diagnosis must be differentiated from Self-Concept, Disturbance in; Thought Process Altered; Nutrition, Altered; Individual Coping, Ineffective; and Anxiety. Many of these same alterations may exist, and may not necessarily contribute to altered role-relationship patterns, although it is a likely possibility. A critical element needed for individualized consideration for each patient is emphasized to best determine how the potential for social isolation might become actual. It is not appropriate, for example, to judge that all patients recovering from surgical intervention need to have visitors limited, nor is it appropriate to assume that all patients recovering from surgery need to have visitors to best meet goals for return to normal activities. In each of these instances a critical element would be a subjective component addressing a desire for usual social activities despite limitations for the same to occur.

Additionally, any alterations in thought process should be further explored to determine if there are related mental health alterations which may assume greater priority. An example of this might be an altered social process carried to extreme, as in phobia of crowds.

OBJECTIVES

1. Will identify at least (number) ways to increase social interaction by (date).

AND/OR

2. Will participate in social activities at least weekly by (date).

TARGET DATE

A target date range of 2–7 days would be acceptable depending on the exact social interaction chosen.

NURSING ORDERS

ADULT HEALTH

1. Encourage patient to verbalize feelings of isolation and aloneness.
2. Provide feedback and support.
3 Encourage visits from family and significant others.
4. Encourage patient to participate in diversional activities, especially those involving groups.
5. Encourage patient to identify and use support systems and groups.
   a. Transportation
   b. Clothing
   c. Communications
   d. Day care centers
   e. Church groups
   f. Telephone help line
   g. Pets
   h. Wheelchair groups

CHILD HEALTH

1. Provide opportunities for expression of feelings about desired social activity by spending 15–20 minutes per shift during waking hours with patients and family.
2. Determine what obstacles are perceived by patient and family in pursuit of desired social activities.
3. Identify what realistic patterns for socialization are applicable for patient and family in collaboration with same.
4. Collaborate with health professionals and related paraprofessionals to assist in meeting realistic goals for patient and family socialization, such as:
   a. Clinical nurse specialist
   b. Family therapist
   c. Psychiatrist or psychologist
   d. Social worker
   e. Play therapist
   f. Pediatrician and subspecialists
   g. Social worker
   h. Legal counselor
5. Assess for contributory related factors to best consider social activity pattern.
6. Identify support groups to assist in realization of desired social activities.

7. Assess patient's and family's perception of the effect desired social activities may have on current role-relationship pattern.
8. Assist patient and family to identify the effect desired social activities may have on family dynamics.
9. Provide appropriate opportunities for assessment of young child's perceptions of situational needs and how he or she views self.
10. Assist patient to develop schedule for consideration of desired social activities at least 2 days before dismissal from hospital.
11. Provide for appropriate follow-up appointment as needed previous to dismissal from hospital.

WOMEN'S HEALTH

Sexually Transmitted Diseases Herpes Genitalis, Syphilis, Chlamydia, Gonorrhea, AIDS)

(Note: For detailed nursing orders see Chapter 10. The following nursing orders apply to the social isolation the patient feels who has these diseases.)

1. Assure client of confidentiality.
2. Refer for counseling to:
   a. Support groups
   b. Professional
      (1) Clinics
         (a) Public health
         (b) Private
      (2) Nurse specialists
      (3) Physicians
3. Provide a nonjudgmental atmosphere to:
   a. Encourage verbalization of concerns.
      (1) Recurrent nature of disease, especially herpes, and chlamydia
      (2) Lack of cure for disease (AIDS)
      (3) Economics in treating disease
      (4) Social stigma associated with disease
      (5) Opportunity for entrance into health care system
   b. Encourge honesty in answers to such questions as:
      (1) Multiple sexual partners
         (a) Identify contacts
      (2) Describing sexual behavior
4. Encourage client to seek treatment from health care providers.
5. Encourage honest communciation with sexual partners.
6. Inform client of services available for support:
   a. Support Groups
      (1) National Association of People with AIDS
         Washington, DC 20035
         (202) 483-797
      (2) Herpes Resources Information
         Box 100
         Palo Alto, CA 94302
   b. Telephone hot lines
      (1) National AIDS Hot Line
         (800) 342-AIDS
      (2) National VD Hotline
         (800) 227-8922
         in California, (800) 982-5883

    c. Special medical facilities, such as hospital for AIDS.

MENTAL HEALTH

1. If delusions and or hallucinations are present, refer to Thought Process, Altered (Chapter 7) for detailed interventions.
2. If social isolation is related to client's feelings of powerlessness, refer to Powerlessness (Chapter 8) for detailed care plan.
3. Discuss with client his or her perception of the source of the social isolation and have him or her list those things he or she has tried to resolve the situation.
4. Have client list those persons in the environment that are considered family, friends, and acquaintances. Then have client note how many interactions per week occur with each person. Have client identify what interferes with feeling connected with these persons. This activity should be implemented by the primary nurse. Note schedule for this interaction here.
5. When contributing factors have been identified, develop a plan to alter these factors. This could include:
    a. Assertiveness training;
    b. Role playing difficult situations;
    c. Teaching client relaxation techniques to reduce anxiety in social situations. (Note plan and schedule for implementation here.)
6. Develop a list of those things the client finds rewarding and provide these rewards as client successfully completes progressive steps in treatment plan. This schedule should be developed with the client. Note schedule for rewards and the kinds of behavior to be rewarded here.
7. Consult with occupational therapist if client needs to learn specific skills to facilitate social interactions (e.g., cooking skills so friends can be invited to dinner; craft skills so client can join others in social interactions around these activities; dancing).
8. Provide client with those prostheses necessary to facilitate social interactions (e.g., hearing aids, eyeglasses). Note here assistance needed from nursing staff in providing these to client. Also note where they are to be stored while not in use.
9. Include client in group activities on the unit; assign client activities that can be easily accomplished and that will provide positive social reinforcement from other persons involved in the activities. This could include things like having client assume reponsibility for preparing a part of a group meal or for serving a portion of a meal, etc.
10. Role play with client those social interactions identified as most difficult. This will be done by primary nurse. Note schedule for this activity here.
11. Discuss with client those times it would be appropriate to be alone and develop a plan for coping with these times in a positive manner (e.g., client will develop a list of books to read, music to listen to, community activities to attend).
12. When client is demonstrating socially inappropriate behavior, keep interactions to a minimum and escort to a place way from group activities.
13. When inappropriate behavior stops, discuss the behavior with the client and develop a list of alternative kinds of behavior for the client to use in situations where the inappropriate behavior is elicited. Note those kinds of behavior that are identified as problematic here with the action to be taken if they are demonstrated (e.g., client will spend a time out in seclusion or sleeping area).
14. Develop a schedule of gradually increasing time for client in group activities (e.g., client will spend (number) minutes in the group dining hall during meal times or will spend (number) minutes in a group game twice a day). Note specific goals for client here.
15. Primary nurse will spend 30 minutes once a day with client discussing client's reactions to social interactions and in assisting client with reality testing social interactions (e.g., what others might mean by silence, or various nonverbal and common verbal expressions). This time can also be used to discuss relationship roles and client's specific concerns about relationships.

16. Assign client a room near areas with high activity.
17. If negative self-concept affects interactions with others, refer to Self-Concept, Disturbance in (Chapter 8) for detailed care plan.
18. Assign one staff person to the client each shift and have this person interact with client every 30 minutes.
19. Be open and direct with client in interactions, and avoid verbal and nonverbal behavior that requires interpretation from client.
20. Have client tell staff his or her interpretation of interactions.
21. Have client identify those activities in the community that are of interest and would provide opportunities for interactions with others. List client's interest here.
22. Develop with the client a plan for making contact with the identified community activities before discharge.
23. When client demonstrates tolerance for group interactions, schedule time for the client to participate in a therapy group that provides opportunities for feedback about relationship behavior from peers and for listening to the thoughts and feelings of peers.
24. Arrange at least 1 hour a week for client to interact with support system in the presence of the primary nurse. This will allow the nurse to assess and facilitate these interactions.
25. Discuss with support system ways in which they can facilitate client interaction.
26. Model for support system and for client those kinds of behavior that facilitate communication (see Smitherman, 1981, for a review of communication skills or Watzlawick, Beavin, & Jackson, 1967, for basic information related to system communication).
27. Limit the amount of time client can spend alone in room. This should be a gradual alteration and should be done in steps that can easily be accomplished by client. Note specific schedule for client here (e.g., client will spend 5 minutes per hour out in day area) Have staff person remain with client during these times until client demonstrates an ability to interact with others.
28. Refer client to appropriate community agencies:
    a. Visiting nurse
    b. Occupational therapist
    c. Social services
    d. Sheltered workshops
    e. Adult day care
    f. Meals on Wheels
    g. Church groups
    h. Social groups that share interest with the client
    i. Mental health nurse clinician

HOME HEALTH

1. Involve patient and family in planning and implementing strategies to reduce social isolation:
   a. Family conference
   b. Mutual goal setting
   c. Communication
2. Assist family and patient with life-style adjustments that may be required:
   a. Promote social interaction
   b. Provide transportation
   c. Provide activities to keep busy during lonely times
   d. Provide communication alternatives for those with sensory deficit
   e. Assist with disfiguring illness (e.g., enterstomal therapist, prothesis manufacturer)
   f. Control incontinence or provide absorbent undergarments when socializing
   g. Promote self-worth
   h. Promote self-care

    i. Develop and utilize support groups
    j. Use pets
    k. Establish regular telephone contact
    l. Inform of volunteer programs in community that person could work for
3. Consult with or refer to assistive resources as indicated:
    a. Enterstomal therapist
    b. Occupational therapist
    c. Visting nurse
    d. Social service
    e. Physician
    f. Self-help groups such as Reach to Recovery, I Can Cope, Ostomy Association, etc.
    g. Church groups
    h. Civic groups
    i. Day care or respite care
    j. Senior citizen centers
    k. Community groups that contact the homebound
    l. Home teaching program
    m. Interactive computer

EVALUATION
OBJECTIVE 1

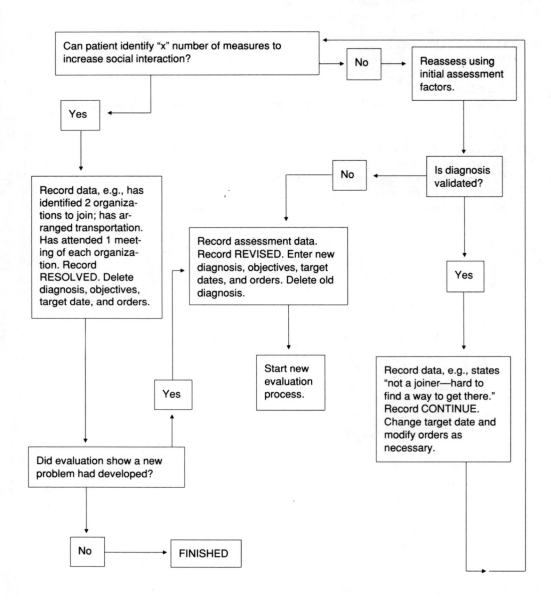

OBJECTIVE 2

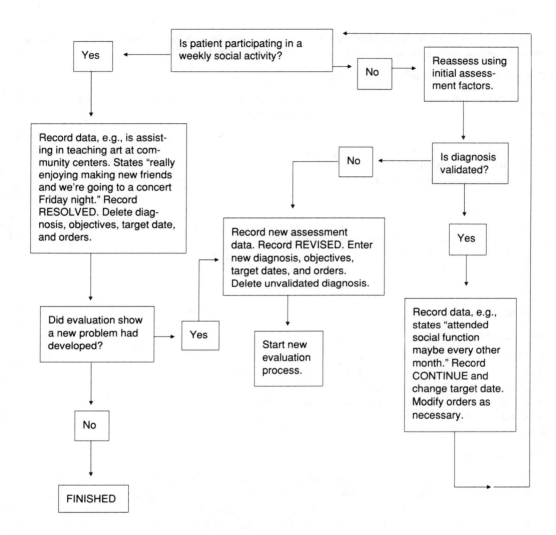

Is patient participating in a weekly social activity?

Yes

No

Reassess using initial assessment factors.

Record data, e.g., is assisting in teaching art at community centers. States "really enjoying making new friends and we're going to a concert Friday night." Record RESOLVED. Delete diagnosis, objectives, target date, and orders.

No

Is diagnosis validated?

Record new assessment data. Record REVISED. Enter new diagnosis, objectives, target dates, and orders. Delete unvalidated diagnosis.

Yes

Did evaluation show a new problem had developed?

Yes

Start new evaluation process.

Record data, e.g., states "attended social function maybe every other month." Record CONTINUE and change target date. Modify orders as necessary.

No

FINISHED

Verbal Communication, Impaired

DEFINITION

The state in which an individual experiences a decreased or absent ability to use or understand language in human interaction (NANDA, 1987, p. 57)

DEFINING CHARACTERISTICS (NANDA, 1987, p. 57)

The nurse will review the initial pattern assessment for the following defining characteristics to determine the diagnosis of Verbal Communication Impaired.

1. Major defining characteristics
   a. Is unable to speak dominant language
   b. Speaks or verbalizes with difficulty
   c. Does not or cannot speak
   d. Stutters
   e. Slurs words
   f. Has difficulty forming words or sentences
   g. Has difficulty expressing thought verbally
   h. Verbalizes inappropriately
   i. Has dyspnea
   j. Is disoriented
2. Minor defining characteristics
   None given.

RELATED FACTORS (NANDA, 1987, p. 57)

1. Decrease in circulation to brain
2. Physical barrier (brain tumor, tracheostomy, intubation)
3. Anatomical defect, cleft palate
4. Psychological barriers (psychosis, lack of stimuli)
5. Cultural difference
6. Developmental or age-related

DIFFERENTIATION

Verbal Communication, Impaired should be differentiated from Social Isolation and Sensory-Perceptual Alteration or Deficit. Social Isolation can occur because of the reduced ability or inability of an individual to use language as a means of communication. It makes no difference if the individual cannot communicate because of physical problems or because of not understanding the language; some form of social isolation will usually occur. However, the primary cause of the impairment will provide the nurse a clue as to which of the above diagnoses is the correct one to use in a specific situation.

The capacity of the individual to communicate is validated, which differentiates this pattern from Sensory-Perceptual Alteration or Deficit. It is important that the nurse dealing with these clients distinguish receptive from expressive communication deficits.

OBJECTIVES

1. Will verbalize satisfaction with communication process by (date).

AND/OR

2. Will communicate in a clear manner via (state specific method, e.g., orally, esophageal speech, computer, etc.) by (date).

TARGET DATE

The target date for resolution of this diagnosis will be long-range. However, 7 days would be appropriate for initial evaluation.

NURSING ORDERS

ADULT HEALTH

1. Maintain a patient, calm approach.
2. Allow adequate time for communication.
3. Do not interrupt the patient or attempt to finish sentences for him or her.
4. Ask questions that require short answers or a nod of the head; anticipate needs.
5. Provide materials that can be used to assist in communication (e.g., magic slate, flash cards, pad and pencil, ''Speak and Spell'' computer toy, pictures, letter board).
6. Assure patient that parenteral therapy does not interfere with patient's ability to write.
7. Answer call bell promptly rather than using the intercom system.
8. Inform family and significant others and other health care personnel of the effective ways patient communicates.
9. Initiate referral to speech therapist if appropriate.
10. Initiate referrals to support agencies such as Lost Chord Club or New Voice Club as appropriate.
11. Discuss use of electronic voice box, esophageal speech.
12. Encourage patient to have recordings made for reaching police, fire department, doctor or emergency medical services if impaired verbal communication is a long-term condition.

CHILD HEALTH

1. Monitor patient's potential for speech according to subjective and objective components to include the following:
    a. Reported or documented previous speech capacity or potential
    b. Health history for evidence of cognitive, sensory, perceptual, or neurologic dysfunction
    c. Actual auditory documentation of speech potential
    d. Assessment done by speech specialist
    e. Patterns of speech of parents and significant others
    f. Cultural meaning attached to speech
    g. Any related trauma or pathophysiology
    h. Parental perception of child's status, especially in instances of congential anomaly such as cleft lip or palate
    i. Identification of dominant language and secondary languages heard or spoken in family.
2. Assist the patient and parents to understand needed explanations for procedures, treatments, and equipment to be used in nursing care.
3. In the absence of speech, provide for alternate form of communication, such as writing or agreed-upon nod or other body language.
4. Encourage feelings to be expressed by taking time to understand possible attempts at speech. Use pictures if necessary for young children.
5. Assist the patient and family in relearning communication to be used in instances of cerebrovascular accident (CVA) or related long-term etiology in which actual potential for speech may be unknown through use of:
    a. Speech therapist
    b. Occupational therapist
    c. Play therapist
    d. Computer augmentative communication specialist
    e. Clinical nurse specialist
    f. Pediatrician

g. Neurologist or neurosurgeon

h. Psychologist or psychiatrist

6. Encourage family participation in care of patient as situation allows.

7. Assist family to identify support groups to assist in future coping.

8. Assist patient and family in determining the impact altered verbal communication may have for family functioning.

9. Provide information for long-term medical follow-up as indicated, especially for congenital anomalies.

10. Assist in identification of appropriate financial support if child is able to qualify for same according to state and federal legislation.

11. Monitor for potential for related alterations in role-relationship patterns as a result of altered verbal communication.

12. Monitor for potential for related alterations in self-concept or coping patterns as a result of altered verbal communication.

13. Provide appropriate patient and family teaching for care of patient if permanent tracheostomy or related prosthetic is to be used to include:

a. Appropriate number or size of tracheostomy tube

b. Appropriate duplication of size of tracheostomy tube in place in event of accidental dislodging or loss

c. Appropriate administration of oxygen via trach adapter

d. Appropriate suctioning technique, sterile and nonsterile

e. Appropriate list of supplies and how to procure them

f. Resources for actual care in emergency, with list of numbers including ambulance and nearest hospital

g. Appropriate indications for notification of physician

(1) Bleeding from tracheostomy

(2) Coughing out or dislodging of tracheostomy

(3) Difficulty in passing catheter to suction tracheostomy

(4) Fever above 101°F

h. Appropriate daily hygiene of tracheostomy

i. Caution regarding use of regular gauze or other substances which might be inhaled or ingested through tracheostomy

j. Need for humidification of tracheostomy

(Note: These may vary slightly according to physician's plan or actual patient status.)

WOMEN'S HEALTH

This nursing diagnosis will pertain to women the same as to any other adult. The reader is referred to the other sections (Adult Health, Home Health, and Mental Health).

MENTAL HEALTH

1. If impaired communication is related to alterations in physiology or surgical alterations, refer to Adult Health for detailed care plans.

2. Establish a calm, reassuring environment.

3. Provide client with a private environment if experiencing high levels of anxiety to assist client in focusing on relevant stimuli.

4. Communicate with client in clear, concise language.

5. Speak slowly to client.

6. Do not shout.

7. Face client when talking to him or her.

8. Role model agreement between verbal and nonverbal behavior.

9. Spend 30 minutes twice a day with client discussing communication patterns. Note schedule for these interactions here with the person responsible for them. This time could also include, as the client progresses:
   a. Constructive confrontation about the effects of the dysfunctional communication patterns on relationships.
   b. Role playing appropriate communication patterns
   c. Pointing out to client the lack of agreement between verbal and nonverbal behavior and context
   d. Helping client to understand purpose of dysfunctional communication patterns
   e. Developing alternative ways for client to have needs met
10. Develop, with the client's assistance, a reward program for appropriate communication patterns and for progress on goals. Note the kinds of behavior to be rewarded and schedule for reward here.
11. Instruct client in assertive communication techniques and practice these in daily interactions with the client. Note here those assertive skills client is to practice and how these are to be practiced (e.g., each medication is to be requested by the client in an assertive manner).
12. Provide the client with positive verbal rewards for appropriate communication.
13. Sit with client while another client is asked for feedback about an interaction.
14. Keep interactions brief and goal-directed when client is communicating in dysfunctional manner.
15. Spend an extra 5 minutes in interactions in which client is communicating clearly, and inform client of this reward of time.
16. Reward improvement in client's listening behavior. This can be evaluated by having the client repeat what has just been heard. Provide clarification for the differences between what was heard and what was said.
17. Have support system participate in one interaction per week with the client in the presence of a staff member. The staff member will facilitate communication between the client and the support system. Note time for these interactions here with the name of the staff person responsible for this process.
18. Arrange for client to participate in a therapeutic group in which feedback on communication can be gained from peers and client can observe peers' patterns of interactions. Note schedule for these groups here.
19. Request that client clarify unclear statements or communications in private language.
20. Teach client to request clarification on confusing communications. This may be practiced with role play.
21. Include client in unit activities and assign appropriate tasks to client. These should require a level of communication the client can easily achieve so that a positive learning experience can occur. Note level of activity appropriate for client here.
22. If communication problems evolve from a language difference have someone who understands the language orient the client to the unit as soon as possible and answer any questions the client might have.
23. Use nonverbal communication to interact with client when there is no one available to translate.
24. Obtain information about nonverbal communication in the client's culture and about appropriate psychosocial behavior. Alter interactions and expectations to fit these beliefs as they fit the client. Note here that information that is important in providing daily care for this client.
25. Determine if the client understands any English and if so how is it best understood (i.e., written, spoken).
26. If client does not understand English, determine if a language other than the one from the culture of origin is spoken. Perhaps a common language for staff and client can be found (e.g., few people other than Navajos speak Navajo but some older Navajos also speak Spanish).

27. Do not shout when talking with someone who speaks another language. Speak slowly and concisely.
28. Use pictures to enhance nonverbal communication.
29. If a staff member does not speak the client's language arrange for a translator to visit with the client at least once a day to answer questions and provide information. Have a schedule for the next day available so this can be reviewed with the client and information can be provided about complex procedures. Have a staff member remain with the client during these interactions to serve as a resource person for the translator. Allow time for the client to ask questions and express feelings. Note schedule for these visits here with the name of the translator.

HOME HEALTH

1. Involve patient and family in planning and implementing strategies to decrease, prevent, or cope with impaired verbal communication.
   a. Family conference
   b. Group discussion
   c. Mutual goal setting
   d. Communication
2. Teach patient and family appropriate information regarding the care of a person with impaired verbal communication:
   a. Use of pencil and paper, alphabet letters, head signals, sign language, pictures, flash cards, computer
   b. Use of repetition
   c. Facing the person when communicating
   d. Using simple, one-step commands
   e. Allowing time for person to respond
   f. Use of drawing, painting, coloring, singing, exercising
   g. Identifying tasks the person with impaired verbal communication can do well
   h. Decreasing external noise
3. Assist patient and family in life-style adjustments that may be required:
   a. Stress management
   b. Changing role functions and relationships
   c. Learning a foreign language
   d. Acknowledging and coping with frustration with communication efforts
   e. Obtaining necessary supportive equipment (e.g., hearing aid, special telephone, artificial larynx)
4. Consult with or refer to appropriate assistive resources as required:
   a. Speech therapist
   b. Rehabilitation
   c. Psychiatric nurse clinician
   d. Physician
   e. Visiting nurse
   f. Language education
   g. Support groups
   h. Stress management training
   i. Self-help groups
   j. Social service

EVALUATION
OBJECTIVE 1

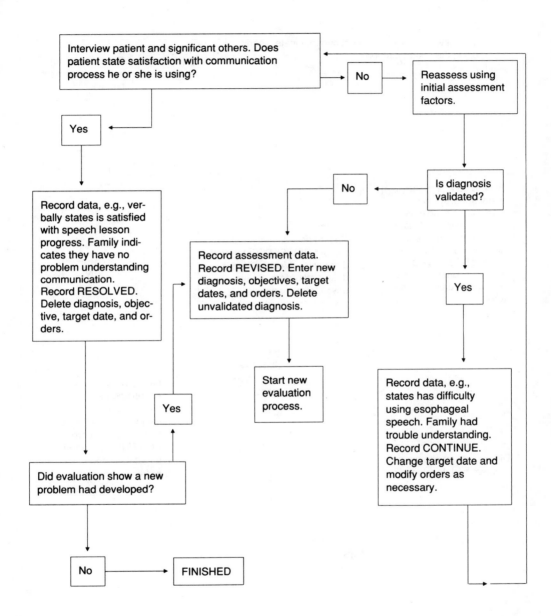

OBJECTIVE 2

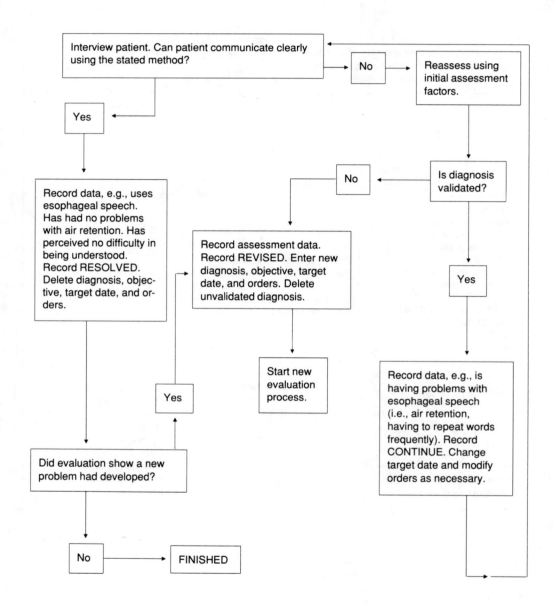

Violence, Potential for

DEFINITION

A state in which an individual experiences behaviors that can be physically harmful either to the self or others (NANDA. 1987, p 110).

DEFINING CHARACTERISTICS (NANDA, 1987, p 110).

The nurse will review the initial pattern assessment for the following defining characteristics to determine the diagnosis of Violence for Potential.

1. Major defining characteristics
   a. Body language
   b. Clenched fists, tense facial expression, rigid posture, tautness indicating effort to control
   c. Hostile, threatening verbalizations: boasting of or prior abuse of others
   d. Increased motor activity: pacing, excitement, irritability, agitation
   e. Overt and aggressive acts: goal-direction destruction of objects in environment
   f. Possessions of destructive means: gun, knife, weapon
   g. Rage
   h. Self-destructive behavior; active, aggressive suicidal acts
   i. Suspicion of others, paranoid ideation, delusions, hallucinations
   j. Substance abuse or withdrawal
2. Minor defining characteristics
   a. Increasing anxiety levels
   b. Fear of self or others
   c. Inability to verbalize feelings
   d. Repetition of verbalizations
   e. Continued complaints, requests, and demands
   f. Anger
   g. Provocative behavior: argumentative, dissatisfied, overreactive, hypersensitive
   h. Vulnerable self-esteem
   i. Depression (specifically active, aggressive, suicidal acts

RELATED FACTORS (NANDA, 1987, p. 111)

1. Antisocial character
2. Battered women
3. Catatonic excitement
4. Child abuse
5. Manic excitement
6. Organic brain syndrome
7. Panic states
8. Rage reactions
9. Suicidal behavior
10. Temporal lobe epilepsy
11. Toxic reactions to medication

DIFFERENTIATION

It is important to note that a single cue does not constitute a pattern for potential abuse, but a cluster of cues does. An individual with a potential for violence will affect family patterns and role-relationship patterns. Assessment of the family for the potential for abuse or violence includes observation of prenatal, labor and delivery, childhood, adolescent, and later-life dynamics. All other role-relationship patterns may contribute to this potential or actual violence pattern. Of particular note would be Parenting, Altered. Additionally, any individual experiencing alterations in coping or self-concept would also be at risk for violence. Evidence suggests a potential for violence also exists related to care for the elderly and those individuals who are handicapped and unable to speak for themselves.

Violence, Potential for should also be differentiated from Rape Trauma Syndrome. Rape Trauma Syndrome deals with the client who has already experienced violence. Violence, Potential for deals with the client who is in danger of being a victim of violence or creating the violence for another. The nurse who deals with these patients should be aware not only of the client's perceptions and feelings but of the social and family factors that are present which could lead to violence.

OBJECTIVES

1. Will demonstrate at least (number) alternative methods for releasing anger by (date).

AND/OR

2. Will identify factors that contribute to potential for violence by (date).

TARGET DATE

For the sake of all concerned, the patient should begin to demonstrate progress within 3–5 days. To totally control violent behavior may take several months.

NURSING ORDERS

ADULT HEALTH

1. Monitor for signs of anger or distress.
2. Accept anger of patient but do not participate in it.
3. Remain calm; set limits on patient's behavior, reduce environmental stimuli.
4. Encourage patient to verbalize angry feelings rather than physically demonstrating them.
5. Let the patient know that he or she has control of own actions; he or she is responsible for own actions. Help patient identify situations that interfere with his or her control.
6. Provide a safe environment; restrain or seclude as needed.
7. Encourage patient to identify alternate methods of dealing with anger.
8. Observe for signs of suicide.
9. Give medications as ordered (tranquilizer, sedative, etc.)
10. Refer to psychiatric nurse clinician (see mental health nursing orders for more detailed interventions).

CHILD HEALTH

1. Assist patient and family to describe usual patterns of role-relationship activities.
2. Monitor for precipitating or triggering events which seem to recur as the pattern for violence is explored.
3. Assist the patient and family to describe own perception of the actual or potential violence pattern.
4. Provide opportunities for expression of emotions related to the violence appropriate for age and developmental capacity (e.g., toddler: dolls, puppets, or other noninvasive methods).
5. Provide appropriate collaboration for long-term follow-up regarding appropriate intervention to include:
   a. Family therapist
   b. Legal counsel
   c. Social worker
   d. Child protective services
   e. Clinical nurse specialist
   f. Pediatrician or medical specialists
   g. Play therapist

   h. Community health nurse

   i. Psychiatrist or psychologist

6. Provide for role-taking by parents in a supportive manner when possible.
7. Provide consistency in caregivers to best develop a trust for nursing staff during hospitalization.
8. Provide for confidentiality and privacy.
9. Ensure that discussions regarding child and family be carried out with objectivity.
10. Address appropriate authorities as needed for protection of child and family members to include security or police members according to institutional policy.
11. Provide support in determining usual coping patterns and how these may be enhanced to deal with altered role-relationship pattern of violence.
12. Assist in plans for placement, transitional placement, or dismissal to return home for family.
13. Assist in identification of specific resources for long-term planning as appropriate to include the following:

   a. Crisis nurseries

   b. Parents Anonymous

   c. Lay therapy for role modeling

   d. Residential treatment centers

   e. Women's protective services

   f. Hot lines

   g. Special preschool programs

   h. Halfway community programs

14. Maintain objectivity in documentation of parent-child interactions.

WOMEN'S HEALTH

(Note: Women will have the same nursing orders as those applied to adult health, mental health, and home health in all those various situations and settings. The following nursing orders relate directly to the abused and battered woman.)

1. Provide a quiet, secure atmosphere to facilitate verbalization of:

   a. Fears

   b. Anger, rage

   c. Guilt

   d. Shame

2. Provide information on options available to client.
3. Assist the client in raising her self-esteem by:

   a. Asking permission to do nursing tasks;

   b. Involving client in decision making;

   c. Providing client with choices;

   d. Letting client ask questions;

   e. Assuring client of confidentiality.

4. Assist client in reviewing and understanding family dynamics.
5. Assess the client's employment status or job training needs.
6. Assess the client's personal relationships with:

   a. Men

   b. Children

   c. Other women

7. Assist with arrangements for child care.
8. Encourage planning for economic and financial needs.

   a. Housing

   b. Job

   c. Child care

   d. Food

e. Clothing
f. School for the children
9. Assist in obtaining legal assistance for protection and prosecution.
10. Assist in obtaining immediate financial assistance for:
a. Shelter
b. Food
c. Clothing
d. Child care
11. Assist client in identifying life-style adjustments that each decision could entail.
12. Encourage development of community and social network systems such as:
a. Family
b. Friends, relatives
c. Neighbors
d. Community agencies
e. Coworkers
f. Church
13. Assist client in evaluating her:
a. Economic situation
(1) Housing
(2) Others dependent on her
(a) Parents
(b) Children
(c) Siblings
(3) Job opportunities
b. Health status
14. Assess present problems and provide appropriate nursing care.
15. Be alert for cues which might indicate battering such as:
a. Hesitancy in providing detailed information about injury and how it occurred
b. Inappropriate affect for the situation
c. Delayed reporting of symptoms
d. Types and sites of injuries such as bruises to head, throat, chest, breast, or genitals
e. Inappropriate explanation
f. Increased anxiety in presence of the batterer (Griffith-Kenney, 1986, pp. 214–215)
16. Encourage client to set short-term and long-term goals for self.
17. List modifications or changes in life-style that must be considered.

MENTAL HEALTH

1. If aggressive behavior is resulting from toxic substances, consult with physician for medication and detoxification procedure.
2. Observe client every 15 minutes during detoxification, assessing vital signs and mental status until condition is stable.
3. Place client in quiet environment for detoxification.
4. Eliminate enviornmental stimuli that affect client in a negative manner. This could include staff, family, and other clients.
5. Provide a calm, reassuring environment.
6. Observe client's use of physical space and do not invade client's personal space.
7. If it is necessary to have physical contact with the client, explain this need to the client in brief, simple terms before approaching.
8. Remove unnecessary clutter and excess stimuli from the environment.
9. Talk with client in calm, reassuring voice.

10. Do not make sudden moves.
11. Remove persons that irritate the client from the environment. Remember the best intervention for violent behavior is prevention. Observe client carefully for signs of increasing anxiety and tension.
12. If increase in tension is noted, talk with client about feelings.
13. Help client attach feelings to appropriate persons and situations (e.g., "your boss really made you angry this time").
14. Suggest to client alternative behavior for releasing tension (e.g., "you really seem tense right now, let's go to the gym so you can use the punching bag" or "let's go for a walk").
15. Provide medication as ordered and observe client for signs of side effects, especially orthostatic hypotension.
16. Do not assume physical postures that are perceived as threatening to the client.
17. Answer questions in an open, direct manner.
18. Orient client to reality in interactions. Use methods of indirect confrontation that do not pose a personal threat to client. Do not agree with delusions (e.g., "I do not hear voices other than yours or mine" or "this is the mental health unit at [name] Hospital").
19. Refer to Thought Processes, Altered (Chapter 7) for detailed interventions for delusions and hallucinations.
20. Assign one staff member to be primary caregiver to client to facilitate the development of a therapeutic relationship.
21. Introduce self to client and call client by name.
22. Assist client in identifying potential problem behavior with feedback about his or her behavior.
23. Inform client before any attempts to make physical contact are made in the process of normal provision of care (e.g., explain to client you would like to assist him or her with dressing, would this be O.K.?).
24. Have client talk about angry feelings toward self and others.
25. Contract with client to talk with staff member when he or she feels an increase in internal tension or anger.
26. Set limits on inappropriate behavior and discuss these limits with the client. Note these limits here as well as the consequences for these kinds of behaviors. This information should be very specific so the intervention is consistent from shift to shift.
27. If conflict occurs between client and someone else, sit with them as they resolve the conflict in an appropriate manner. The nurse will serve as a facilitator during this interaction.
28. Discuss tension reduction techniques with client and develop a plan for client to learn these techniques and apply them in difficult situations. Note the plan here.
29. Develop with the client a reward system for appropriate behavior. Note reward system here.
30. Talk with client about the differences between feelings and behavior. Role play with client, attaching different kinds of behavior to feelings of anger.
31. Help client in determining if the feeling being experienced is really anger. Explain that at times of high stress we can misinterpret feelings and must be very careful not to express the wrong feeling. Anger may be relabeled anxiety, frustration, etc. Placing other names on the feeling may open new behavior possibilities to the client. If this were anger, lashing out would be appropriate but since it is anxiety, it is more appropriate to relax.
32. When client is capable, assign to group in which feelings can be expressed and feedback can be obtained from peers. Note schedule for group activity here. This should also provide client with role models of how to cope with feelings in a different manner.
33. Review with client consequences of inappropriate behavior and assess the gains of this behavior over the costs.
34. Accept all threats of aggressive behavior as serious.
35. Remind staff to not take aggressive acts personally even if they appear to be directed at one staff member.

36. Provide client with positive verbal feedback about positive behavior changes.
37. Do not place client in frustrating experiences without a staff member to support client during the experience.
38. If client is suicidal place in a room with another client.
39. Remove locks from bathroom and bedroom doors.
40. Remove potential weapons from the environment. Sharp objects should never be left unsupervised in client care areas.
41. Provide client with opportunities to regain self-control without aggressive interventions by giving client choices that will facilitate control (e.g., "would you like to take some medication now or spend some time with a staff member in your room," or "we can help you into seclusion or you can walk there on your own").
42. Provide client with opportunities to maintain dignity.
43. Assure client that you will not allow him or her to harm self or someone else.
44. Reinforce this by having more staff present than necessary to physically control client if necessary. Persons from other areas of the institution may be needed in these situations. If others are used they should be trained in proper procedures.
45. If potential for physical aggression is high:
    a. Place one staff member in charge of the situation
    b. As primary person attempts to talk client down, other staff member should remove other clients and visitors from the situation
    c. Other staff member should remove potential weapons from the environment in an unobtrusive manner. This could include pool cues and balls, chairs, flower vases, books, etc.
    d. Avoid sudden movements
    e. Never turn back on client
    f. Maintain eye contact (this should not be direct, for this can be perceived as threatening to the client) and watch client's eyes for cues about potential targets of attack
    g. Do not attempt to subdue client without adequate assistance
    h. Put increased distance between client and self
    i. Tell client of the concern in brief, concise terms
    j. Suggest alternative behavior
    k. Help client focus aggression away from staff
    l. Encourage client to discuss concerns
46. If talking does not resolve the situation:
    a. Have additional assistance prepared for action (at least 4 persons should be present)
    b. Have those who are going to be involved in the intervention remove any personal items that could harm client or self (i.e., glasses, guns, long earrings, necklaces, bracelets)
    c. Have seclusion area ready for client, remove glass objects and sharp objects, and open doors for easy entry
    d. Briefly explain to client what is going to happen and why
    e. Use method practiced by intervention team to place client in seclusion or restraints
    f. Protect self with blankets, arms bent in front of body to protect head and neck
    g. Be prepared to leave the situation and be aware of location of exits
47. See Physical Mobility, Impaired (Chapter 5) for care of client in seclusion or restraints.
48. Discuss the violent episode with the client when control has been regained. Answer questions client has about the situation and provide client with opportunities to express thoughts and feelings about the episode.
49. Inform client of the behavior that is necessary to be released from seclusion or restraints.

HOME HEALTH

1. Teach patient and family appropriate monitoring of signs and symptoms of the potential for violence:

    a. Substance abuse
    b. Increased stress
    c. Social isolation
    d. Hostility
    e. Increased motor activity
    f. Disorientation to person, place, and time
    g. Disconnected thoughts
    h. Clenched fists
    i. Throwing objects
    j. Verbalizations of threats to self or others

2. Assist patient and family in life-style adjustments that may be required:
    a. Recognition of feelings of anger or hostility
    b. Developing coping strategies to express anger and hostility in acceptable manner: exercise, sports, art, music, etc.
    c. Prevention of harm to self and others
    d. Treatment of substance abuse
    e. Management of debilitating disease
    f. Coping with loss
    g. Stress management
    h. Decreasing sensory stimulation
    i. Provision of safe environment: removal of weapons, toxic drugs, etc.
    j. Development and use of support network

3. Involve patient and family in planning and implementing strategies to reduce the potential for violence:
    a. Family conference
    b. Mutual goal setting
    c. Communication

4. Assist patient and family to set criteria to help them to determine when intervention of law enforcement officials or health professionals is required.

5. Consult with or refer to assistive resources as appropriate:
    a. Police
    b. Psychiatric nurse clinician
    c. Shelter
    d. Crisis counseling
    e. Suicide prevention
    f. Family counseling
    g. Physician
    h. Group therapy
    i. Social support networks
    j. Emergency room
    k. Visiting nurse
    l. Social service
    m. Religious counseling

EVALUATION
OBJECTIVE 1

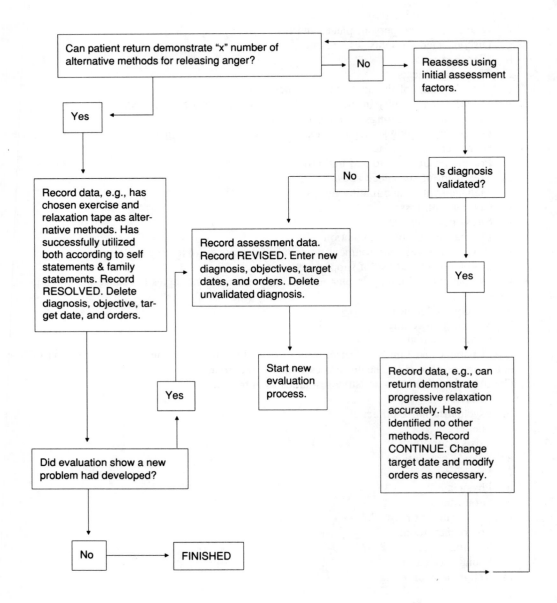

OBJECTIVE 2

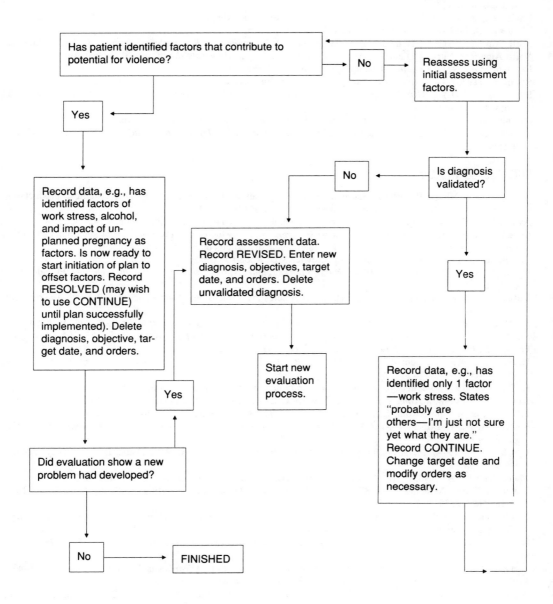

REFERENCES

Griffith-Kenney, J. (1986). *Contemporary women's health: A nursing advocacy approach.* Menlo Park, CA: Addison-Wesley.
Kneisl, C., & Wilson, H. (1984). *Handbook of psychosocial nursing care.* Menlo Park, CA: Addison-Wesley.
Murdock, G. (1949). *Social structure.* New York: Macmillan.
North American Nursing Diagnosis Association. (1987). *Taxonomy I with complete diagnosis.* St. Louis: Author.
North American Nursing Diagnosis Association. (1988). *Proposed nursing diagnoses.* St. Louis: Author.
Patterson, G. (1971). *Families.* Champaign, IL: Research Press.
Rubin, R. (1970). Cognitive style in pregnancy. *American Journal of Nursing, 3,* 502–508.
Shibutani, T. (ED.). (1970). *Human nature and collective behavior: Papers in honor of Herbert Blumer.* Englewood Cliffs, NJ: Prentice-Hall.
Smitherman, C. (1981). *Nursing actions for health promotion.* Philadelphia: F. A. Davis.
Watzlawick, P., Beavin, J., & Jackson, D. (1967). *Pragmatics of human communication.* New York: W. W. Norton.

SUGGESTED READINGS

Atwood, J., & Hinds, P. (1986). Heuristic heresy: Application of reliability and validity criteria to products of grounded theory. *Western Journal of Nursing Research.* 8 (2), 135–154.
Avant, K. (1979). Nursing diagnosis: Maternal attachment. *Advances in Nursing Science, 2,* 45–55.
Brazelton, T. B. (1983). *Infants and mothers: Differences in development.* New York: Delta/Seymour Lawrence.
Carpenito, L. (1983). *Nursing diagnosis.* Philadelphia: J. B. Lippincott.
Crittendon, R. (1983). *Discharge planning.* Bowie, MD: Robert J. Brady.
Doenges, M., & Moorhouse, M. (1986). *Nurse's pocket guide: Nursing diagnoses with interventions.* Philadelphia: F. A. Davis.
Dufault, K., & Martocchio, B. (1985). Hope: Its spheres and dimensions. *Nursing Clinics of North America, 20* (2), 379–391.
Fogel, E. I., & Woods, N. F. (1981). *Health care of women: A nursing perspective.* St. Louis: C. V. Mosby.
Frank, J.(1968). The role of hope in psychotherapy. *International Journal of Psychiatry, 5,* 383–395.
Fromm, E. (1968). *The resolution of hope.* New York: Harper & Row.
Haber, J., Leach, A., Schudy, S., & Sideleau, B. (1982). *Comprehensive psychiatric nursing* (2nd ed.). New York: McGraw-Hill.
Hadeka, M. (1987). *Clinical judgment in community health nursing.* Boston: Little, Brown.
Humphrey, C. (1986). *Home care nursing handbook.* East Norwalk, CT: Appleton-Century-Crofts.
Jaffe, M., & Skidmore-Roth, L. (1988). *Home health nursing care plans.* St. Louis: C. V. Mosby.
Jensen, M. D., & Bobak, I. M. (1985). *Maternity and gynecologic care: The nurse and the family.* St. Louis: C. V. Mosby.
Lynch, W. F. (1974). *Images of hope: Imagination as healer of the hopeless.* Notre Dame, IN: University of Notre Dame Press.
Maagedenberg, A. (1983). The "violent" patient. *American Journal of Nursing, 83* (3), 402–403.
Maternity Center Association. (1987). *AIDS and pregnancy.* (Available by writing to 48 East 92nd Street, New York, NY 10128, 212–367–7300).
McClelland, E., Kelly, K., & Buckwalter, K. (1984). *Continuity of care: Advancing the concept of discharge planning.* Orlando, FL: Grune & Stratton.
McFarland, G., & Wasli, E. (1986). *Nursing diagnoses and process in psychiatric mental health nursing.* Philadelphia: J. B. Lippincott.
McGee, R. (1984, July). Hope: A factor influencing crisis resolution. *Advances in Nursing Science,* pp. 34–43.
Miller, J. (1985). Inspiring hope. *American Journal of Nursing, 85* (1), 22–25.
National League for Nursing. (1986). *Policies and procedures.* New York: Accreditation Division for Home Care, National League for Nursing.
National League for Nursing. (1988). *Accreditation program for home care and community health: Criteria and standards.* New York: Author.
Neeson, J. D., & May, K. A. (1986). *Comprehensive maternity nursing: Nursing process and the childbearing family.* Philadelphia: J. B. Lippincott.
Reeder, S. J., & Martin, L. L. (1987). *Maternity nursing: Family, newborn and women's health care* (16th ed.). Philadelphia: J. B. Lippincott.
Rinke, L. (1988). *Outcome standards in home health.* New York: National League for Nursing.
Roberts, R. B. (1983). Infant behavior and the transition to parenthood. *Nursing Research, 32,* 213–217.

Schuster, C., & Ashburn, S. (1986). *The process of human development,* (2nd ed.). Boston: Little, Brown.

Sherwen, L. (Ed.). (1984). Alternative parenting patterns: Clinical implications. *Topics in Clinical Nursing, 6* (3), 132.

Steffi, B., & Eide, I. (1978). *Discharge planning handbook.* New York: Charles B. Slack.

Stuart, G., & Sundeen, S. (1988). *Pocket nurse guide to psychiatric nursing.* St. Louis: C. V. Mosby.

Travelbee, J. (1971). *Interpersonal aspects of nursing,* (2nd ed.). Philadelphia: F. A. Davis.

Vaillot, M. (1970). Hope the restoration of being. *American Journal of Nursing, 70* (2), 268–273.

Walsh, J., Persons, C., & Wieck, L. (1987). *Manual of home health care nursing.* Philadelphia: J. B. Lippincott.

Watson, J. (1985). *Nursing: The philosophy and science of caring.* Boulder, CO: Colorado Associated University Press.

Whaley, L. & Wong, D. (1987). Nursing care of infants and children. St. Louis: C.R. Mosby.

Wright, L., & Leahey, M. (1984). *Nurses and families.* Philadelphia: F. A. Davis.

CHAPTER TEN

Sexuality-Reproductive Pattern

Pattern Description

This pattern focuses on the sexual-reproductive aspects of individuals during their life span. Sexuality permeates all aspects of an individual's biologic, psychologic, and sociologic being.

Sexuality patterns involve sex role behavior, gender identification, physiologic and biologic functioning, as well as the cultural and societal expectations of sexual behavior. An individual's anatomic structure identifies sexual status, which determines the social and cultural responses of others toward the individual and in turn, the individual's responsive behavior toward others.

Reproductive patterns involve the capability to procreate, actual procreation, and the ability to express sexual feelings. The success or failure of psychologically and physically expressing sexual feelings and procreating can affect an individual's life-style, health, and self-concept.

The nurse may care for clients who, because of illness, violence, or life-styles, experience alterations or disturbances in their sexual health which affect their sexuality and reproductive patterns.

Pattern Assessment

1. Patient's description of sexual functioning.
   a. Sexual drive
      (1) Degree of arousal
      (2) Decreased
      (3) Absent
      (4) Overly active
   b. Sexual satisfaction
      (1) Ambivalence
      (2) Satisfaction
      (3) Confusion
2. Assessment of development of secondary sexual characteristics.
   a. Physiologic factors
      (1) Girls have:
         (a) Breast growth;
         (b) Pubic hair and axillary hair growth;
         (c) Menstruation;
         (d) Growth of uterus and vagina.
      (2) Boys have:
         (a) Testicular and scrotum enlargement;
         (b) Pubic hair growth;
         (c) Ejaculation;

(d) Enlargement of the penis;
(e) Growth of axillary and facial hair.
(3) Sweating
(4) Fatigue
b. Emotional factors
(1) Bewilderment
(2) Fear
(3) Pride
(4) Concern
(5) Anxiety
(6) Preoccupation with body changes
(7) Role confusion
c. Biologic factors
(1) Capable of reproduction
(2) Irregular menstrual patterns (girls)
(3) Nocturnal emissions (wet dreams) (boys)
(4) Growth—height
(5) Weight
(6) Skin problems such as acne
3. Patient's description of sexual behavior.
a. Attitudes and values
(1) Accepting of own sexuality
(2) Comfortable with own and others' sexuality
(3) Religious views
(4) Moral standards
b. Psychosocial
(1) Marriage
(2) Men's roles
(3) Women's roles
(4) Parenting
(5) Communication between partners
(6) Race and class
c. Psychosexual
(1) Orgasm
(2) Performance
(a) Satisfactory
(b) Fear of failure
(3) Guilt
(4) Anxiety
4. Cultural
a. Dictate acceptable sexual behavior
b. Dictate who performs sexual acts
c. Norms for males
d. Norms for females
e. Active or passive roles for females or males
f. Marital-nonmarital relations
g. Race and class
5. Patient's description of sexual preferences
a. Heterosexual
b. Homosexual
c. Bisexual

6. Determine client's sexual attitudes
   a. Body image
      (1) Physical disabilities
         (a) Ugly or unacceptable
         (b) Uncontrollable
            (i) Physical dependency
            (ii) Spasticity
            (iii) Incontinence
            (iv) Dependent on equipment
               (*a*) braces
               (*b*) wheelchairs
               (*c*) colostomy bags
      (2) Aging
         (a) Looks "old"
            (i) Grey hair
            (ii) Wrinkles
            (iii) Sagging body parts (e.g., breasts, facial features)
            (iv) Osteoporosis
         (b) Presumed to be asexual or not interested
         (c) Stereotyping
            (i) "Old hag"
            (ii) "Old maid"
            (iii) "My old lady" or "My old man"
            (iv) "Dirty old man"
            (v) "Bag lady"
      (3) Youth
         (a) "Skinny not fat"
            (i) Bulemia
            (ii) Anorexia
         (b) Athletic
            (i) Exercise
            (ii) Participant in sports
            (iii) "Body-beautiful"
      (4) Pregnancy
         (a) "Fat"
         (b) "Not interested in sex"
         (c) "Waddles like a duck"
         (d) Enlarged breasts
         (e) Striae (stretch marks) on abdomen, breasts, and thighs
         (f) Chloasma (mask of pregnancy) on face
         (g) Scars (cesarean-section)
   b. Reproductive choices
      (1) Have children
      (2) Not have children
      (3) Infertility
   c. Religious beliefs
      (1) Birth control
      (2) Marriage
      (3) Moral codes
   d. Cultural values
      (1) Women's roles

    (2) Men's roles
    (3) Value old age or not value old age
  e. Environmental factors
    (1) Health (e.g., presence of chronic disease, medications)
    (2) Economics
    (3) Mental status
    (4) Social (e.g., substance abuse)
  f. Peer group values
  g. Family and personal experiences
    (1) Role model
    (2) No role model
    (3) Abusive
    (4) Stable
    (5) Unstable

Conceptual Information

Gender development and sexuality are closely entwined with biologic, psychologic, sociologic, spiritual, and cultural aspects of human life. The biologic sex of an individual is decided at the time of conception, but sexual patterning is influenced from the moment of birth by the actions of those surrounding the individual. From this moment males and females receive messages about who they are and what it means to be masculine or feminine (Woods, 1984).

The sexuality of an individual is composed of biologic sex, gender identity, and gender role. The biologic and psychologic perspectives of culture and society determine how an individual develops sexually, particularly in the sense one has of being male or female (gender identity). Biologic identity begins at the moment of fertilization when chromosomal sex is determined and becomes even more defined at 5–6 weeks of fetal life. At this time the undifferentiated fetal gonads become ovaries (XX, female chromosomal sex), or testes (XY, male chromosomal sex), and hormones finalize the genital appearance between the 7th and 12th weeks. Fetal androgens (testicular hormones) must be present for male reproductive structures to develop from the wolffian ducts. If fetal androgens are not present the fetus will develop female reproductive structures. By the 12th week of fetal life biologic sex is well established (Speroff & Glass, 1984; Woods, 1984).

Reactions by others begin the moment the biologic sex of the fetus or infant is known. Whether the sex of the infant is known before birth or not until the time of birth, the parents and those about them prepare for either a boy or a girl by buying clothes and toys for a boy (color blue, pants, shirts, footballs) or a girl (color pink, frilly dresses, dolls), as well as speaking to the infant differently according to sex. Girls are usually spoken to in a high, sing-song voice: "Oh, isn't she cute!"; while boys are spoken to in a low pitched, matter of fact voice: "Look at that big boy, he will really make a good football player one of these days!" These actions contribute to the infant's gender identity and perception of self. Behavioral responses from the infant are elicited by the parents based on their views of what roles a boy or girl should fulfill.

Gender role is determined by the kinds of sex behavior that are performed by individuals to symbolize to themselves and others that they are masculine or feminine (Fogel & Woods, 1981). Early civilizations assigned roles according to who performed what tasks for survival. Women were relegated to specific roles because of the biologic nature of bearing, raising children, and gathering food. The men were the hunters and soldiers. Advanced technologies, changing mores, birth control, and alternative methods of securing food and raising children have led to changes in roles based on gender in Western society. Gender roles are influenced by cultural, religious, and social pressures. "Gender role stereotypes are culturally assigned clusters of behaviors or attributes covering everything from play activities and personal traits to physical appearance, dress and vocational activities" (Schuster & Ashburn, 1986, p. 320).

As in gender identity, researchers have noticed gender role play in children as young as 13 months. School children are particularly exposed and pressured into gender role stereotyping by parents, teachers, and peers, who demand expected, rigid behavior patterns according to the sex of the child. Molding into gender roles is often accomplished by handling girls and boys differently; little girls are usually handled gently as infants, such as fussing with the baby's hair and telling them how pretty they are; and little boys are usually roughhoused, and are told "what a big boy you are." Sex directional training is also accomplished by such verbalizations as "where's Daddy's girl?" and "big boys don't cry, be a man" (Biddle & Thomas, 1979, p. 355).

Western North American society is moving toward a blending of male and female roles; however, stereotyping still exists. According to Schuster and Ashburn (1986), stereotyping is not all bad, as it can help "reduce anxiety arising from gender differences and may aid in the process of psychic separation from one's parents" (p. 321). Therefore, they conclude that stereotypes can provide structure and facilitate development as well as restrict development and become too rigid and interfere with a child's potential (Schuster & Ashburn, 1986).

One's sexuality is a continuing lifetime process, changing as one matures and progresses through the life cycle. It is impossible to separate an individual's sexuality from his or her development, as sexuality combines the interaction of the biophysical and psychosocial elements of the individual (Molcan & Fickley, 1988).

Developmental Considerations

Infant

Erickson (Schuster & Ashburn, 1986) defines the major task of infancy as the development of trust versus mistrust. The act of the parents nurturing and providing care-taking activities allows the infant to begin experiencing various pleasures and physical sensations such as warmth, pleasure, security, and trust (Woods, 1984), and it is through these acts of nurturing that the infant begins to develop a sense of masculinity or femininity (gender identity). The infant is further molded by the parent's perceptions of sex-appropriate behavior through reward and punishment. Female infants tend to be less aggressive and develop more sensitivity because girls are usually rewarded for "being good," and male infants develop more aggressively and learn to be independent because boys are told that "big boys don't cry" and he learns to comfort himself. By the age of 13 months sexual behavior patterns and differences are in place (Schuster & Ashburn, 1986; Woods, 1984), and core gender identity is theorized to be formed by 18 months (Molcan & Fickley, 1988). "These early behaviors are so critical to one's core gender-identity that children who experience gender reassignment after the age of 2 years are high-risk candidates for psychotic disorders" (Schuster & Ashburn, 1986, p. 321).

The infant who is sexually abused is usually physically traumatized and many times dies. Developmental delays can be recognized in these children by failure to thrive, low weight or no weight gain, lethargy, and flat affect.

Toddler

Neuromuscular control allows toddlers to explore their environment, interact with their peers (Schuster & Ashburn, 1986, Woods, 1984), and develop autonomy and independence (Molcan & Fickley, 1988). Genital organs continue to increase in size but not in function. The toddlers' vocabulary increases, they distinguish between male and female by recognizing clothing and body parts, and they develop pride in their own bodies, especially the genital area, as they become aware of elimination or excretory functions. They need guidance and require parents to set limits as they learn to "hold on" or "let go" in order to achieve a sense of autonomy (Schuster & Ashburn, 1986, Woods, 1984). By the age of 3 they have perfected verbal terms for the sexes, understand the meaning of gender terms, and understand the roles associated with those terms (for example, girl: sister or mother, and boy: brother or father) (Woods, 1984), and receives pleasure from kissing and hugging (Molcan & Fickley, 1988).

The preschooler is busy developing a sense of socialization and purpose. Learning suitable behavior for girls and boys or sex-role behavior is the major task during the preschool years. Preschoolers will often identify with the parent of the same sex while forming an attachment to the parent of the opposite sex. They are inquisitive about sex and are often occupied in exploration of their own bodies and friends' bodies. This will often be exhibited in group games such as "doctor/nurse," urinating "outside," or masturbating (Molcan & Fickley, 1988). The toddlers' concept of their bodies, not as a whole but as individual parts, changes when as preschoolers they begin to develop "an awareness of themselves as individuals, and become more concerned about body integrity and intactness" (Schuster & Ashburn, 1986, p. 227).

It is important to note that 6-year-olds are the age group most subjected to sexual abuse (Ames & Ilg, 1976). How a child handles this experience and his or her future developmental and psychological growth depend largely on the reactions and actions of the significant adult in the child's life (Molcan & Fickley, 1988). Rape which occurs during early childhood may simply be acknowledged by the child as part of the experience of growing up and may have no long-term effects if not repeated. Usually counseling during this developmental age has great effect. All claims of abuse by a child should be investigated and should be handled with someone who has the experience and knowledge to deal with the child and his parents in a professional and understanding manner.

School-Age Child

Play is the most important work of children—it allows them to be curious and investigate social, sexual, and adult behavior. "Through play children learn how to get their needs met and how to meet the needs of others" (Schuster & Ashburn, 1986, p. 304). Different socialization of boys and girls tends to become apparent in play during the school years, with boys engaging in aggressive team play and girls in milder play and forming individual friendships. These activities can lead to stereotyping and exaggeration of gender difference.

Going to school allows children to begin to be more independent and form peer groups of the same sex. Although the peer group becomes very important to them, they need adult direction in learning socially acceptable forms of sexual behavior and when they may engage in them. If they do not receive the information they are seeking, negative feelings and apprehension about sexuality may develop (Woods, 1984).

Great trauma can occur when rape occurs during these years. It is very damaging to the value systems which are being formed. Sexual identity can be disturbed, and sexual confusion can occur.

Adolescent

Puberty, "the period of maturation of the reproductive system" (Schuster & Ashburn, 1986, p. 329), causes profound changes in the individual's sexual anatomy and physiology and is a major developmental crisis for the adolescent. Secondary sex characteristics appear—breasts, pubic hair, and menstruation in girls; testicular enlargement, penile enlargement, pubic hair, ejaculation, and growth of muscle mass in boys. The configuration, contour, and function of the body changes rapidly and dramatically points out sexual differences and the onset of adulthood. These changes bring new feelings that create role confusion and increase awareness of sexual feelings. "The major task of adolescence is the establishment of identity in the face of role confusion" (Woods, 1984, p. 55).

Peer groups have an important influence on the young adolescent (12–15 years), but during late adolescence (16–19 years) the peer group influence lessens and more intimate relationships with the opposite sex develop (Molcan & Fickley, 1988). These relationships can involve a wide range of sexual behavior from exploring behavior to intercourse, sometimes with the result of teenage pregnancy. Exploring behavior can be either with the opposite sex (foreplay and intercourse), the same sex (homosexuality), or self (masturbation). How the teenager views himself or herself sexually will depend on the reassurance and guidance he or she receives from a significant adult in his or her life. The greatest misunderstandings of teenagers involve homosexuality, masturbation, and conception and contraception; and how they are approached, taught, and supported can influence their adult sexuality (Molcan & Fickley, 1988; Woods, 1984).

It is during adolescence, when new experiences of sexual maturity begin, that questions about maleness or femaleness are asked by the individual and concerns arise about "who one is within the peer group" (Woods, 1984, p. 55). Adolescents must evaluate their masculinity and femininity, question and then decide on their gender identity, gender orientation, and gender preference. The adolescent deals not only with physical changes but integrates past experiences and role models with new experiences and new role models into his or her own gender identity.

Violent sexual occurrences during this period of life can devastate a person for the rest of his or her life. Adolescents are dealing with sexual confusion and identification; rape can stop or slow or change this process. Fear and loss of self-esteem can dictate actions and influence the sexual identity and gender expression.

Young Adult

This period of an individual's life (usually 20s and early 30s) is concerned with selecting a vocation, obtaining an education, military service, choosing a partner, building a career, and establishing an intimate relationship. This is a period of maximal sexual self-consciousness, commitment to a relationship, and social legitimization of sexual experiences (Molcan & Fickley, 1988; Schuster & Ashburn, 1986; Woods, 1984). There is a concern with parenting and establishment of the marital relationship.

Rape can slow or stop normal sexual relationships during the adult years. Fear can become the greater part of life for the victim. These years are ones for forming lasting relationships with the opposite sex, marrying, and beginning families. Rape can cause withdrawal from any interaction with the opposite sex; relationships can break up, not only because of the reaction of the victims of rape, but also because of the reactions of the families and spouses of the victims.

Adult

Demands placed on adults by their careers and raising children may interfere with their sexual interest and activity (Woods, 1984). The major task of this period of life is to accent one's own life-style and decisions rather than feeling frustrated and disappointed. "Social pressures and expectations, feedback from significant others and finally self-perception all influence how one evaluates the success of one's life" (Woods, 1984, p. 6).

Although the adult is at the peak of his or her career or profession, physiologic changes begin to influence the adult's life-style. The aging process, illnesses, and menopause (male and female) cause changes in life-styles and everyday activities. Sexual activities can undergo changes because of these physical and physiologic changes; however, the adult who lives a healthy life-style, has good nutrition, exercises, and has an optimistic outlook usually feels good and functions well sexually. Often older adults, just as they have finished raising their children, are faced with the task of caring for their elderly parents.

Older Adult

As in adolescence, dramatic body changes begin in late adulthood and continue into old age. There is no reason that healthy men and women cannot continue to enjoy their sexuality into old age. Women must deal with menopause and post-menopause and men must often deal with impotence; however, with an interested sexual partner, good healthy sexuality can continue.

Older women are viewed by rapists as easy victims. Slowing of physical reactions and disabilities of old age (seeing, hearing, slow gait) keep them from being alert to danger and from reacting quickly. More important, the older woman often views herself as inferior and this contributes to her own victimization (Warner, 1980). Because most women outlive men and face changes in life-styles and economic status, they are reluctant, and often cannot afford, to leave familiar older parts of cities which often change and deteriorate. This may expose them to the accompanying increase in crime rates (Warner, 1980).

Applicable Nursing Diagnoses

Rape Trauma Syndrome

DEFINITION

Forced, violent sexual penetration against the victim's will and consent. The trauma syndrome that develops from this attack or attempted attack includes an acute phase of disorganization of the victim's life-style and a long-term process of reorganization of life style. The syndrome includes three subcomponents: Rape Trauma, Compound Reaction, and Silent Reaction (North American Nursing Diagnosis Association [NANDA], 1987, p. 115).

DEFINING CHARACTERISTICS (NANDA, 1987, pp. 115–117)

The nurse will review the initial pattern assessment for the following defining characteristics to determine the diagnosis of Rape Trauma Syndrome.

1. Rape Trauma
   a. Acute phase
      (1) Emotional reactions (anger, embarrassment, fear of physical violence and death, humiliation, revenge, self-blame)
      (2) Multiple physical symptoms (gastrointestinal irritability, genitourinary discomfort, muscle tension, steep pattern disturbance)
   b. Long-term phase
      (1) Changes in life-style (changes in residence, dealing with repetitive nightmares and phobias, seeking family support, seeking social network support)
2. Compound Reaction
   a. Acute phase
      (1) Same as 1 and 2 of Rape Trauma plus:
      (2) Reactivated symptoms of previous conditions (i.e., physical illness, psychiatric illness, reliance on alcohol or drugs).
   b. Long-term phase
      (1) Same as Rape Trauma
3. Silent Reaction
   a. Major defining characteristics
      (1) Abrupt changes in relationships with men
      (2) Increase in nightmares
      (3) Increased anxiety during interview (i.e., blocking of associations, long periods of silence, minor stuttering, physical distress)
      (4) Pronounced changes in sexual behavior
      (5) No verbalization of the occurrence of rape
      (6) Sudden onset of phobic reactions
   b. Minor defining characteristics
      None given.

RELATED FACTORS (NANDA, 1987, p. 115)

Included in definition of diagnosis.

DIFFERENTIATION

Rape Trauma should be differentiated from Sexual Dysfunction. As stated in the differentiation of Sexual Dysfunction, rape can be the cause of sexual dysfunction in a patient who cannot learn to put into perspective or deal with the rape experience. Rape Trauma is always the result of a violent act and must be dealt with according to the individual situation. Although Sexual Dysfunction can occur as the result of rape, the nurse must deal with the trauma of the rape in order

patient with the sexual dysfunction, which is a symptom of the greater problem of

tify and use at least (number) support systems by (date).

lize (number) positive self-statements related to personal response to the incident

ried physical and emotional impact of rape, a target date of 2–3 days would not valuate for progress.

3. Be supp... of patient's values and beliefs. Maintain nonjudgmental attitude.
4. Use calm, consistent approach.
5. Explain need for medicolegal procedures.
6. Actively listen when patient wants to talk about event. Encourage verbalization of thoughts, feelings, and perceptions of the event. Explore basis for and reality of thoughts, feelings, and perceptions.
7. Refer to rape crisis center.
8. Recognize that patient will proceed at own rate in resolving rape trauma. Do not rush or force patient.
9. Assist patient in activities of daily living after examination.
10. Help identify available support systems and involve significant other as appropriate.
11. Monitor coping in patient and significant other.
12. Assist patient to identify own strengths in dealing with the rape.
13. Respect patient's rights.
14. Provide anticipatory guidance about the long-term effects of rape. Promote self-confidence and self-esteem through positive feedback regarding strengths, plans, reality.
15. Collaborate with other health care professionals as needed.

CHILD HEALTH

1. Attend to physical and health priorities such as lacerations, infection, etc. with appropriate explanations and preparation.
2. Encourage collaboration among health professionals to best address patient's needs to include:
   a. Pediatrician, subspecialists
   b. Pediatric clinical nurse specialist
   c. Play therapist
   d. Child protective services
   e. Legal counsel
   f. Psychiatrist
   g. Community health nurse
   h. Social worker
   i. School counselor
   j. Family therapist
   k. Supportive peer group

    l. Clergyperson
   3. Try to establish trust as dictated by age and circumstances related to rape trauma (with nurse being same sex as patient):
    Infants & Toddlers: Ensure continuity of caregivers; explain procedures with dolls and puppets.
    Preschoolers: Ensure continuity of caregivers, allow patient to perform self-care behavior as ability presents. Use art and methods which deal with general view of what happened, singling out child as not being "cause" of this incident.
    School-Agers: Maintain continuity of care, assist patient to express concerns related to incident. Use appropriate techniques in interviewing to determine extent of sexual dysfunction or potential threat to future functioning.
    Adolescents: Maintain continuity in care. Encourage patient to express how this experience effects own self-identity and future sexual activities. Allow for need for in-depth psychiatric assistance in resolving this crisis for any patients of this age group.
   4. Provide for appropriate privacy and health teaching as care is administered, not to perpetuate fear of recurrence of rape situation (e.g., explain why vaginal area is being examined or medication is being applied). Allow patient to see own anatomy if this seems appropriate as part of health teaching.
   5. Follow up with appropriate documentation and coordination of child protective service needs. Determine if situation involves incest.
   6. Assist patient to deal with residual feelings such as guilt for revealing or identifying assailant (in young children this often must be dealt with within family or extended-family situations) by allowing time of approximately 30 minutes/shift.
   7. Determine to what degree or extent symptoms of physical reactions exist such as:
    a. Pain, body soreness
    b. Disturbances in sleep
    c. Altered eating patterns
    d. Anger
    e. Self-blame
    f. Mood swings
    g. Feelings of helplessness
   8. Encourage family members to assist in care and follow-up of patient's reorganization plans.
    a. Be alert for signs of distress such as refusing to go to school, dreams, nightmares, or verbalized concerns.
    b. Identify ways to gradually resume normal daily schedule.
    c. Assist family to identify how best to resolve and express feelings about the incident.
   9. Arrange for appropriate long-term follow-up before dismissal from hospital.
  10. Administer medications as ordered to alleviate pain, anxiety, or inability to sleep.
  11. Provide for appropriate epidemiologic follow-up in cases of veneral disease.
  12. Carry out appropriate health teaching regarding normal sexual physiology and functioning according to age and developmental capacity.

WOMEN'S HEALTH

   1. Assist the victim through the procedures for provision of necessary health care treatment explain each phase of examination to patient.
    a. History
      (1) List of previous veneral disease
      (2) List of previous pelvic infections
      (3) Any injuries that were present before attack
      (4) Obstetric menstrual history
    b. Physical examination

(1) Remain with the victim at all times
(2) Assist in gathering information to provide proper health and legal care
(3) Secure patient's description of any objects used in the attack and how these objects were used in the attack and inserted into rectum or vagina
c. Maintain sequencing and collection of evidence (chain of evidence)
  (1) Label each specimen with:
    (a) Patient's name
    (b) Patient's hospital number;
    (c) Date and time of collection;
    (d) Area from which specimen was collected
    (e) Collector's name.
  (2) Ensure proper storage and packaging of specimens.
    (a) Clothing and items that are wet (e.g., with blood or semen) should be put in paper bags, not plastic (plastic bags will cause molding of wet items).
    (b) Specimens obtained on microscopic slides or swabs need to be air dried before packaging.
    (c) Comb pubic hair for traces of attacker's pubic hair or other evidence.
      (i) Submit paper towel placed under victim to catch combings, as well as the comb used, along with pubic hair.
      (ii) Pluck (do not cut) 2–3 pubic hairs from the patient, and label properly. These are used for comparison.
  (3) When custody of evidence is transferred to police, be certain written evidence of transfer is properly recorded.
    (a) Signature of individuals involved in transfer
    (b) To whom being transferred
    (c) Date and time
  (4) Take Photographs of injuries or torn clothing
  (5) Have patient forms for release of information to authorities
d. Provide medical treatment and follow-up for:
  (1) Injuries
  (2) Sexually transmitted diseases
    (a) AIDS
    (b) Gonorrhea
    (c) Syphilis
  (3) Pregnancy
2. Report to proper authorities any suspicion of family violence.
3. Refer client for appropriate assistive resources such as:
  a. Medical intervention;
  b. Police intervention;
  c. Psychologic intervention;
  d. Rape crisis center.
4. Provide nonjudgmental atmosphere that allows client to express fears, concerns, and experiences.
5. Identify support system available to the victim.
  a. Family
  b. Nonfamily
    (1) Friends
    (2) People at place of employment
    (3) Formal support system (rape crisis centers)
6. Do not leave the victim alone.

7. Provide privacy for victim and family.

Children

8. Place with someone child trusts; do not leave alone.
9. Assist parents or guardians in signing proper release forms.
10. Use simple language in dealing with child.
11. Use puppets or anatomically correct dolls to help child explain what happened.
12. Be gentle and patient.
13. Look for signs of growth of secondary sex characteristics (important because case may not go to trial until victim is fully developed, and the jury needs to understand that when she was raped she was prepubertal).

Male Rape Victim

14. Provide same considerations as with female victim (usually as result of homosexual relationships; most reported cases are children and early adolescents).
15. Refer to trained male counselor (rape crisis center).

Incest

16. Monitor for inappropriate sexual behavior among family members.
17. Monitor for children who know more about the actual mechanics of sexual intercourse than their developmental age indicates.
18. Monitor for girls who seem to have taken over the mother's role in the home.
19. Monitor for mothers who have withdrawn from the home, either emotionally or physically.

Long Term

20. Evaluate for increased rate of changing residences.
21. Evaluate for reported nightmares, sleep pattern disturbances.
22. Allow client to discuss phobias and frustrations.
23. Allow client to verbalize fears and guilt.
24. Be available and allow client to express difficulties in establishing normal activities of daily living.
25. Let client describe the attack.
26. Assist client in developing a plan of reorganization of activities of daily living.

MENTAL HEALTH

1. Assign a primary care nurse to client. This nurse should be of the sex the client demonstrates most comfort with at the current time.
2. Primary care nurse will remain with the client during the orientation to the unit.
3. Limit visitors as client feels necessary.
4. Answer client's questions openly and honestly.
5. Primary care nurse will be present to provide support for client during medical or legal examinations if the client has not identified another person.
6. Assist client in identifying a support person and arrange for this person to remain with the client as much as necessary. Note the name of this person here.
7. Provide information to the client's support system as the client indicates is needed.
8. Allow client to talk about the incident as much as is desired. Sit with client during these times and encourage expression of feelings.
9. Communicate to client that his or her response is normal. This could include expressions of anger, fear, discomfort with persons of the opposite sex, discomfort with sexuality, personal blame, etc.
10. Inform client that rape is a physical assult rather than a sexual act and that rapists choose victims without regard for age, physical appearance, or manner of dress.

11. Assist client in developing a plan to return to activities of daily living. The plan should begin with steps that are easily accomplished so that the client can regain a sense of personal control and power. Note the steps of the plan here.

12. Provide positive social rewards for the client's accomplishment of established goals. Note here the kinds of behavior that are to be rewarded and the rewards to be used.

13. Provide the client with opportunities to express anger at the assailant in a constructive manner (i.e., talking about fantasies of revenge, use of punching bag or pillow, physical activity, etc.).

14. When client can interact with small groups, arrange for client's involvement in a therapeutic group that provides interaction with peers. Note time of group meetings here.

15. Involve client in unit activities. Assign client activities that can be easily accomplished. Note client's level of functioning here along with those tasks that are to be assigned to the client.

16. Primary nurse will spend (number) minutes with client twice a day to focus on expression of feelings related to the rape. Encourage client not to close these feelings off too quickly. Assist client in reducing stress in other life situations while healing emotionally from the rape experience.

17. Assist client in developing a plan to reduce life stressors so emotional healing can continue. Note this plan here with the support needed from the nursing staff in implementing this plan.

18. Primary nurse will meet with client and primary support person once per day to facilitate their discussion of the rape. If the client is involved in an ongoing relationship, such as a marriage, this interaction is very important. The support person should be encouraged to express his or her thoughts and feelings in a constructive manner. If it is assessed that the rape has resulted in potential long-term relationship difficulties such as rejection or sexual problems, refer to couple therapy.

19. Refer client to appropriate community support groups and assist with contacting these before discharge. These systems could include:
    a. Rape crisis center;
    b. Outpatient mental health services;
    c. Visiting nurse;
    d. Family therapy;
    e. Mental health nurse clinical specialist;
    f. Legal aid.

HOME HEALTH

1. During the acute phase, the nurse will see that appropriate assessment, law enforcement involvement, and treatment of physical injuries or sexually transmitted diseases is provided.

2. Assist patient and family in life-style changes that may be needed.
    a. Treatment for physical injuries or sexually transmitted disease
    b. Testimony in court
    c. Protection
    d. Coping with terror, nightmares, or fear
    e. Coping with alterations in sexual response to significant others
    f. Development and use of support networks
    g. Stress management
    h. Changing phone number or moving
    i. Traveling with companion
    j. Strategies for prevention of rape

3. Assist patient and family in planning and implementing strategies for resolution of rape trauma syndrome.
    a. Communication
    b. Mutual sharing and trust

   c. Problem solving
4. Consult with or refer to assistive resources as appropriate
   a. Rape crisis center
   b. Law enforcement
   c. Physician
   d. Emergency room
   e. Psychiatric nurse clinician
   f. Self-help group
   g. Sexual counseling
   h. Marriage and family therapy
   i. Attorney
   j. Temporary shelter

EVALUATION
OBJECTIVE 1

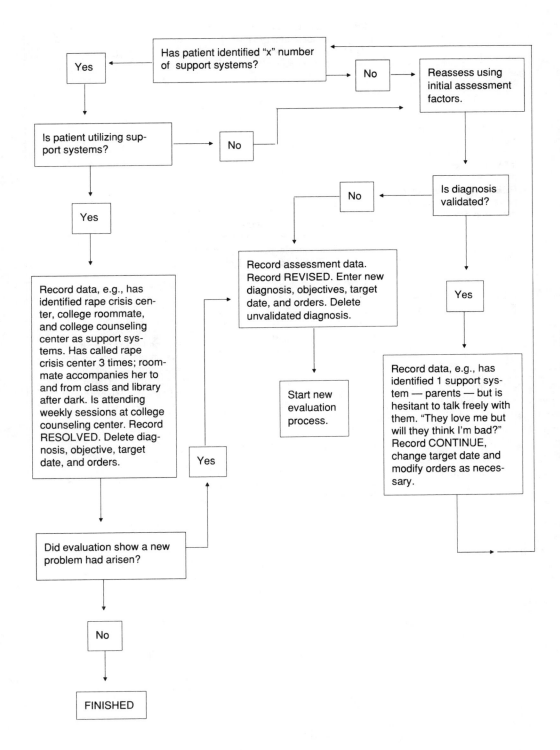

OBJECTIVE 2

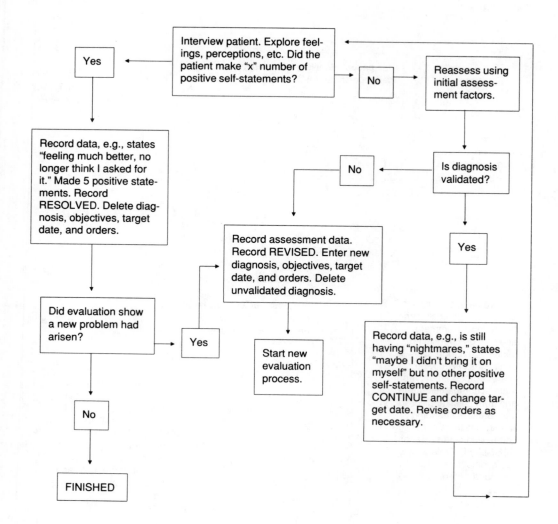

Sexual Dysfunction

DEFINITION

The state in which an individual experiences a change in sexual function that is viewed as unsatisfying, unrewarding, or inadequate (NANDA, 1987, p. 66).

DEFINING CHARACTERISTICS (NANDA, 1987, p. 66)

The nurse will review the initial pattern assessment for the following defining characteristics to determine the diagnosis of Sexual Dysfunction.

1. Major defining characteristics
   a. Verbalization of problem
   b. Alterations in achieving perceived sex role
   c. Actual or perceived limitation imposed by disease or therapy
   d. Conflicts involving values
   e. Alteration in achieving sexual satisfaction
   f. Inability to achieve desired satisfaction
   g. Seeking confirmation of desirability
   h. Alteration in relationship with significant other
   i. Change of interest in self and others
2. Minor defining characteristics
   None given.

RELATED FACTORS (NANDA, 1987, p. 66)

1. Biopsychosocial alteration of sexuality
2. Ineffectual or absent role models
3. Physical abuse
4. Psychosocial abuse (e.g., harmful relationships)
5. Vulnerability
6. Values conflict
7. Lack of privacy
8. Lack of significant other
9. Altered body structure or function (pregnancy, recent childbirth, drugs, surgery, anomalies, disease process, trauma, radiation)
10. Misinformation or lack of knowledge

DIFFERENTIATION

Sexual Dysfunction should be differentiated from Sexuality Patterns, Altered; and Rape Trauma Syndrome: Compound and Silent Reaction. Sexual Dysfuntion deals with the patient's perceived problems in sexual functioning. These problems can be caused by actual pathophysiological problems or conflicts within the patient's own value system. Sexuality Patterns, Altered can be the result of Sexual Dysfunction, but does not mean that it is necessarily a problem to the patient. Sexuality Patterns, Altered can be compatible with the patient's life-style for whatever reason, and create no concerns or problems for the patient.

Rape Trauma Syndrome: Compound and Silent Reaction can result in Sexual Dysfunction because of the patient's inability to deal with the violence, trauma, and life-style changes as a result of rape. The key here is for the nurse to closely ascertain the cause of the Sexual Dysfunction and to determine if it is the result of the patient's perception of sexuality in general, pathophysiology, or trauma.

OBJECTIVES

1. Will have decreased complaints of sexual dysfunction by (date).

AND/OR

2. Will report return as near as possible to previous levels of sexual functioning by (date).

TARGET DATE

Depending on the patient's perception of the sexual dysfunction, target dates may range from 1 week to several months.

NURSING ORDERS

ADULT HEALTH

1. Facilitate communication between patient and partner by providing at least (number) minutes/day for privacy to communicate.
2. Encourage patient and partner to talk about concerns and problems during conference.
3. Clarify misconceptions as needed.
4. Be nonjudgmental in your attitudes.
5. Respect patient's values and attitudes about sexuality and sexual functioning.
6. Talk with patient and partner about alternate ways to attain sexual satisfaction. Provide factual informational material.
7. Discuss alternate ways to express sexuality.
8. Provide accurate information on effects of disease or treatment on sexual functioning.
9. Implement measures to improve self-concept.
10. Provide privacy.
11. Teach patient importance of adequate rest before and after sexual activity.
12. If dyspareunia is a problem, teach patient and significant other to:
    a. Use adequate amounts of water-soluble lubricant to increase comfort and reduce trauma;
    b. Use vaginal steroid cream to ease dryness and inflammation;
    c. Take sitz baths for perineal comfort.
13. If impotence is a problem, advise patient to:
    a. Consult with physician regarding a complete physical examination;
    b. Consult with sex therapist;
    c. Consider penile prothesis.

CHILD HEALTH

1. Monitor for all potential contributory factors, including:
    a. Specific events;
    b. Value conflicts;
    c. Role model deficit;
    d. Related health issues;
    e. Physiologic condition;
    f. Psychologic condition;
    g. Previous unresolved conflict.
2. Discuss realistic expectations of the nurse-patient relationship in terms child will understand.
3. Determine how the child views his or her sexual dysfunctioning.
4. Provide education, as needed, regarding underlying body structure, physiologic function, adverse effects of medication (such as steroidal hirsutism), or sexual-related activity.
5. Allow patient and family input into plan of care.
6. Address peer support needs as appropriate.
7. Adapt plan of care according to child's daily activities.
8. Provide referral to related health team members as necessary to address child's needs, such as:
    a. Clinical nurse specialist
    b. Pediatrician, subspecialist

   c. Psychiatrist
   d. Psychologist
   e. Family therapist
   f. Social worker
9. Make appropriate referral to community resource or support groups, such as "ostomy" groups, American Cancer Society.

WOMEN'S HEALTH

(Note: Nothing was found in the literature relating to sexual dysfunction in lesbian women. The following refers to those who have a heterosexual relationship.)

1. Obtain detailed sexual history.
2. Determine who the client is:
   a. Female
   b. Male
   c. Couple or partners
3. Review communication skills between partners.
4. Ascertain couple's knowledge of:
   a. Sexual performance
      (1) Anatomy and physiology
         (a) Female
         (b) Male
   b. Orgasm
      (1) Female
      (2) Male
      (3) Anticipatory performance anxiety
   c. Unrealistic romantic ideas
   d. Rigid religious conformity
   e. Negative conditioning in formative years
   f. Erection and ejaculation
   g. Stimulation
   h. Arousal
   i. Sexual anxiety
      (1) Fear of failure
      (2) Demand for performance
      (3) Fear of rejection
5. Dispel sexual myths and fallacies or misinformation about sexuality by:
   a. Allowing client to talk about beliefs and practices in a nonthreatening atmosphere;
   b. Providing correct information;
   c. Answering questions in an honest manner;
   d. Referring to the appropriate agencies or health care providers.
6. Obtain description of current problem.
   a. Psychological
   b. Physical
   c. Social
7. Explore past treatments and results of those treatments.
8. Determine type of sexual dysfunction.
   a. General
      (1) Lack of erotic feeling
      (2) Lack of sexual responses
      (3) No pleasure in sexual act
         (a) Consider it an ordeal

    (b) Avoidance
    (c) Frustration
    (d) Disappointment
    (e) Fear
    (f) Disgust
    (4) No physiologic responses
        (a) Lubrication
        (b) Genital vasoconstriction
  b. Orgasmic difficulties
    (1) Sexually responsive but cannot complete sexual response cycle
        (a) Situational
            (i)   Inhibited
            (ii) Disappointed
            (iii) Disinterested
        (b) Physiologic
            (i)   Lack of lubrication
            (ii) Impotence
            (iii) Interference with sexual response cycle
        (c) Psychologic
            (i)   Ambivalence
            (ii) Guilt
            (iii) Fear
  c. Vaginismus (tight closing of vaginal muscle with any attempt at penetration)
    (1) Fear of vaginal penetration
    (2) Spasm of vaginal muscle
    (3) Frustration
    (4) Fear of inadequacy
    (5) Guilt
    (6) Pain
    (7) Prior sexual trauma
    (8) Strict religious code
    (9) Rape
  d. Dyspareunia (painful intercourse)
9. Discuss consequences of sexual acts and situations in an honest and nonthreatening manner.
10. Collaborate with appropriate therapists.

MENTAL HEALTH

(Note: If sexual dysfunction is related to physiologic limitations, loss of body part, or impotence, refer to Adult Health care plan. If dysfunction is related to ineffective coping or poor social skills, initiate the following plan.)

1. Set limits on the inappropriate expression of sexual needs. Note the kinds of behavior to be limited and the consequences for inappropriate behavior here (e.g., when client approaches staff member with sexually provocative remarks the staff member will use constructive confrontation and discontinue the interaction. See Wilson & Kneisl, 1984, Appendix C). Inform client of these limits.
2. Assign primary care nurse to client on each shift. The primary care nurse will:
   a. Spend 30 minutes with the client twice per shift to develop a relationship and then begin to explore with the client the effects this behavior has on others and the needs that are being met by the behavior.
   b. Assist client in identifying environmental stimuli that provoke sexual behavior and in developing alternative responses to these stimuli in inappropriate situations.

    c. Develop with the client a list of alternative kinds of behavior to meet the needs currently being met by the sexual behavior. (Note alternative behavior patterns here with plan for implementing them).

    d. Provide client with information about appropriate sexual behavior, i.e., what are "normal" sexual expressions, what are appropriate ways to meet sexual needs (intercourse with appropriate person or masturbation at suitable time in an appropriate place, etc.).

    e. Role play with client those social situations that have been identified as problematic. These could include setting limits on other's inappropriate behavior toward the client or situations in which the client needs to practice appropriate social responses.

    f. Assist client in appropriate labeling of feelings and needs (e.g., anxiety may be inappropriately labeled as sexual tension).

3. Plan a private time and place for client. Inform client that this can be used for appropriate sexual expression. Note this here.

4. If client begins inappropriate sexual behavior while involved in group activities remove client from group to a private place and explain to client purpose of this. Inform client that he or she may return to the group when (the limit set by the care team will be noted here).

5. If sexual behavior results from anxiety refer to Anxiety for detailed care plan.

6. Assign client tasks in unit activities that are appropriate for client's level of comfort with group interaction (e.g., if client is uncomfortable with persons of opposite sex assign a task that requires involvement with a same-sex group or involvement with an opposite-sex staff member who can begin a relationship). Note client's specific needs and assignments here.

7. Recognize and support client's feelings (e.g., "you sound confused").

8. Engage client in a socialization group once a day at (note time here). This should provide the client with an opportunity to interact with peers in an environment that provides feedback to the client in a supportive manner.

9. Arrange a consultation with occupational therapist to assist client in developing needed social skills (e.g., cooking skills, skills at games that require socialization, etc.).

10. Provide an environment that does not stimulate inappropriate sexual behavior (e.g., staff member indirectly encourages client's behavior with dress or verbal comments or other clients interact with client in a sexual manner).

11. Sit with client (number) minutes once a shift to discuss nonsexually related information.

12. Provide positive social rewards for appropriate behavior (the rewards as well as the kinds of behavior to be rewarded should be noted here).

13. Evaluate the effects of the client's current medication on sexual behavior and consult with physician as needed for necessary alterations.

14. Develop a structured daily activity schedule for the client and provide client with this information.

15. Schedule time for client to engage in physical activity. This activity should be developed with the client's assistance and could include walking, jogging, basketball, cycling, dancing, "soft" aerobics, etc. A staff member should participate with the client in these activities to provide positive social reinforcement. Note schedule and type of activity here.

16. Refer client to appropriate community support groups and assist with making arrangements for the client to contact these before discharge. These systems could include:

    a. Visiting nurse

    b. Outpatient mental health services

    c. Family therapist

    d. Sex therapist

    e. Mental health clinical nurse specialist

    f. Social services

HOME HEALTH

1. Involve patient and significant in planning and implementing strategies for reducing sexual dysfunction and enhancing sexual relationship.
   a. Communication
   b. Mutual sharing and trust
   c. Problem solving
2. Assist patient and significant with life-style adjustments that may be required by:
   a. Providing accurate and appropriate information regarding contraception;
   b. Providing time and privacy for development and improvement of sexual relationship;
   c. Teaching stress management;
   d. Providing information regarding sexuality and clarifying myths regarding sexuality;
   e. Exploring strategies for coping with disabling injury or disease;
   f. Using massage;
   g. Using touch;
   h. Treating substance abuse;
   i. Exercising regularly;
   j. Coping with changes in role functions and role relationships;
   k. Using water soluble lubricants;
   l. Obtaining treatment for physical problems (e.g., vaginal infections, penile discharge, etc.);
   m. Teaching changes accompanying pregnancy;
   n. Teaching side effects of medications.
3. Consult with or refer to assistive resources as indicated.
   a. Sex therapist
   b. Marriage and family counselor
   c. Physican
   d. Social service
   e. Stress management classes
   f. Psychiatric nurse clinician
   g. Rehabilition for special injury
   h. Planned Parenthood

EVALUATION
OBJECTIVE 1

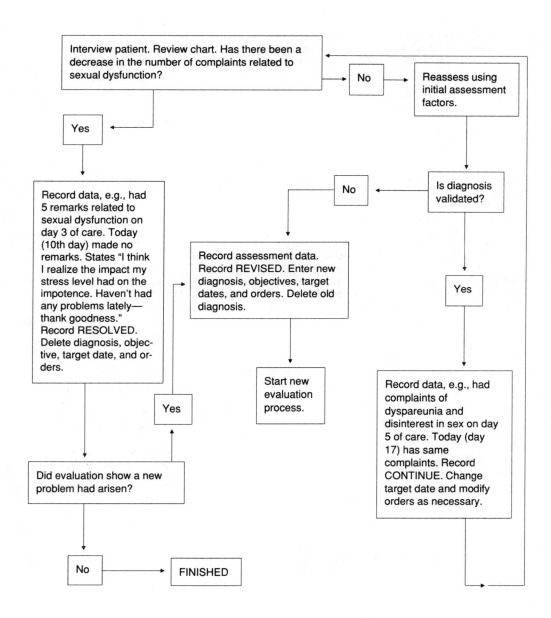

OBJECTIVE 2

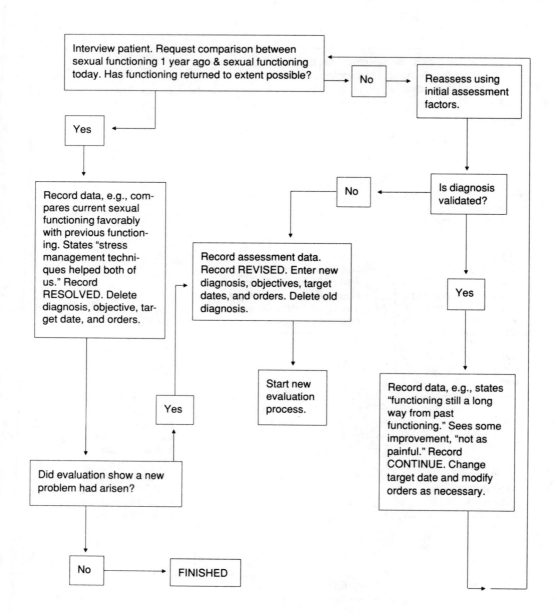

Sexuality Patterns, Altered

DEFINITION

The state in which an individual expresses concern regarding his or her sexuality (NANDA, 1987, p. 69.

DEFINING CHARACTERISTICS (NANDA, 1987, p. 69)

The nurse will review the initial pattern assessment for the following defining characteristics to determine the diagnosis of Sexuality Patterns, Altered.

1. Major defining characteristics
   a. Reported difficulties, limitations, or changes in sexual behavior or activities.
2. Minor defining charcteristics
   None given.

RELATED FACTORS (NANDA, 1987, p. 69)

1. Knowledge or skill deficit about alternative responses to health-related transitions, altered body function or structure, illnesses, or medical problems.
2. Lack of privacy.
3. Lack of significant other.
4. Ineffective or absent role models.
5. Conflicts with sexual orientation or variant preferences.
6. Fear of pregnancy or of acquiring a sexually transmitted disease.
7. Impaired relationship with a significant other.

DIFFERENTIATION

Sexuality Patterns, Altered can be confused with Sexual Dysfunction and life-styles different from heterosexual norms. These disruptions in sexual feelings and functioning can be long-term such as in the chronically ill, the terminally ill, or a disabled person who has no understanding partner; or short-term such as during a pregnancy or an illness. The changes in sexual behavior can have underlying physical, psychological, or social causes. The individual may resolve the crisis by himself or herself or may need to be referred for professional help. Nursing diagnoses such as Self-Concept, Disturbance in (Body-Image); Injury, Potential for (Trauma); Infection, Potential for; Comfort Altered: Pain and Chronic Pain; Fear; Anxiety; Grieving, Dysfunctional; and Role Performance, Altered can affect sexual feelings and functioning in both men and women.

OBJECTIVES

1. Will identify at least (number) factors contributing to altered sexual pattern by (date).

AND/OR

2. Will verbalize fewer complaints regarding altered sexual pattern by (date).

TARGET DATE

Because of the extremly personal nature of sexuality, the patient may be reluctant to express needs or problems in this area. For this reason a target date of 5–7 days would be acceptable.

NURSING ORDERS

ADULT HEALTH

1. Establish therapeutic and trusting relationship with patient and significant others.
2. Actively listen to patient's and significant other's efforts to talk about fears or changes in body image affecting sexuality or altered sexual preferences.
3. Help patient and significant other to understand that sexuality does not necessarily mean intercourse.

4. Discuss alternate methods for expressing sexuality, including masturbation.
5. Do not be judgmental with patient or significant other.
6. Provide privacy and time for patient and significant other to be alone if so desired.
7. Identify community support groups that may help with specific problems.
8. Monitor for contributory etiologic components and provide appropriate education and follow-up.

CHILD HEALTH

1. Monitor for contributory etiologic components.
2. Address other primary nursing needs, especially physiologically related and self-image related.
3. Encourage child and family to verbalize perception of altered sexual functioning.
4. Assist patient and family to identify how the desired sexual function may be attained.
5. Include appropriate collaboration with other health team members as needed to include:
    a. Surgeon or pediatrician
    b. Clinical nurse specialist
    c. Psychiatrist
    d. Play therapist
    e. Occupational therapist
    f. Physical therapist
6. Provide attention to developmentally appropriate role modeling for age and situation.
7. Encourage peer support during hospitalization as appropriate.
8. Address educational needs for teaching of procedures, care, or therapy plans upon discharge.
9. Allow for appropriate follow-up after dismissal via referral to local support groups.
10. Administer medications as ordered with monitoring of potential side effects.
11. Plan for potential long-term nursing follow-up.

WOMEN'S HEALTH

1. Assist the client to describe her sexuality and understanding of sexual functioning as it relates to her life-style and life-style decisions.
2. Allow client time to discuss sexuality and sex-related problems in a nonthreatening atmosphere.
3. Assist client in listing life-style adjustments that need to be made.
4. Identify significant others in client's life.
5. Involve significant others, if so desired, by client in discussion and problem-solving activities regarding sexual adjustments.
6. Provide atmosphere that allows client to discuss freely the following issues:
    a. Partner choice
    b. Sexual orientation
    c. Sexual roles
7. Assist client in identifying life-style adjustments to each different cycle of reproductive life:
    a. Puberty
    b. Pregnancy
    c. Menopause
    d. Post-menopause
8. Discuss pregnancy and the changes that will occur during pregnancy:
    a. Sexuality
    b. Mood swings
    c. Alternative methods of intercourse during pregnancy
        (1) Positions
        (2) Frequency
        (3) Effects on baby
        (4) Effects on pregnancy

    d. Fears about sexual changes
  9. Obtain complete sexual history.
 10. Note patient's mental state.
    a. Anxious
    b. Frightened
    c. Ambivalent
 11. Assist client facing surgery or body structure changes in identifying life-style adjustments that may be needed.
 12. Allow client to grieve loss of body image.
 13. Reassure client that she can still participate in sexual activities.
 14. Assure confidentiality for patient with sexually transmitted diseases.
 15. Encourage verbalization of concerns with sexually transmitted diseases.
    a. Recurrent nature of disease, especially herpes and chlamydia.
    b. Lack of cure for disease (AIDS).
    c. Economics in treating disease.
    d. Social stigma associated with disease.
 16. Encourage honesty in answers to such questions as:
    a. Multiple sex partners.
    b. Describing sexual behavior.
 17. Encourage honest communication with sexual partner(s). (See Chapter 9 for AIDS hot line telephone number).

MENTAL HEALTH

(Note: If alteration is related to altered body function or structure or illness, refer to Adult Health care plan.)

1. Assign primary care nurse who is comfortable discussing sexually related material with client.
2. Primary nurse will spend (number) minutes (number) times a day with client discussing issues related to diagnosis. These discussions will include:
    a. Client's thoughts and feelings about alteration;
    b. Other stressors and concerns in the client's life that could affect sexual patterns;
    c. Client's perceptions of partner's responses;
    d. Client's perceptions of self as a sexual person without a partner;
    e. Client's perceptions of social or cultural expectations;
    f. Client's thoughts and feelings about sexuality.
3. If alteration is related to lack of information, develop a teaching plan and note teaching plan here.
4. If alteration is related to problems with the significant other, arrange a meeting with client and significant other to discuss the perceptions each has about the problem. If these difficulties are related to a lack of information, develop a teaching plan and note it here. If alteration is related to long-term problems in the relationship or if alteration is only one of several problems, refer to marriage and family therapist or clinical nurse specialist.
5. Arrange private time for client and partner to discuss relationship issues, including sexuality. Note time and place arranged for this discussion here.
6. During interactions with client and significant other, have them express feelings about their relationship. These should be both positive and negative feelings.

HOME HEALTH

1. Monitor for factors contributing to altered sexuality patterns by (date).
2. Involve appropriate family members (e.g., significant or parents of child) in planning, implementing, and promoting reduction or elimination of altered sexuality patterns:
    a. Communication

   b. Mutual sharing and trust
   c. Problem solving
   d. Sex education
3. Assist patient and family with life-style adjustments that may be required:
   a. Accurate and appropriate information regarding sexuality and contraception
   b. Providing time and privacy for development and improvement of sexual relationship
   c. Stress management
   d. Coping with loss of sexual partner
   e. Accurate and appropriate information regarding sexually transmitted diseases
   f. Accurate and appropriate information regarding sexual orientation (e.g., homosexuality, heterosexuality, transexuality, etc.).
   g. Coping with physical disability
   h. Side effects of medical treatments
4. Consult with assistive resources as indicated:
   a. Sex therapist
   b. Health educator
   c. Marriage and family counselor
   d. Nurse
   e. Physician
   f. Psychiatric nurse clinician
   g. Contraceptive counselor
   h. Singles groups
   i. Sex educator
   j. Occupational therapist
   k. Physical therapist
   l. Support groups

EVALUATION
OBJECTIVE 1

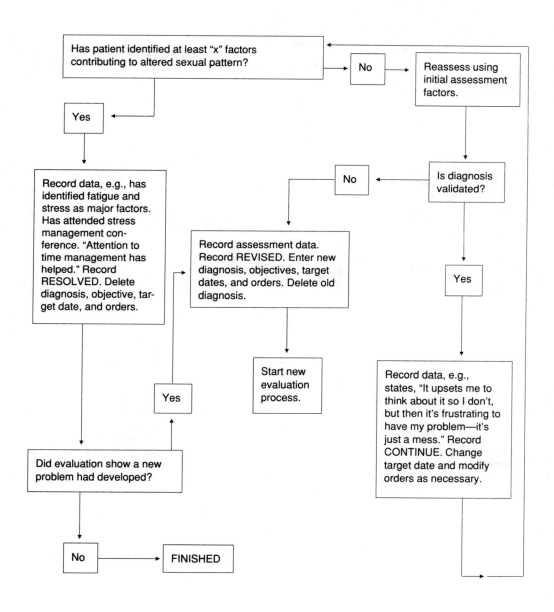

OBJECTIVE 2

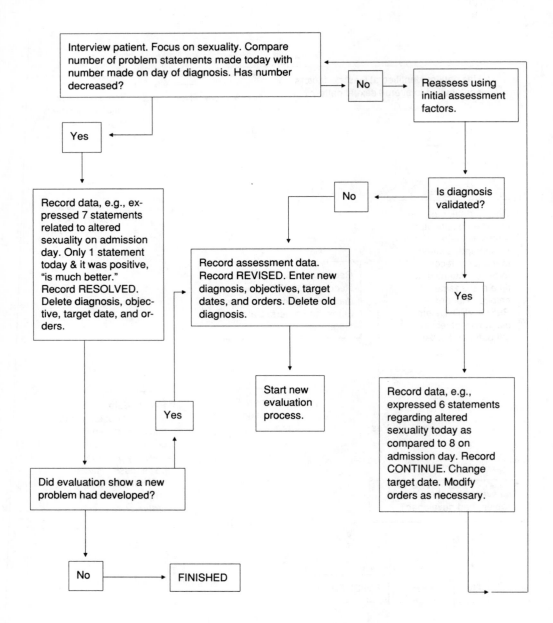

REFERENCES

Ames, L. B., & Ilg, F. L. (1976). *Child behavior*. New York: Dell.

Biddle, B. J., & Thomas, E. J. (1979). *Role theory: Concepts and research*. Huntington, NY: Robert E. Drieger.

Fogel, C. I., & Woods, N. F. (1981). *Health care of women: A nursing perspective*. St. Louis: C. V. Mosby.

Molcan, K. L., & Fickley, B. S. (1988). Sexuality and the life cycle. in S. G. Poorman (Ed.), *Human sexuality and the nursing process*. Norwalk, CT Appleton & Lange.

North American Nursing Diagnosis Association. (1987). *Taxonomy I with complete diagnosis*. St. Louis: Author.

Schuster, C. S. & Ashburn, S. S. (1986). *The process of human development: A holistic life-span approach* (2nd ed.). Boston: Little, Brown.

Speroff, L., & Glass, R. H. (1984). *Clinical gynecologic endrocrinology and infertility* (3rd ed.). Baltimore: Williams & Wilkins.

Warner, C. G. (1980). *Rape and sexual assault: Management and intervention*. Germantown, MD: Aspen Systems.

Wilson, H. S., & Kneisel, C. (1984). *Psychiatric nursing* (2nd ed.). Menlo Park, CA: Addison-Wesley.

Woods, N. F. (1984). *Human sexuality in health and illness*. St. Louis: C. V. Mosby.

SUGGESTED READINGS

Agulera, D. C., & Messick, J. M. (1982). *Crisis intervention* (4th ed.). St. Louis: C. V. Mosby.

AIDS and Pregnancy. (1987). New York, New York: Maternity Center Association.

Antognoli-Toland, P. (1985). Comprehensive program for examination of sexual assault victims by nurses: A hospital-based project in Texas. *Journal of Emergency Nursing, 11* (3), 132–135.

Carpenito, L. (1983). *Nursing diagnosis*. Philadelphia: J. B. Lippincott.

Crittendon, R. (1983). *Discharge planning*. Bowie, MD: Robert J. Brady.

Doenges, M., & Moorhouse, M. (1985). *Nurse's pocket guide: Nursing Diagnosis with interventions*. Philadelphia: F. A. Davis.

Foley, T. S. (1983). Counseling the victim of rape. In G. W.Stuart & S. Sundeen (Eds), *Principles and practice of psychiatric nursing* (pp. 836–865). St. Louis: C. V. Mosby.

Griffith-Kenney, J. (1986). *Contemporary women's health: A nursing advocacy approach*. Menlo Park, CA Addison-Wesley.

Haber, J., Hoskins, P., Leach, A., & Sideleau, B. (1987). *Comprehensive psychiatric nursing* (3rd ed.). New York: McGraw-Hill.

Hadeka, M. (1987). *Clinical judgment in community health nursing*. Boston: Little, Brown.

Hogan, R. (1985). *Human sexuality: A nursing perspective*. East Norwalk, CT: Appleton-Century-Crofts.

Humphrey, C. (1986). *Home care nursing handbook*. East Norwalk, CT: Appleton-Century-Crofts.

Jaffe, M., & Skidmore-Roth, L. (1988). *Home health nursing care plans*. St. Louis: C. V. Mosby.

Kolly, K. (1985 August). Victim, *Nursing 85*, p. 72.

McClelland, E., Kelly, K.,& Buckwalter, K. (1984). *Continuity of care: Advancing the concept of discharge planning*. Orlando, FL: Grune & Stratton.

McFarland, G., & Wasli, E. (1986). *Nursing diagnosis and process in psychiatric mental health nursing*. Philadelphia: J. B.Lippincott

National League for Nursing. (1986). *Policies and procedures*. New York: Accreditation Division for Home Care, National League for Nursing.

National League for Nursing. (1988). *Accreditation program for home care and community health: Criteria and standards*. New York: Author.

North American Nursing Diagnosis Association. (1988). *Proposed nursing diagnoses*. St. Louis: Author.

Poorman, S. G. (1988). *Human sexuality and the nursing process*. Norwalk, CT: Appleton & Lange.

Rinke, L. (1988). *Outcome standards in home health*. New York: National League for Nursing.

Schultz, J., & Dark, S. (1982). *Manual of psychiatric nursing care plans*. Boston: Little, Brown.

Steffi, B., & Eide, I. (1978). *Discharge planning handbook*. New York: Charles B. Slack.

Stuart, G., & Sundeen, S. (1987). *Principles and practice of psychiatric nursing* (3rd ed.). St. Louis: C. V. Mosby.

Stuart, G. & Sundeen, S. (1988). *Pocket nurse guide to psychiatric nursing*. St. Louis: C .V. Mosby.

Ten common sex problems: Do they affect you? (1987) *Women's Health Watch, 2* (1), 8–9.

Walsh, J., Persons, C., & Weick, L. (1987). *Manual of home health care nursing*. Philadelphia: J. B. Lippincott.

Whaley, L. & Wong, D. (1987). *Nursing care of infants & children*. St. Louis: C.V. Mosby.

CHAPTER ELEVEN

Coping–Stress Tolerance Pattern

Pattern Description

Stress has been defined as the response of the body or the system to any demand made on it. (Sutterley, 1979). This response can be both physiologic and psychosocial. Since demands are synonymous with living, stress has been defined as "life itself" (Sutterley, 1979, p. 1). The system's (individual, family, or community) ability to respond to these demands has an effect on the well-being of the system. Stress tolerance pattern refers to the system's usual manner of responding to stress or to the amount of stress previously experienced. This includes the stress response history of the individual, family, or community (Gordon, 1987). Coping has been defined as "efforts to master conditions of harm, threat or challenge when a routine or automatic response is not readily available" (Ziemer, 1982, p. 4). Thus, the coping pattern is the system's pattern of responding to nonroutine threats. The client's ability to respond to stress is affected by a complex interaction of physical, social, and emotional well-being. Assessment of this pattern focuses on gaining an understanding of the interaction of these factors within the system. Interventions are related to maximizing the system's well-being (Sutterley, 1979; Ziemer, 1982).

Pattern Assessment

(Note: Client refers to individual, family, or community as appropriate)

1. Describe client's mental status and cognitive functioning (for a detailed description of this process see Pattern Assessment, Chapter 8).
2. Assess client's past coping behavior by discussing past stresses and how these were managed.
3. Describe client's cognitive appraisal or perception of the situation.
4. Assess client's nutritional status.
5. Assess client's exercise and physical activity patterns.
6. Assess client's support system.
7. Assess client's sleep-rest patterns.
8. Assess client's environment for potential stressors such as improper lighting, excessive noise, hazardous or toxic substances, and radiation.
9. Describe cultural values related to the situation (e.g., attitudes about abortion, homosexuality, discrimination, or working women).
10. Assess client's perception of the situation.
11. Assess client's perception of self.
12. Assess client's developmental level of functioning.
13. Assess client's philosophy of living.
14. Assess client's health hazards and awareness of these (e.g., awareness of and use of seat belts, knowledge and use of firearms) (Gordon, 1987; Sutterley, 1979; Ziemer, 1982).

15. Assess client's financial situation.
16. Assess client's readiness to address concerns and alternative ways of coping.

Conceptual Information

To understand coping one must first understand the concept of stress; coping is the system's attempt to adapt to stress. An understanding of these concepts and their relationship is crucial for the promotion of well-being. Research has clearly demonstrated that undue stress can be related to major health problems if inappropriate coping is present.

Stress has been defined as the body's nonspecific response to any demand placed upon it (Sutterley, 1979). These demands can be any situation that would require the system to adapt. For the individual this could include anything from getting out of bed in the morning to experiencing the loss resulting from a major environmental disaster. Stress is life.

The body's physiologic response to stress involves activation of the autonomic nervous system. The symptoms of this activation can include sweating, tachycardia, tachypnea, nausea, and tremors. This process has been labeled the general-adaptation syndrome (GAS) by Selye (Frain & Valiga, 1979) and occurs in three stages. These stages are alarm reaction, resistance, and exhaustion. The alarm stage mobilizes the system's defense forces by initiating the autonomic nervous system response. The system is prepared for "fight or flight." In the resistance stage, the system fights back and adapts, and normal functioning returns. If the stress continues, and all attempts of the system to adapt fail, exhaustion occurs, and the system is at risk for experiencing major disorganization.

Frain and Valiga (1979) describe four levels of psychophysiologic stress responses. The first level comprises the day-to-day stressors that all systems experience as a part of living. This stress calls upon the self-regulating processes of the system for adaptation. Intrasystem coping mechanisms are used and the system does not require assistance from outside sources to adapt. Level 2 comprises less-routine or new experiences encountered by the system. The system experiences a mild alarm reaction that is not prolonged. The individual system might experience a mild increase in heart rate, sensations of bladder fullness and increased frequency of urination, temporary insomnia, tachypnea, anxiety, fear, guilt, shame, or frustration. Some outside assistance may be necessary to facilitate adaptation. This assistance could be identifying stressors and strengths, or encouraging the individual to solve problems. Level 3 consists of the moderate amount of stress that occurs when a persistent stress is encountered or when a new situation is perceived as threatening. Emergency adaptation processes are activated. The individual would experience tachycardia, palpitations, tremors, weakness, cool pale skin, headache, oliguria, vomiting, constipation, and increased susceptibility to infections. This level of stress usually requires assistance from a professional helper. This assistance can include identifying problems and coping strengths, teaching, performing tasks for the client, or altering the environment to facilitate coping. When the system cannot adapt to a stressful situation with assistance, a severe degree of stress is experienced. This is labeled level 4. This occurs when all coping strategies are exhausted. Intervention at this level requires the assistance of professionals who have the skills to assist with the development of unique coping strategies.

Since stress is life itself, adaptation to reduce the effects of stress on the system is imperative. To begin this process it is important to understand those factors that can influence the system's ability to respond to stress. Stress can arise from biophysical, chemical, psychosocial, and cultural sources. The basic health of the affected system improves the ability to respond to these stressors. Response to the biophysical-chemical stressors can be improved by improving the condition of the biological system. This would include proper nutrition, appropriate amounts of rest, appropriate levels of exercise, and reduced exposure of the system to toxic chemicals (Sutterley, 1979).

Sutterley (1979) indicates that a great deal of psychosocial-cultural stress evolves from a philosophy of life that is impossible to fulfill. This would indicate that a great deal of stress arises from the perception of events, not in the events themselves. This is compounded by the social and cultural influences on the system. The sociocultural influences could include the cultural attitudes about age, body appearance, and family roles and the social approaches to assistance for working mothers, advancement in employment status, etc. The system's beliefs about these social-cultural stressors can affect the degree to which the stressors affect the system. If the stressor is perceived as unnatural or impossible to adapt to, the system's stress level will be increased. Response to the psychosocial-cultural stressors can be improved with attitude assessment and interventions that reduce the physiologic response to psychosocial stressors.

Coping has been defined as behavior (conscious and unconscious) that a system uses to change a situation for the better or to manage the stress-resultant emotions (Mengel, 1982). These kinds of behavior can occur on the biologic, psychologic, and social levels. Effective coping uses biologic, psychologic, and social resources in attempts to manage the situation.

Antonovsky (Ziemer, 1982) presents a model for coping that addresses the biologic, psychologic, and sociocultural aspects of this process. He indicates that systems have generalized resistance resources (GRRs) to facilitate coping. GRRs are those characteristics of the system that can facilitate effective tension management. Genetic characteristics that provide increased resistance to the effects of stressors are considered physical and biochemical GRRs. These GRRs can include levels of immunity, nutritional status, and the adaptability of the neurologic system. Valuative and attitudinal GRRs describe consistent features of the system's coping behavior. This could include personality characteristics and the system's perception of the stressor. The more flexible, rational, and long-term these are, the more effective they are as GRRs. Interpersonal-relational GRRs include social support systems and can provide an important resource in managing stress. Finally, those cultural supports that facilitate coping are referred to as macrosociocultural GRRs. Macro-sociocultural GRRs could include religions, rites of passage, and governmental structures.

Effective coping can occur when the system has a strong physiologic base combined with adequate psychosociocultural support. This implies that any intervention that addresses coping behavior should address each of these areas. Interventions that have been applied to this process include therapeutic touch, kinesiology, meditation, relaxation training, hypnosis, family therapy, nutritional counseling, massage, and physical exercise.

Developmental Considerations

The number of resources available to the system greatly affects its ability to cope with stressors. This indicates a need to maximize physical, cognitive, and psychosocial development. Cross-cultural research has identified those characteristics that are common to individuals who are perceived as mature and capable of coping effectively. These characteristics include an ability to anticipate consequences; calm, clear thinking; potential fulfillment; problem solving that is orderly and organized; predictability; purposefulness; realisticness; reflectiveness; strong convictions; and implacability (Schuster & Ashburn, 1986). The development of these characteristics are maximized in environments that provide children with a loving, warm environment; respect and acceptance for personal interests, ideas, needs, and talents; stable role models; challenges that foster development of competence and responsibility; opportunities to explore all of their feelings; a variety of experiences, opportunities for age-appropriate problem solving and the knowledge that they must live with the consequences of their decisions; opportunities to develop commitments to others; and encouragement in the development of their own standards, values, and goals (Schuster & Ashburn, 1986).

According to developmental stages, there are some specific etiologies and symptom clusters:

Infant

Interactions with significant others are the primary source of the infant's response to trauma. If the significant other is supportive and consistent, the effects of the event on the infant are minimized. Events that separate infants from their significant others also pose a threat to this age group. Primary symptoms are disruptions in physiologic responses.

The chronic diseases place this age group at special risk. Since the development of coping behavior is limited at this age, the primary caregivers (usually the parents) provide the child with the support to cope. If the caregivers cannot provide the proper supports, then the child is affected. Chronic illness in the child places an extreme stress on the family and can result in divorce. Support for the parents is crucial in supporting the child's coping.

Toddler and Preschooler

Responses of significant others are still the primary supports for the child in this age group. Thus, as for the infant, the response of significant others or separation from these persons can have an effect on the child in this age group. In addition, threats to body integrity pose a special threat to this age group. Traumatic events that inflict physical damage on this age group place the child at greatest risk. Regression is the primary symptom and coping behavior. This can be frustrating to caregivers who expect the child to assist in a time of crisis with age-appropriate developmental behavior when the child may regress to a very dependent stage. Other methods used by young children in coping include denial, repression, and projection. Coping may be more difficult because adults may not recognize that young children can experience crisis and will, therefore, not provide assistance with the coping process (Smitherman, 1981).

School-age Child

Symptoms include problems with school performance, withdrawal from family and peers, behavioral regression, and physical problems related to anxiety and aggressive behavior to self or others. Coping behavior includes that used by the younger child, only in a more effective manner. This age group may find a great deal of support from siblings during crisis. Situations that can precipitate crisis in this age group include school entry, threats to body image, peer problems, and family stress such as divorce or death of a loved one (Smitherman, 1981).

Chronic disease or disability also affects the adjustment of this age group. Again, the primary support for adaptation comes from the primary caregivers, usually the parents.

Adolescent

The adolescent demonstrates more adult-like coping behavior. Symptoms of stress include anxiety, increased physical activity, increased daydreaming, increased apathy, change in mood cycles, alteration in sleeping patterns, aggressive behavior directed at self or others, and physical symptoms associated with anxiety. Crisis-producing situations can include role changes, peer difficulties, threats to body integrity, rapidly changing body functioning, conflict with parents, personal failures, sexual awareness, and school demands (Smitherman, 1981).

Response to traumatic events is similar to that of adults (see Pattern Assessment). Etiologies for this age group are also similar to those for adults. Specific events that place this age group at greater risk are those that affect the peer group and could have effects on body image or sexual functioning. Coping behavior is adult-like. This age group may find support from peers especially useful in facilitating coping. Coping may also be affected by limited life experience and impulsive behavior.

Illnesses that threaten body image could result in difficulties in adjustment. Peers again provide a primary support system and can have a great impact on the adolescent's acceptance. Educating significant peers about the client's situation could facilitate their acceptance of the client and in turn facilitate the client's adjustment to the change in health status. Adjustment could also be facilitated by involving the client in a support group composed of peers with similar alterations.

Young Adult

Symptoms of problems with coping include changes in performance of roles at home and at work, aggressive behavior directed at the self or to others, and physical symptoms associated with anxiety and denial. Changes in role performance might include loss of interest in sexual relationships or withdrawal from the community. Situations that might tax the coping abilities of the young adult include balancing increasing role responsibilities; dealing with threats to the self or to body integrity; leaving home; and making career choices (Smitherman, 1981; Carpenito, 1983).

Alterations in health status that affect the ability of role performance place this age group at risk for impaired adjustment. This could include loss of ability to function in job responsibilities. Behavior can include regression, but this does not necessarily indicate that the client is experiencing impaired adjustment.

Adult

Coping resources have broadened for this age group due to past successful coping experiences and the possible addition of adult children as supports during crisis. Symptoms of difficulties with coping are similar to those of the young adult. Age-related stressors include increased loss, including significant others and physical functioning; role changes such as job loss and the leaving of adult children; aging parents; career pressures; cultural role expectations (Smitherman, 1981).

Older Adult

Symptoms of extreme stress in this age group may be overlooked and attributed to senility. These symptoms include withdrawal, decreased functioning, increased physical complaints, and aggressive behavior. Coping behavior is affected by decreased function of hearing, vision, and mobility as well as loss of support systems and other resources. These problems can be balanced by life experience that has provided the individual with many situations of successful coping to fall back on during stressful times. Situations that place this age group at risk are multiple losses, decreased physical functioning, increased dependence, retirement, relocation, and loss of respect due to cultural attitudes.

The effects of multiple losses related to alteration in health status and the losses of support systems place the older adult at risk for impaired adjustment. In the absence of illness affecting cognitive functioning the older adult maintains formal operational thinking and can assume responsibility for making decisions related to alterations in health status. This ability combined with life experience can facilitate creative problem solving with the support of health care personnel (Dixon & Dixon, 1984).

The following is a presentation of the developmental framework of the family life cycle as described by Elizabeth Carter and Monica McGoldrick (1980).

Between families: The unattached young adult—the process of this level is accepting parent-child separation. The individual must separate from family of origin and develop intimate peer relationships and a career.

The joining of families through marriage: The newly married couple—the process of this level involves commitment to a new system. The individuals form a marital system and realign relationships with extended families and friends to include spouse.

The family with young children: The task faced is to accept a new generation of members into the system. The marital system adjusts to make space for the child(ren) and assumes parent roles. Another relignment takes place to include parenting and grandparenting roles.

The family with adolescents: The family task is to increase flexibility of family boundaries to include children's independence. The parent-child relationships shift to allow the adolescents to move in and out of the system. The parents refocus on midlife marital and career issues, and there is a beginning shift toward concerns for the older generation.

The family in later life: Accepting the shifting of generational roles is the task of this stage. The system maintains individual and couple functioning and interests in conjunction with physiologic decline. There is an exploration of new role options with more support for a more central role for the middle generation. The system also makes room of the wisdom and experience for the elderly to support the older generation without overprotecting them. This stage will also include coping with the deaths of significant others and preparation for death.

Specific problems can arise in family coping when the family developmental cycle or expectations do not correspond with the developmental tasks of individual family members. There are three stages that are nodal points in family development.

The joining of families through marriage requires a new commitment to a new system. If the separation from the parent is not successful then, the new family does not have an opportunity to form its own identity, combining the experiences both bring into this new relationship. Symptoms of unsuccessful resolution of this stage could result in the marital partners returning home to their parents when conflict arises or an ongoing struggle over loyalties to families of origin.

The second major shift occurs when children enter the system. The new role of parent is assumed and the couple boundaries must be opened to accept the child. Unsuccessful resolution of this stage could result in physical or emotional abuse of the child. If there is a developmental delay in the parents and they are not ready to assume the responsibilities that accompany parenthood, family dysfunction can occur.

A family with adolescents is faced with the task of increasing flexibility to include children's independence. This may require a major shift in family rules. This is also influenced by the parent's perception of the adolescent and the environment. If the adolescent is seen as being competent, and the environment that the adolescent interacts in is seen as safe, then it will be much easier for the family to provide the necessary shifts in relationships. When this stage is not resolved successfully the adolescent may enhance behavior that highlight his or her differences with the family to force separation, or the frequency and intensity of family conflict may increase. Unsuccessful resolution of this stage may indicate that the family has overly rigid boundaries to the external world and individual boundaries that are overly permeable.

Applicable Nursing Diagnoses

Adjustment, Impaired

DEFINITION

The state in which the individual is unable to modify his or her life-style or behavior in a manner consistent with a change in health status (North American Nursing Diagnosis Association (NANDA, 1987, p. 72).

DEFINING CHARACTERISTICS (NANDA, 1987, p. 72)

The nurse will review the initial pattern assessment for the following defining characteristics to determine the diagnosis of Adjustment, Impaired.

1. Major defining characteristics
   a. Verbalization of nonacceptance of health status change
   b. Nonexistent or unsuccessful ability to be involved in problem solving or goal setting
2. Minor defining characteristics
   a. Lack of movement toward independence
   b. Extended period of shock, disbelief, or anger regarding health status change
   c. Lack of future-oriented thinking

RELATED FACTORS (NANDA, 1987, p. 72)

1. Disability requiring change in life-style
2. Inadequate support systems
3. Impaired cognition
4. Sensory overload
5. Assault to self-esteem
6. Altered locus of control
7. Incomplete grieving

DIFFERENTIATION

Adjustment, Impaired should be differentiated from Individual Coping, Ineffective; Powerlessness; Self-Concept, Disturbance in; Sensory-Perceptual Alteration; Spiritual Distress; Thought Process, Altered; Grieving, Dysfunctional; and Anxiety.

Individual Coping, Ineffective, results from the client's inability to cope appropriately with stress. Adjustment, Impaired is the client's inability to adjust to a specific disease process. If the client's behavior is related to the adjustment to a specific disease process, the diagnosis would be Adjustment, Impaired; however, if the behavior is related to coping with general life stressors, the diagnosis would be Individual Coping, Ineffective.

Powerlessness would be an appropriate diagnosis or co-diagnosis if the client demonstrates the belief that personal action cannot affect or alter the situation. Adjustment, Impaired may result from Powerlessness. If this is the situation then the appropriate primary diagnosis would be Powerlessness.

Self-Concept, Disturbance in can affect the client's perception of his or her ability to adjust to an alteration in health status. If it appears the client's inability to adjust is related to self-concept, then the appropriate primary diagnosis would be Self-Concept, Disturbance in.

Sensory-Perceptual Alteration can affect the individual's ability to adjust to an alteration in health status. If it is determined that perceptual alterations are affecting the client's ability to adapt, then the appropriate primary diagnosis would be Sensory-Perceptual Alteration.

Spiritual Distress is a questioning of one's life principles or values rather than questioning the self or one's ability to adapt to an alteration in health status. If the client's concerns are focused only on the value-belief system, then the appropriate diagnosis would be Spiritual Distress.

Thought Process, Altered can inhibit the client's ability to adapt effectively to an alteration in health status. If the inability to adapt to the alteration is related to an alteration in thought processes, then the appropriate primary diagnosis would be Thought Process, Altered.

Grieving, Dysfunctional can have a strong effect on the client's ability to adjust to an alteration in health status. This differentiation is complicated by the fact that a normal response to an alteration in health status can be grief. If, however, the client is not reporting a sense of loss then the appropriate diagnosis would be, Adjustment, Impaired. If the client reports a sense of loss with the appropriate defining characteristics, then the appropriate diagnosis would be Grieving. If the grieving is prolonged or exceptionally severe (see Grieving, Dysfunctional for a detailed description) then an appropriate co-diagnosis with Adjustment, Impaired would be Grieving, Dysfunctional.

Anxiety presents with a nonspecific threat. If the threat is identified as the alteration in health status, then the appropriate diagnosis would be Adjustment, Impaired.

OBJECTIVES

1. Will verbalize increased adaptation to change in health status by (date).

AND/OR

2. Will return demonstrate measures necessary to increase independence by (date).

TARGET DATE

Adjustment to a change in health status will require time; therefore, an acceptable initial target date would be no sooner than 7–10 days following the date of diagnosis.

NURSING ORDERS

ADULT HEALTH

1. Establish a therapeutic relationship with patient and significant others.
2. Explain the disease process and prognosis to patient.
3. Encourage patient to ask questions about health status.
4. Encourage patient to participate in own care.
5. Encourage patient to express feelings about disease process and prognosis.
6. Identify previous coping mechanisms and assist patient to find new ones.
7. Help patient find alternatives or modifications in previous life-style behavior.
8. Encourage independence in self-care activities.
9. Refer to psychiatric nurse clinician. (See Mental Health nursing orders for more detailed interventions.)

CHILD HEALTH

1. Monitor for all possible etiologic factors via active listening as appropriate for child (who, what, where, when) regarding first feeling of not being able to adjust.
2. Help the child to realize it is normal to need some time and assistance in adjusting to changes.
3. Explore the child's and family's previous coping strategies.
4. Identify ways the child can feel better about coping with the needed adjustment, including reinforcement of desired behavior.
5. Assist the child and family in creating realistic goals for coping.
6. Collaborate with related health team members as needed, especially:
   a. Pediatrician
   b. Pediatric clinical nurse specialist

    c. Psychiatrist
    d. Psychologist
    e. Play therapist
    f. Social worker
    f. Family therapist
    h. Clergy
7. Provide clear and simple explanations for procedures.
8. Address educational needs related to health care.
9. Deal with other primary care needs promptly.
10. Provide for post-hospitalization follow-up with home care as needed.
11. Assist patient and family in identification of community resources to offer support.

WOMEN'S HEALTH

1. Provide a nonjudgmental atmosphere to allow client to express concerns of:
    a. Self-image as a father
    b. Relationship with his father
    c. Self-responsibility
    d. Feelings about wife's or partner's pregnancy
    e. Concerns about wife's or partner's safety
2. Refer to appropriate support groups.
    a. Childbirth education classes
    b. Health care providers
        (1) Perinatal nurses or nurse practitioners
        (2) Certified nurse midwife
        (3) Physician's office
            (a) Obstetricians
            (b) Family practitioner
    c. Psychiatric counseling (if signs of pseudocyesis appear)
3. Accurately record physical symptoms described by expectant father.
    a. Fatigue
    b. Weight gain
    c. Nausea, vomiting
    d. Headaches
    e. Backaches
    f. Food cravings
4. Monitor men experiencing the above symptoms to identify those men experiencing Couvade syndrome.
5. Support and guide the men through the changes being experienced.
6. Assure expectant couple that:
    a. Expectant fathers can suffer physical symptoms during partner's pregnancy;
    b. Pregnancy affects both partners;
    c. Fathers also have emotional needs during pregnancy.
7. When counseling with expectant fathers be alert for symptoms listed in the "Index of Suspicion for the Couvade Syndrome" (Viken, 1982, pp. 40–42):
    a. Affects males only
    b. Wives are pregnant usually, in the 3rd or 9th month of gestation
    c. Symptoms are confined to GI or GU system, notable exceptions are toothache and skin growths
    d. Anxiety, affective disturbances are common
    e. Physical findings are minimal

f. Laboratory and x-ray testing yields, normal results
g. Patient makes no connection between his symptoms and his wife's pregnancy

Depression Postpartum, Puerperal Psychosis

8. Allow client to express fears related to care and health of infant.
   a. Less-than-perfect infant
   b. Low-birth-weight infant
   c. Wrong sex
   d. Fussy infant
9. Complications during pregnancy, delivery, or postpartum.
10. Provide nonjudgmental atmosphere for client to discuss family situation:
    a. Partner's lack of sexual interest
    b. Any illnesses or problems with older children
    c. Marital status
    d. Planned or unplanned pregnancy
    e. Birth experience
       (1) Disappointment in experience
          (a) Unexpected C-section
          (b) Medications administered during labor
          (c) Any unexpected occurrences
    f. Isolation during postpartum
       (1) Unable to return to work immediately
       (2) No adults available to talk to during day
       (3) Unable to complete daily activities
          (a) Fatigue
          (b) Demands of infant
          (c) Uncooperative partner
       (4) Lack of support system
          (a) Other mothers in same situation
          (b) No immediate or extended family
          (c) No support groups available

MENTAL HEALTH

1. Discuss with client his or her perception of the current alteration in health status. This should include information about the coping strategies that have been attempted and his or her assessment of what has made them ineffective in promoting adaptation.
2. Provide client with clocks and calendars to promote orientation and involvement in the environment.
3. Give client information about the care that is to be provided, including times for treatments, medicines, groups, and other therapy.
4. Assign client appropriate tasks during unit activities. These should be at a level that can easily be accomplished. Provide client with positive verbal support for completing the task. Gradually increase the difficulty of the tasks as the client's abilities increase. The client's current level of functioning, as well as the tasks assigned, should be noted here.
5. Sit with client (number) minutes (number) times per day at (specific times listed) to discuss current concerns and feelings.
6. Provide client with familiar needed objects. These should be noted here. These should assist the client in identifying a personal space over which he or she feels some control. This space is to be respected by the staff and the client's permission should be obtained before altering this environment.
7. Provide client with an environment that will optimize sensory input. This could include hearing

aids, eyeglasses, pencil and paper, decreased noise in conversation areas, appropriate lighting (these interventions should indicate an awareness of sensory deficit as well as sensory overload, and the specific interventions for this client should be noted here, e.g., place hearing aid in when client awakens and remove before bedtime [9:00 p.m.]).

8. Communicate to client an understanding that all coping behavior to this point has been his or her best effort and asking for assistance at this time is not failure—a complex problem often requires some outside assistance in resolution.

9. Call client by the name he or she has identified as the preferred name with each interaction. Note this name on the care plan.

10. Have client dress in "street clothing." This should be items of clothing that have been brought from home and in which the client feels comfortable.

11. Provide client with opportunities to make appropriate decisions related to care at his or her level of ability. This may begin as a choice between two options and then evolve into more complex decision making. It is important that this be at the client's level of functioning so confidence can be built with successful decision-making experiences. Note those decisions that the client has made here.

12. Provide client with primary care nurse on each shift. Nurse will spend 30 minutes once per shift at (note time here) developing a relationship with the client. This time could be spent answering client's questions about the hospital, about daily routines, etc., or providing the client with a backrub.

13. Identify with client methods of anxiety reduction. The specific method selected by the client should be noted here. For the first 3 days the staff should remain with the client during a 30-minute practice of the selected method. The method should be practiced 30 minutes three times a day at (note times here). (See Anxiety, Chapter 8, for specific instructions about anxiety reduction methods.)

14. Provide positive social reinforcement and other behavioral rewards for demonstration of adaptation (those things that the client finds rewarding should be listed here with a schedule for use. The kinds of behavior that the team are to be rewarding should also be listed with the appropriate reward).

15. Assist client in identifying support systems and in developing a plan for their use. The support systems identified should be noted along with the plan for their use.

16. Schedule a meeting with the identified support system to assist them in understanding the alterations in the client's health. Provide time to answer any questions they may have. Note the time for this meeting here and the person responsible for this meeting.

17. Provide client with group interaction with (number) persons, (number) minutes, (number) times per day at (times of day). (This activity should be graded with client's ability, e.g., on admission client may tolerate one person for 5 minutes. If the interactions are brief the frequency should be high, e.g., 5-minute interactions should occur at 30-minute intervals. If client is meeting with a large client group this may occur only once a day. The larger groups should include persons who are more advanced in adapting to their alterations and persons who may be less advanced).

18. Make available items necessary for client to groom self. Have these items adapted as necessary to facilitate client use. List those items that are necessary here along with any assistance that is necessary from the nursing staff. Assign one person per day to be responsible for this assistance. Provide positive social reinforcement for client's accomplishments in this area.

19. Set an appointment to discuss with client and significant others effects of the loss or change on their relationship (time and date of appointment and all follow-up appointments should be listed here). Note person responsible for these meetings.

20. Monitor nurse's nonverbal reactions to loss or change and provide client with verbal information when necessary to establish nurse's acceptance of the change.

21. If nursing staff is having difficulty coping with the client's alterations, schedule a staff meeting where these issues can be discussed. An outside clinical nurse specialist may be useful in facilitating these meetings. Schedule ongoing support meetings as appears necessary.
22. Utilize constructive confrontation if necessary to include:
    a. "I" statements;
    b. Relationship statements that reflect nurse's reaction to the interaction;
    c. Responses that will assist client in understanding, such as paraphrasing and validation of perceptions.
23. When a relationship has been developed the primary care nurse will spend 30 minutes twice a day at (time) and (time) with the client discussing thoughts and feelings related to the alteration in health status. These discussions could include memories that have been activated by this alteration, client's fears and concerns for the future, client's plans for the future before the alteration in health status, client's perceptions of how this alteration will affect daily life, client's perceptions of how this alteration will affect the lives of significant others, etc.
24. Provide client with information about care and treatment. Give information in concise terms appropriate to the client's level of understanding. Note those areas that client needs the most information in here with a plan for providing this information.
25. Do not argue with client while he or she is experiencing an alteration in thought process (refer to Thought Process, Altered, Chapter 7, for related care plan).
26. Develop with the client a very specific behavioral plan for adapting to the alteration in health status. Note that plan here. This plan should include achievable goals so the client will not become frustrated.
27. Refer client to occupational therapy to develop the necessary adaptations to the occupational role. Note time for these meetings here.
28. Schedule time for the client and his or her support system to be together without interruptions. The times for these interactions should be noted here.
29. If client is disoriented, orient to reality as needed and before attempting any teaching activity. Provide client with clocks and calendars and refer to day, date, and time in each interaction with this client.
30. Refer client to appropriate assistive resources as indicated
    a. Visiting nurse
    b. Nutritionist
    c. Social services
    d. Family therapist
    e. Psychiatric nurse clinician
    f. Physical therapist
    g. American Cancer Society
    h. American Heart Association
    i. Other groups related to the client's specific diagnosis
    j. Spiritual counselor
31. Note those referrals made here with the name of the contact person.

HOME HEALTH

1. Monitor for factors contributing to impaired adjustment (e.g., psychologic, social, economic, spiritual, environmental, etc.).
2. Involve patient and family in planning, implementing, and promoting reduction or elimination of impaired adjustment:
    a. Family conference
    b. Mutual goal sharing
    c. Communication
    d. Support for caregiver

    e. Problem solving
3. Assist patient and family in life-style adjustments that may be required:
    a. Stress management
    b. Development and use of support networks
    c. Treatment for disability
    d. Appropriate balance of dependence and independence
    e. Grief counseling
    f. Change in role functions
    g. Treatment for cognitive impairment
    h. Provision of comfortable and safe environment
    i. Activities to increase self-esteem
4. Consult with or refer to appropriate assistive resources as indicated:
    a. Psychiatric nurse clinician
    b. Mental health center
    c. Stress management training
    d. Financial counselor
    e. Physician
    f. Social services
    g. Family counselor
    h. Support groups
    i. Occupational therapist

EVALUATION
OBJECTIVE 1

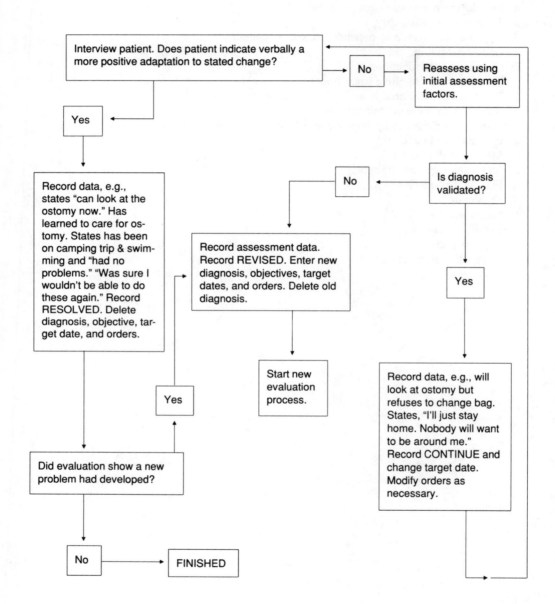

OBJECTIVE 2

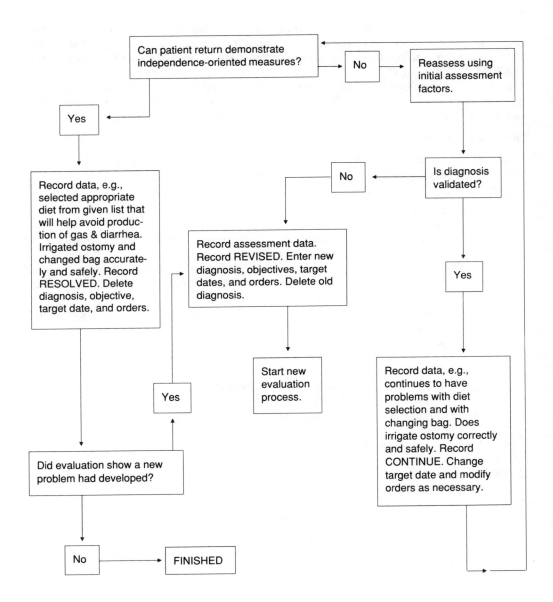

Family Coping, Ineffective: Compromised and Disabling

DEFINITION

Compromised: Insufficient, ineffective, or compromised support, comfort, assistance, or encouragement usually by a supportive primary person (family member or close friend); client may need it to manage or master adaptive tasks related to his or her health challenge (NANDA, 1987, p. 76).

Disabling: Behavior of significant person (family member or other primary person) that disables his or her own capacities and the client's capacities to effectively address tasks essential to either person's adaptation to the health challenge (NANDA, 1987, p. 74).

DEFINING CHARACTERISTICS (NANDA, 1987, pp. 74,76)

The nurse will review the initial pattern assessment for the following defining characteristics to determine the diagnosis of Family Coping, Ineffective.

1. Compromised
   a. Major defining characteristics
      (1) Subjective
         (a) Client expresses or confirms a concern or complaint about significant other's response to his or her health problem.
         (b) Significant person describes preoccupation with personal reactions (e.g., fear, guilt, anticipatory grief, anxiety) to client's illness or disability or to other situational or developmental crises.
         (c) Significant person describes or confirms inadequate understanding or knowledge base which interferes with effective assistive or supportive behavior.
      (2) Objective
         (a) Significant person attempts assistive or supportive behavior with less than satisfactory results.
         (b) Significant person withdraws or enters into limited or temporary personal communication with the client at the time of need.
         (c) Significant person displays protective behavior disproportionate (too little or too much) to the client's abilities or need for autonomy.
   b. Minor defining characteristics
      None given.
2. Disabling
   a. Major defining characteristics
      (1) Neglectful care of the client in regard to basic human needs or illness treatment
      (2) Distortion of reality regarding the client's health problem, including extreme denial about its existence or severity
      (3) Intolerance
      (4) Rejection
      (5) Abandonment
      (6) Desertion
      (7) Carrying on usual routines, disregarding client's needs
      (8) Psychosomaticism
      (9) Taking on illness signs of client
      (10) Decisions and actions by family which are detrimental to economic or social well-being
      (11) Agitation, depression, aggression, hostility
      (12) Impaired restructuring of a meaningful life for self, impaired individualization, prolonged overconcern for client

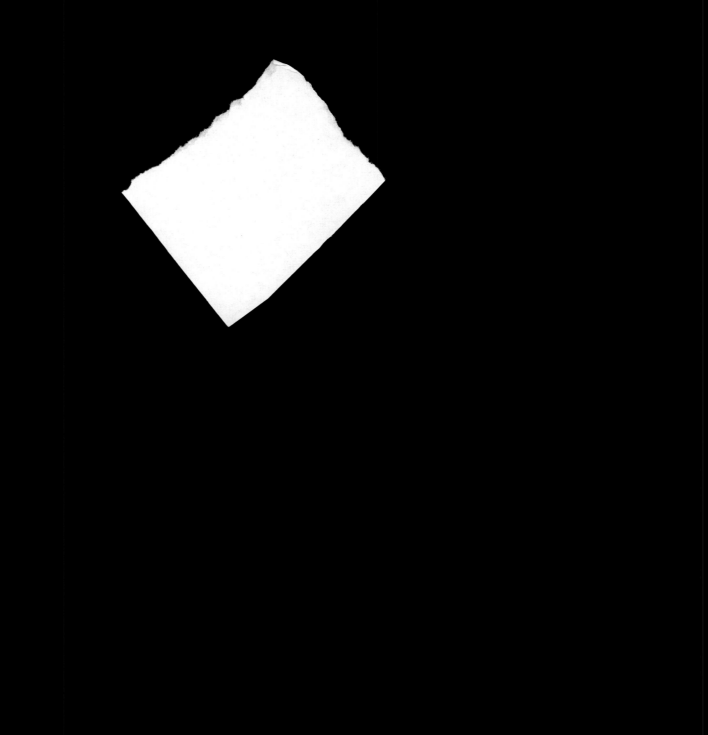

(13) Neglectful relationships with other family members

(14) Client's development of helpless, inactive dependence

  b. Minor defining characteristics

  None given.

RELATED FACTORS (NANDA, 1987, pp. 74,75,77)

1. Compromised
   a. Inadequate or incorrect information or understanding by a primary person
   b. Temporary preoccupation by a significant person who is trying to manage emotional conflicts and personal suffering and is unable to perceive or act effectively in regard to client's needs
   c. Temporary family disorganization and role changes
   d. Other situational or developmental crises or situations the significant person may be facing
   e. Little support provided by client, in turn, for primary person
   f. Prolonged disease or disability progression that exhausts supportive capacity of significant people
2. Disabling
   a. Significant person with chronically expressed feelings of guilt, anxiety, hostility, despair, etc.
   b. Dissonant discrepancy of coping styles for dealing with adaptive tasks by the significant person and client or among significant people
   c. Highly ambivalent family relationships
   d. Arbitrary handling of family's resistance to treatment, which tends to solidify defensiveness as it fails to deal adequately with underlying anxiety

DIFFERENTIATION

This diagnosis should be differentiated from Family Process, Altered; Family Coping, Potential for Growth; and Parenting, Altered. One should also differentiate between compromised and disabling dysfunction.

Compromised dysfunction reflects the family that cannot provide appropriate support to the identified patient. This problem removes a possible support system from the client. If the family dysfunction results in the dysfunction of the identified patient, then the diagnosis is Disabling. Because this diagnosis is used to describe family processes it may be difficult at times to differentiate between compromised and disabling because there is not an identified patient or the effects of the family patterns on the client cannot be determined. When this is the situation, the diagnosis can be made as Family Coping, Ineffective.

Family Coping, Potential for Growth is appropriate for families that are coping well with current stressors and are in a position to enhance their coping abilities. Family Coping, Ineffective describes a family that has a deficit in coping abilities that threatens the family's existence.

Parenting, Altered refers to an inability to fulfill the parenting role. This dysfunction is circumscribed and time-limited when contrasted with Family Coping, Ineffective.

OBJECTIVES

1. Will initiate a plan to cope with (the identified stressor) by (date).

AND/OR

2. Will identify the effects current coping strategies have on the family by (date).

TARGET DATE

The target dates should reflect the complexity and power of the system. Four-week intervals would be appropriate to assess for progress.

NURSING ORDERS

ADULT HEALTH

1. Encourage and assist family and significant others to verbalize their needs, fears, feelings, and concerns.
2. Provide accurate information about the situation.
3. Include family and significant others in decision making and plan of care.
4. Assist family and significant others to identify and explore alternatives to dealing with the situation.
5. Assist family and significant others to identify sources of community support that could assist them to cope with their feelings and to supply relief when needed.
6. Encourage family to provide time for themselves.
7. Initiate referral to psychiatric clinical nurse specialist as needed.

CHILD HEALTH

1. Encourage child and family to express feelings and fears by allotting 30 minutes per shift for this purpose.
2. Review family dynamics previous to crisis.
3. Encourage family members to participate in child's care, including bathing, feeding, comfort, and diversional activity.
4. Provide education to all family members regarding child's illness, prognosis, and special needs as appropriate.
5. Involve health team members in collaboration for care to include:
   a. Pediatrician
   b. Pediatric subspecialist
   c. Clinical nurse specialist
   d. Psychologist
   e. Psychiatrist
   f. Occupational therapist
   g. Physical therapist
   h. Social worker
   i. Family therapist
   j. Play therapist
   k. Child protective services
   l. Legal counsel
   m. Community health nurse
   n. Clergy
6. Provide referral to appropriate community resources for support purposes (e.g., State Crippled Children).
7. Provide for home discharge planning at least 5 days prior to discharge.
8. Make referral for home health care as needed.

MENTAL HEALTH

1. Role model effective communication by:
   a. Seeking clarification;
   b. Demonstrating respect for individual family members and the family system;
   c. Listening to expression of thoughts and feelings;
   d. Setting clear limits;
   e. Being consistent;
   f. Communicating with the individual being addressed in a clear manner;
   g. Encouraging sharing of information among appropriate system subgroups.
2. Demonstrate an understanding of the complexity of system problems by:

   a. Not taking sides in family disagreements;
   b. Providing alternative explanations of behavior patterns that recognize the contributions of all persons involved in the problem, including health care providers if appropriate;
   c. Requesting the perspective of multiple family members on a problem or stressor.
3. Determine risk for physical harm and refer to appropriate authorities if risk is high (child protective services, battered women's centers, police).
4. Assist family in developing behavioral short-term goals by:
   a. Asking what changes they would expect to see when the problem is improved;
   b. Having them break the problem into several parts that combine to form the identified stressor or crisis;
   c. Setting a time limit of 1 week to accomplish a task (e.g., ''What could you do this week to improve the current situation?'').
5. Develop with family a priority list.
6. Begin work with the presenting problem and enlist the system's assistance in resolving concerns.
7. Include assessment data in determining how to work on the presenting problem (e.g., if behavioral controls for a child are requested, the nurse can develop a plan for teaching and implementing them in the home that includes both parents).
8. Encourage communication between family members by:
   a. Having family members discuss alternatives to the problem in the presence of the nurse;
   b. Having each family member indicate how he or she might help resolve the problem;
   c. Having each family member indicate how he or she contributes to the maintenance of the problem or how he or she does not help the identified patient change behavior;
   d. Spending time having the family members give each other positive feedback.
9. Support the development of appropriate subgroups by:
   a. Presenting problems to the appropriate subsystems for discussion (e.g., if the problem involves a discussion of how the sexual functioning of the marital couple will change as a result of illness, this issue should be discussed with the husband and wife);
   b. Providing an opportunity for the children to discuss their concerns with their parents;
   c. Supporting appropriate generational boundaries (e.g., parent's attempts to exclude children from parental roles).
10. Develop direct interventions that instruct a family to do something different or not to do something (if direct interventions are not successful and reassessment indicates they were presented appropriately, this may indicate the family system is having unusual problems with the change process and should be referred to an advanced practitioner for further care).
11. Provide experiences for the family to learn how they can think differently about the problem (e.g., a job loss can be seen as an opportunity to reevaluate family goals, focus on interpersonal closeness, and enhance family problem-solving skills).
12. Provide opportunities for the expression of a range of affect; this can mean laughing and crying together. This validates family members' emotions and helps them to identify the appropriateness of their affective responses. This may require that the nurse ''push'' the family to express feelings with the skills of confrontation or providing feedback (Kneisl & Wilson, 1984; Wright & Leahey, 1984).
13. Develop a teaching plan to provide the family with information that will enhance their problem solving.
14. Assist family with interactions with other systems by:
   a. Providing information about the system;
   b. Maintaining open communication between nurse and other agencies or systems;
   c. Having family identify what their relationship is with the system and how they could best achieve the goals they have for their interactions with this system.
15. Provide constructive confrontation to the family about problematic coping behavior (see Kneisl

& Wilson, 1984, for guidelines on constructive confrontation). Those kinds of behavior identified by the treatment team as problematic should be listed here.

16. Teach family methods to reduce anxiety and practice and discuss the use of these methods with the family (number) times per week. (This should be done at least once a week until family members are using this as a coping method.) This could include deep muscle relaxation, physical exercise, family games that require physical activity, cycling, etc. (Those methods selected by the family should be listed here with the time schedule for implementation.) The family should be given "homework" related to the practice of these techniques at home on a daily basis.

17. Provide family with the information about proper nutrition that was indicated as missing on the assessment. This should include time spent on discussing how proper nutrition can fit the family life-style. (This teaching plan should be listed here.) A "homework" assignment related to the necessary pattern change should be given. This should involve all of the family members. Make an assignment that has high potential for successful completion by the family.

18. If a homework assignment is not completed do not chastise the family. Indicate that the nurse misjudged the complexity of the task and assess what made it difficult for the family to complete the task. Develop a new, less complex task based on this information. If a family continues not to complete tasks they may need to be referred to an advanced practitioner for continued care.

19. Monitor family's desire for spiritual counseling and refer to appropriate resources. The name of the resource person should be listed here.

20. Assist family in identifying support systems and in developing a plan for their use. This plan should be recorded here.

21. Refer family to community resources as necessary for continued support. These could include:
    a. Visiting nurse
    b. Psychiatric nurse clinician
    c. Physician
    d. Family therapist
    e. Physical therapist
    f. Nutritionist
    g. Social services
    h. Financial counselor
    i. Specific illness-related support groups

WOMEN'S HEALTH

Single Mothers

1. Review the physical, mental, social, and economic status of the single mother, taking into account if she is:
   a. Widowed;
   b. Divorced;
   c. Single and a parent by choice;
   d. Single and a parent not by choice.

2. Identify support system available to the single mother.
   a. Family
   b. Nonfamily
      (1) Friends
      (2) People at place of employment
      (3) Formal support systems

3. Identify social system available to the single mother.
   a. Social contacts other than friends or family
      (1) Church

    (2) Community organizations

    (3) Professional organizations

    (4) Support groups

4. Review client's perception of employment status
   a. Educational level and skills
   b. Job opportunities or none
   c. Opportunity for improvement or none
5. Identify child care requirements
   a. Age of children
   b. Custody of children
   c. Child support
      (1) Financial
      (2) Emotional
6. Suggest strategies for exposing children to male role models (Griffith-Kenney, 1986, p. 319).
   a. Assign to classes with male teachers
   b. Assistance from brothers or grandparents
   c. Involve children in sports (coaches usually are male)

HOME HEALTH

1. Involve patient and family in planning and implementing strategies to improve family coping:
   a. Crisis management
   b. Mutual goal setting
   c. Communication
   d. Family conference
   e. Problem solving
2. Assist family and patient in life-style adjustments that may be required.
   a. Stress management
   b. Altering past ineffective coping strategies
   c. Treatment for substance abuse
   d. Treatment for physical illness
   e. Appropriate use of denial
   f. Avoiding scapegoating
   g. Activities of daily family living
   h. Financial concerns
   i. Change in geographic or sociocultural location
   j. Potential for violence
   k. Identify family strengths
   l. Obtain temporary assistance: housekeeper, sitter, temporary placement outside home, etc.
   m. Development and use of support networks
3. Consult with and refer to assistive resources as appropriate
   a. Psychiatric nurse clinician
   b. Physician
   c. Marriage and family therapy
   d. Women's protective service
   e. Child protective service
   f. Social service
   g. Financial counselor
   h. Community support networks (e.g., church, welcome wagon, volunteer groups)

EVALUATION
OBJECTIVE 1

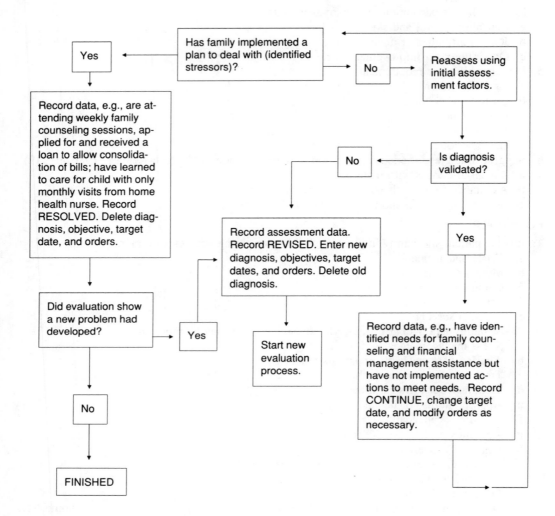

OBJECTIVE 2

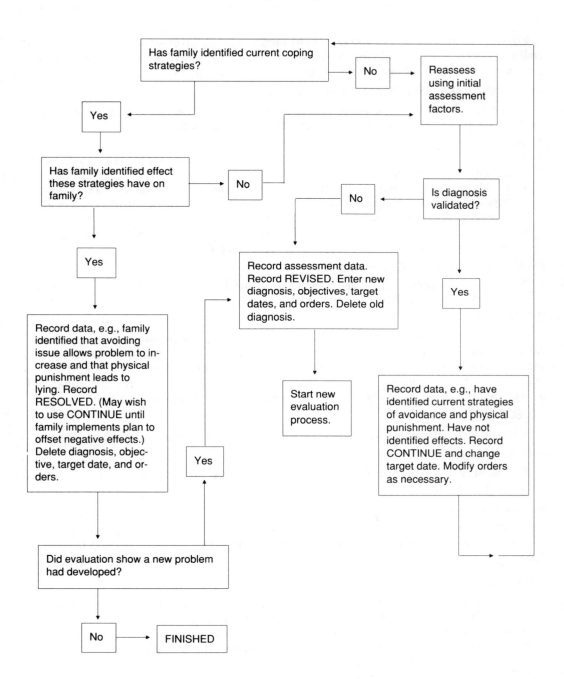

Family Coping, Potential for Growth

DEFINITION

Effective management of adaptive tasks by family member involved with the client's health challenge, who now is exhibiting desire and readiness for enhanced health and growth in regard to self and in relation to the client (NANDA, 1987, p. 78).

DEFINING CHARACTERISTICS (NANDA, 1987, p. 78)

The nurse will review the initial pattern assessment for the following defining characteristics to determine the diagnosis of Family Coping, Potential for Growth.

1. Major defining characteristics
   a. Family member attempting to describe growth impact of crisis on his or her own values, priorities, goals, or relationships.
   b. Family member moving in direction of health-promoting and enriching life-style which supports and monitors maturational processes, audits and negotiates treatment program, and generally chooses experiences which optimize wellness.
   c. Individual expressing interest in making contact on a one-to-one basis or on a mutual-aid group basis with another person who has experienced a similar situation.

RELATED FACTORS (NANDA, 1987, p. 78)

1. Needs are sufficiently gratified and adaptive tasks are effectively addressed to enable goals of self-actualization to surface.

DIFFERENTIATION

This diagnosis should be differentiated from Family Coping, Ineffective and Family Process, Altered. Family Coping, Potential for Growth addresses the family that is currently handling stresses well and that is in a position to enhance their coping abilities. The other nursing diagnoses related to family functioning address various aspects of family dysfunction. If any dysfunction is present Family Coping, Potential for Growth would not be the diagnosis of choice.

OBJECTIVES

1. Will verbalize satisfaction with current progress toward family goals by (date).

AND/OR

2. Will identify at least (number) community groups that can provide family with useful input and output by (date).

TARGET DATE

Depending on the family size and the commitment of each member toward growth, the target date could range from weeks to months. A reasonable initial target date would be 2 weeks.

NURSING ORDERS

ADULT HEALTH

1. Provide opportunities for family and significant others to discuss patient's condition and treatment modalities by scheduling at least one family session every other day.
2. Include family and significant others in planning and providing care.
3. Provide instruction as needed in supportive and assistive behavior for patient.
4. Answer questions clearly and honestly.
5. Refer family and significant others to support groups and resources as indicated.

CHILD HEALTH

1. Identify how the child views the current crisis.
2. Identify family coping patterns.

3. Identify child's previous coping patterns.
4. Identify current coping strategies for child and family.
5. Assist child in identifying ways the current crisis or situation can enhance his or her coping for future needs.
6. Identify appropriate health members who can assist in providing support for growth potential:
   a. Pediatrician
   b. Subspecialists
   c. Clinical nurse specialist
   d. Psychologist
   e. Psychiatrist
   f. Clergyman
   g. Social worker
   h. Legal counsel
   i. Occupational therapist
   j. Physical therapist
   k. Community health nurse
7. Offer educational instruction to meet patient's and family's needs related to health care.
8. Provide referral to groups for support within the community.
9. Allow for sufficient time while in hospital to reinforce necessary skills for care, such as range of motion exercises.
10. Make appropriate referrals for home health care as needed.

WOMEN'S HEALTH

1. Encourage participation of significant others in preparation for birth.
   a. Spouse
   b. Boyfriend
   c. Partner
   d. Children
   e. In-laws
   f. Grandparents
   g. Others that are important to the individual
2. Discuss childbirth and the changes that will occur in the family unit.
3. Encourage woman and partner (significant other) to attend childbirth education classes or parenting classes in preparation for the birthing experience.
4. Encourage client to list family life-style adjustments that need to be made.
5. Involve significant others in discussion and problem solving activities regarding family adjustments to the newborn.
6. Encourage client to consider how she will manage a newborn and working.
7. Encourage expectant couple to explore child care before it is needed.
8. Assist client in setting goals for herself and the family related to:
   a. Child care
   b. Working
   c. Household responsibilities
   d. Social network
   e. Support groups

MENTAL HEALTH

1. Talk with family to identify their goals and concerns.
2. Assist family in identifying strengths.
3. Refer family to appropriate community support groups. These could include:
   a. Alcoholics Anonymous

   b. AlAnon
   c. Support groups for families with cancer
   d. Support groups for parents who have lost a child
   e. Parents Without Partners
   f. Mother's Day Out programs
   g. Community centers that have support groups for families with small children
   h. Parenting classes
   i. Couples communication or marriage enrichment programs
 4. Teach family those skills necessary to provide care to an ill member.
 5. Talk with family about the role flexibility necessary to cope with an ill member and how this may be affecting their family.
 6. Provide family with information about normal developmental stages and anticipatory guidance related to these stages.
 7. Discuss with family normal adaptive responses to an ill family member and relate this to their current functioning.
 8. Support appropriate family boundaries by providing information to the appropriate family subgroup.
 9. Model effective communication skills for family by using active listening skills, "I" messages, problem solving skills, and open communication without secrets.
10. Spend 1 hour with family on a weekly basis providing them with the opportunity to practice communication skills and to share feelings (if this is an identified goal).
11. Arrange 1-hour appointments with client weekly for 1 month to assess progress on the established goals. The need for continued follow-up can be decided at the end of the last scheduled visit.
12. Accept family's decisions about goals for care.
13. Discuss with family the role nutrition has in health maintenance and develop a family nutritional plan. Consult with nutritionist as necessary.
14. Discuss with family the role exercise has in improving ability to cope with stress and assist in the development of a family exercise plan. Consult with physical therapist as necessary.
15. Refer family to community resources as necessary for continued support. These could include:
   a. Visiting nurse
   b. Physician
   c. Psychiatric nurse clinician
   d. Family therapist
   e. Physical therapist
   f. Nutritionist
   g. Social services
   h. Financial counselor

HOME HEALTH

1. Involve patient and family in planning and implementing strategies to enhance health and growth:
   a. Family conference
   b. Mutual goal setting
   c. Communication
   d. Education
2. Assist family and patient in life-style adjustments that may be required:
   a. Provide information related to health promotion.
   b. Provide information related to expected growth and development milestones, both individual and family.
   c. Assist in development and use of support networks.

3. Consult with and refer to assistive resources as appropriate.
    a. Community resources (e.g., colleges and universities, extension service, recreation facilities, parks and recreation)
    b. Cooking classes
    c. Marriage enrichment
    d. Volunteer agencies such as Lion's Club, Altrusa, etc.

EVALUATION
OBJECTIVE 1

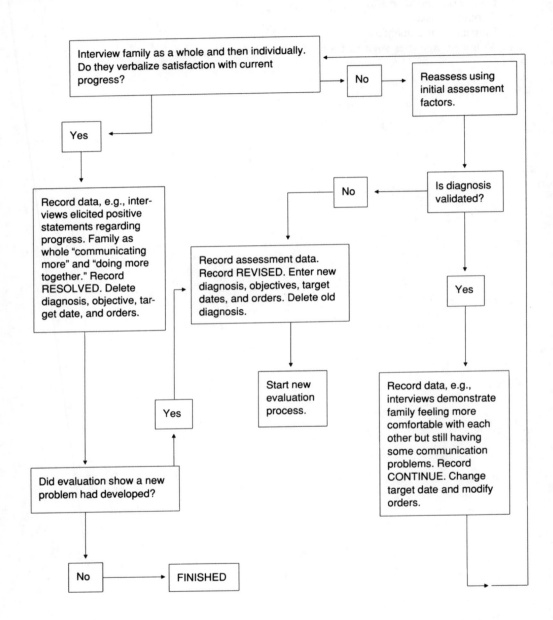

Interview family as a whole and then individually. Do they verbalize satisfaction with current progress?

No → Reassess using initial assessment factors.

Yes

Record data, e.g., interviews elicited positive statements regarding progress. Family as whole "communicating more" and "doing more together." Record RESOLVED. Delete diagnosis, objective, target date, and orders.

No ← Is diagnosis validated?

Record assessment data. Record REVISED. Enter new diagnosis, objectives, target dates, and orders. Delete old diagnosis.

Yes

Start new evaluation process.

Yes

Record data, e.g., interviews demonstrate family feeling more comfortable with each other but still having some communication problems. Record CONTINUE. Change target date and modify orders.

Did evaluation show a new problem had developed?

No → FINISHED

OBJECTIVE 2

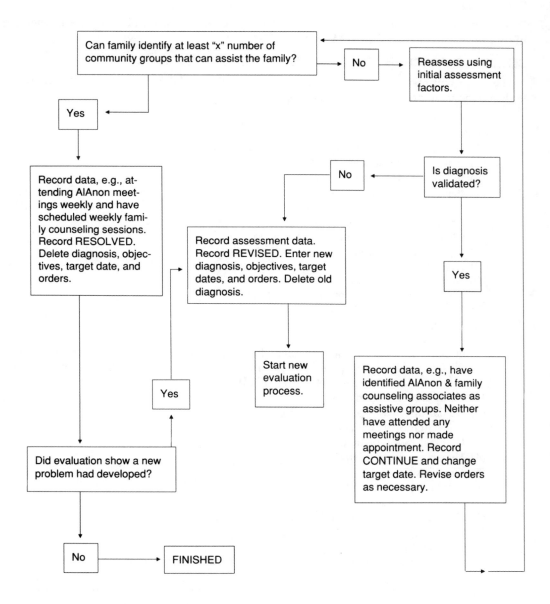

Individual Coping, Ineffective

DEFINITION

Impairment of adaptive behavior and problem-solving abilities of a person in meeting life's demands and roles (NANDA, 1987, p. 71).

DEFINING CHARACTERISTICS (NANDA, 1987, p. 71)

The nurse will review the initial pattern assessment for the following defining characteristics to determine the diagnosis of Individual Coping, Ineffective.

1. Ineffective Individual Coping
   a. Major defining characteristics
      (1) Verbalization of inability to cope or inability to ask for help
      (2) Inability to meet role expectations
      (3) Inability to meet basic needs
      (4) Inability to solve problems
      (5) Alteration in societal participation
      (6) Inappropriate use of defense mechanisms
      (7) Change in usual communication patterns
      (8) Verbal manipulation
      (9) High illness rate
      (10) High rate of accidents
      (11) Destructive behavior toward self and others
   b. Minor defining characteristics
      None given.
2. Defensive Coping
   a. Definition: The state in which an individual repeatedly projects falsely positive self-evaluation based on a self-protective pattern which defends against underlying perceived threats to positive self-regard (NANDA, 1988).
   b. Major defining characteristics
      (1) Denial of obvious problems and weaknesses
      (2) Projection of blame and responsibility
      (3) Rationalization of failures
      (4) Hypersensitivity to slight or criticism
      (5) Grandiosity
   c. Minor defining characteristics
      (1) Superior attitude toward others
      (2) Difficulty establishing and maintaining relationships
      (3) Hostile laughter or ridicule of others
      (4) Difficulty in reality-testing perception
      (5) Lack of follow-through or participation in treatment or therapy
3. Ineffective Denial
   a. Definition: The state of a conscious or unconscious attempt to disavow the knowledge or meaning of an event to reduce anxiety or fear to the detriment of health (NANDA, 1988).
   b. Major defining characteristics
      (1) Delays seeking or refuses health care attention to the detriment of health
      (2) Does not perceive personal relevance of symptoms or danger
   c. Minor defining characteristics
      (1) Uses home remedies (self-treatment) to relieve symptoms
      (2) Does not admit fear of death or invalidism
      (3) Minimizes symptoms

(4) Displaces source of symptoms to other organs
(5) Unable to admit impact of disease on life pattern
(6) Makes dismissive gestures or comments when speaking of distressing events
(7) Displaces fear of impact of the condition
(8) Displays inappropriate affect

RELATED FACTORS (NANDA, 1987, p. 71)

1. Situational crises
2. Maturational crisis
3. Personal vulnerability

DIFFERENTIATION

Individual Coping, Ineffective should be differentiated from Powerlessness; Violence, Potential for; Self-Concept, Disturbance in; Sensory-Perceptual Alteration; Spiritual Distress; Thought Process, Altered; Grieving, Dysfunctional; and Anxiety (Kelley, 1985, p. 209).

Anxiety is often the primary diagnosis. Individual Coping, Ineffective would be used if the client demonstrates an inability to cope appropriately with the anxiety in an appropriate amount of time. If the client is demonstrating anxiety with appropriate coping, then the diagnosis would be Anxiety. Individual Coping, Ineffective would only be used if the client could not adapt to the anxiety.

Violence, Potential for would be the appropriate diagnosis if the aggressive behavior of the client poses the threat of physical or psychologic harm. This would be the primary diagnosis if the risk of harm was high. If the client's risk for violence is assessed to be very low, then this would be the secondary diagnosis with Individual Coping, Ineffective being the primary diagnosis. In this situation the diagnosis of Violence, Potential for would serve as a reminder to care providers of the potential for this behavior.

Self-Concept, Disturbance in is the appropriate primary diagnosis if the client is experiencing a disturbance in self-perception, including body image, self-esteem, or personal identity. If adaptation to the disturbance is impaired because of the client's lack of adaptive behavior or problem solving skills, the diagnosis would be Individual Coping, Ineffective.

Sensory-Perceptual Alteration is the disruption of sensory stimuli recognition or interpretation. If coping abilities are affected by alterations in sensory input, then Sensory-Perceptual Alteration would be the appropriate primary diagnosis.

Spiritual Distress is a disturbance in the client's belief or value system. If the client indicates an inability to cope with this disruption, then the appropriate diagnosis would be Individual Coping, Ineffective.

Thought Process, Altered can effect the individual's ability to cope and if these alterations are present with ineffective individual coping, then the primary diagnosis should be Thought Process, Altered. Effective problem solving is inhibited as long as this disruption in thinking is present.

Grieving, Dysfunctional is the appropriate diagnosis if the client's behavior is related to resolving a loss or change. The loss can be actual or perceived. If the client demonstrates an inability to manage this process, then the appropriate diagnosis would be Individual Coping, Ineffective.

Powerlessness can produce a personal perception that would result in Individual Coping, Ineffective. If one perceives that one's own actions cannot influence the situation, then Powerlessness would the primary diagnosis.

OBJECTIVES

1. Will describe implementation of a plan to cope with the identified stressors by (date).

AND/OR

2. Will return demonstrate at least (number) new coping strategies by (date).

TARGET DATE

A realistic target date, considering assessment and teaching time, would be 7 days from the date of diagnosis.

NURSING ORDERS

ADULT HEALTH

1. Assist patient to identify and explore specific situations that are creating stress and possible alternatives for dealing with the situation by allowing at least 1 hour per shift for interviewing and teaching.
2. Help the patient to evaluate which methods he or she has used which either have not been successful or have been only partially successful.
3. Maintain consistency in approach and teaching.
4. Encourage participation in care.
5. Encourage support from family and significant others.
6. Initiate referral to psychiatric clinical nurse specialist as needed.
7. Provide diversional activities.
8. Assist patient to maintain activities of daily living to degree possible.
9. Assist patient to identify and use available support systems.
10. Monitor for and reinforce behavior suggesting effective coping.

CHILD HEALTH

1. Establish a trusting relationship with the child and respective family by allowing time (30 minutes) per shift for verbalization of concerns.
2. Identify need for collaboration with related health team members to include:
   a. Pediatrician
   b. Clinical nurse specialist
   c. Psychiatrist
   d. Psychologist
   e. Social worker
   f. Play therapist
   g. Family therapist
   h. School teacher
   i. Occupational therapist
   j. Physical therapist
3. Encourage patient and family to verbalize feelings and perception of situation.
4. Reinforce appropriate behavior of choosing or coping by verbal praise.
5. Assist the patient and family in setting realistic goals.
6. Provide appropriate attention to primary nursing needs.
7. Offer education to provide clarification of information as needed regarding any health-related needs.
8. Determine appropriate developmental baseline behavior versus actual coping behavior.
9. Once contributing factors and usual adaptive coping behavior are determined, begin to formulate individualized plan of care directed at reestablishing usual coping as possible according to situation.
10. Administer medications as ordered, including sedatives.
11. Set aside time each shift (specify) to deal with how child and parents feel about the defensive behavior. This may require art, puppetry, or related expressive dynamics.
12. Provide feedback with support for progress. When progress is not occurring, provide reflective referral back to child and parent as applicable.
13. Provide ongoing information regarding child's health status which could affect defensive behavior by child or parents.

14. Allow for misperceptions by staff, child, and family and make attempts to clarify any mis-communication or misperception.
15. Throughout defensive coping period, monitor and ensure child's safety.
16. Determine disciplinary plans for all to abide by with safety in mind.
17. Provide appropriate reality confrontation according to readiness of child and parents.
18. Provide for discharge planning with reinforcement of value of follow-up appointments as needed.
19. Identify, along with patient and family, resources to assist in coping, including support groups.
20. Provide for home care upon return to home setting as needed.

WOMEN'S HEALTH

1. Identify groups at high risk for ineffective individual coping.
   a. Women
   b. Single women
   c. Single parents (female)
   d. Minority women
   e. Women with the superwoman syndrome
   f. Lesbians
2. Identify situations which place client at high risk for ineffective individual coping.
   a. Unwanted or unplanned pregnancy
   b. Unhappy home situation (marriage)
   c. Demands at work
   d. Demands of children or spouse
3. Assist client in identifying typical stressors:
   a. At home
   b. At work
   c. Socially
   d. During an average day
4. Assist client in identifying life-style adjustments that may be made to lower stress levels.
5. Assist client in identifying factors which contribute to ineffective coping.
   a. Depression
   b. Guilt (blaming self)
   c. Assuming helplessness
   d. Passive acceptance of traditional feminine role
   e. Anger toward self and others
      (1) Aggressive behavior
      (2) Suicide
      (3) Substance abuse
         (a) Drugs
         (b) Alcohol
         (c) Food
            (i)   Anorexia
            (ii) Bulimia
            (iii) Obesity
   f. Failure to make time for self
      (1) Relaxation
      (2) Pleasure
      (3) Nurture
      (4) Self-care
6. Assist client in developing problem-solving skills to modify stressors.
7. Assist client in identifying negative and positive responses to stressors.

8. Assist client in developing an individual plan of stress management.
   a. Relaxation techniques
   b. Assertiveness training
   c. Support groups
   d. Individual self-care
9. Involve significant others in discussion and problem solving activities.
10. Provide a nonjudgmental atmosphere that allows the client to discuss her feelings about the pregnancy, including such areas as:
    a. Their life-style
    b. Children
    c. Their support systems
11. Explore client's use of what she perceives are contraceptives.
    a. Method
       (1) Pills
       (2) Mechanical devices
       (3) Diaphragm
       (4) Withdrawal
       (5) Feminine hygiene products
       (6) Douching
       (7) Foaming (spermicides)
       (8) Rhythm
12. Explore client's lack of contraceptive use due to:
    a. Ignorance
    b. "It won't happen to me" syndrome
    c. Guilt—"If I use the pill then I am not good"
    d. Spontaneity
    e. Excitement due to risk
    f. Loneliness
    g. Crisis or pressure
    h. Uncertainty in sex role relationships
    i. Self-image

MENTAL HEALTH

1. Determine client's functional abilities and developmental level for the adaptation of all future interventions (the results of this assessment should be noted here).
2. Discuss with client his or her perception of the current crisis and stressors. This should include information about the coping strategies that the client has attempted and his or her assessment of what has made them ineffective in resolving this stressor or crisis.
3. Assist client in developing an appropriate time frame for the resolution of the situation. (Often when experiencing a crisis the individual has the perception that resolution must take place immediately.) This could include, as appropriate to the client's situation:
   a. Informing client that any difficulty that has taxed his or her resources as much as this one has will take an extended time to resolve because it must be complex;
   b. That a situation that is as important as this one is to the individual's future deserves a well-thought-out answer and that a decision should not be made hastily;
   c. Assisting client in determining the source of the time pressure and the appropriateness of this time frame;
   d. Assisting client in developing an appropriate perspective on the time frame. One question that could be useful: "What would be the worst that could happen if this problem is not resolved by (client's time frame here)?
4. Provide a quiet, nonstimulating environment or an environment that does not add additional

stress to an already overwhelmed coping ability (potential environmental stressors for this client should be listed here with the plan for reducing them in this environment).

5. Sit with client (number) minutes (number) time per day at (specific times listed) to discuss current concerns and feelings.

6. Assist client with setting appropriate limits on aggressive behavior by (see Violence, Potential For Chapter 9, for detailed care plan if this is an appropriate diagnosis):
   a. Decreasing environmental stimulation as appropriate (this might include a secluded environment);
   b. Providing client with appropriate alternative outlets for physical tension (this should be stated specifically and could include walking, running, talking with a staff member, using a punching bag, listening to music, or doing a deep muscle relaxation sequence) (number) times per day (state specific times) or when increased tension is observed. These outlets should be selected with the client's input.

7. Orient client to date, time, and place. Provide clocks, calendars, bulletin boards. Make references to this information in daily interactions with the client. The frequency needed for this client should be noted here (e.g., every 2 hours, every day, three times a day).

8. Provide client with familiar or needed objects. These should be noted here.

9. Provide client with an environment that will optimize sensory input. This could include hearing aids, eyeglasses, pencil and paper, decreased noise in conversation areas, appropriate lighting (these interventions should indicate an awareness of sensory deficit as well as sensory overload, the specific interventions for this client should be noted here, e.g., place hearing aid in when client awakens and remove before bedtime [9:00 PM.]).

10. Provide client with achievable tasks, activities, and goals (these should be listed here). These activities should be provided with increasing complexity to give client an increasing sense of accomplishment and mastery.

11. Communicate to client an understanding that all coping behavior to this point has been his or her best effort and asking for assistance at this time is not failure; a complex problem often requires some outside assistance in resolution (this will assist client to maintain self-esteem and diminish feelings of failure).

12. Provide client with opportunities to make appropriate decisions related to care at his or her level of ability. This may begin as a choice between two options and then evolve into more complex decision making. It is important that this be at the client's level of functioning so confidence can be built with successful decision making experiences.

13. Provide client with a primary care nurse on each shift.

14. When relationship has been developed with primary care nurse, this person will sit with client (minutes, begin with 30 and increase as client's ability to concentrate improves) per shift to discuss concerns about sexual issues, fears, and anxieties.

15. Provide constructive confrontation for client about problematic coping behavior (see Kneisl & Wilson, 1984 for guidelines on constructive confrontation). Those kinds of behavior identified by the treatment team as problematic should be listed here.

16. Provide client with information about care and treatment. Give information in concise terms appropriate to the client's level of understanding.

17. Identify with client methods for anxiety reduction. Those specific methods selected should be listed here.

18. Assist client with practice of anxiety reduction techniques and remind client to implement these techniques when level of anxiety is increasing.

19. Provide client with opportunities to test problem solutions either with role plays or by applying them to graded real life experiences.

20. Assist client to revise problem solutions if they are not effective (this will assist learning that no solution is perfect or final and problem solving is a process of applying various alternatives and revising them as necessary).

21. Allow client to discover and develop solutions that best fit his or her concerns. The nurse's role is to provide assistance and feedback and to encourage creative approaches to problem behavior.
22. Teach client skills that facilitate problem solving such as assertive behavior, goal setting, relaxation, evaluation, information gathering, requesting assistance, and early identification of problem behavior. Those skills that are identified by the treatment team as being necessary should be listed here with the teaching plan. This should include a schedule of the information to be provided and identification of the person responsible for providing the information.
23. Spend (number) minutes two times per day with client role playing and practicing problem solving and implementation of developed solutions. This will be the responsibility of the primary care nurse.
24. Assist client in identifying those problems he or she cannot control or resolve and in developing coping strategies for these situations. This may involve alteration of the client's perception of the problem.
25. Monitor client's desire for spiritual counseling and refer to appropriate resources.
26. Provide positive social reinforcement and other behavioral rewards for demonstration of adaptive problem solving. (Those things that the client finds rewarding should be listed here with a schedule for use. The kinds of behavior that are to be rewarded should also be listed).
27. Assist client in identifying support systems and in developing a plan for their use.
28. Refer to appropriate assistive resources as indicated, e.g.,
    a. Visiting nurse
    b. Nutritionist
    c. Social services
    d. Psychiatric nurse clinician
    e. Occupational therapist
    f. Physical therapist
29. The following interventions relate to the client who is experiencing problems related to organic brain dysfunction:
    a. Maintain a consistent environment; do not move furniture or personal belongings.
    b. Remove hazardous objects from the environment such as loose rugs or small items on the floor.
    c. Provide environmental cues to assist client in locating important places such as the bathroom, own room, or the dining room.
    d. Do not argue with client about details of recent past.
    e. Avoid situations that result in aggressive behavior by redirecting client's attention.
    f. Provide a constant daily routine and a homelike atmosphere, to include:
       (1) Personal belongings
       (2) Music
       (3) Social mealtimes with assistance with meal preparation; this can often provide appetite cues to the client and stimulate memories
    g. Provide group experiences that explore current events, seasonal changes, reminiscence, and organizing life experiences.
30. The following interventions relate to the client who is experiencing Defensive Coping.
    a. Approach client in a positive, nonjudgmental manner.
    b. Focus any feedback on client's behavior.
    c. Provide an opportunity for client to share his or her perspectives and feelings.
    d. Use "I" statements (e.g., I feel angry when I see you breaking the window).
    e. Develop a trusting relationship with the client before using confrontation or requesting major changes in behavior (see Haber, Hoskins, Leach, & Sideleau, 1987; or Stuart & Sundeen, 1987, for information on the development of a trusting relationship).

f. Provide positive reinforcement for client when issues are addressed (those things that are reinforcing for this client should be noted here).

g. When client's defenses increase, reduce anxiety in situation (see Anxiety, Chapter 8, for precise information on anxiety control).

h. Determine the kinds of behavior by staff members that increase client's defensive coping and note them here with a plan to decrease them.

i. Be clear and direct with client.

j. If defensive coping is related to alteration in self-concept refer to the appropriate nursing diagnosis for interventions.

k. Reduce or eliminate environmental stressors or threats.

l. Arrange time for client to be involved in activity that is enjoyed and provides client with positive emotional experiences. Note activity and time for this activity here.

31. The following interventions are for the client experiencing Denial.

a. Determine if current use of denial is appropriate in the current situation.

b. If denial is determined to be inappropriate, initiate the following interventions.

   (1) Provide a safe, secure environment.

   (2) Allow client time to express feelings.

   (3) Provide a positive, nonjudgmental environment.

   (4) Develop a trusting relationship with client before presenting threatening information.

   (5) Present information in a clear, concise manner.

   (6) Determine which kinds of staff behavior reinforce denial and note them here with alternative behavior.

   (7) Utilize "I" messages and reflect on client's behavior (see Kneisl & Wilson, 1984, for information on constructive confrontation).

   (8) Present client with information that demonstrates inconsistencies between thoughts and feelings, between thoughts and behavior and between thoughts about others and their perceptions of the situation.

   (9) Arrange for client to participate in a group that will provide feedback from peers regarding the stressful situation.

  (10) Present client with differences between his or her perceptions and the nurses' perceptions with "I" messages.

  (11) Do not agree with client's perceptions that are related to denial.

  (12) Schedule time for client and support system to discuss issues related to the current problem (note this time here with the name of the staff person responsible for this session).

  (13) Assist support system in learning constructive ways of coping with the client's denial.

  (14) Schedule time for client to be involved in positive esteem-building activity (this activity should be selected with client input). Note activity and schedule for this activity here.

  (15) Provide positive feedback for client addressing concerns in a direct manner (note those things that are rewarding for the client here).

  (16) Determine needs that are being met with denial. Establish and present client with alternative kinds of behavior for meeting these needs. Note alternatives here.

  (17) Refer client to appropriate support systems in the community.

HOME HEALTH

1. Involve patient and family in planning and implementing strategies to improve individual coping:

a. Family conference

b. Mutual goal setting

    c. Communication

    d. Problem solving

2. Assist family and patient in life-style adjustments that may be required:

    a. Stress management

    b. Development and use of support networks

    c. Alteration of past ineffective coping strategies

    d. Treatment for substance abuse

    e. Treatment for physical illness

    f. Activities to increase self-esteem: exercise, stress management

    g. Temporary assistance: babysitter, housekeeper, secretarial support, etc.

    h. Identification of signs and symptoms of illness.

    i. Recognition of hazards and benefits of home remedies, self-diagnosis, and self-prescribing.

3. Consult with and refer to assistive resources as appropriate:

    a. Psychiatric nurse clinician

    b. Physician

    c. Marriage and family therapist

    d. Support group

EVALUATION
OBJECTIVE 1

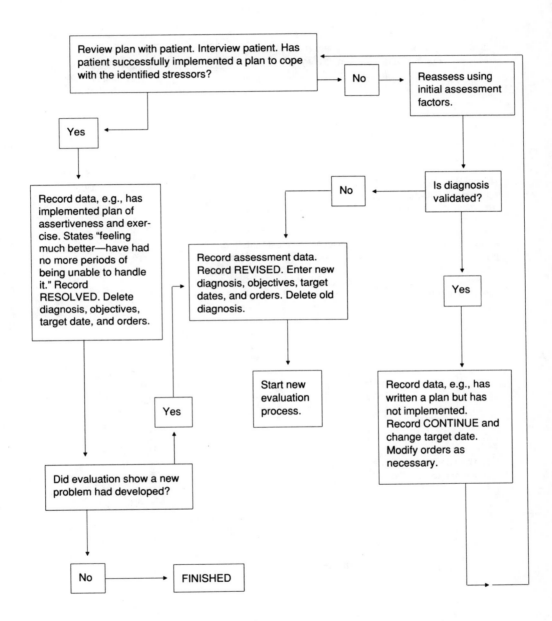

OBJECTIVE 2

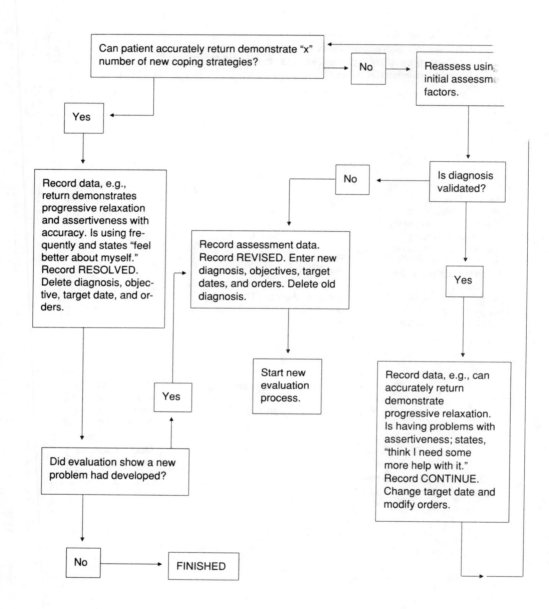

Post-Trauma Response

DEFINITION

The state of an individual experiencing a sustained painful response to an unexpected extraordinary life event (NANDA, 1987, p. 113).

DEFINING CHARACTERISTICS (NANDA, 1987, p. 13)

The nurse will review the initial pattern assessment for the following defining characteristics to determine the diagnosis of Post-Trauma Response.

1. Major defining characteristics
   a. Reexperience of the traumatic event which may be identified in cognitive, affective, or sensorimotor activities (flashbacks, intrusive thoughts, repetitive dreams or nightmares, excessive verbalization of survival guilt or guilt about behavior required for survival).
2. Minor defining characteristics
   a. Psychic or emotional numbness (impaired interpretation of reality, confusion, dissociation or amnesia, vagueness about traumatic event, constricted affect).
   b. Altered life-style (self-destructiveness, such as substances abuse, suicide attempt or other acting out behavior, difficulty with interpersonal relationships, development of phobia regarding trauma, poor impulse control or irritability, and explosiveness).

RELATED FACTORS (NANDA, 1987, p. 113)

1. Disasters
2. Wars
3. Epidemics
4. Rape
5. Assault
6. Torture
7. Catastrophic illness or accident

DIFFERENTIATION

Post-Trauma Response should be differentiated from Anxiety; Individual Coping, Ineffective; Disturbance in; Thought Process, Altered; Self Concept, Disturbance in; Grieving, Dysfunctional; Social Interaction, Impaired; and Rape Trauma Syndrome.

Anxiety may be the initial diagnosis given to the individual. As the relationship with the client progresses, it may become evident that the source of the anxiety is a traumatic event. If this is the case, then the diagnosis of Post-Trauma Response would be added to the diagnosis of anxiety. As long as the symptoms of Anxiety are predominant this would be the primary diagnosis.

The initial diagnosis that may be given to the individual would be Individual Coping, Ineffective. If, however, the symptoms are related to a response to an overwhelming traumatic event, then the diagnosis would be Post-Trauma Response. Individual Coping, Ineffective is used when the symptoms do not relate to the individual's having experienced an *overwhelming* traumatic event.

Some of the symptoms of Post-Trauma Response are similar to Self-Concept, Disturbance in. When the symptoms occur in an individual that has experienced a traumatic event the primary diagnosis would be Post-Trauma Response. When the individual has not experienced a trauma, then the primary diagnosis would be, Self-Concept Disturbance in.

Post-Trauma Response can produce symptoms similar to Thought Process, Altered. If these alterations are present in the client that has experienced a traumatic event, then the primary diagnosis would be Post-Trauma Response. If the disruption in thinking persists after intervention has begun for Post-Trauma Response, then Thought Process, Altered should be reconsidered as a diagnosis.

Grieving, Dysfunctional is the appropriate diagnosis if the client's behavior is related to resolving a loss or change and this loss or change is not the result of an *overwhelming* traumatic event. If it is the result of a traumatic event then the appropriate diagnosis would be Post-Trauma Response.

Social Interaction, Impaired would be the appropriate diagnosis if the client is demonstrating an inability to establish or maintain stable, supportive relationships and has not experienced an *overwhelming* traumatic event. If the client has experienced a traumatic event and is also demonstrating other symptoms related to Post-Trauma Response, then this would be the appropriate diagnosis.

Rape Trauma Synmrome is the appropriate diagnosis if the individual's symptoms are related to a rape. If the symptoms are related to another *overwhelming* traumatic event or if the rape occured in conjunction with another *overwhelming* traumatic event, then the appropriate diagnosis would be Post-Trauma Response.

OBJECTIVES

1. Will demonstrate return to pre-trauma behavior by (date).

AND/OR

2. Will report decrease in signs and symptoms of post-trauma response by (date).

TARGET DATE

Due to the highly individualized and personalized response to trauma, target dates will have to be highly individualized and based on initial assessment. A reasonable initial target date would be 7 days.

NURSING ORDERS

ADULT HEALTH

1. Establish a therapeutic relationship.
2. Encourage patient to express feelings about event.
3. Help patient to see the event realistically.
4. Help patient identify support groups that have previously experienced the same or similar traumatic event.
5. Initiate a psychiatric nursing consultation.
6. Help patient to identify diversional activities to activate when he or she feels he or she is going to reexperience the event.
7. Orient patient to reality.
8. Engage patient in social interactions with nurses or with other support groups.
9. Teach patient relaxation and stress management techniques.

CHILD HEALTH

1. Monitor for details surrounding the incident causing post-trauma response.
2. Allow for developmental needs in encouraging child to express feelings about trauma.
   a. Play for infants
   b. Puppets, dolls for toddlers
   c. Stories or play for preschoolers
3. Deal appropriately with other primary nursing needs.
4. Provide for one-on-one care and continuity as possible with staff to enhance trust.
5. Encourage patient and family to note positive outcomes of experience.
6. Review previous coping skills.
7. Address educational needs according to situation.
8. Allow for visitation by family and significant others.
9. Refer appropriately for continuity and follow-up after discharge from hospital.
10. Provide for diversional activity of child's choice.

11. Allow for potential sleep disturbances. Provide favorite toy or security object. Offer adequate comforting such as by holding infant on waking.
12. Make appropriate referral for psychologic needs.
13. Provide for follow-up for delayed post-trauma response up to 1–2 years after the trauma.
14. Provide reassurance that child is not being punished, and is not responsible for trauma.

WOMEN'S HEALTH

This nursing diagnosis will pertain to the woman the same as to any other adult. The reader is referred to Rape Trauma Syndrome (Chapter 10) and to other sections (Adult Health, Home Health, and Mental Health) for specific nursing orders and objectives pertaining to women and Post-Trauma Response.

MENTAL HEALTH

1. Assign a primary care nurse to the client and assign the same staff member to the client each day on each shift.
2. Begin appropriate anxiety reducing interventions if this is a significant problem for the client (see Anxiety, Chapter 8, for detailed intervention strategies and assessment criteria).
3. Discuss with client his or her perception of the current situation and stressors. This should include information about the coping strategies that the client has attempted and his or her assessment of what has made them ineffective in resolving this situation.
4. Provide a quiet, nonstimulating environment or an environment that does not add additional stress to an already overwhelmed coping ability. (Potential environmental stressors for this client should be listed here with the plan for reducing them in this environment.)
5. Sit with client (number) minutes (number) times a day at (specific times listed) to discuss the traumatic event. Person responsible for this activity should be listed here. This should be the nurse who has established a relationship with the client.
6. Assist client with setting appropriate limits on aggressive behavior by (see Violence, Potential for, Chapter 9, for detailed care plan if this is an appropriate diagnosis):
    a. Decreasing environmental stimulation as appropriate (this might include a secluded environment or a time out);
    b. Providing client with appropriate alternative outlets for physical tension (this should be stated specifically and could include walking, running, talking with staff member, using a punching bag, listening to music, doing a deep muscle relaxation sequence) (number) times per day at (state specific times) or when increased tension is observed. These outlets should be selected with the client's input. Those outlets that the client selects should be listed here;
    c. Talking with client about past situations that resulted in loss of control and discussing alternative ways of coping with these situations. (Persons responsible for this discussion should be noted here. This will not be accomplished in one discussion, the time and date for the initial discussion should be noted with the times and dates for follow-up discussions).
7. Once the symptoms have been identified and linked to the traumatic event, the primary nurse will sit with client (number) minutes (begin with 30 and increase as client's ability to concentrate improves) per shift to discuss the traumatic event. These discussions should include:
    a. The uniqueness of the situation and that one could not plan for the behavior that might be needed during this time.
    b. Ways of evaluating behavior, including moral and ethical standards, may be inappropriate for the unique situation of a traumatic event.
    c. Details of the event as the individual remembers them and the thoughts and feelings that occur with these memories.
    d. Meaning of life since the event and the implications this has for the future.

e. If feelings become extreme such as with rage or despondency, then the client should focus on thoughts rather than feelings about the event.

8. Provide constructive confrontation for client about problematic coping behavior. (See Kneisl & Wilson, 1984, for guidelines on constructive confrontation). Those kinds of behavior identified by the treatment team as problematic should be listed here with the selected method of confrontation.

9. Provide client with information about care and treatment.

10. Provide client with opportunities to make appropriate decisions related to care at his or her level of ability. This may begin as a choice between two options and then evolve into more complex decision making. It is important that this be at the client's level of functioning so confidence can be built with successful decision making experiences. Those decisions that the client has made should be noted.

11. Provide positive social reinforcement and other behavioral rewards for demonstration of adaptive problem solving and coping. (Those things that the client finds rewarding should be listed here with a schedule for use. Those kinds of behavior that are to be rewarded should also be listed.)

12. Assist client in identifying support systems and in developing a plan for their use. This plan should be noted here.

13. Inform significant others of the relationship between client's behavior and the traumatic event. Discuss with them their thoughts and feelings about the client's behavior. Person responsible for these discussions should be noted here with the schedule for the discussion times. This should also include information about the importance of supporting the client in discussing the event and how this might be facilitated. The concerns the significant others have about their response to this sharing should be discussed as well as planning for the types of information they might be exposed to.

14. When client develops a degree of comfort discussing the traumatic event, meetings between the client and significant others should be scheduled. Content of these meetings should include:
    a. Opportunities for the client to share thoughts and feelings about the event.
    b. Opportunities for the significant others to share their thoughts and feelings about client's behavior.
    c. Sharing of thoughts and feelings related to other events in the relationship as they surface as important topics of discussion during the meetings.
    d. Sharing of caring thoughts and feelings with each other.

15. Arrange for client to attend support group meetings with others who have experienced similar traumas. The times and days for these meetings should be noted here with any special arrangements that are needed to facilitate client's attendance (e.g., transportation to group meeting place). This could include veterans groups, groups for survivors of natural disasters, victim's groups, etc.

16. Schedule client involvement in unit activities. Note client responsibilities in these activities here with times the client will be involved in the activity.

17. Refer to appropriate community resources as indicated:
    a. Visiting nurse
    b. Social services
    c. Psychiatric nurse clinician
    d. Occupational therapist
    e. Physical therapist
    f. Veterans groups
    g. Red Cross
    h. Battered women's centers
    i. Community mental health center
    j. Parents Anonymous

k. Alcoholics or Narcotics Anonymous

l. Religious or spiritual counselors

HOME HEALTH

1. Monitor for factors contributing to post-trauma response.
2. Teach patient and family appropriate monitoring of signs and symptoms of Post-Trauma Response:
   a. Flashbacks
   b. Nightmares
   c. Survival guilt
   d. Confusion
   e. Amnesia
   f. Constricted affect
   g. Substance abuse
   h. Suicide attempt
   i. Poor impulse control
3. Assist patient and family in life-style adjustments that may be required:
   a. Recognition of feelings
   b. Prevention of harm to self or others
   c. Treatment of substance abuse
   d. Provision of safe environment
   e. Development and use of support network
   f. Prevention of further trauma
   g. Role changes
   h. Treatment of injuries
4. Involve patient and family in planning and implementing strategies to reduce or eliminate post-traumatic response:
   a. Family conference
   b. Communication
   c. Mutual goal setting
   d. Family members response to traumatic event
5. Consult with assistive resources as indicated:
   a. Psychiatric nurse clinician
   b. Psychiatrist
   c. Support groups such as Viet Nam Vets, Rape Crisis, etc.
   d. Law enforcement officials
   e. Attorney
   f. Crisis counselor
   g. Suicide prevention
   h. Family counselor
   i. Social service
   j. Social support networks

EVALUATION
OBJECTIVE 1

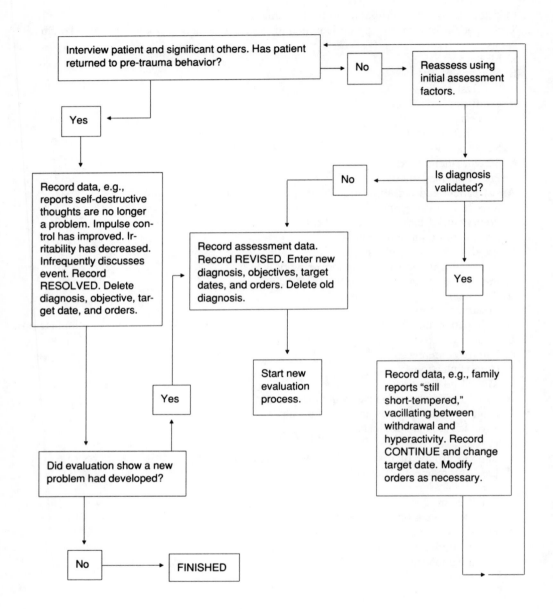

OBJECTIVE 2

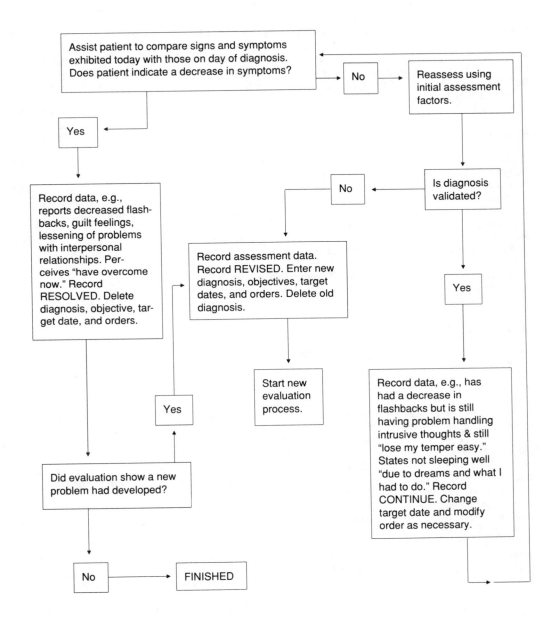

REFERENCES

Carpenito, L. (1983). *Nursing diagnosis: Applications to clinical practice*. Philadelphia: J. B. Lippincott.

Carter, E., & McGoldrick, M. (Eds.). (1980). *The family life cycle*. New York: Gardner Press.

Dixon, J., & Dixon, J. P. (1984). An evolutionary-based model of health and viability. *Advances in Nursing Science, 6* (3), 1–18.

Frain, M., & Valiga, T. (1979). The multiple dimensions of stress. *Topics in Clinical Nursing, 1*, (1), 43–52.

Gordon, M. (1987). *Manual of nursing diagnosis 1986–1987*. New York: McGraw-Hill.

Griffith-Kenney, J. (1986). *Contemporary women's health: A nursing advocacy approach*. Menlo Park, CA: Addison-Wesley.

Haber, J., Hoskins, P., Leach, A., & Sideleau, B. (1987). *Comprehensive psychiatric nursing* (3rd Ed.). New York: McGraw-Hill.

Kelly, M. A. (1985). *Nursing diagnosis source book: Guidelines for clinical application*. East Norwalk, CT: Appleton-Century-Crofts.

Kneisl, C., & Wilson, H. (1984). *Handbook of psychosocial nursing care*. Menlo Park, CA: Addison-Wesley.

Mengel, A. (Ed.). (1982). Coping. *Topics in Clinical Nursing, 4* (2), 80–82.

North American Nursing Diagnosis Association. (1987). *Taxonomy I with complete diagnosis*. St. Louis: Author.

North American Nursing Diagnosis Association. (1988). *Proposed nursing diagnoses*. St. Louis: Author.

Schuster, C., & Ashburn, S. (1986). *The process of human development* (2nd ed.). Boston: Little, Brown.

Smitherman, C. (1981). *Nursing actions for health promotion*. Philadelphia: F. A. Davis.

Stuart, G., & Sundeen, S. (1987). *Principles and practice of psychiatric nursing* (3rd ed.). St. Louis: C. V. Mosby.

Sutterley, D. (1979). Stress in health: A survey of self regulation modalities. *Topics in Clinical Nursing, 1* (1), 1–30.

Viken, R. M. (1982). The modern couvade syndrome. *The Female Patient, 7*, 40/41–40/42.

Wright, L., & Leahey, M. (1984). *Nurses and families*. Philadelphia: F. A. Davis.

Ziemer, M. (1982). Coping behavior: A response to stress. *Topics in Clinical Nursing, 4* (2), 4–12.

SUGGESTED READINGS

Adams, M. (1982). PTSD: An inpatient treatment unit. *American Journal of Nursing, 82* (11), 1704–1705.

Aguilera, D., & Messick, J. (1982). *Crisis intervention: Theory and methodology*. (4th ed.). St. Louis: C. V. Mosby.

American Psychiatric Association. (1980). *Diagnostic and statistical manual of mental disorders* (3rd ed.). Washington, DC: Author.

Baer, C. (Ed.) (1986). Patient Compliance: Issues and outcomes. *Topics in Clinical Nursing, 7* (4), 32–36.

Carpenito, L. (1987). *Handbook of nursing diagnosis* (2nd ed.). Philadelphia: J. B. Lippincott.

Crittendon, R. (1983). *Discharge planning*. Bowie, MD: Robert J. Brady.

Furey, J. (1982). For some, the war rages on. *American Journal of Nursing, 82* (11), 1695–1696.

Garvey, M. J. (1984). Postpartum depression. *The Journal of Reproductive Medicine, 29* (2), 113–116.

Hadeka, M. (1987). *Clinical judgment in community health nursing*. Boston: Little, Brown.

Hoff, L. (1984). *People in crisis* (2nd ed.). Menlo Park, CA: Addison-Wesley.

Humphrey, C. (1986). *Home care nursing handbook*. East Norwalk, CT: Appleton-Century-Crofts.

Huppenbauer, S. (1982). PTSD: A portrait of the problem. *American Journal of Nursing, 82* (11), 1699–1703.

Jaffe, M., & Skidmore-Roth, L. (1988). *Home health nursing care plans*. St. Louis: C. V. Mosby.

Jimenez, S. L. M. (1979). Beating the blues. *American Baby, 16*, 24.

Kendell, R. E., Mackenzie, W. E., West, C., McGuire, R. J., & Cox, J. L. (1986). Day-to-day mood changes after childbirth: Further Data. *Obstetrical and Gynecological Survey, 41* (2), 88–90.

Lamb, G. S., & Lipkin, M. (1982). Somatic symptoms of expectant fathers. *MCN: The American Journal of Maternal Child Nursing, 7* (2), 110–115.

Lambert, V., & Lambert C. (1985). *Psychosocial care of the physically ill* (2nd ed.). Englewood Cliffs, NJ: Prentice-Hall.

McClelland, E., Kelly, K., & Buckwalter, K. (1984). *Continuity of care: Advancing the concept of discharge planning*. Orlando, FL: Grune & Stratton.

Mozley, P. D. (1985). Predicting postpartum depression. *Contemporary Ob/GYN*, 173–176,179.

Mullis, M. (1984). Vietnam: The human fallout. *Journal of Psychosocial Nursing, 22* (2), 27–31.

National League for Nursing. (1986). *Policies and procedures*. New York: Accreditation Division for Home Care, National League for Nursing.

National League for Nursing. (1988). *Accreditation program for home care and community health: Criteria and standards*. New York: Author.

Norman, E. (1982). PTSD: The victim who survived. *American Journal of Nursing, 82* (11), 1696–1698.

Rawlins, R., & Heacock, P. (1988). *Clinical manual of psychiatric nursing.* St. Louis: C. V. Mosby.

Rinke, L. (1988). *Outcome standards in home health.* New York: National League for Nursing.

Schoolcraft, V. (1987). Grappling with illness during hospitalization. In J. Haber, P. Hoskins, A. Leach, & B. Sideleau (Eds.), *Comprehensive psychiatric nursing* (3rd ed.). New York: McGraw-Hill.

Schultz, J., & Dark, S. (1982). *Manual of psychiatric nursing care plans.* Boston: Little, Brown.

Shehan, C. (1987). Spouse support and Vietnam veterans' adjustment to post-traumatic stress disorder. *Family Relations, 36,* 55–60.

Steffi, B., & Eide, I. (1978). *Discharge planning handbook.* New York: Charles B. Slack.

Valiga, T. (Ed.). (1980). Education for self-care. *Topics in Clinical Nursing, 2* (2), 10–16.

Walsh, F. (Ed.). (1982). *Normal family processes.* New York: The Guilford Press.

Whaley, L. & Wong, D. (1987). *Nursing care of infants & children.* St. Louis: C.V. Mosby.

CHAPTER TWELVE

Value-Belief Pattern

Pattern Description

The nurse may care for patients who, because of health alterations, experience disturbances in their individual value-belief systems. These alterations may take a form ranging from being disturbed to being demolished. These disturbances can be manifested by the inability to practice formal religious directions, such as attending church or following a specific diet, to being totally unable to manage their own spiritual needs and live within a certain spiritual structure. Conversely, religion can affect physical or emotional well-being if the practice of the religion results in spiritual distress. An individual's value-belief system can contribute to alterations in health just as alterations in health can contribute to disturbances in the individual's values and beliefs. The nurse must individualize care to help minimize spiritual distress while meeting the specific needs of the individual patient within his or her value-belief system.

The value-belief pattern looks specifically at how physical illness can interfere with the individual's ability to practice religion and maintain beliefs, values, and spiritual life; as well as how a person's judgment and the meaning of life for himself or herself can affect or interfere with health care practices.

Pattern Assessment

1. Patient's description of values or life beliefs:
   a. Philosophical basis
   b. Theological basis
   c. Goals
   d. Ideas
   e. Opinions
   f. Actions
2. Patient's description of his or her sense of worth:
   a. Significant people
   b. Materialness
   c. Usefulness
   d. Merit
   e. Perception of being loved
3. Patient's or family's description of usual religious practices and the importance of these practices to them:
   a. Dietary practices
   b. Mode of worship
   c. Symbols necessary
   d. Environment
   e. Restrictions
4. Patient or family expresses fear, uncertainty, or anger at life's circumstances and indicates a relationship to beliefs and values (e.g., punishment, testing).

5. Patient or family requests specific spiritual help:
   a. Asking for their religious or cultural leaders.
      (1) Pastor
      (2) Priest
      (3) Rabbi
      (4) Guru
      (5) Shaman
      (6) Curandera
      (7) Chief
      (8) Family leader
   b. Asking for placement or removal of religious objects in room.
   c. Asking for specific dietary items or refusal to eat specific foods.
   d. Refusing specific treatments (e.g., blood transfusions).
   e. Requesting a change in usual hospital routine because of religious holiday.
   f. Requesting personnel to save all body parts taken from patient (e.g., amputated limbs, fingernails, hair).
   g. Describing hygiene or personal habits that have religious connotations (e.g., undergarments, head coverings).
6. Patient's description of the impact that health alteration has had on level of spiritual functioning (e.g., disbelief, anger, fear, resentment).
7. Patient's or family's description of religious involvement (e.g., overinvolvement that could signify use of religion as an ineffective coping mechanism).

Conceptual Information

The faith, belief, or value system of a person can be described as the predominating force which provides the vital direction to that person's existence. This predominating force can be a faith in a supreme being or God, a belief in one's self, or a belief in others. By this, it is conceptualized that each person must find his or her place in the world, nature, and in relationships with other beings. This faith, belief, or value system is exhibited by the individual in the form of organized religion, attitudes, and actions related to the individual's sense of what is right, cultural beliefs, and the individual's internal motivations.

All persons have some philosophical orientation to life which assists in constructing their reality, regardless of whether or not they practice a formal religion. Spirituality is interwoven into a person's cultural background, beliefs, and individual value system. This spirituality is what gives life meaning and allows the person to function in a more total manner. These beliefs and values influence a person's behavior and attitudes toward what is right and what is wrong, and what life-style they practice.

Many authors stress that not only must the nurse take into consideration the patient's beliefs and value system, but must also recognize his or her own beliefs and values (Carpenito, 1983; Gordon, 1982, Potter and Perry, 1985). The nurse must know about or develop resources to assist with understanding the different beliefs and religious practices of groups encountered in practice settings.

Studies have shown that the value of specific rituals such as prayer to the individuals who practice them is not affected by the fact that they can or cannot be proven scientifically (Carpenito, 1983; Stoll, 1979). Potter and Perry (1985) quote Margaret Newman in describing the impact of values and beliefs: "When as much emphasis is placed on the symbolic and intuitive as on the analytical, consciousness develops more fully." Newman concludes, "the expansion of consciousness is what life and, therefore, health is all about and health can coexist with illness and even encompass it as a meaningful aspect" (p. 404). This can be seen in those individuals who consider suffering, illness, and even death as having "meaning in life" or as "God's will."

Many individuals believe that the only value of life, and the source of strength and power, is the will of the individual and that there is no need for assistance from the outside. Stoll (1979) quotes Duncan, who described this focus as "a person's authority within himself." This focus may actually revolve around his "work, physical activity, or even himself—I can do anything I want to when I want to" (pp. 1574–1575). In discussing the value of life, Bayles (1980) describes three predominant indicators that must be considered when judging the value of continued life: "mental capacity, physical capacity and pain" (p. 2226). Bayles states that for most of us, "life is not intrinsically valuable to the possessor of it; instead, it is the quality of conscious life that is important" (p. 2226).

Because of the conscious, subconscious, and unconscious components of the value-belief system, nurses must be continually alert for disruptions in the system. Awareness of and respect for the impact and influence values and beliefs have on the patient cannot be overemphasized in providing quality care for the patient.

Developmental Considerations

The geographic, social, political, and home environment in which he or she lives has a major effect on how a person develops, how he or she will view his or her health, and how he or she formulates his or her spirituality, values, and beliefs. The values a person holds influence all facets of life. How one perceives the world about him or her, as well as his or her basic philosophy, guides all interactions with others and ultimately reflects a person's individuality.

Infant

The infant is totally dependent on the parents and those about him or her and is busy building trust or mistrust according to Erickson (1978). Unable at this age to form values or distinguish spirituality, the infant is a mirror image of those about him or her. The parent's method of interaction, communicating, and fulfilling the emotional and physiologic needs of the infant forms the basis for value development.

Toddler and Preschooler

The toddler imitates those about him or her: parents, siblings, and other adults. The toddler develops by mimicking observed behavior and receiving either positive or negative reinforcement. Values begin to form as the toddler begins to become aware of others and to interact with those around him or her. Values become known to individuals through the process of social cognition, which begins in early childhood. Chandler (1977) quotes Piaget, who wrote:

"The responsibility for development in general and the acquisition of knowledge in particular, neither arises from objects nor from the subject, but from the interaction . . . between the subject and those objects (p. 95)

School-Age Child

The school-age child begins to be influenced by peers outside the family structure and begins to question and make choices. The school-age child actively participates in his or her own moral development. Kohlberg, (1981) another cognitive developmentalist, based his theory of moral reasoning on Piaget's work. Kohlberg states that the individual's reasoning develops through various stages, beginning in the school-age years. He further states that play is the major mechanism of learning throughout the school-age years. As a result of his research, Kohlberg formulated six stages in the development of moral reasoning.

Adolescent

The adolescent searches for his or her own identity and begins to practice values that are separate and yet congruent with his or her family units. The adolescent is constantly questioning, trying, and searching for the 'truth of life' and for his or her identity in the scheme of things. He or she sees values as being either 'black or white' and there can be no overlapping. The adolescent is still struggling with his or her own independence and formulating his or her own values, beliefs, and spirituality.

Young Adult

Young adults are constantly examining, reformulating and changing their values, beliefs, and spirituality. Often they change completely the values and beliefs they developed during adolescence, although it is important to note that they often keep the basic values and beliefs they learned during their young years with their families.

Adult

Adults usually strengthen the values and beliefs they have formed according to their life experiences. The young adult is continually exploring and trying to see if his or her value system fits within his or her life-style. They are busy teaching children the values and beliefs that they wish their children to adopt for their lives.

Older Adult

Older adults find great solace in their spirituality and the values and beliefs they have formed through a lifetime. They are often not willing to change and indeed have a narrow focus in what comforts them and in what they believe in.

Applicable Nursing Diagnoses

Spiritual Distress (Distress of Human Spirit)

DEFINITION

Disruption in the life principle which pervades a person's entire being and which integrates and transcends one's biological and psychosocial nature (North American Nursing Diagnosis Association [NANDA], 1987, p. 70).

DEFINING CHARACTERISTICS (NANDA, 1987, p. 70)

The nurse will review the initial pattern assessment for the following defining characteristics to determine the diagnosis of Spiritual Distress.

1. Major defining characteristics
   a. Expresses concern with meaning of life and death and belief systems
   b. Expresses anger toward God
   c. Questions meaning of suffering
   d. Verbalizes inner conflict about beliefs
   e. Verbalizes concern about relationship with deity
   f. Questions meaning of own existence
   g. Is unable to participate in usual religious practices
   h. Seeks spiritual assistance
   i. Questions moral and ethical implications of therapeutic regimen
   j. Uses gallows humor
   k. Displaces anger toward religious representatives
   l. Describes nightmares or sleep disturbances
   m. Has alteration in behavior or mood evidenced by anger, crying, withdrawal, preoccupation, anxiety, hostility, apathy, etc.

RELATED FACTORS (NANDA, 1987, p. 70)

1. Separation from religious or cultural ties
2. Challenged belief and value systems (e.g., due to moral or ethical implications of therapy, due to intense suffering)

DIFFERENTIATION

It is very difficult to differentiate value-belief disturbances from other diagnoses because the very fiber of what makes the individual is intertwined with his or her physical and spiritual being. As in sleep pattern disturbance, one possible differentiation is Individual Coping, Ineffective. Many individuals use religion or beliefs as a means of bargaining in unwanted life situations or denying his or her role in the situation by blaming it on a superior being. Others will find their source of strength and hope from their beliefs in a superior being or God and are able to live fully functional lives despite physical handicaps.

Differentiation must be based on the assessment of the individual and his or her usual religious practices, beliefs, and values compared to the current attitudes and practices. The best means of differentiation relies on attention to what the patient is saying.

OBJECTIVES

1. Will verbalize sense of spiritual peace by (date).

AND/OR

2. Will describe at least (number) support systems to use when conflict with spirituality arises by (date).

TARGET DATE

Because of the largely subconscious nature of spiritual beliefs and values, it is recommended the target date be at least 5 days from the date of admission.

NURSING ORDERS

ADULT HEALTH

1. Assist patient to identify and define his or her own values particularly in relation to health and illness, through use of value clarification techniques such as sentence completion, rank ordering excercises, and completion of health-value scale.
2. Demonstrate respect for and acceptance of patient's value and spiritual system by not judging, moralizing, or advising changes in values or religious practices.
3. Assist patient to develop problem-solving behavior through practice of problem-solving techniques.
4. Adapt nursing therapeutics as necessary to incorporate values and religious beliefs.
5. Schedule appropriate rituals as necessary (e.g., baptism, confession, etc.).
6. Collaborate with dietitian regarding dietary prescriptions or restrictions.
7. Arrange visits from needed support persons (e.g., pastor, rabbi, priest, prayer group).
8. Provide privacy for religious practices and rituals.
9. Encourage family to bring significant symbols to patient.
10. Plan to spend at least 15 minutes with patient twice a day to allow verbalization, questioning, counseling, and support on a one-to-one basis.

CHILD HEALTH

1. Support the patient in attaining or maintaining spiritual integrity according to specific identified needs and developmental level.
   a. Allow for appropriate privacy.
   b. Allow time for self-reflection.
   c. Allow time for prayer and practice of worship as permitted within surrounding environment.
   d. Provide assistance, as requested by patient or family, in referral to clergy, chaplains, or other spiritual leaders.
   e. Support the child in expressing feelings about spiritual distress and related factors through use of open-ended questions and providing time for this at least twice a day.
   f. Act as advocate for the child and family when they are expressing differing beliefs from that of the staff, institution, or significant others.
2. Answer value-belief related questions honestly according to patient's developmental level and after conferring with parents.
3. Adapt policies and procedures to meet value-belief needs of patient and family (e.g., extended visiting hours, permission to substitute plasma expanders for blood).

Additional Information

As was mentioned in Conceptual Information, the spirituality of a child is formed in the early years of life. As with values, spirituality is a learned process with modification and reinforcement taking place as a result of socialization throughout the life span. Depending on the child's age and developmental capacity, appropriate assessment and intervention should be planned and carried out to the best extent possible in meeting the individual's needs representing the spiritual domain. An additional problem in child health is that the value-belief preferences of the parental dyad must also be considered and incorporated into planning care.

WOMEN'S HEALTH

1. Assist patient in adapting religious practices to current situation.
2. Adjust hospital routines to the extent possible to assist patient adaptation.
3. Allow mother and family to express feelings at the less-than-perfect pregnancy outcome: